DOSAGE
CALCULATIONS

NINTH EDITION

Gloria D. Pickar, EdD, RN

Group President & Chief Academic Officer
EmbanetCompass
Orlando, Chicago, Toronto

Former Academic Dean
Seminole State College of Florida
Sanford, Florida

Amy Pickar Abernethy, MD

Associate Professor of Medicine and Nursing
Duke University
Durham, North Carolina

gpercocco@stratford.ed

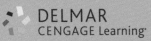

DELMAR
CENGAGE Learning

Australia • Brazil • Japan • Korea • Mexico • Singapore • Spain • United Kingdom • United States

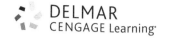

Dosage Calculations, Ninth Edition
Gloria D. Pickar, EdD, RN
and Amy Pickar Abernethy, MD

Vice President, Editorial: Dave Garza

Executive Editor: Stephen Helba

Senior Acquisitions Editor: Maureen Rosener

Managing Editor: Marah Bellegarde

Senior Product Manager: Elisabeth F. Williams

Editorial Assistant: Samantha Miller

Vice President, Marketing: Jennifer Baker

Marketing Director: Wendy E. Mapstone

Executive Marketing Manager: Michele McTighe

Associate Marketing Manager: Scott A. Chrysler

Production Manager: Andrew Crouth

Content Project Manager: Allyson Bozeth

Senior Art Director: Jack Pendleton

For product information and technology assistance, contact us at
Cengage Learning Customer & Sales Support, 1-800-354-9706
For permission to use material from this text or product,
submit all requests online at **www.cengage.com/permissions.**
Further permissions questions can be e-mailed to
permissionrequest@cengage.co

Library of Congress Control Number: 2011926858

ISBN-13: 978-1-4390-5847-3
ISBN-10: 1-4390-5847-4

Delmar
5 Maxwell Drive
Clifton Park, NY 12065-2919
USA

Cengage Learning is a leading provider of customized learning solutions with office locations around the globe, including Singapore, the United Kingdom, Australia, Mexico, Brazil, and Japan. Locate your local office at: **international.cengage.com/region**

Cengage Learning products are represented in Canada by Nelson Education, Ltd.

To learn more about Delmar, visit **www.cengage.com/delmar**
Purchase any of our products at your local college store or at our preferred online store **www.cengagebrain.com**

Notice to the Reader

ited States of America
3 12 11

Contents

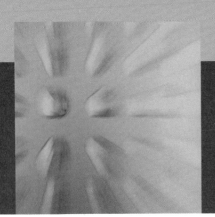

Preface

Introduction

Dosage Calculations, ninth edition, offers a clear and concise method of calculating drug dosages. The text is directed to students and professionals who want to increase their comfort level with mathematics and also to faculty members who prefer the formula method for calculating dosages. Along with the companion text, *Dosage Calculations: A Ratio-Proportion Approach,* third edition, the content has been classroom tested and reviewed by well over 1 million faculty and students, who report that it has helped allay math anxiety and promote confidence in their ability to perform accurate calculations. As one reviewer noted, "I have looked at others [texts], and I don't feel they can compare."

The only math prerequisite is the ability to do basic arithmetic. For those who need a review, *Chapters 1* and *2* offer an overview of basic arithmetic calculations with extensive exercises for practice. The text teaches the learner to use a Three-Step Approach for calculating dosages.

1. Convert measurements to the same system and same size units.

2. Consider what dosage is reasonable.

3. Calculate using the formula method.

Dosage Calculations, ninth edition, is based on feedback from users of the previous editions and users of other dosage calculations texts. The new edition also responds to changes in the health care field and includes the introduction of new drugs, replacement of outdated drugs, and discussion of new or refined methods of administering medications. The importance of avoiding medication errors is highlighted by the incorporation of applied critical thinking skills in clinical reasoning scenarios based on patient care situations, and a chapter on preventing medication errors. Clinical reasoning content has been expanded considering the Quality and Safety Education for Nurses (QSEN: www.qsen.org) competencies that take into account the complexity of nursing work. Learners and faculty will find QSEN

principles incorporated throughout: stacking, mindfulness, sensemaking, anticipating, memory aids, and work-arounds. To better prepare graduates for licensure examinations, test items patterned after NCLEX-RN and NCLEX-PN have been added for frequent practice.

Organization of Content

The text is organized in a natural progression of basic to more complex information. Learners gain self-confidence as they master content in small increments with ample review and reinforcement. Many learners claim that while using this text, they did not fear math for the very first time.

The seventeen chapters are divided into four sections.

Section 1 starts with a *Pretest* patterned after examinations often used by hospitals and health care agencies to evaluate the readiness of new graduates to prepare and administer medications. Learners can both evaluate their level of knowledge as they begin their study of dosage calculations and test their learning with the same examination as a posttest. This is followed by a mathematics diagnostic evaluation and a thorough mathematics review in *Chapters 1* and *2*. The *Mathematics Diagnostic Evaluation* allows learners to determine their computational strengths and weaknesses to guide them through the review of the *Section 1* chapters. *Chapters 1* and *2* provide a review of basic arithmetic skills, including fractions, decimals, ratios, percents, and simple equations, with numerous examples and practice problems to ensure that students can apply the procedures.

Section 2 includes *Chapters 3* through *9*. This section provides essential information that makes up the foundation for accurate dosage calculations and safe medication administration including medicine orders, labels, and equipment. *Chapters 3* and *4* introduce the three systems of measurement: metric, household, and apothecary. The metric system of measurement is emphasized because of its standardization in the health care field and the household system is included because of its implications for care at home. Apothecary measure and conversions can be found in Appendix B, as the apothecary system is outdated and no longer recommended for use in health care. International, or 24-hour, time and Fahrenheit and Celsius temperature conversions are presented in *Chapter 5.*

In *Chapter 6,* students learn to recognize and select appropriate equipment for the administration of medications based on the drug, dosage, and method of administration. Emphasis is placed on interpreting syringe calibrations to ensure that the dosage to be administered is accurate. All photos and drawings have been enhanced for improved clarity with updates from state-of-the-art technology and information systems.

Chapter 7 presents the common abbreviations used in health care so that learners can become proficient in interpreting medical orders. The content on computerized medication administration records has been updated and expanded for this edition.

It is essential that learners be able to read medication labels to calculate dosages accurately. This skill is developed by having readers interpret the medication labels provided beginning in *Chapter 8.* These labels represent current commonly prescribed medications and are presented in full color and actual size (except in a few instances where the label is enlarged to improve readability). Some labels have been substituted with generic simulated labels to demonstrate critical calculations. This ensures that the entire range of medications seen in practice is presented, and gives the learners the experience with actual generic drugs. A full list of all labels in the text can be found in the ***Drug Label Index***.

Chapter 9 has been expanded and directs the learner's attention to the risks and responsibilities inherent in receiving medication prescriptions, transcribing orders, and administering medications. It provides the rationale for the patient's rights to safe medication administration and identifies the common causes of medication errors, including safe methods to prevent them. Throughout the text, care is taken to comply with standards and recommendations for medical notation available at the time of publication by The Joint Commission and The Institute for Safe Medication Practices. The *Official "Do Not Use" List* is emphasized. Learners are directed to stay abreast of these standards as they evolve to best ensure patient safety and prevent medication administration errors. More resources and tools for error prevention are presented, such as Tall Man letters to avoid mistaken identity of look-alike/sound-alike drugs.

In ***Section 3,*** students learn and practice the skill of dosage calculations applied to patients across the life span.

Chapters 10 and *11* guide the learner to apply all the skills mastered in previous chapters to achieve accurate oral and injectable drug dosage calculations. The authors used QSEN quality and safety competencies as a guide for the development of realistic and challenging medication scenarios which simulate the complexity of various factors that challenge learners as they interpret, retrieve, prepare, calculate, and administer medications. Safety competencies are incorporated to ensure learners carefully consider each aspect of the medication administration process for safe practice. Students learn to think through each problem logically for the right answer and then to apply the formula method for calculations to double-check their thinking. When this logical but unique system is applied every time to every problem, experience has shown that decreased math anxiety and increased accuracy result.

High-alert drugs, such as insulin and heparin, are thoroughly presented. Insulin types, species, and manufacturers have been updated with a description of insulin action time and the addition of U-500 insulin, including the difference between administering U-500 in the hospital and at home. The 70/30 and 50/50 insulins and the insulin pen are also thoroughly explained.

Chapter 12 introduces the concepts of solutions. Users learn the calculations associated with diluting solutions and reconstituting injectable drugs. This chapter provides a segue to intravenous calculations by fully describing the preparation of solutions. With the expanding role of the nurse and other health care workers in the home setting, clinical calculations for home care, such as nutritional feedings, are also emphasized.

Chapter 13 covers the calculation of pediatric and adult dosages and concentrates on the body weight method. Emphasis is placed on verifying safe dosages and applying concepts across the life span.

Chapter 14 introduces ratio-proportion and dimensional analysis methods of calculating dosages for faculty who may prefer these methods. Ample *Review Sets* and *Practice Problems* provide exposure to these methods, giving the learner an opportunity to sample other calculation methods and choose the one preferred.

Section 4 presents advanced clinical calculations applicable to both adults and children. Intravenous administration calculations are presented in Chapters *15* through *17.* Coverage reflects the greater application of IVs in drug therapy. Shortcut calculation methods are presented and explained fully. More electronic infusion devices are included. Heparin and saline locks, types of IV solutions, IV monitoring, IV administration records, and IV push drugs are included in *Chapter 15.* Pediatric IV calculations are presented in *Chapter 16,* and obstetric, heparin, insulin, and critical care IV calculations are covered in *Chapter 17.* Ample problems help students master the necessary calculations. Additional attention is directed to the clinical reasoning skills required to safely administer high-alert medications according to standard protocols.

Procedures in the text are introduced using *Rule* boxes and several *Examples*. Many examples use *Clinical Simulations* to guide learners through clinical reasoning and critical calculations. Key concepts are summarized and highlighted in *Quick Review* boxes before each set of *Review Problems* to give learners an opportunity to review major concepts prior to working through the problems. *Math Tips* provide memory joggers to assist learners in accurately solving problems. Learning is reinforced by *Practice Problems* that conclude each chapter. The importance of calculation accuracy and patient safety is emphasized by patient scenarios that require careful and accurate consideration. *Clinical Reasoning Skills* scenarios allow learners to apply critical thinking to analyze and resolve medication administration errors at the end of each chapter beginning with Section 2. Additional scenarios accompany each chapter's *Practice Problems* to further emphasize accuracy and safety.

Information to be memorized is identified in *Remember* boxes, and *Caution* boxes alert learners to critical procedures and information.

Section Self-Evaluations found at the end of each section provide learners with an opportunity to test their mastery of chapter objectives prior to proceeding to the next section. Two *Posttests* at the conclusion of the text serve to evaluate the learner's overall skill in dosage calculations. The first *Posttest* refers the learner back to the *Essential Skills Evaluation Pretest* from the beginning of the text, which covers essential skills commonly tested by employers. The second posttest, the *Comprehensive Skills Evaluation,* serves as a comprehensive examination covering all 17 chapters. Both are presented in a case study format to simulate actual clinical calculations.

An *Answer Key* at the back of the text provides all answers and solutions to selected problems in the *Pretest, Review Sets, Practice Problems, Section Self-Evaluations,* and *Posttests. Appendix A Study Guide* provides essential abbreviations, equivalents, rules, and formulas from each clinical chapter, and *Appendix B Apothecary System* describes apothecary conversions. Both a general content *Index* and a *Drug Label Index* conclude the text.

Features of the Ninth Edition

- Content is divided into four main sections to help learners better organize their studies.

- Measurable objectives at the beginning of each chapter emphasize the content to be mastered.

- More than 2,700 problems are included for learners to practice their skills and reinforce their learning, reflecting current drugs and protocols.

- *Clinical Reasoning Skills* apply critical thinking to real-life patient care situations to emphasize the importance of accurate dosage calculations and the avoidance of medication errors.

- Full color is used to make the text more user friendly, enhance presentation, and improve readability. Chapter elements, such as *Rules, Math Tips, Cautions, Remember* boxes, *Quick Reviews, Examples,* and *Summaries* are color-coded for easy recognition and use. Color also highlights *Review Sets* and *Practice Problems.*

- Color has been added to selected syringe drawings throughout the text to *simulate a specific amount of medication,* as indicated in the example or problem. Because the color used may not correspond to the actual color of the medications named, *it must not be used as a reference for identifying medications.*

- Photos and drug labels are presented in full color. Special attention is given to visual clarity with some labels enlarged to ensure legibility.

- The *Math Review* brings learners up to the required level of basic math competence.

- SI conventional metric system notation is used (apothecary and household systems of measurement are introduced; apothecary measure can be found in Appendix B).

- *Rule* boxes draw the learner's attention to pertinent instructions.

- *Remember* boxes highlight information to be memorized.

- *Quick Review* boxes summarize critical information throughout the chapters before *Review Sets* are solved.

- *Caution* boxes alert learners to critical information.

- *Math Tips* serve to point out math shortcuts and reminders.

- Each new topic or skill presented is followed by *Review Sets* with end-of-chapter *Practice Problems* to assess understanding and skills and to reinforce learning.

- Many problems are included involving the interpretation of syringe scales to ensure that the proper dosage is administered. Once the dosage is calculated, the learner is directed to draw an arrow on a syringe at the proper value.

- Many more labels of current and commonly prescribed medications are presented, including a few simulated labels to help users learn how to select the proper information required to determine correct dosage. There are over 375 labels included.

■ Hundreds of *Examples* are included to demonstrate the $\frac{D}{H} \times Q = X$, ratio-proportion, or dimensional analysis methods of calculating dosages.

■ The addition of the ratio-proportion and dimensional analysis methods gives learners and instructors a choice of which method they prefer to use.

■ Abbreviations, measurements, acronyms, and symbols follow The Joint Commission "Do Not Use" List and ISMP standards.

■ Clear instructions are included for calculating IV medications administered in milligram per kilogram per minute.

■ Clinical situations are simulated using actual medication labels, syringes, physician order forms, various medication storage and retrieval systems, and medication administration records.

■ The Pretest, Section Evaluations, Chapter Practice Problems, and Posttests include scenarios that simulate substantial aspects of real-world clinical calculation situations.

■ An *Essential Skills Evaluation Pretest* and *Posttest* simulate exams commonly administered by employers for new hires, assess prior knowledge, and evaluate learning of essential calculation skills. A *Comprehensive Skills Evaluation* evaluates the learner's overall comprehension in preparation for a level or program assessment.

■ *Appendix A Study Guide* summarizes the most frequently used abbreviations, equivalents, and formulas from each chapter. Learners can refer to this valuable study tool for solving problems which will reinforce remembering essential information.

■ General *Index* facilitates learner and instructor access to content and skills, and the *Drug Index* facilitates access to all labels used in the text.

New to the Ninth Edition

■ *Quality and Safety in Nursing Education* (QSEN) principles and competencies have been adapted to reduce the risk of medication errors and improve patient safety.

■ *Clinical simulations* provided in examples and test questions develop clinical reasoning and calculation skills.

■ Section Examinations include test items formatted like graduate licensure examinations, such as the *NCLEX-RN and NCLEX-PN exams*.

■ Content on *high-alert drugs,* such as heparin and insulin, has been extensively augmented, including safety concerns with the increased use of *insulin pens* in hospitals. *U-500 insulin* content and calculations have been expanded, including conversions for preparation using both U-100 and 1 mL syringes.

■ New questions are added throughout to reflect current drugs and protocols.

■ Photographs of state-of-the-art equipment are replaced and updated, including the latest medication storage and retrieval systems.

■ Apothecary calculations have been deleted within the text and evaluation items, consistent with current standards. Apothecary measure has been moved to Appendix B.

■ Learners apply critical thinking to prevent medication errors in *Clinical Reasoning Skills* scenarios based on QSEN principles.

■ Dosage calculations scenarios have been expanded to incorporate each step of the medication administration process: interpretation of order, acquisition of drug information, retrieval of drug, dosage calculation, dose measurement, preparation, and administration.

■ Learners are purposely directed to be mindful of the seriousness of their clinical practice and the value of *safety alerts* to prevent errors.

■ *Appendix A Study Guide* summarizes essential rules, formulas, abbreviations, and equivalents to facilitate problem solving and reinforce learning.

■ *Appendix B Apothecary System* gives common units, abbreviations, and symbols of the original dosage measurement system, for faculty and students interested in comparing and converting between apothecary and metric measure.

■ A *Drug Label Index* has been added presenting both generic and brand names to facilitate identification of all drug labels presented in the text.

■ Online course formats are available in **Blackboard** and **Angel** so that students can access their *Dosage Calculations* course content, practice activities, communications, and assessments through the Internet.

■ An exciting new *Premium Website* with *Practice Software* is available, offering a glossary review, chapter tutorials, interactive exercises, and hundreds of practice problems.

Learning Package for the Student

WebTutor Advantage Plus on Blackboard (ISBN 978-1-4390-5850-3) and Angel (ISBN 978-1-4390-5847-9)

WebTutor Advantage Plus course cartridges (in both Blackboard and Angel formats) accompany this new edition of *Dosage Calculations*. These online courses offer must-have classroom management tools such as chats and calendars, as well as additional content resources, including class notes, lecture slides, student quizzes, frequently asked questions, a glossary, and more.

Premium Website (ISBN 978-1-1335-9210-5)

The **Premium Website** can be accessed by users of the text at **www.CengageBrain.com.** Enter your passcode, found in the front of the book, and the Premium Website will be added to your bookshelf. Here you can access the engaging *Practice Software*, which includes:

- A user-friendly menu structure to immediately access the program's items.

- A bank of several hundred questions for practice and to reinforce the content presented in the text.

- A tutorial for each chapter outlining instructions and approaches to safe and accurate dosage calculation.

- *Quizzes, Pretest,* and *Posttest* that operate within a tutorial mode, which allows two tries before the correct answer is provided.

- Interactive exercises that ask you to fill a medicine cup or draw back a syringe to the correctly calculated dose.

- A comprehensive glossary of terms and drug names with definitions and pronunciations.

- Drop-down calculator available at a click of a button, as used on the NCLEX-RN™ and -PN examinations.

Teaching Package for the Instructor (ISBN 978-1-4390-5848-0)

The *Instructor Resources (IR) to Accompany Dosage Calculations,* ninth edition, contains a variety of tools to help instructors successfully prepare lectures and teach within this subject area. The following components in the *IR* are free to adopters of the text:

- A **Solutions Manual** includes answers and step-by-step solutions for every question in the *Pretest, Math Evaluation, Review Sets, Practice Problems, Section Evaluations,* and *Posttests* from the book.

- The **Computerized Test Bank** includes approximately 500 additional questions not found in the book for further assessment. The software also allows for the creation of test items and full tests, as well as coding for difficulty level.

- Lecture slides created in **PowerPoint®** offer a depiction of administration tools and include calculation tips helpful to classroom lecture of dosage calculations.

- An **Image Library** is an invaluable digital resource of dozens of figures, labels, and syringes from the text. With the Image Library, you can search for, copy, and save images to easily paste into slide presentations or other learning tools.

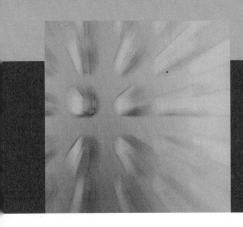

Acknowledgments

Contributor

Maureen D. Tremel, MSN, ARNP
Professor of Nursing
Seminole State College of Florida
Sanford, Florida

Reviewers

Michele Bach, MS
Professor
Engineering, Mathematics, and Sciences
Kansas City Kansas Community College
Kansas City, Kansas

Lou Ann Boose, RN, MSN
Professor
Harrisburg Area Community College
Harrisburg, Pennsylvania

Irene Colson Coons, RN, MSN, CNE
Professor
College of Southern Nevada
Las Vegas, Nevada

Jacqueline Sayre Dorsey, RN, MS, ANP
Assistant Professor
Monroe Community College
Rochester, New York

Patricia Van Tine, RN, MA
Theory Instructor
Vocational Nursing Program
American Career College
Los Angeles, California

Accuracy Reviewers

Beverly Meyers, MEd, MAT
Professor, Mathematics and Science
Jefferson College
Hillsboro, Missouri

Julie E. Pickar
Freelance Copy Editor and Proofreader
Maitland, Florida

From the Authors

We wish to thank our many students and colleagues who have provided inspiration and made contributions to the production of the text. We are particularly grateful to Maureen Tremel for her careful attention to researching and updating information; to Julie Pickar and Beverly Meyers for their careful attention to accuracy; to Maureen Rosener, Elisabeth Williams, Allyson Bozeth, Brian Davis, and Samantha Miller for their careful attention to deadlines and details; and to Roger Pickar and Steve Abernethy for their careful attention to us and our families.

Gloria D. Pickar, EdD, RN
Amy Pickar Abernethy, MD

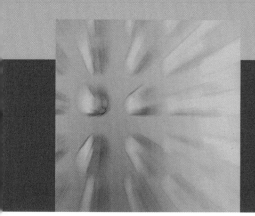

Introduction to the Learner

The accurate calculation of drug dosages is an essential skill in health care. Paracelsus (1493–1591), often referred to as the father of pharmacology, recognized that the difference between a poison, narcotic, hallucinogen, and medicine is dosage. Serious harm to the patient can result from incorrect interpretation or transcription of a medication order, retrieving the wrong drug, or a mathematical error during the calculation and subsequent administration of a drug dosage. It is the responsibility of those administering drugs to precisely and efficiently carry out medical orders and to recognize unsafe dosages and prescriptions.

Learning to calculate drug dosages need not be a difficult or burdensome process. *Dosage Calculations,* ninth edition, provides an uncomplicated, easy-to-learn, easy-to-recall Three-Step Approach to dosage calculations. Once you master this method, you will be able to consistently compute dosages with accuracy, ease, and confidence.

The text is a self-study guide that is divided into four main sections. The only mathematical prerequisite is the basic ability to add, subtract, multiply, and divide whole numbers. A review of fractions, decimals, percents, simple equations, ratios, and proportions is included. You are encouraged to work at your own pace and seek assistance from a qualified instructor as needed.

Each procedure in the text is introduced by several *Examples.* Key concepts are summarized and highlighted throughout each chapter, to give you an opportunity to review the concepts before working the problems. Ample *Review* and *Practice Problems* are given to reinforce your skill and confidence.

Before calculating the dosage, you are asked to consider the reasonableness of the computation. More often than not, the correct amount can be estimated in your head. Many errors can be avoided if you approach dosage calculation in this logical fashion. The mathematical computation can then be used to double-check your thinking. Answers to all problems and step-by-step solutions to select problems are included at the back of the text.

Many photos and drawings are included to demonstrate key concepts and equipment. Drug labels and measuring devices (for example, syringes) are included to give a simulated "hands-on" experience outside of the clinical setting or laboratory. *Clinical Reasoning Skills* emphasize the importance of dosage calculation accuracy, and medication scenarios provide opportunities to analyze and prevent errors.

This text has helped hundreds of thousands of learners just like you to feel at ease about math and to master dosage calculations. I am interested in your feedback. Please write to me to share your reactions and success stories.

Gloria D. Pickar, EdD, RN
gpickar@cfl.rr.com

Dedicated to Julie,
in recognition of the importance of preventing errors.

Using This Book

■ Concepts are presented from simple to complex, in small increments, followed by solved *Examples* and a *Quick Review*. *Review Sets* and *Practice Problems* provide opportunities for you to reinforce your learning.

Refer to the following label to identify the specific drug information described in questions 16 through 21.

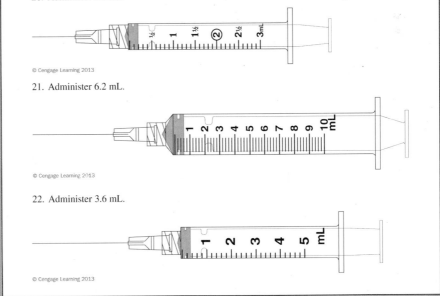

16. Generic name _____

17. Brand name _____

18. Dosage strength _____

19. Route of administration _____

20. National Drug Code _____

21. Manufacturer _____

■ All syringes are drawn to full size, providing accurate scale renderings to help you master the reading of injectable dosages.

20. Administer 1.1 mL.

© Cengage Learning 2013

21. Administer 6.2 mL.

© Cengage Learning 2013

22. Administer 3.6 mL.

© Cengage Learning 2013

■ Photos and drug labels are presented in full color; actual size labels help prepare you to read and interpret content in its true-life format.

FAMOTIDINE INJECTION

NDC 55390-028-10
FOR INTRAVENOUS USE ONLY AFTER DILUTION.
USUAL DOSAGE: See package insert.

*Each mL contains 10 mg of famotidine and the following inactive ingredients: L-aspartic acid 4 mg, mannitol 20 mg, and Water for Injection, q.s., 1 mL. Benzyl alcohol 0.9% added as preservative.

Store at 2° to 8°C (36° to 46°F).

40 mg/4 mL*

20 mg/2 mL
4 mL TWO-DOSE VIAL
Rx ONLY

Manufactured for:
Bedford Laboratories™
Bedford, OH 44146

FAMPV04

Used with permission from Bedford Laboratories.

MATH TIP

Notice that to multiply 2 by 1,000, you are moving the decimal three places to the right. This is a shortcut. Sometimes to complete this operation, you add zeros to hold the places equal to the number of zeros in the equivalent. In this case, 1 g = 1,000 mg, so you add three zeros:
$2 \times 1,000 = 2.000. = 2,000$

- *Math Tip* boxes provide you with clues to essential computations.

CAUTION

If any of the seven parts is missing or unclear, the order is considered incomplete and is therefore not a legal drug order.

- *Caution* boxes alert you to critical information and safety concerns.

RULE

The formula method to calculate IV flow rate for manually-regulated IVs ordered in mL/h or for a prescribed number of minutes is:

$$\frac{V}{T} \times C = R$$

$\frac{\text{Volume (mL)}}{\text{Time (min)}} \times \text{Calibration or drop factor (gtt/mL)} = \text{Rate (gtt/min)}$

- *Rule* boxes highlight and draw your attention to important formulas and pertinent instructions.

REMEMBER

The Six Rights of safe and accurate medication administration are as follows:

The *right patient* must receive the *right drug* in the *right amount* by the *right route* at the *right time*, followed by the *right documentation*.

- *Remember* boxes highlight information that you should memorize.

QUICK REVIEW

Look again at Steps 1 through 3 as a valuable dosage calculation checklist.

Step 1	Convert	Be sure that all measurements are in the same system and all units are the same size.
Step 2	Think	Carefully estimate the reasonable amount of the drug that you should administer.
Step 3	Calculate	$\frac{D}{H} \times Q = X$ $\frac{D \text{ (desired)}}{H \text{ (have)}} \times Q \text{ (quantity)} = X \text{ (amount)}$

- *Quick Review* boxes summarize critical information that you will need to know and understand to safely prepare and administer medications.

SUMMARY

At this point, you should be quite familiar with the equivalents for converting within the metric and household systems and from one system to another. From memory, you should be able to recall quickly and accurately the equivalents for conversions. If you are having difficulty understanding the concept of converting from one unit of measurement to another, review this chapter and seek additional help from your instructor.

Consider the two Clinical Reasoning Skills scenarios, and work the Practice Problems for Chapter 4. Concentrate on accuracy. One error can be a serious mistake when calculating the dosages of medicines or performing critical measurements of health status.

- *Summary* boxes draw out key information from the chapter as a self-check and review tool.

EXAMPLE 4 ■

Convert: 0.15 kg to g

Equivalent: 1 kg = 1,000 g; therefore, conversion factor is 1,000 g/kg

THINK: Larger ↓ Smaller → Multiply (×)

Multiply by 1,000 g/kg: $0.15 \text{ kg} \times 1,000 \text{ g/kg} = 150 \text{ g}$
or move decimal point 3 places to the right
0.15 kg = 0.150. = 150 g (1 zero is added to complete the operation)

- *Examples* walk you step-by-step through each calculation process, using different conversions, medications, and methods, to ensure that your mastery of the process is complete.

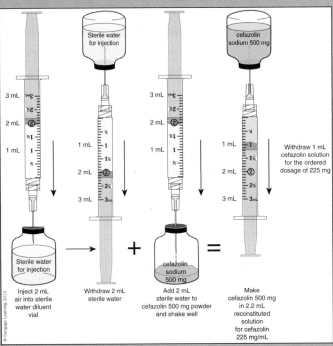

■ *Illustrations* simulate critical dosage calculation and dose preparation skills.

■ *Clinical Reasoning Skills* apply critical thinking to real-life patient care situations emphasizing the importance of accurate dosage calculations and the avoidance of medication errors. As an added benefit, clinical reasoning scenarios present prevention strategies so that you can learn how to avoid these errors in practice.

CLINICAL REASONING SKILLS

Many insulin errors occur when the nurse fails to clarify an incomplete order. Let's look at an example of an insulin error when the order did not include the type of insulin to be given.

ERROR

Failing to clarify an insulin order when the type of insulin is not specified.

Possible Scenario

Suppose the physician who intended for a patient to receive NPH U-100 insulin wrote an insulin order this way:

Humulin U-100 insulin 50 units subcut a.c. breakfast   INCORRECT

Because the physician did not specify the type of insulin, the nurse assumed it was regular insulin and noted that on the medication administration record. Suppose the patient was given the regular U-100 insulin instead of the insulin intended by the physician. Several hours later, the patient develops signs of hypoglycemia (low blood glucose), including shakiness, tremors, confusion, and sweating.

Potential Outcome

A stat blood glucose would likely reveal a dangerously low glucose level. The patient would be given a glucose infusion to increase the blood sugar. The nurse may not realize the error until she and the doctor check the original order and find that the incomplete order was filled in by the nurse. When the doctor did not specify the type of insulin, the nurse assumed that the physician meant regular, which is short-acting, when in fact intermediate-acting NPH insulin was desired.

Prevention

This error could have been avoided by remembering all the essential components of an insulin order: brand or generic name, type of insulin (such as regular or NPH), supply dosage, the amount to give in units, and the frequency. When you fill in an incomplete order, you are essentially practicing medicine without a license. This would be a clear malpractice incident. It does not make sense to put yourself and your patient in such jeopardy. A simple phone call would clarify the situation for everyone involved. Further, the nurse should have double-checked the dosage with another licensed practitioner. Had the nurse done so, the error could have been discovered prior to administration.

Review Set 13

Convert each of the following to the equivalent unit indicated.

1. 500 mL = _____ L		16. 0.75 L = _____ mL	
2. 0.015 g = _____ mg		17. 5,000 mL = _____ L	
3. 8 mg = _____ g		18. 1 L = _____ mL	
4. 10 mg = _____ g		19. 1 g = _____ mg	
5. 60 mg = _____ g		20. 3,000 mL = _____ L	
6. 300 mg = _____ g		21. 23 mcg = _____ mg	
7. 0.2 g = _____ mg		22. 1.05 g = _____ kg	
8. 1.2 g = _____ mg		23. 18 mcg = _____ mg	
9. 0.0025 kg = _____ g		24. 0.4 mg = _____ mcg	
10. 0.065 g = _____ mg		25. 2,625 g = _____ kg	

■ *Review Sets* are inserted after each new topic, to encourage you to stop and check your understanding of the material just presented.

■ *Practice Problems* round out each chapter. This is your opportunity to put your skills to the test, to identify your areas of strength, and also to acknowledge those areas in which you need additional study.

PRACTICE PROBLEMS—CHAPTER 11

Calculate the amount you will prepare for 1 dose. Indicate the syringe you will select to measure the medication.

1. Order: Dilaudid 4 mg slow IV push (over 10 min) IV q.4h p.r.n., severe pain

   Supply: Dilaudid 10 mg/mL

   Give: _____ mL   Select: _____ syringe

2. Order: morphine sulfate 15 mg slow IV push (over 5 min) stat

   Supply: morphine sulfate 10 mg/mL

   Give: _____ mL   Select: _____ syringe

SECTION 4 SELF-EVALUATION

Chapter 15—Intravenous Solutions, Equipment, and Calculations

1. Which of the following IV solutions is normal saline? _____ 0.45% NaCl

   _____ 0.9% NaCl _____ D₅W

2. What is the solute and concentration of 0.9% NaCl? _____

3. What is the solute and concentration of 0.45% NaCl? _____

Use the following information to answer questions 4 and 5.

Order: D₅ 0.45% NaCl 1,000 mL IV q.8h

4. The IV solution contains _____ g dextrose.

■ *Essential Skills Pretest, Section Self-Evaluations* and two *Posttests* test your mastery of concepts and critical calculation skills.

■ *Clinical Simulations* provide opportunities to practice your clinical reasoning combined with dosage calculation skills for safe and accurate medication administration.

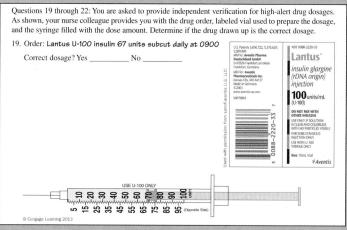

Questions 19 through 22: You are asked to provide independent verification for high-alert drug dosages. As shown, your nurse colleague provides you with the drug order, labeled vial used to prepare the dosage, and the syringe filled with the dose amount. Determine if the drug drawn up is the correct dosage.

19. Order: Lantus U-100 insulin 67 units subcut daily at 0900

   Correct dosage? Yes _____ No _____

■ *NCLEX-RN and NCLEX-PN* alternate test items give you an opportunity to practice answering questions formatted like these licensure examinations.

54. **NCLEX** *Drag-and-Drop / Ordered-Response* item:

Copy the tasks from the box onto the list in the proper sequence to *safely reconstitute an antibiotic powder with 2 mL diluent in order to administer 1 mL of the reconstituted drug.*

| Add 2 mL sterile water to the antibiotic powder. |
| Inject 2 mL air into the vial of sterile water. |
| Mix the powder and sterile water. |
| Withdraw 1 mL antibiotic solution. |
| Withdraw 2 mL sterile water. |
| Gather information about the drug. |

Answer:

_____

_____

_____

_____

_____

_____

■ *Drug Index* identifies each label in the text as a quick reference.

Drug Label Index

■ *Online Practice Software* is offered as your built-in learning tutor. As you study each chapter, be sure to also work with the online study tool. This valuable resource will help you verify your understanding of key rules and calculations.

■ *Online Resources* are available at your fingertips. Visit the **Premium Website** and **WebTutor Advantage** *Plus* components for valuable course content, exercises, class notes, and case studies.

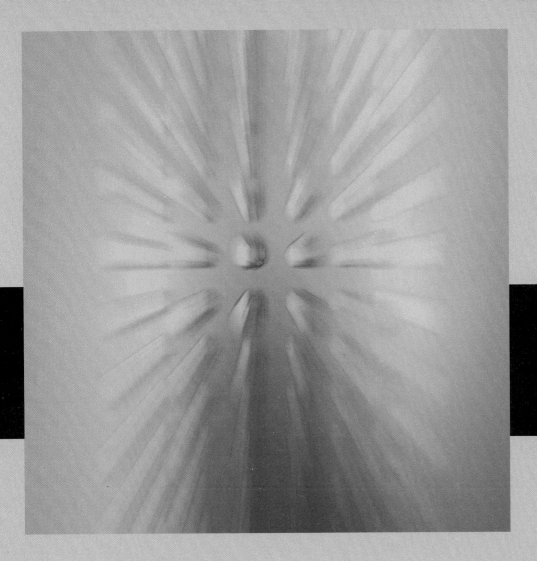

Pretest and Mathematics Review

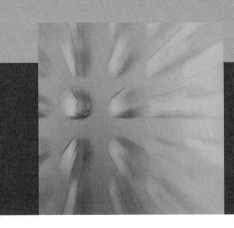

Essential Skills Evaluation: Pretest

Record your answers on the Essential Skills Evaluation: Pretest Answer Sheet on page 21. Do not record your answers on the test itself. You will refer back to this Essential Skills Evaluation as an essential skills posttest when you conclude your studies.

As you begin the study of safe dosage calculation, consider that you bring previous knowledge from life experiences. Perhaps you have worked or volunteered in a health care setting or administered medication to a family member or friend. This essential skills pretest will help you identify dosage calculation skills you already possess and highlight skills that you will learn and master as you work through the text. Take this pretest now, but do not be concerned if there are many questions you are unable to answer. That is to be expected. Use scrap paper to work the problems rather than writing on the test pages so that you can take this test again once you have completed this course of study. Separate answer sheets are provided following the pretest and again following Section 4 (as a posttest) for you to record your answers. Comparing your answers from the pretest with those of the posttest will allow you to measure your improvement and see what material you may need to revisit with your instructor.

The Essential Skills Evaluation is designed to be similar to the type of entry-level test given by hospitals and health care agencies during orientation for new graduates and new employees. It excludes the advanced calculation skills presented in Chapters 16 and 17. A more comprehensive skills evaluation will be available at the end of the text, to measure mastery of the full range of dosage calculation skills presented in all 17 chapters of the text.

Locate the Essential Skills Evaluation: Pretest Answer Sheet, gather some scratch paper, and let's get started!

Instructions for questions 1 through 19:

Throughout your assigned shift on a busy adult medical unit, you will give medications to a group of patients. The following labels represent the medications available on the medical unit to fill the orders given. Calculate the amount you will administer for one dose, and identify the frequency of administration of each dose. For solutions, mark an arrow on the syringe to indicate the correct volume. When multiple syringes are provided, choose the most appropriate one to mark.

1. Order: Calan 40 mg p.o. t.i.d.

   Give: _____ tablet(s)   Frequency: _____

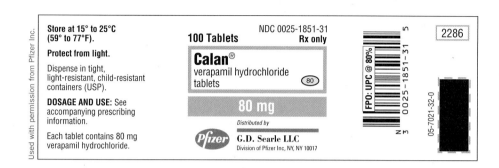

2. Order: clonazepam 1.5 mg p.o. b.i.d.

   Give: _____ tablet(s)   Frequency: _____

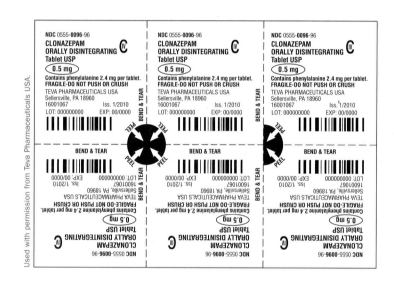

3. Order: atomoxetine 20 mg p.o. daily

   Choose: _____ mg capsules   Give: _____ capsule(s)   Frequency: _____

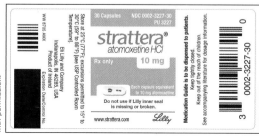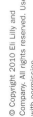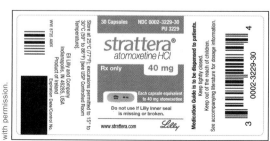

A   B

4. Order: **Lortab 2.5 mg p.o. q.3h, p.r.n., moderate pain** (ordered according to dose of hydrocodone)

Give: _____ tablet(s)

Frequency: _____

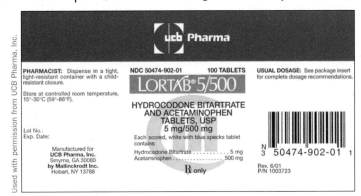

5. Order: **levothyroxine 0.3 mg p.o. q.AM**

Give: _____ tablet(s)

Frequency: _____

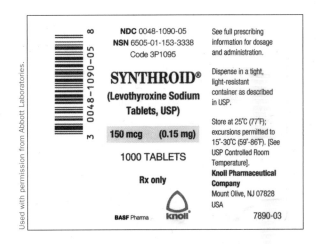

6. Order: **amoxicillin and clavulanate potassium 100 mg p.o. q.8h** (ordered according to dose of amoxicilin)

Give: _____ mL   Frequency: _____

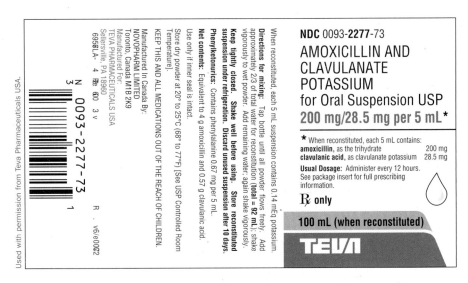

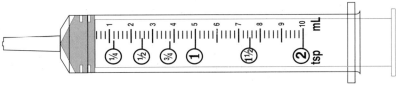

7. Order: promethazine 12.5 mg IV q.4h p.r.n., nausea

   Give: _____ mL (Use label A.)

   Frequency: _____

© Cengage Learning 2013

8. Order: promethazine 40 mg IM stat

   Give: _____ mL (Use label B.)

   Frequency: _____

© Cengage Learning 2013

9. Order: morphine sulfate 4 mg slow IV push q.4h p.r.n., severe pain

   Give: _____ mL   Frequency: _____

© Cengage Learning 2013

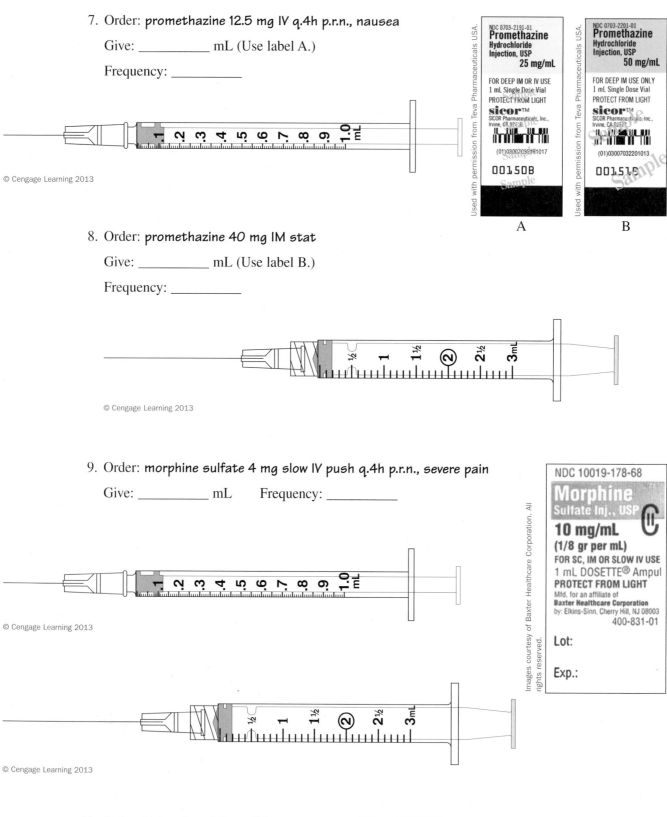

10. Order: butorphanol 3 mg IM stat

    Give: _____ mL

    Frequency: _____

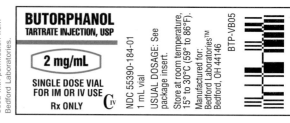

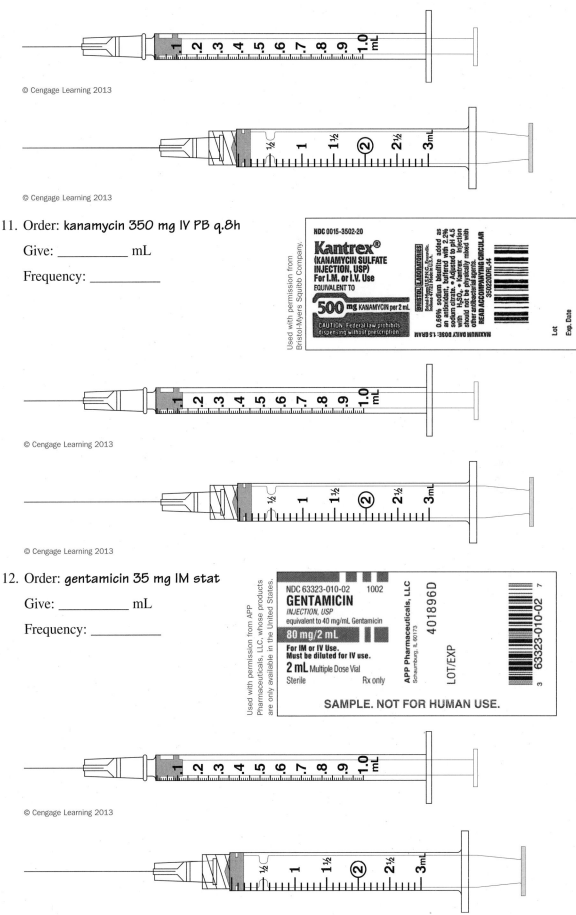

© Cengage Learning 2013

© Cengage Learning 2013

11. Order: kanamycin 350 mg IV PB q.8h

Give: _____ mL

Frequency: _____

© Cengage Learning 2013

© Cengage Learning 2013

12. Order: gentamicin 35 mg IM stat

Give: _____ mL

Frequency: _____

© Cengage Learning 2013

© Cengage Learning 2013

13. Order: glycopyrrolate 200 mcg IV stat

    Give: _____ mL

    Frequency: _____

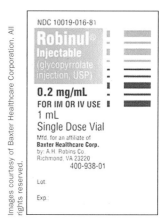

NDC 10019-016-81

Robinul
Injectable
(glycopyrrolate
injection, USP)

0.2 mg/mL
FOR IM OR IV USE

1 mL
Single Dose Vial

Mfd. for an affiliate of
Baxter Healthcare Corp.
by: A.H. Robins Co.
Richmond, VA 23220
400-938-01

Lot.

Exp.

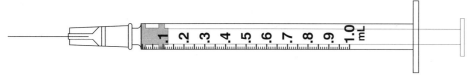

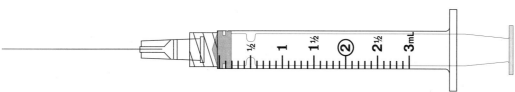

14. Order: digoxin 0.125 mg IV q.AM

    Give: _____ mL

    Frequency: _____

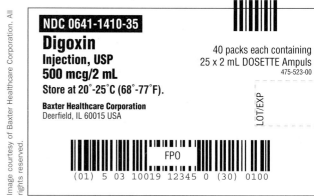

NDC 0641-1410-35

Digoxin
Injection, USP
500 mcg/2 mL
Store at 20°-25°C (68°-77°F).

Baxter Healthcare Corporation
Deerfield, IL 60015 USA

40 packs each containing
25 x 2 mL DOSETTE Ampuls
475-523-00

LOT/EXP

FPO

(01) 5 03 10019 12345 0 (30) 0100

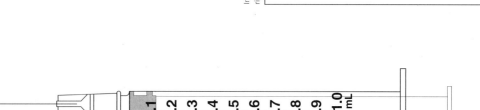

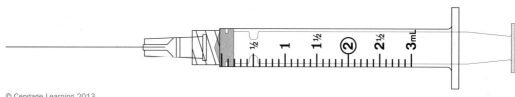

15. Order: doxycycline 80 mg IV PB q.12h

Give: _____ mL

Frequency: _____

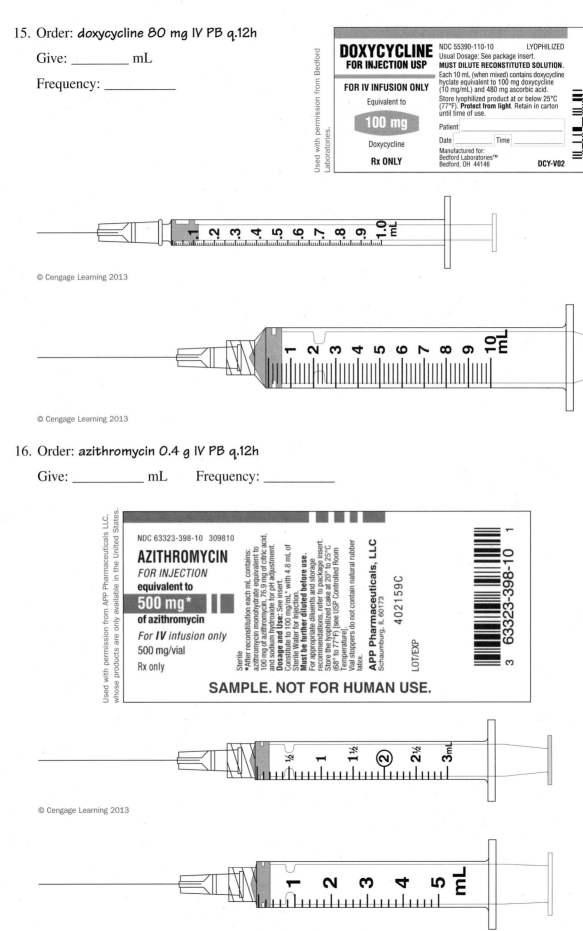

DOXYCYCLINE
FOR INJECTION USP

FOR IV INFUSION ONLY

Equivalent to

100 mg

Doxycycline

Rx ONLY

NDC 55390-110-10   LYOPHILIZED
Usual Dosage: See package insert.
MUST DILUTE RECONSTITUTED SOLUTION.
Each 10 mL (when mixed) contains doxycycline
hyclate equivalent to 100 mg doxycycline
(10 mg/mL) and 480 mg ascorbic acid.
Store lyophilized product at or below 25°C
(77°F). **Protect from light.** Retain in carton
until time of use.

Patient _____
Date _____ Time _____
Manufactured for:
Bedford Laboratories™
Bedford, OH 44146   **DCY-V02**

Used with permission from Bedford Laboratories.

© Cengage Learning 2013

© Cengage Learning 2013

16. Order: azithromycin 0.4 g IV PB q.12h

Give: _____ mL   Frequency: _____

Used with permission from APP Pharmaceuticals LLC, whose products are only available in the United States.

NDC 63323-398-10   309810

AZITHROMYCIN

FOR INJECTION

equivalent to

500 mg*

of azithromycin

For IV infusion only

500 mg/vial

Rx only

Sterile
*After reconstitution each mL contains:
azithromycin monohydrate equivalent to
100 mg of azithromycin, 76.9 mg of citric acid,
and sodium hydroxide for pH adjustment.
Dosage and Use: See insert.
Constitute to 100 mg/mL* with 4.8 mL of
Sterile Water for Injection.
Must be further diluted before use.
For appropriate diluents and storage
recommendations, refer to package insert.
Store the lyophilized cake at 20° to 25°C
(68° to 77°F) [see USP Controlled Room
Temperature].
Vial stoppers do not contain natural rubber
latex.

APP Pharmaceuticals, LLC
Schaumburg, IL 60173

402159C

LOT/EXP

3 63323-398-10 1

SAMPLE. NOT FOR HUMAN USE.

© Cengage Learning 2013

© Cengage Learning 2013

17. Order: **phenytoin 50 mg IV push q.8h** (administer at the rate recommended on the label)

Give: _____ mL at _____ mL/min, which equals _____ mL per 15 sec

Frequency: _____

Dosage–See package insert.

℞ only

Manufactured by:
Parkedale Pharmaceuticals, Inc.
Rochester, MI 48307

For:
PARKE-DAVIS
Div of Warner-Lambert Co
Morris Plains, NJ 07950 USA

N 0071-4475-45
STERI-VIAL®
Dilantin®
(Phenytoin Sodium Injection, USP)
ready/mixed
250 mg in 5 mL
5 mL

Do not exceed
50 mg/minute IV
IM/IV (no infusion)

© 1997-'98, Warner-Lambert Co.

4475G233

Used with permission from Pfizer Inc.

© Cengage Learning 2013

© Cengage Learning 2013

18. Order: **ranitidine 35 mg in 100 mL D$_5$W IV PB over 20 minutes q.6h**

Add: _____ mL to the IV PB bag, and set the drip rate on the tubing to _____ gtt/min

Frequency: _____

RANITIDINE
INJECTION, USP

50 mg/2 mL

25 mg/mL*

NDC 55390-616-10   2 mL STERILE vial
*Each mL contains ranitidine 25 mg (as the hydrochloride) with phenol 5 mg as preservative.
Rx ONLY

Mfg for: Bedford Laboratories™
Bedford, OH 44146   **RNPV02**

Used with permission from Bedford Laboratories.

© Cengage Learning 2013

No. 4967
VENOSET® Piggyback
Primary I.V. Set, Vented, 80 Inch   **15** DROPS/mL
ABBOTT LABORATORIES, NORTH CHICAGO, IL 60064, USA

Used with permission from Abbott Laboratories.

19. Order: Novolin N NPH U-100 insulin 46 units c̄ Novolin R regular U-100 insulin 22 units subcut daily ā breakfast

You will give _____ units total.   Frequency: _____

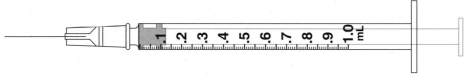

Refer to the following information to answer questions 20 through 24.

One of your assigned patients, Mrs. Betty Smedley, ID# 532729, with a history of osteoarthritis, is postop following a total hip replacement. She received a bolus of morphine sulfate by the epidural route in the recovery room at 1000 hours and has medication orders for breakthrough pain and other comfort measures. Refer to the medication administration record (MAR) on page 12 to answer the questions regarding administration of medication to Mrs. Smedley.

20. Mrs. Smedley had 60 mg of ketorolac at 1500 hours. At 2130 hours, she is complaining of severe pain again. How much ketorolac in the prefilled syringe will you give her now? Give _____ mL.

21. Mrs. Smedley is complaining of itching. What p.r.n. medication would you select, and how much will you administer? Select _____ and give _____ mL. Draw an arrow on the appropriate syringe to indicate how much you will give.

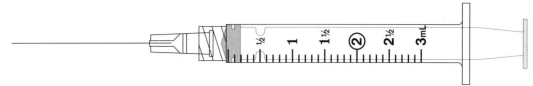

© Cengage Learning 2013

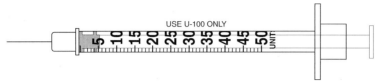

© Cengage Learning 2013

09/15/xx		**MEDICATION ADMINISTRATION RECORD**			PAGE: 1
0826					REPT: PHR20B

CHECKED BY: - - - - - - - - - - - - - - -

2ND	241		DIAGNOSIS: 71590		DIET: Regular
217A	532729		ALLERGIES: NKA		ADMIT: 09/15/xx
	Smedley, Betty		NOTES:		WT: 154 lb
			DX: OSTEOARTHRITIS-UNSPEC		

ADMINISTRATION PERIOD: 0730 09/15/xx TO 0729 09/16/xx					

ORDER # DRUG NAME, STRENGTH, DOSAGE FORM DOSE RATE ROUTE SCHEDULE	START	STOP	TIME PERIOD 0730 TO 1529	TIME PERIOD 1530 TO 2329	TIME PERIOD 2330 TO 0729
NURSE:					
• • • PRNs FOLLOW • • •		• • • PRNs FOLLOW • • •			
264077 TYLENOL 325 MG TABLET PRN **650 MG** ORAL Q4H/PRN FOR TEMP GREATER THAN 101 F	0930 09/15/xx			2110 GP	
264147 KETOROLAC 60 MG 2mL SYRINGE PRN **60 MG** IM PRN GIVE 60 MG FOR BREAKTHROUGH PAIN X1 DOSE THEN 30 MG Q6H/PRN	0930 09/15/xx		1500 MS		
264148 KETOROLAC 60 MG 2mL SYRINGE PRN **30 MG** IM Q6H/PRN GIVE 6 HOURS AFTER 60 MG DOSE FOR BREAK- THROUGH PAIN.	0930 09/15/xx				
264151 INAPSINE 2.5 MG/ML AMPULE PRN **SEE NOTE** IV Q6H/PRN SAME AS DROPERIDOL; DOSE IS 0.625 MG TO 1.25 MG (0.5-1.0 ML) FOR NAUSEA	0930 09/15/xx				
264152 BENADRYL 50 MG/ML AMPULE PRN **35 MG** IV Q4H/PRN FOR ITCHING	0930 09/15/xx				
264153 NARCAN 0.4 MG/ML AMPULE PRN **0.4 MG** IV PRN FOR RR LESS THAN 8 AND IF PT. IS UNAROUSABLE	0930 09/15/xx				

INITIALS	SIGNATURE	INITIALS	SIGNATURE		NOTES
GP	G. Pickar, R.N.				
MS	M. Smith, R.N.				

217A	Betty Smedley	AGE: 73	SEX: F	PHYSICIAN: J. Physician, MD
	ID# 532729			

22. At 2400, Mrs. Smedley's respiratory rate (RR) is 7, and she is difficult to arouse. What medication is indicated? _____ Give _____ mL. Draw an arrow on the syringe to indicate how much of this medication you will give.

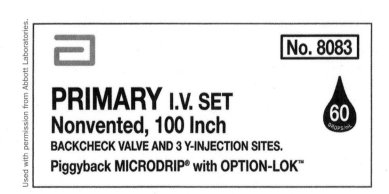

© Cengage Learning 2013

23. Mrs. Smedley had her last dose of Tylenol at 2110 hours. It is now 0215 hours, and her temperature is 39°C. Is Tylenol indicated? _____

    Explain: _____

    _____

24. How many tablets of Tylenol should she receive for each dose? _____ tablet(s)

Refer to the following information to answer questions 25 through 29.

Another of your assigned patients, Mr. John Beck, ID# 768342, with a history of insulin-dependent diabetes, is admitted to the medical unit with asthma. Refer to the medication administration record (MAR) on page 15 and all labels provided to answer the questions regarding administration of medication to Mr. Beck.

25. Theophylline is supplied in a solution strength of 80 mg per 15 mL. How much theophylline will you add to prepare the 50 mL piggyback bag? _____ mL

    Set the drip rate on the manually regulated IV tubing at _____ gtt/min.

No. 8083

PRIMARY I.V. SET
Nonvented, 100 Inch
BACKCHECK VALVE AND 3 Y-INJECTION SITES.
Piggyback MICRODRIP® with OPTION-LOK™

60 DROPS/mL

Used with permission from Abbott Laboratories.

26. An infusion pump, calibrated in whole mL/h, becomes available, and you decide to use it for Mr. Beck's IV. To administer the theophylline by infusion pump, set the pump at _____ mL/h.

27. Reconstitute the Solu-Medrol with _____ mL diluent, and give _____ mL.

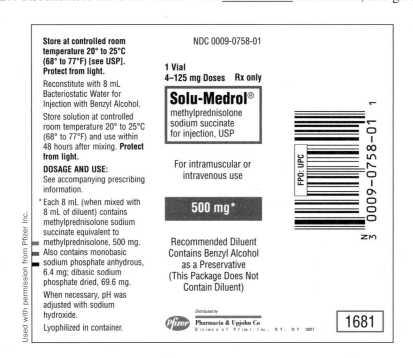

28. Mealtimes are 8 AM, 1 PM, and 6 PM. Using international time, give _____ tablet(s) of Carafate per dose each day at _____, _____, and _____ hours.

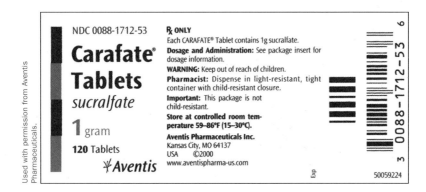

29. At 0730, Mr. Beck's blood sugar is 360. You will give him _____ units of insulin by the _____ route. Draw an arrow on the appropriate syringe to indicate the correct dosage.

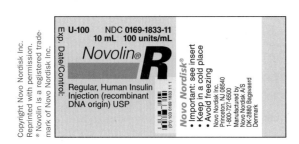

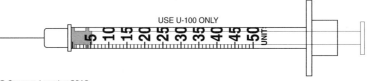

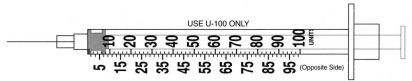

USE U-100 ONLY

5 10 20 30 40 50 60 70 80 90 100 UNITS

5 15 25 35 45 55 65 75 85 95 (Opposite Side)

© Cengage Learning 2013

.1 .2 .3 .4 .5 .6 .7 .8 .9 1.0 mL

© Cengage Learning 2013

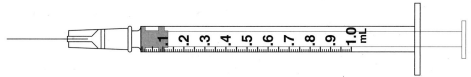

MEDICATION ADMINISTRATION RECORD

PAGE _____ of _____

ORIGINAL ORDER DATE	DATE STARTED/RENEWED	MEDICATION - DOSAGE	ROUTE	SCHEDULE 11-7	7-3	3-11	DATE 3-10-xx 11-7	7-3	3-11	DATE 3-11-xx 11-7	7-3	3-11	DATE 3-12-xx 11-7	7-3	3-11	DATE 3-13-xx 11-7	7-3	3-11
3-10-xx	3-10	Theophylline 100 mg in 50 mL D₅W x 30 min q.6h	IV PB	12 6	12	6		GP 12	MS 6	JJ12 JJ6								
3-10-xx	3-10	Solu-Medrol 125 mg q.6h	IV	12 6	12	6		GP 12	MS 6	JJ12 JJ6								
3-10-xx	3-10	Carafate 1 g 60 min ac	PO		7 12	5		GP7 GP12	MS5									
3-10-xx	3-10	Novulin R Regular U-100 insulin 30 min ac per sliding scale: Blood sugar Units 0-150 0 units 151-250 8 units 251-350 13 units 351-400 18 units greater than 400 Call M.D.	sub-cut		7:30 11:30	5:30		GP7:30 GP11:30	MS5:30									

PRN

INJECTION SITES

B - RIGHT ARM
C - RIGHT ABDOMEN
D - RIGHT ANTERIOR THIGH
G - LEFT ARM
H - LEFT ABDOMEN
J - LEFT ANTERIOR THIGH
L - LEFT BUTTOCKS
M - RIGHT BUTTOCKS

DATE GIVEN	TIME	INT.	ONE - TIME MEDICATION - DOSAGE	RT.	11-7	7-3	3-11	11-7	7-3	3-11	11-7	7-3	3-11	11-7	7-3	3-11
					SCHEDULE			DATE			DATE			DATE		

SIGNATURE OF NURSE ADMINISTERING MEDICATIONS

11-7		JJ J.Jones LPN
7-3	GP G.Pickar, RN	
3-11	MS M.Smith, RN	

DATE GIVEN	TIME	INT.	MEDICATION-DOSAGE-CONT.	RT.

RECOPIED BY:

CHECKED BY:

LITHO IN U.S.A. K6508 (7-92) D395538

Beck, John
ID #768342

ALLERGIES:

602-31 (7-xx) (MPC# 1355)

(1)

ORIGINAL COPY

© Cengage Learning 2013

Refer to the following information to answer questions 30 through 32.

You are working in the health department pediatric clinic. Your first patient, Jimmy Bryan, a 22 lb child, is brought to the clinic by his mother and diagnosed with otitis media, an ear infection. Answer the following questions to determine the safe dosage, and administer the correct dose amount.

30. The nurse practitioner orders amoxicillin 100 mg p.o. q.8h for Jimmy. To reconstitute the amoxicillin, add _____ mL water.

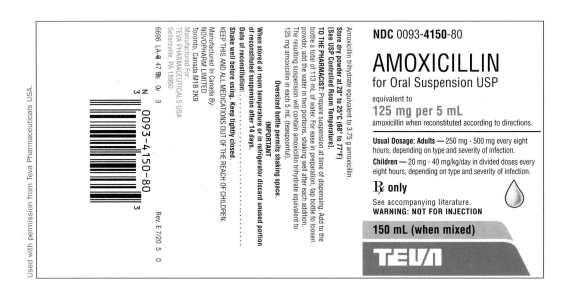

31. Is Jimmy's amoxicillin order safe and reasonable? _____ Explain: _____

_____

32. The nurse practitioner asks you to give Jimmy 1 dose of the amoxicillin stat. You will give Jimmy _____ mL.

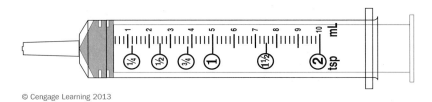

© Cengage Learning 2013

Refer to the following information to answer questions 33 and 34.

Your next patient, Marcus Williams, is a 4-year-old, 40 lb preschooler being treated for an upper respiratory infection. The nurse practitioner prescribes amoxicillin clavulanate 240 mg p.o. q.8h based on the amoxicillin dose of the combination medication.

33. According to a drug reference, the recommended dosage of amoxicillin is 40 mg/kg/day in divided doses q.8h. Will the ordered dosage provide the recommended dosage for Marcus? _____
    Explain: _____

34. If the order is the correct recommended dosage, how much would you administer for 1 dose?

Give: _____ mL

If it is not the recommended dose, what would you do next?

_____

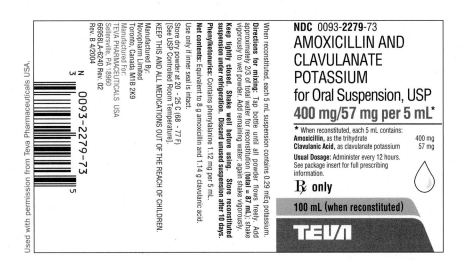

Refer to the following information to answer questions 35 through 37.

Your third patient seen at the pediatric clinic is Alexandra Martin, a 6-year-old, 62 lb school-age child with a fever of 39.6°C. The nurse practitioner orders **acetaminophen 300 mg p.o. stat.** For hyperthermia in children, the recommended dosage of acetaminophen is 10 to 15 mg/kg p.o. q.4h, not to exceed 5 doses per day.

35. Alexandra's mother is not familiar with Celsius measurements and asks what the temperature is in Fahrenheit. What will you tell her? _____ °F

36. What is the safe single dosage range of acetaminophen for Alexandra? _____ mg/dose to _____ mg/dose

37. Acetaminophen is available in the clinic supply as a suspension of 80 mg per 2.5 mL. How many mL will you administer for this dose? _____ mL

Refer to the following information to answer questions 38 through 40.

Your patient, Jill Jones, a 16-year-old, 110 lb adolescent, is admitted to the medical unit. She has a history of a duodenal ulcer, and her current problem is abdominal pain. Answer the following questions regarding a safe ordered dose of IV medication, infusion rate, and intake and output.

38. The physician orders **cimetidine 250 mg q.6h.** According to a drug reference, the recommended dosage range of cimetidine is 20 to 30 mg/kg/day in 4 divided doses. What is the recommended single dosage range for Jill? _____ mg/dose to _____ mg/dose. Will the order provide the recommended dosage? _____

39. The pharmacy has supplied a vial of cimetidine 300 mg per 2 mL and a D$_5$W 50 mL IV PB bag, with instructions to infuse over 20 min. Add _____ mL of cimetidine to the IV PB bag, and set the manual drip rate at _____ gtt/min.

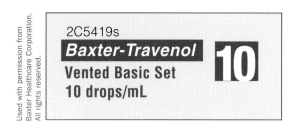

2C5419s
Baxter-Travenol **10**
Vented Basic Set
10 drops/mL

40. Jill is on strict intake and output measurements. Calculate the 8-hour total fluid intake for documentation in the metric system.

Time	Oral Intake	Time	IV Intake
0800	Gelatin 4 fl oz Water 3 fl oz	0800	50 mL
1000	Water 3 fl oz		
1300	Apple juice 16 fl oz	1400	50 mL

What is her total fluid intake for the 8-hour shift? _____ mL

41. The following day the physician orders **washed, packed red blood cells 2 units (600 mL) IV to infuse in 4 hours.** The manually regulated IV tubing has a drop factor of 10 gtt/mL. You will set the IV drip rate to _____ gtt/min.

Refer to the following information to answer questions 42 through 49.

Mr. Ralph Callahan, a 52 year old, has just returned to the surgical unit, following abdominal surgery, with a patient-controlled analgesic (PCA) pump started at 1430. The medication cartridge in the pump contains morphine sulfate 50 mg per 50 mL, set for patient administration at **1 mg q.10 min p.r.n.**

42. Mr. Callahan may self-administer _____ mL every 10 minutes.

43. If he attempts and receives 5 doses this hour, he would receive _____ mg per _____ mL of morphine.

44. Based on the amount of morphine in the syringe in the PCA pump, how many total doses can Mr. Callahan receive? _____ dose(s)

45. If he receives 5 doses every hour, at what time would he finish receiving his morphine dosage? _____ hours or _____ in traditional AM/PM time.

46. Postop orders for Mr. Callahan include *ceftriaxone 0.5 g IV q.8h.*

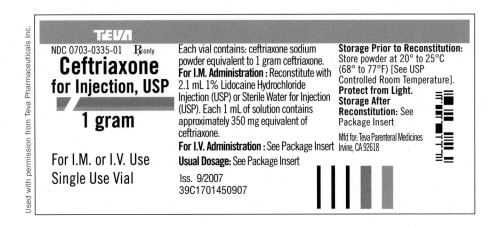

The supplied medication needs to be reconstituted prior to use. Administration instructions include:

Intravenous Administration

Ceftriaxone for injection, USP should be administered intravenously by infusion over a period of 30 minutes. Concentrations between 10 mg/mL and 40 mg/mL are recommended; however, lower concentrations may be used if desired. Reconstitute vials with an appropriate IV diluent (see **COMPATIBILITY AND STABILITY**).

Vial Dosage Size	Amount of Diluent to be Added
250 mg	2.4 mL
500 mg	4.8 mL
1 g	9.6 mL
2 g	19.2 mL

After reconstitution, each 1 mL of solution contains approximately 100 mg equivalent of ceftriaxone. Withdraw entire contents and dilute to the desired concentration with the appropriate IV diluent.

The total volume of the ceftriaxone after reconstitution is _____ mL.

47. The resulting dosage strength of ceftriaxone is _____ mg per _____ mL.

48. Give _____ mL of ceftriaxone.

49. You reconstituted the drug at 1500 on 1/30/xx. The package insert for ceftriaxone states: "Reconstituted solution is stable at room temperature for 24 hours and refrigerated for 3 days." Prepare a reconstitution label for the ceftriaxone.

50. Describe the clinical reasoning you would use to prevent this medication error.

   Possible Scenario
   Order: *dexamethasone 4 mg IV q.6h*

   Day 1 Supply: dexamethasone 4 mg/mL

   Student nurse prepared and administered 1 mL.

   Day 2 Supply: dexamethasone 10 mg/mL

   Student nurse prepared 1 mL.

   Potential Outcome
   On Day 2, the student's instructor asked the student to recheck the order, think about the action, check the calculation, and provide the rationale for the amount prepared. The student was alarmed at the possibility of administering two-and-a-half times the prescribed dosage. The student insisted that the pharmacy should consistently supply the same unit dosage. The instructor advised the student of the possibility that different pharmacy technicians could be involved or possibly the original supply dosage was not available.

   Prevention

   _____

   _____

After completing these problems, see pages 581–587 to check your answers. Give yourself 2 points for each correct answer.

Perfect score = 100   My score = _____

Minimum mastery score = 90 (45 correct)

1. Give: _____ tablet(s)   Frequency: _____

2. Give: _____ tablet(s)   Frequency: _____

3. Choose: _____ mg capsules   Give: _____ capsule(s)   Frequency: _____

4. Give: _____ tablet(s)   Frequency: _____

5. Give: _____ tablet(s)   Frequency: _____

6. Give: _____ mL   Frequency: _____

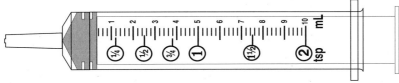

© Cengage Learning 2013

7. Give: _____ mL   Frequency: _____

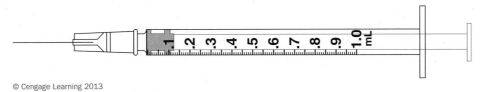

© Cengage Learning 2013

8. Give: _____ mL   Frequency: _____

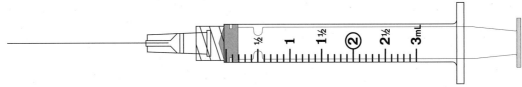

© Cengage Learning 2013

9. Give: _____ mL   Frequency: _____

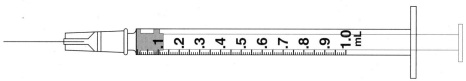

© Cengage Learning 2013

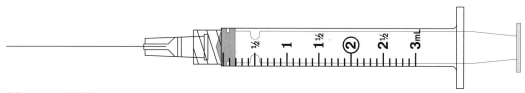

© Cengage Learning 2013

10. Give: _____ mL   Frequency: _____

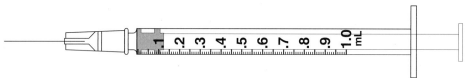

© Cengage Learning 2013

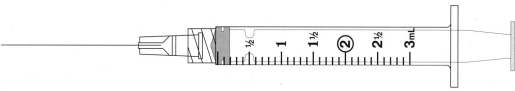

© Cengage Learning 2013

11. Give: _____ mL   Frequency: _____

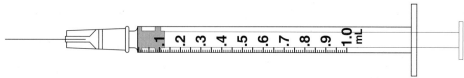

© Cengage Learning 2013

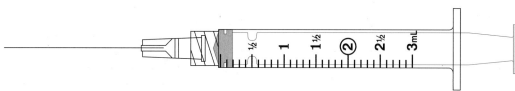

© Cengage Learning 2013

12. Give: _____ mL   Frequency: _____

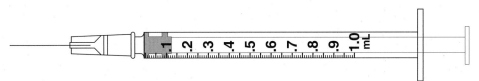

© Cengage Learning 2013

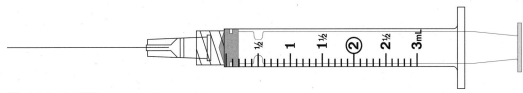

© Cengage Learning 2013

13. Give: _____ mL   Frequency: _____

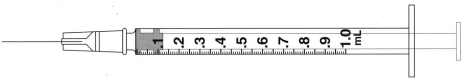

© Cengage Learning 2013

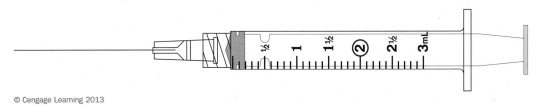

© Cengage Learning 2013

14. Give: _____ mL   Frequency: _____

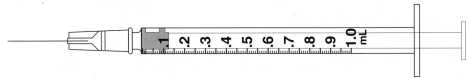

© Cengage Learning 2013

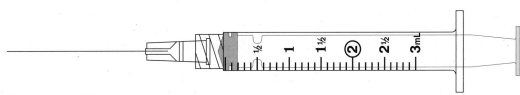

© Cengage Learning 2013

15. Give: _____ mL   Frequency: _____

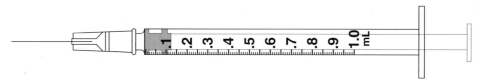

© Cengage Learning 2013

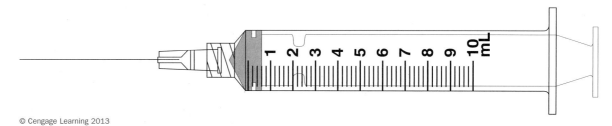

© Cengage Learning 2013

16. Give: _____ mL   Frequency: _____

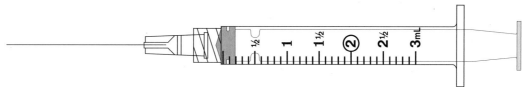

© Cengage Learning 2013

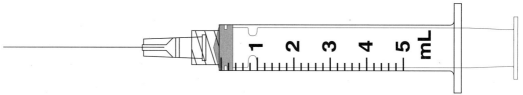

© Cengage Learning 2013

17. Give: _____ mL at _____ mL/min, which equals _____ mL per 15 sec

    Frequency: _____

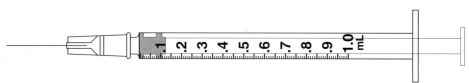

© Cengage Learning 2013

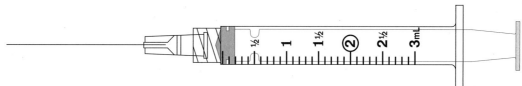

© Cengage Learning 2013

18. Add: _____ mL to the IV PB bag, and set the drip rate on the tubing to _____ gtt/min

    Frequency: _____

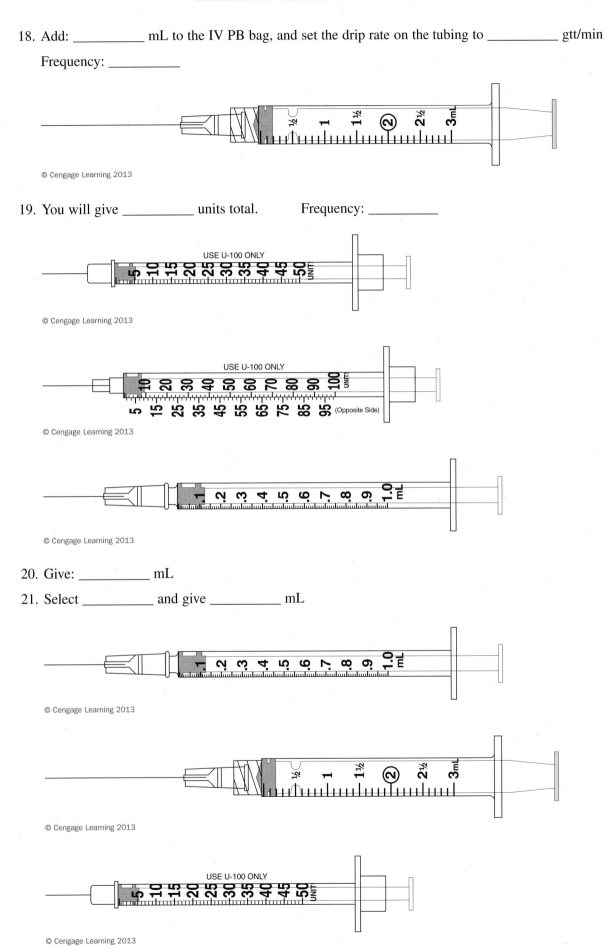

© Cengage Learning 2013

19. You will give _____ units total.　　Frequency: _____

© Cengage Learning 2013

© Cengage Learning 2013

© Cengage Learning 2013

20. Give: _____ mL

21. Select _____ and give _____ mL

© Cengage Learning 2013

© Cengage Learning 2013

© Cengage Learning 2013

22. Medication: _____   Give: _____ mL

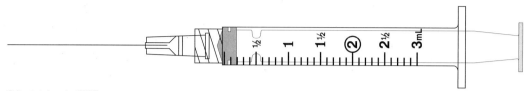

© Cengage Learning 2013

23. Yes or No: _____   Explain: _____

_____

24. _____ tablet(s)

25. _____ mL; _____ gtt/min

26. _____ mL/h

27. _____ mL diluent; give _____ mL

28. _____ tablet(s); _____, _____, and _____ hours

29. _____ units; _____ route

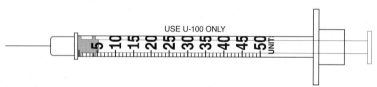

© Cengage Learning 2013

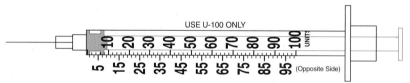

© Cengage Learning 2013

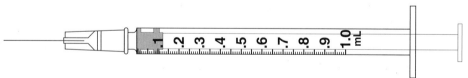

© Cengage Learning 2013

30. _____ mL

31. Yes or No: _____   Explain: _____

_____

32. _____ mL

33. Yes or No: _____   Explain: _____

_____

34. _____ mL   Next Action: _____

35. _____ °F

36. _____ mg/dose to _____ mg/dose

37. _____ mL

38. _____ mg/dose to _____ mg/dose; Yes or No: _____

39. _____ mL; _____ gtt/min

40. _____ mL

41. _____ gtt/min

42. _____ mL

43. _____ mg; _____ mL

44. _____ dose(s)

45. _____ hours; _____ (AM/PM)

46. _____ mL

47. _____ mg per _____ mL

48. _____ mL

49.

50. **Prevention:** _____

_____

After completing these problems, see pages 581–587 to check your answers. Give yourself
2 points for each correct answer.

Perfect score = 100   My score = _____

Minimum mastery score = 90 (45 correct)

MATHEMATICS DIAGNOSTIC EVALUATION

As a prerequisite objective, *Dosage Calculations* takes into account that you can add, subtract, multiply, and divide whole numbers. You should have a working knowledge of fractions, decimals, ratios, percents, and basic problem solving as well. This text reviews these important mathematical operations, which support all dosage calculations in health care.

Set aside $1\frac{1}{2}$ hours in a quiet place to complete the 50 items in the following diagnostic evaluation. You will need scratch paper and a pencil to work the problems.

Use your results to determine your computational strengths and weaknesses to guide your review. A minimum score of 86 is recommended as an indicator of readiness for dosage calculations. If you achieve that score, you may proceed to Chapter 3. However, note any problems that you answered incorrectly, and use the related review materials in Chapters 1 and 2 to refresh your skills.

This mathematics diagnostic evaluation and the review that follows are provided to enhance your confidence and proficiency in arithmetic skills, thereby helping you to avoid careless mistakes when you perform dosage calculations.

Good luck!

Directions

1. Carry answers to three decimal places and round to two places.

   (Examples: 5.175 = 5.18; 5.174 = 5.17)

2. Express fractions in lowest terms.

   (Example: $\frac{6}{10} = \frac{3}{5}$)

Mathematics Diagnostic Evaluation

1. $1{,}517 + 0.63 =$ _____

2. Express the value of $0.7 + 0.035 + 20.006$ rounded to two decimal places. _____

3. $9.5 + 17.06 + 32 + 41.11 + 0.99 =$ _____

4. $\$19.69 + \$304.03 =$ _____

5. $93.2 - 47.09 =$ _____

6. $1{,}005 - 250.5 =$ _____

7. Express the value of $17.156 - 0.25$ rounded to two decimal places. _____

8. $509 \times 38.3 =$ _____

9. $\$4.12 \times 42 =$ _____

10. $17.16 \times 23.5 =$ _____

11. $972 \div 27 =$ _____

12. $2.5 \div 0.001 =$ _____

13. Express the value of $\frac{1}{4} \div \frac{3}{8}$ as a fraction reduced to lowest terms. _____

14. Express $\frac{1{,}500}{240}$ as a decimal. _____

15. Express 0.8 as a fraction. _____

16. Express $\frac{2}{5}$ as a percent. _____

17. Express 0.004 as a percent. _____

18. Express 5% as a decimal. _____

19. Express $33\frac{1}{3}\%$ as a ratio in lowest terms. _____

20. Express 1:50 as a decimal. _____

21. $\frac{1}{2} + \frac{3}{4} =$ _____

22. $1\frac{2}{3} + 4\frac{7}{8} =$ _____

23. $1\frac{5}{6} - \frac{2}{9} =$ _____

24. Express the value of $\frac{1}{100} \times 60$ as a fraction. _____

25. Express the value of $4\frac{1}{4} \times 3\frac{1}{2}$ as a mixed number. _____

26. Identify the fraction with the greatest value: $\frac{1}{150}, \frac{1}{200}, \frac{1}{100}$. _____

27. Identify the decimal with the least value: 0.009, 0.19, 0.9. _____

28. $\frac{6.4}{0.02} =$ _____

29. $\frac{0.02 + 0.16}{0.4 - 0.34} =$ _____

30. Express the value of $\frac{3}{12 + 3} \times 0.25$ as a decimal. _____

31. 8% of 50 = _____

32. $\frac{1}{2}\%$ of 18 = _____

33. 0.9% of 24 = _____

Find the value of X. Express your answer as a decimal.

34. $\frac{1:1,000}{1:100} \times 250 = X$ _____

35. $\frac{300}{150} \times 2 = X$ _____

36. $\frac{2.5}{5} \times 1.5 = X$ _____

37. $\frac{1,000,000}{250,000} \times X = 12$ _____

38. $\frac{0.51}{1.7} \times X = 150$ _____

39. $X = (82.4 - 52)\frac{3}{5}$ _____

40. $\frac{\frac{1}{150}}{\frac{1}{300}} \times 1.2 = X$ _____

41. Express 2:10 as a fraction in lowest terms. _____

42. Express 2% as a ratio in lowest terms. _____

43. If five equal medication containers contain a total of 25 tablets, how many tablets are in each container? _____

44. A person is receiving 0.5 milligrams of a medication four times a day. What is the total amount of milligrams of medication given each day? _____

45. If 1 kilogram equals 2.2 pounds, how many kilograms does a 66-pound child weigh? _____

46. If 1 kilogram equals 2.2 pounds, how many pounds are in 1.5 kilograms? (Express your answer as a decimal.) _____

47. If 1 centimeter equals $\frac{3}{8}$ inch, how many centimeters are in $2\frac{1}{2}$ inches? (Express your answer as a decimal.)   _____

48. If 2.5 centimeters equal 1 inch, how long in centimeters is a 3-inch wound?   _____

49. This diagnostic test has a total of 50 problems. If you incorrectly answer 5 problems, what percentage will you have answered correctly?   _____

50. For every 5 female student nurses in a nursing class, there is 1 male student nurse. What is the ratio of female to male student nurses?   _____

After completing these problems, see pages 587–588 to check your answers. Give yourself 2 points for each correct answer.

Perfect score = 100   My score = _____

Minimum readiness score = 86 (43 correct)

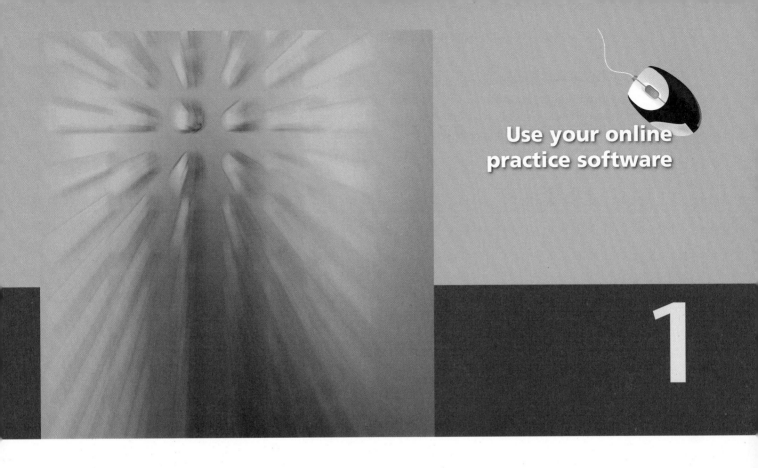

1

Fractions and Decimals

OBJECTIVES

Upon mastery of Chapter 1, you will be able to perform basic mathematical computations essential for clinical calculations that involve fractions and decimals. Specifically, you will be able to:

- Compare the values of fractions and decimals.
- Convert between mixed numbers and improper fractions, and between reduced and equivalent forms of fractions.
- Add, subtract, multiply, and divide fractions and decimals.
- Round a decimal to a given place value.
- Read and write out the values of decimal numbers.

Health care professionals need to understand fractions and decimals to be able to interpret and act on medical orders, read prescriptions, and understand patient records and information in health care literature. The most common system of measurement used in prescription, dosage calculation, and administration of medications is the metric system. The metric system is international, and it is the most precise system of measurement. Metric measure is based on decimals. Occasionally, you will see fractions used in apothecary and household measures in dosage calculations. The method of solving dosage problems in this book relies on expressing relationships in fractional form. Therefore, proficiency with fractions and decimals will add to your success with a variety of medical applications.

FRACTIONS

A *fraction* indicates a portion of a whole number. There are two types of fractions: *common fractions,* such as $\frac{1}{2}$ (usually referred to simply as *fractions*) and *decimal fractions,* such as 0.5 (usually referred to simply as *decimals*).

A fraction is an expression of division, with one number placed over another number ($\frac{1}{4}, \frac{2}{3}, \frac{4}{5}$). The bottom number, or *denominator,* indicates the total number of equal-sized parts into which the whole is divided. The top number, or *numerator,* indicates how many of those parts are considered. The fraction may also be read as *the numerator divided by the denominator.*

EXAMPLE ■

$\frac{1}{4}$ $\frac{\text{numerator}}{\text{denominator}}$

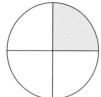

The whole is divided into four equal parts (denominator), and one part (numerator) is considered.

© Cengage Learning 2013

$\frac{1}{4} = 1$ part of 4 parts, or $\frac{1}{4}$ of the whole.

The fraction $\frac{1}{4}$ may also be read as *1 divided by 4.*

MATH TIP
The *d*enominator begins with *d* and is *d*own below the line in a fraction.

Types of Fractions

There are four types of fractions: proper, improper, mixed numbers, and complex.

Proper Fractions

Proper fractions are fractions in which the value of the numerator is less than the value of the denominator. The value of the proper fraction is less than 1.

RULE
Whenever the numerator is less than the denominator, the value of the fraction must be less than 1.

EXAMPLE ■

$\frac{5}{8}$ is less than 1

Improper Fractions

Improper fractions are fractions in which the value of the numerator is greater than or equal to the value of the denominator. The value of the improper fraction is greater than or equal to 1.

RULE
Whenever the numerator is greater than the denominator, the value of the fraction must be greater than 1.

EXAMPLE ■

$\frac{8}{5}$ is greater than 1

RULE
Whenever the numerator and denominator are equal, the value of the improper fraction is always equal to 1; a nonzero number divided by itself is equal to 1.

EXAMPLE ■

$\frac{5}{5} = 1$

Mixed Numbers

When a whole number and a proper fraction are combined, the result is referred to as a *mixed number*. The value of the mixed number is always greater than 1.

EXAMPLE ■

$1\frac{5}{8} = 1 + \frac{5}{8}$ $1\frac{5}{8}$ is greater than 1

Complex Fractions

Complex fractions include fractions in which the numerator, the denominator, or both contain a fraction, decimal, or mixed number. The value may be less than, greater than, or equal to 1.

EXAMPLES ■

$\frac{\frac{5}{8}}{\frac{1}{2}}$ is greater than 1 $\frac{\frac{5}{8}}{2}$ is less than 1 $\frac{1\frac{5}{8}}{\frac{1}{5}}$ is greater than 1 $\frac{\frac{1}{2}}{\frac{2}{4}} = 1$

To perform dosage calculations that involve fractions, you must be able to convert among these different types of fractions and reduce them to lowest terms. You must also be able to add, subtract, multiply, and divide fractions. Review these simple rules of working with fractions. Continue to practice until the concepts are crystal clear and automatic.

Equivalent Fractions

The value of a fraction can be expressed in several ways. This is called *finding an equivalent fraction*. In finding an equivalent fraction, both terms of the fraction (numerator and denominator) are either multiplied or divided by the same nonzero number.

MATH TIP
In an equivalent fraction, the form of the fraction is changed, but the value of the fraction remains the same.

EXAMPLES ■

$\frac{2}{4} = \frac{2 \div 2}{4 \div 2} = \frac{1}{2}$ $\frac{1}{3} = \frac{1 \times 3}{3 \times 3} = \frac{3}{9}$

Reducing Fractions to Lowest Terms

When calculating dosages, it is usually easier to work with fractions using the smallest possible numbers. Finding these equivalent fractions is called *reducing the fraction to the lowest terms* or *simplifying the fraction*.

RULE

To reduce a fraction to lowest terms, divide both the numerator and denominator by the largest nonzero whole number that will go evenly into both the numerator and the denominator.

EXAMPLE ▪

Reduce $\frac{6}{12}$ to lowest terms.

6 is the largest number that will divide evenly into both 6 (numerator) and 12 (denominator).

$\frac{6}{12} = \frac{6 \div 6}{12 \div 6} = \frac{1}{2}$ in lowest terms

Sometimes this reduction can be done in several steps. Always check a fraction to see if it can be reduced further.

EXAMPLE ▪

$\frac{5,000}{20,000} = \frac{5,000 \div 1,000}{20,000 \div 1,000} = \frac{5}{20}$ (not in lowest terms)

$\frac{5}{20} = \frac{5 \div 5}{20 \div 5} = \frac{1}{4}$ (in lowest terms)

MATH TIP

If neither the numerator nor the denominator can be divided evenly by a nonzero number other than 1, then the fraction is already in lowest terms.

Enlarging Fractions

RULE

To find an equivalent fraction in which both terms are larger, multiply both the numerator and the denominator by the same nonzero number.

EXAMPLE ▪

Enlarge $\frac{3}{5}$ to the equivalent fraction in tenths.

$\frac{3}{5} = \frac{3 \times 2}{5 \times 2} = \frac{6}{10}$

Conversion

It is important to be able to convert among different types of fractions. Conversion allows you to perform various calculations with greater ease and permits you to express answers in simplest terms.

Converting Mixed Numbers to Improper Fractions

RULE

To change or convert a mixed number to an improper fraction with the same denominator, multiply the whole number by the denominator and add the numerator. This value becomes the numerator, while the denominator remains the same as it was in the fraction of the initial mixed number.

EXAMPLE ■

$$2\frac{5}{8} = \frac{(2 \times 8) + 5}{8} = \frac{16 + 5}{8} = \frac{21}{8}$$

Converting Improper Fractions to Mixed Numbers

RULE

To change or convert an improper fraction to an equivalent mixed number or whole number, divide the numerator by the denominator. Any remainder becomes the numerator of a proper fraction that should be reduced to lowest terms.

EXAMPLES ■

$$\frac{8}{5} = 8 \div 5 = 1\frac{3}{5}$$

$$\frac{10}{4} = 10 \div 4 = 2\frac{2}{4} = 2\frac{1}{2}$$

Comparing Fractions

In calculating some drug dosages, it is helpful to know when the value of one fraction is greater or less than another. The relative sizes of fractions can be determined by comparing the numerators when the denominators are the same or comparing the denominators if the numerators are the same.

RULE

If the denominators are the same, the fraction with the smaller numerator has the lesser value.

EXAMPLE ■

Compare $\frac{2}{5}$ and $\frac{3}{5}$

Denominators are both 5

Numerators: 2 is less than 3

$\frac{2}{5}$ has a lesser value

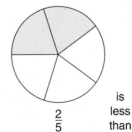

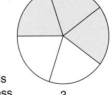

$\frac{2}{5}$ is less than $\frac{3}{5}$

RULE

If the numerators are the same, the fraction with the smaller denominator has the greater value.

EXAMPLE ▪

Compare $\frac{1}{2}$ and $\frac{1}{4}$

Numerators are both 1

Denominators: 2 is less than 4

$\frac{1}{2}$ has a greater value

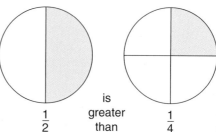

$\frac{1}{2}$ is greater than $\frac{1}{4}$

© Cengage Learning 2013

Note: A smaller denominator means the whole has been divided into fewer pieces, so each piece is larger.

QUICK REVIEW

- Proper fraction: numerator is less than denominator; value is less than 1. Example: $\frac{1}{2}$

- Improper fraction: numerator is greater than denominator; value is greater than 1. Example: $\frac{4}{3}$

  Or numerator = denominator; value = 1. Example: $\frac{5}{5}$

- Mixed number: whole number + a fraction; value is greater than 1. Example: $1\frac{1}{2}$

- Complex fraction: numerator and/or denominator are composed of a fraction, decimal, or mixed number; value is less than, greater than, or = 1.

  Example: $\dfrac{\frac{1}{2}}{\frac{1}{50}}$

- Any nonzero number divided by itself = 1. Example: $\frac{3}{3} = 1$

- To reduce a fraction to lowest terms, divide both terms by the largest nonzero whole number that will divide both the numerator and denominator evenly. Value remains the same.

  Example: $\frac{6}{10} = \frac{6 \div 2}{10 \div 2} = \frac{3}{5}$

- To enlarge a fraction, multiply both terms by the same nonzero number. Value remains the same.

  Example: $\frac{1}{12} = \frac{1 \times 2}{12 \times 2} = \frac{2}{24}$

- To convert a mixed number to an improper fraction, multiply the whole number by the denominator and add the numerator; use original denominator in the fractional part.

  Example: $1\frac{1}{3} = \frac{(1 \times 3) + 1}{3} = \frac{3 + 1}{3} = \frac{4}{3}$

- To convert an improper fraction to a mixed number, divide the numerator by the denominator. Express any remainder as a proper fraction reduced to lowest terms.

  Example: $\frac{21}{9} = 21 \div 9 = 2\frac{3}{9} = 2\frac{1}{3}$

- When numerators are equal, the fraction with the smaller denominator is greater.

  Example: $\frac{1}{2}$ is greater than $\frac{1}{3}$

- When denominators are equal, the fraction with the larger numerator is greater.

  Example: $\frac{2}{3}$ is greater than $\frac{1}{3}$

Review Set 1

1. Circle the *improper* fraction(s).

$$\frac{2}{3} \qquad 1\frac{3}{4} \qquad \frac{6}{6} \qquad \frac{7}{5} \qquad \frac{16}{17} \qquad \frac{\frac{1}{9}}{\frac{2}{3}}$$

2. Circle the *complex* fraction(s).

$$\frac{4}{5} \qquad 3\frac{7}{8} \qquad \frac{2}{2} \qquad \frac{9}{8} \qquad \frac{8}{9} \qquad \frac{\frac{1}{100}}{\frac{1}{150}}$$

3. Circle the *proper* fraction(s).

$$\frac{1}{4} \qquad \frac{1}{14} \qquad \frac{14}{1} \qquad \frac{14}{14} \qquad \frac{144}{14}$$

4. Circle the *mixed* number(s) *reduced to the lowest terms.*

$$3\frac{4}{8} \qquad \frac{2}{3} \qquad 1\frac{2}{9} \qquad \frac{1}{3} \qquad 1\frac{1}{4} \qquad 5\frac{7}{8}$$

5. Circle the pair(s) of *equivalent* fractions.

$$\frac{3}{4}=\frac{6}{8} \qquad \frac{1}{5}=\frac{2}{10} \qquad \frac{3}{9}=\frac{1}{3} \qquad \frac{3}{4}=\frac{4}{3} \qquad 1\frac{4}{9}=1\frac{2}{3}$$

Change the following mixed numbers to improper fractions.

6. $6\frac{1}{2} =$ _____

7. $1\frac{1}{5} =$ _____

8. $10\frac{2}{3} =$ _____

9. $7\frac{5}{6} =$ _____

10. $102\frac{3}{4} =$ _____

Change the following improper fractions to whole numbers or mixed numbers; reduce to lowest terms.

11. $\frac{24}{12} =$ _____

12. $\frac{8}{8} =$ _____

13. $\frac{30}{9} =$ _____

14. $\frac{100}{75} =$ _____

15. $\frac{44}{16} =$ _____

Enlarge the following fractions to the number of parts indicated.

16. $\frac{3}{4}$ to eighths _____

17. $\frac{1}{4}$ to sixteenths _____

18. $\frac{2}{3}$ to twelfths _____

19. $\frac{2}{5}$ to tenths _____

20. $\frac{2}{3}$ to ninths _____

Circle the correct answer.

21. Which is larger? $\frac{1}{150}$ or $\frac{1}{100}$

22. Which is smaller? $\frac{1}{1,000}$ or $\frac{1}{10,000}$

23. Which is larger? $\frac{2}{9}$ or $\frac{5}{9}$

24. Which is smaller? $\frac{3}{10}$ or $\frac{5}{10}$

25. A patient is supposed to drink a 10 fluid ounce bottle of magnesium citrate prior to his X-ray study. He has been able to drink 6 fluid ounces. What portion of the liquid remains? (Express your answer as a fraction reduced to lowest terms.) _____

26. If 1 medicine bottle contains 12 doses, how many full and fractional bottles of medicine are required for 18 doses? (Express your answer as a fraction reduced to lowest terms.) _____

27. A respiratory therapy class consists of 24 men and 36 women. What fraction of the students in the class are men? (Express your answer as a fraction reduced to lowest terms.) _____

28. A nursing student answers 18 out of 20 questions correctly on a test. Write a proper fraction (reduced to lowest terms) to represent the portion of the test questions that were answered correctly.

_____

29. A typical dose of Children's Tylenol contains 160 milligrams of medication per teaspoonful. Each 80 milligrams is what part of a typical dose? _____

30. In question 29, how many teaspoons of Children's Tylenol would you need to give an 80 milligram dose? _____

After completing these problems, see page 588 to check your answers.

If you answered question 30 correctly, you can already calculate a dosage! In this text you will learn additional steps to focus on safety during calculations.

Addition and Subtraction of Fractions

To add or subtract fractions, all the denominators must be the same. You can determine the least common denominator by finding the smallest whole number into which all denominators will divide evenly. Once the least common denominator is determined, convert the fractions to equivalent fractions with the least common denominator. This operation involves *enlarging the fractions,* which we examined in the last section. Let's look at an example of this important operation.

EXAMPLE ▪

Find the equivalent fractions with the least common denominator for $\frac{3}{8}$ and $\frac{1}{3}$.

1. Find the smallest whole number into which the denominators 8 and 3 will divide evenly. The least common denominator is 24.

2. Convert the fractions to equivalent fractions with 24 as the denominator.

$$\frac{3}{8} = \frac{3 \times 3}{8 \times 3} = \frac{9}{24} \qquad \frac{1}{3} = \frac{1 \times 8}{3 \times 8} = \frac{8}{24}$$

You have enlarged $\frac{3}{8}$ to $\frac{9}{24}$ and $\frac{1}{3}$ to $\frac{8}{24}$. Now both fractions have the same denominator. Finding the least common denominator is the first step in adding or subtracting fractions.

RULE

To add or subtract fractions:

1. Convert all fractions to equivalent fractions with the least common denominator.

2. Add or subtract the numerators, place that value in the numerator, and use the least common denominator as the denominator.

3. Convert to a mixed number and/or reduce the fraction to lowest terms, if possible.

MATH TIP
To add or subtract fractions, no calculations are performed on the denominators once they are all converted to equivalent fractions with the least common denominators. Perform the mathematical operation (addition or subtraction) on the *numerators* only, and use the least common denominator as the denominator of the answer. Never add or subtract denominators.

Adding Fractions

EXAMPLE 1 ■

$\frac{3}{4} + \frac{1}{4} + \frac{2}{4}$

1. Find the least common denominator. This step is not necessary in this example, because the fractions already have the same denominator.

2. Add the numerators, and use the common denominator: $\frac{3 + 1 + 2}{4} = \frac{6}{4}$

3. Convert to a mixed number, and reduce to lowest terms: $\frac{6}{4} = 1\frac{2}{4} = 1\frac{1}{2}$

EXAMPLE 2 ■

$\frac{1}{3} + \frac{3}{4} + \frac{1}{6}$

1. Find the least common denominator: 12. The number 12 is the smallest number that 3, 4, and 6 will all equally divide into.

   Convert to equivalent fractions in twelfths. This is the same as enlarging the fractions.

   $\frac{1}{3} = \frac{1 \times 4}{3 \times 4} = \frac{4}{12}$

   $\frac{3}{4} = \frac{3 \times 3}{4 \times 3} = \frac{9}{12}$

   $\frac{1}{6} = \frac{1 \times 2}{6 \times 2} = \frac{2}{12}$

2. Add the numerators, and use the common denominator: $\frac{4 + 9 + 2}{12} = \frac{15}{12}$

3. Convert to a mixed number, and reduce to lowest terms: $\frac{15}{12} = 1\frac{3}{12} = 1\frac{1}{4}$

Subtracting Fractions

EXAMPLE 1 ■

$\frac{15}{18} - \frac{8}{18}$

1. Find the least common denominator. This is not necessary in this example, because the denominators are the same.

2. Subtract the numerators, and use the common denominator: $\frac{15 - 8}{18} = \frac{7}{18}$

3. Reduce to lowest terms. This is not necessary here, because no further reduction is possible.

EXAMPLE 2 ▪

$1\frac{1}{10} - \frac{3}{5}$

1. Find the least common denominator: 10. The number 10 is the smallest number that both 10 and 5 will equally divide into.

   Convert to equivalent fractions in tenths:

   $1\frac{1}{10} = \frac{11}{10}$ Note: First convert mixed numbers into improper fractions for computations.

   $\frac{3}{5} = \frac{3 \times 2}{5 \times 2} = \frac{6}{10}$

2. Subtract the numerators, and use the common denominator: $\frac{11 - 6}{10} = \frac{5}{10}$

3. Reduce to lowest terms: $\frac{5}{10} = \frac{1}{2}$

   Let's review one more time how to add and subtract fractions.

QUICK REVIEW

To add or subtract fractions:

■ Convert to equivalent fractions with the least common denominator.

■ Add or subtract the numerators; place that value in the numerator. Use the least common denominator as the denominator of the answer.

■ Convert the answer to a mixed number and/or reduce to lowest terms, if possible.

Review Set 2

Add, and reduce the answers to lowest terms.

1. $7\frac{4}{5} + \frac{2}{3} =$ _____

2. $\frac{3}{4} + \frac{2}{3} =$ _____

3. $4\frac{2}{3} + 5\frac{1}{24} + 7\frac{1}{2} =$ _____

4. $\frac{3}{4} + \frac{1}{8} + \frac{1}{6} =$ _____

5. $12\frac{1}{2} + 20\frac{1}{3} =$ _____

6. $\frac{1}{4} + 5\frac{1}{3} =$ _____

7. $\frac{1}{7} + \frac{2}{3} + \frac{11}{21} =$ _____

8. $\frac{4}{9} + \frac{5}{8} + 4\frac{2}{3} =$ _____

9. $34\frac{1}{2} + 8\frac{1}{2} =$ _____

10. $\frac{12}{17} + 5\frac{2}{7} =$ _____

11. $\frac{6}{5} + 1\frac{1}{3} =$ _____

12. $\frac{1}{4} + \frac{5}{33} =$ _____

Subtract, and reduce the answers to lowest terms.

13. $\frac{3}{4} - \frac{1}{4} =$ _____

14. $8\frac{1}{12} - 3\frac{1}{4} =$ _____

15. $\frac{1}{8} - \frac{1}{12} =$ _____

16. $100 - 36\frac{1}{3} =$ _____

17. $355\frac{1}{5} - 55\frac{2}{5} =$ _____

18. $\frac{1}{3} - \frac{1}{6} =$ _____

19. $2\frac{3}{5} - 1\frac{1}{5} =$ _____

20. $14\frac{3}{16} - 7\frac{1}{8} =$ _____

21. $25 - 17\frac{7}{9} =$ _____

22. $4\frac{7}{10} - 3\frac{9}{20} =$ _____

23. $48\frac{6}{11} - 24 =$ _____

24. $1\frac{2}{3} - 1\frac{1}{12} =$ _____

25. A patient weighs 50 pounds on admission and 48 pounds on day 3 of his hospital stay. Write a fraction, reduced to lowest terms, to express the fraction of his original weight that he has lost.

_____

26. A patient is on strict recording of fluid intake and output, including measurement of liquids used to prepare medications. A nursing student mixed the 8 AM medication with $2\frac{1}{2}$ fluid ounces of juice and the 8 PM medication with $3\frac{1}{3}$ fluid ounces of water. What is the total amount of liquid the patient consumed with medications? _____

27. An infant has grown $\frac{1}{2}$ inch during his first month of life, $\frac{1}{4}$ inch during his second month, and $\frac{3}{8}$ inch during his third month. How much did he grow during his first 3 months? _____

28. The required margins for your term paper are $1\frac{1}{2}$ inches at the top and bottom of a paper that has 11 inches of vertical length. How long is the vertical area available for typed information?

_____

29. A stock clerk finds that there are $34\frac{1}{2}$ pints of hydrogen peroxide on the shelf. If the fully stocked shelf held 56 pints of hydrogen peroxide, how many pints were used?

_____

30. Your 1-year-old patient weighs $20\frac{1}{2}$ pounds. At birth, she weighed $7\frac{1}{4}$ pounds. How much weight has she gained in 1 year? _____

After completing these problems, see pages 588–589 to check your answers.

Multiplication of Fractions

To multiply fractions, multiply numerators (for the numerator of the answer) and multiply denominators (for the denominator of the answer) to arrive at the *product,* or result.

When possible, *cancellation of terms* simplifies and shortens the process of multiplication of fractions. Cancellation (like reducing to lowest terms) is based on the fact that the division of both the numerator and denominator by the same nonzero whole number does not change the value of the resulting number. In fact, it makes the calculation simpler, because you are working with smaller numbers.

EXAMPLE ■

$\frac{1}{3} \times \frac{250}{500}$ (numerator and denominator of $\frac{250}{500}$ are both divisible by 250)

$$= \frac{1}{3} \times \frac{\overset{1}{\cancel{250}}}{\underset{2}{\cancel{500}}} = \frac{1}{3} \times \frac{1}{2} = \frac{1}{6}$$

Also, a numerator and a denominator of any of the fractions involved in the multiplication may be cancelled when they can be divided by the same number. This is called *cross-cancellation.*

EXAMPLE ▪

$$\frac{1}{8} \times \frac{8}{9} = \frac{1}{\overset{}{\underset{1}{8}}} \times \frac{\overset{1}{8}}{9} = \frac{1}{1} \times \frac{1}{9} = \frac{1}{9}$$

RULE

To multiply fractions:

1. Cancel terms, if possible.

2. Multiply numerators for the numerator of the answer, and multiply denominators for the denominator of the answer.

3. Reduce the result *(product)* to lowest terms, if possible.

EXAMPLE 1 ▪

$$\frac{3}{4} \times \frac{2}{6}$$

1. Cancel terms: Divide 2 and 6 by 2

$$\frac{3}{4} \times \frac{\overset{1}{2}}{\underset{3}{6}} = \frac{3}{4} \times \frac{1}{3}$$

Divide 3 and 3 by 3

$$\frac{\overset{1}{3}}{4} \times \frac{1}{\underset{1}{3}} = \frac{1}{4} \times \frac{1}{1}$$

2. Multiply numerators and denominators:

$$\frac{1}{4} \times \frac{1}{1} = \frac{1}{4}$$

3. Reduce to lowest terms. This is not necessary here, because no further reduction is possible.

EXAMPLE 2 ▪

$$\frac{15}{30} \times \frac{2}{5}$$

1. Cancel terms: Divide 15 and 30 by 15

$$\frac{\overset{1}{15}}{\underset{2}{30}} \times \frac{2}{5} = \frac{1}{2} \times \frac{2}{5}$$

Divide 2 and 2 by 2

$$\frac{1}{\underset{1}{2}} \times \frac{\overset{1}{2}}{5} = \frac{1}{1} \times \frac{1}{5}$$

2. Multiply numerators and denominators:

$$\frac{1}{1} \times \frac{1}{5} = \frac{1}{5}$$

3. Reduce to lowest terms. This is not necessary here, because no further reduction is possible.

MATH TIP
When multiplying a fraction by a nonzero whole number, first convert the whole number to a fraction with a denominator of 1; the value of the number remains the same.

EXAMPLE 3 ■

$\frac{2}{3} \times 4$

1. No terms to cancel. (You cannot cancel 2 and 4, because both are numerators. To do so would change the value.) Convert the whole number to a fraction.

$$\frac{2}{3} \times 4 = \frac{2}{3} \times \frac{4}{1}$$

2. Multiply numerators and denominators:

$$\frac{2}{3} \times \frac{4}{1} = \frac{8}{3}$$

3. Convert to a mixed number.

$$\frac{8}{3} = 8 \div 3 = 2\frac{2}{3}$$

MATH TIP
To multiply mixed numbers, first convert them to improper fractions, and then multiply.

EXAMPLE 4 ■

$3\frac{1}{2} \times 4\frac{1}{3}$

1. Convert: $3\frac{1}{2} = \frac{7}{2}$

$\qquad\qquad 4\frac{1}{3} = \frac{13}{3}$

Therefore, $3\frac{1}{2} \times 4\frac{1}{3} = \frac{7}{2} \times \frac{13}{3}$

2. Cancel: not necessary. No numbers can be cancelled.

3. Multiply: $\frac{7}{2} \times \frac{13}{3} = \frac{91}{6}$

4. Convert to a mixed number: $\frac{91}{6} = 15\frac{1}{6}$

Division of Fractions

The division of fractions uses three terms: *dividend, divisor,* and *quotient.* The *dividend* is the fraction being divided, or the first number. The *divisor,* the number to the right of the division sign, is the fraction the dividend is divided by. The *quotient* is the result of the division. To divide fractions, the divisor is inverted and the operation is changed to multiplication. Once inverted, the calculation is the same as for multiplication of fractions.

EXAMPLE ▪

$$\frac{1}{4} \quad \div \quad \frac{2}{7} \quad = \quad \frac{1}{4} \quad \times \quad \frac{7}{2} \quad = \quad \frac{7}{8}$$

↑ **Dividend** ↑ **Divisor** ↑ **÷ Changed to ×** ↑ **Inverted Divisor** ↑ **Quotient**

RULE

To divide fractions:

1. Invert the terms of the divisor; change ÷ to ×.

2. Cancel terms, if possible.

3. Multiply the resulting fractions.

4. Convert the result (quotient) to a mixed number, and/or reduce to lowest terms, if possible.

EXAMPLE 1 ▪

$\frac{3}{4} \div \frac{1}{3}$

1. Invert divisor, and change ÷ to ×: $\frac{3}{4} \div \frac{1}{3} = \frac{3}{4} \times \frac{3}{1}$

2. Cancel: not necessary. No numbers can be cancelled.

3. Multiply: $\frac{3}{4} \times \frac{3}{1} = \frac{9}{4}$

4. Convert to mixed number: $\frac{9}{4} = 2\frac{1}{4}$

EXAMPLE 2 ▪

$\frac{2}{3} \div 4$

1. Invert divisor, and change ÷ to ×: $\frac{2}{3} \div \frac{4}{1} = \frac{2}{3} \times \frac{1}{4}$

2. Cancel terms: $\frac{\overset{1}{\cancel{2}}}{3} \times \frac{1}{\underset{2}{\cancel{4}}} = \frac{1}{3} \times \frac{1}{2}$

3. Multiply: $\frac{1}{3} \times \frac{1}{2} = \frac{1}{6}$

4. Reduce: not necessary; already reduced to lowest terms.

MATH TIP

To divide mixed numbers, first convert them to improper fractions.

EXAMPLE 3 ▪

$1\frac{1}{2} \div \frac{3}{4}$

1. Convert: $\frac{3}{2} \div \frac{3}{4}$

2. Invert divisor, and change ÷ to ×: $\frac{3}{2} \times \frac{4}{3}$

3. Cancel: $\dfrac{\overset{1}{\cancel{3}}}{\underset{1}{\cancel{2}}} \times \dfrac{\overset{2}{\cancel{4}}}{\underset{1}{\cancel{3}}} = \dfrac{1}{1} \times \dfrac{2}{1}$

4. Multiply: $\dfrac{1}{1} \times \dfrac{2}{1} = \dfrac{2}{1}$

5. Simplify: $\dfrac{2}{1} = 2$

MATH TIP
Multiplying complex fractions also involves the division of fractions.

In the next example the divisor is the same as the denominator, so you will invert the denominator and multiply. Multiplying complex fractions can be confusing—take your time and study this carefully.

EXAMPLE 4 ▪

$\dfrac{\frac{1}{150}}{\frac{1}{100}} \times 2$

1. Convert: Express 2 as a fraction. $\dfrac{\frac{1}{150}}{\frac{1}{100}} \times \dfrac{2}{1}$

2. Rewrite complex fraction as division: $\dfrac{1}{150} \div \dfrac{1}{100} \times \dfrac{2}{1}$

3. Invert divisor, and change $\div$ to $\times$: $\dfrac{1}{150} \times \dfrac{100}{1} \times \dfrac{2}{1}$

4. Cancel: $\dfrac{1}{\underset{3}{\cancel{150}}} \times \dfrac{\overset{2}{\cancel{100}}}{1} \times \dfrac{2}{1} = \dfrac{1}{3} \times \dfrac{2}{1} \times \dfrac{2}{1}$

5. Multiply: $\dfrac{1}{3} \times \dfrac{2}{1} \times \dfrac{2}{1} = \dfrac{4}{3}$

6. Convert to mixed number: $\dfrac{4}{3} = 1\dfrac{1}{3}$

This example appears difficult at first, but when solved logically, one step at a time, it is just like the others.

QUICK REVIEW
- To *multiply* fractions, cancel terms, multiply numerators, and multiply denominators.
- To *divide* fractions, invert the divisor, cancel terms, and multiply.
- Convert results to a mixed number and/or reduce to lowest terms, if possible.

Review Set 3

Multiply, and reduce the answers to lowest terms.

1. $\dfrac{3}{10} \times \dfrac{1}{12} =$ _____   3. $\dfrac{5}{8} \times 1\dfrac{1}{6} =$ _____

2. $\dfrac{12}{25} \times \dfrac{3}{5} =$ _____   4. $\dfrac{1}{100} \times 3 =$ _____

5. $\dfrac{\frac{1}{6}}{\frac{1}{4}} \times \dfrac{\frac{3}{2}}{\frac{2}{3}} =$ _____

9. $\dfrac{3}{4} \times \dfrac{2}{3} =$ _____

6. $\dfrac{\frac{1}{150}}{\frac{1}{100}} \times 2\frac{1}{2} =$ _____

10. $4\frac{2}{3} \times 5\frac{1}{24} =$ _____

7. $\dfrac{30}{75} \times 2 =$ _____

11. $\dfrac{3}{4} \times \dfrac{1}{8} =$ _____

8. $9\frac{4}{5} \times \dfrac{2}{3} =$ _____

12. $12\frac{1}{2} \times 20\frac{1}{3} =$ _____

Divide, and reduce the answers to lowest terms.

13. $\dfrac{3}{4} \div \dfrac{1}{4} =$ _____

19. $2\frac{1}{2} \div \dfrac{3}{4} =$ _____

14. $6\frac{1}{12} \div 3\frac{1}{4} =$ _____

20. $\dfrac{\frac{1}{20}}{\frac{1}{3}} =$ _____

15. $\dfrac{1}{8} \div \dfrac{7}{12} =$ _____

21. $\dfrac{1}{150} \div \dfrac{1}{50} =$ _____

16. $\dfrac{1}{33} \div \dfrac{1}{3} =$ _____

22. $\dfrac{7}{8} \div 1\frac{1}{2} =$ _____

17. $5\frac{1}{4} \div 10\frac{1}{2} =$ _____

23. $\dfrac{\frac{3}{5}}{\frac{3}{4}} \div \dfrac{\frac{4}{5}}{1\frac{1}{9}} =$ _____

18. $\dfrac{1}{60} \div \dfrac{1}{2} =$ _____

24. The nurse is maintaining calorie counts (or counting calories) for a patient who is not eating well. The patient ate $\frac{3}{4}$ of a large apple. If one large apple contains 80 calories, how many calories were consumed? _____

25. How many seconds are there in $9\frac{1}{3}$ minutes? _____

26. A bottle of Children's Tylenol contains 20 teaspoons of liquid. If each dose for a 2-year-old child is $\frac{1}{2}$ teaspoon, how many doses for a 2 year old are available in this bottle? _____

27. The patient needs to take $1\frac{1}{2}$ tablets of medication 3 times per day for 7 days. Over the 7 days, how many tablets will the patient take? _____

28. The nurse aide observes that the patient's water pitcher is $\frac{1}{3}$ full. If the patient drank 850 milliliters of water, how many milliliters does the pitcher hold? (Hint: The 850 milliliters does not represent $\frac{1}{3}$ of the pitcher.) _____

29. A pharmacist weighs a tube of antibiotic eye ointment and documents that it weighs $\frac{7}{10}$ of an ounce. How much would 75 tubes weigh? _____

30. A patient is taking a liquid antacid from a 16 fluid ounce bottle. If the patient takes $\frac{1}{2}$ fluid ounce every 4 hours while awake beginning at 7 AM and ending with a final dose at 11 PM, how many full days would this bottle last? (Hint: First, draw a clock.) _____

After completing these problems, see page 589 to check your answers.

DECIMALS

Decimal Fractions and Decimal Numbers

Decimal fractions are fractions with a denominator of 10, 100, 1,000, or any power of 10. At first glance, they appear to be whole numbers because of the way they are written. But the numeric value of a decimal fraction is always less than 1.

EXAMPLES ▪

$0.1 \quad = \frac{1}{10}$

$0.01 \quad = \frac{1}{100}$

$0.001 = \frac{1}{1,000}$

 Decimal numbers are numeric values that include a whole number, a decimal point, and a decimal fraction. Generally, decimal fractions and decimal numbers are referred to simply as *decimals*.

EXAMPLES ▪

4.67 and 23.956

 Nurses and other health care professionals must have an understanding of decimals to be competent at dosage calculations. Medication orders and other measurements in health care primarily use metric measure, which is based on the decimal system. Decimals are a special shorthand for designating fractional values. They are simpler to read and faster to use when performing mathematical computations.

MATH TIP

When dealing with decimals, think of the decimal point as the center that separates whole and fractional amounts. The position of the numbers in relation to the decimal point indicates the place value of the numbers.

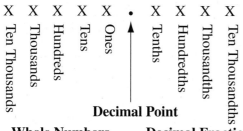

MATH TIP

The words for all decimal fractions end in *th(s)*.

EXAMPLES ▪

0.001 = one thousand*th*

0.02 = two hundred*ths*

0.7 = seven ten*ths*

RULE

The decimal number is read by stating the whole number first, the decimal point as *and,* and then the decimal fraction by naming the value of the last decimal place.

EXAMPLE ▪

Look carefully at the decimal number 4.125. The last decimal place is thousandths. Therefore, the number is read as *four and one hundred twenty-five thousandths.*

$$\underset{\substack{\text{Ones} \\ \text{Tenths} \\ \text{Hundredths} \\ \text{Thousandths}}}{4 \;.\; 1 \quad 2 \quad 5}$$

EXAMPLES ▪

The number 6.2 is read as *six and two tenths.*

The number 10.03 is read as *ten and three hundredths.*

MATH TIP

Given a decimal fraction (whose value is less than 1), the decimal number is read alone, without stating the zero. However, the zero is written to emphasize the decimal point. In fact, since 2005, this is a requirement by the accrediting body for health care organizations, The Joint Commission (2010), when writing decimal fractions in medical notation.

EXAMPLE ▪

0.125 is read as *one hundred twenty-five thousandths.*

A set of rules governs the decimal system of notation.

RULE

The whole number value is controlled by its position to the left of the decimal point.

EXAMPLES ▪

10.1 = ten and one tenth. The whole number is *10.*

1.01 = one and one hundredth. The whole number is *1.*

Notice that the decimal point's position completely changes the numeric value.

RULE

The decimal fraction value is controlled by its position to the right of the decimal point.

EXAMPLES ▪

25.1 = twenty-five and one tenth. The decimal fraction is *one tenth.*

25.01 = twenty-five and one hundredth. The decimal fraction is *one hundredth.*

MATH TIP
Each decimal place is counted off as a power of 10 to tell you which denominator is expected.

EXAMPLE 1 ■

437.5 = four hundred thirty-seven and **five tenths** $(437 + \frac{5}{10})$

One decimal place indicates *tenths*.

EXAMPLE 2 ■

43.75 = forty-three and **seventy-five hundredths** $(43 + \frac{75}{100})$

Two decimal places indicate *hundredths*.

EXAMPLE 3 ■

4.375 = four and **three hundred seventy-five thousandths** $(4 + \frac{375}{1,000})$

Three decimal places indicate *thousandths*.

RULE
Zeros added after the last digit of a decimal fraction do not change its value and are not necessary, except when a zero is required to demonstrate the level of precision of the value being reported, such as for laboratory results.

EXAMPLE ■

$0.25 = 0.25\mathbf{0}$

Twenty-five hundredths equals two hundred fifty thousandths.

CAUTION
When writing decimals, eliminate unnecessary zeros at the end of the number to avoid confusion. The Joint Commission (2010) forbids the use of trailing zeros for medication orders or other medication-related documentation and cautions that, in such cases, the decimal point may be missed when an unnecessary zero is written. This is part of The Joint Commission's *Official "Do Not Use" List* for medical notation, which will be discussed again in Chapters 3 and 9.

Because the last zero does not change the value of the decimal, it is not necessary. For example, the required notation is 0.25 rather than 0.250 and 10 not 10.0, which can be misinterpreted as 250 and 100, respectively, if the decimal point is not clear.

RULE
Zeros added before or after the decimal point of a decimal number *may* change its value.

EXAMPLES ■

$0.125 \neq$ (is not equal to) $\mathbf{0.0}125$

$1.025 \neq \mathbf{10}.025$

However, .6 = **0**.6 and 12 = 12.**0**, but you should write 0.6 (with a leading decimal) and 12 (without a trailing zero).

Comparing Decimals

It is important to be able to compare decimal amounts, noting which has a greater or lesser value.

CAUTION
A common error in comparing decimals is to overlook the decimal place values and misinterpret higher numbers for greater amounts and lower numbers for lesser amounts.

MATH TIP
You can accurately compare decimal amounts by aligning the decimal points and adding zeros so that the numbers to be compared have the same number of decimal places. Remember that adding zeros at the end of a decimal fraction for the purposes of comparison does not change the original value.

EXAMPLE 1 ▪

Compare 0.125, 0.05, and 0.2 to find which decimal fraction is largest.

Align decimal points and add zeros.

$0.125 = \frac{125}{1,000}$ or one hundred twenty-five thousandths

$0.05\mathbf{0} = \frac{50}{1,000}$ or fifty thousandths

$0.2\mathbf{00} = \frac{200}{1,000}$ or two hundred thousandths

Now it is easy to see that 0.2 is the greatest amount and 0.05 is the least. But at first glance, you might have been tricked into thinking that 0.2 was the least amount and 0.125 was the greatest amount. This kind of error can have dire consequences in dosage calculations and health care.

EXAMPLE 2 ▪

Suppose 0.5 microgram of a drug has been ordered. The recommended maximum dosage of the drug is 0.25 microgram, and the minimum recommended dosage is 0.125 microgram. Comparing decimals, you can see that the ordered dosage is not within the recommended range.

0.125 microgram (recommended minimum dosage)

0.25**0** microgram (recommended maximum dosage)

0.5**00** microgram (ordered dosage)

Now you can see that 0.5 microgram is outside the allowable limits of the recommended dosage range of 0.125 to 0.25 microgram for this medication. In fact, it is twice the recommended maximum dosage.

CAUTION
It is important to eliminate possible confusion and avoid errors in dosage calculation. To avoid overlooking a decimal point in a decimal fraction and thereby reading the numeric value as a whole number, always place a zero to the left of the decimal point to emphasize that the number has a value less than 1. This is another of The Joint Commission's requirements. The Joint Commission's *Official "Do Not Use" List* (2010) prohibits writing a decimal fraction that is less than 1 without a leading zero. This important concept will be emphasized again in Chapters 3 and 9.

EXAMPLES ■

0.425, **0**.01, or **0**.005

Conversion between Fractions and Decimals

For dosage calculations, you may need to convert decimals to fractions and vice versa.

RULE

To convert a fraction to a decimal, divide the numerator by the denominator.

MATH TIP

Make sure the numerator is inside the division sign and the denominator is outside. You will avoid reversing the numerator and the denominator in division if you write down the number you read first and put the division sign around that number, with the second number written outside the division sign. This will work regardless of whether it is written as a fraction or as a division problem (such as $\frac{1}{2}$ or $1 \div 2$).

EXAMPLE 1 ■

Convert $\frac{1}{4}$ to a decimal.

$$\frac{1}{4} = 4\overline{)1.00} = 0.25$$
$$\begin{array}{r} .25 \\ \underline{8} \\ 20 \\ \underline{20} \end{array}$$

EXAMPLE 2 ■

Convert $\frac{2}{5}$ to a decimal.

$$\frac{2}{5} = 5\overline{)2.0} = 0.4$$
$$\begin{array}{r} .4 \\ \underline{2.0} \end{array}$$

RULE

To convert a decimal to a fraction:

1. Express the decimal number as a whole number in the numerator of the fraction.

2. Express the denominator of the fraction as the number 1 followed by as many zeros as there are places to the right of the decimal point.

3. Reduce the resulting fraction to lowest terms.

EXAMPLE 1 ■

Convert 0.125 to a fraction.

1. Numerator: 125

2. Denominator: 1 followed by 3 zeros = 1,000

3. Reduce: $\frac{125}{1,000} = \frac{1}{8}$

EXAMPLE 2 ■

Convert 0.65 to a fraction.

1. Numerator: 65

2. Denominator: 1 followed by 2 zeros = 100

3. Reduce: $\frac{65}{100} = \frac{13}{20}$

MATH TIP

State the complete name of the decimal, and write the fraction that has the same name, such as $0.65 = $ "sixty-five hundredths" $= \frac{65}{100}$.

QUICK REVIEW

- In a decimal number, whole number values are to the left of the decimal point and fractional values are to the right.

- Zeros added to a decimal fraction before the decimal point of a decimal number less than 1 or at the end of the decimal fraction do not change the value (except when a zero is required to demonstrate the level of precision of the reported value). Example: $.5 = \mathbf{0.5} = 0.50$. However, using the leading zero is the only acceptable notation (such as 0.5).

- In a decimal number, zeros added before or after the decimal point *may* change the value. Example: $1.5 \neq 1.05$ and $1.5 \neq 10.5$.

- To avoid overlooking the decimal point in a decimal fraction, *always* place a zero to the left of the decimal point.

  Example:
  $.5 \leftarrow$ Avoid writing a decimal fraction this way; it could be mistaken for the whole number *5*.

  Example:
  $\mathbf{0.5} \leftarrow$ This is the required method of writing a decimal fraction with a value less than 1.

- The number of places in a decimal fraction indicates the power of 10.

  Examples:
  $0.5 = $ five tenths
  $0.05 = $ five hundredths
  $0.005 = $ five thousandths

- Compare decimals by aligning decimal points and adding zeros at the end.

  Example:
  Compare 0.5, 0.05, and 0.005.
  $\mathbf{0.500} = $ five hundred thousandths (greatest)
  $\mathbf{0.050} = $ fifty thousandths
  $\mathbf{0.005} = $ five thousandths (least)

- To convert a fraction to a decimal, divide the numerator by the denominator.

- To convert a decimal to a fraction, express the decimal number as a whole number in the numerator and the denominator as the correct power of 10. Reduce the fraction to lowest terms.

  Example:
  $$0.04 = \frac{4 \text{ (numerator is a whole number)}}{100 \text{ (denominator is 1 followed by 2 zeros)}} = \frac{\overset{1}{\cancel{4}}}{\underset{25}{\cancel{100}}} = \frac{1}{25}$$

Review Set 4

Complete the following table of equivalent fractions and decimals. Reduce fractions to lowest terms.

Fraction	Decimal	The decimal number is read as:
1. $\frac{1}{5}$	_____	_____

Fraction	**Decimal**	**The decimal number is read as:**
2. _____	_____.85_____	eighty-five hundredths
3. _____	1.05	_____
4. _____	0.006	_____
5. $10\frac{3}{200}$	_____	_____
6. _____	1.9	_____
7. _____	_____	five and one tenth
8. $\frac{4}{5}$	_____	_____
9. _____	250.5	_____
10. $33\frac{3}{100}$	_____	_____
11. _____	0.95	_____
12. $2\frac{3}{4}$	_____	_____
13. _____	_____	seven and five thousandths
14. $\frac{21}{250}$	_____	_____
15. _____	12.125	_____
16. _____	20.09	_____
17. _____	_____	twenty-two and twenty-two thousandths
18. _____	0.15	_____
19. $1,000\frac{1}{200}$	_____	_____
20. _____	_____	four thousand eighty-five and seventy-five thousandths

21. Change 0.017 to a four-place decimal. _____

22. Change 0.2500 to a two-place decimal. _____

23. Convert $\frac{75}{100}$ to a decimal. _____

24. Convert 0.045 to a fraction reduced to lowest terms. _____

Circle the correct answer.

25. Which is largest?   0.012   0.12   0.021

26. Which is smallest?   0.635   0.6   0.063

27. True or false?   0.375 = 0.0375

28. True or false?   2.2 grams = 2.02 grams

29. True or false?   6.5 ounces = 6.500 ounces

30. For a certain medication, the safe dosage should be greater than or equal to 0.5 gram but less than or equal to 2 grams. Circle each dosage that falls within this range.

   0.8 gram   0.25 gram   2.5 grams   1.25 grams

After completing these problems, see page 589 to check your answers.

Addition and Subtraction of Decimals

The addition and subtraction of decimals is similar to the addition and subtraction of whole numbers. There are two simple but essential rules that are different. Health care professionals must use these two rules to perform accurate dosage calculations for some medications.

RULE

To add and subtract decimals, line up the decimal points.

CAUTION

In final answers, eliminate unnecessary zeros at the end of a decimal to avoid confusion.

EXAMPLE 1 ▪

1.25 + 1.75 = 1.25
       + 1.75
        3.00 = 3

EXAMPLE 3 ▪

3.54 + 1.26 = 3.54
       + 1.26
        4.80 = 4.8

EXAMPLE 2 ▪

1.25 − 0.13 = 1.25
       − 0.13
        1.12

EXAMPLE 4 ▪

2.54 − 1.04 = 2.54
       − 1.04
        1.50 = 1.5

RULE

To add and subtract decimals, add zeros at the end of decimal fractions if necessary to make all decimal numbers of equal length.

EXAMPLE 1 ▪

3.75 − 2.1 = 3.75
       − 2.10
        1.65

EXAMPLE 3 ▪

5.25 − 3.6 = 5.25
       − 3.60
        1.65

EXAMPLE 2 ▪

Add 0.9, 0.65, 0.27, 4.712
   0.900
   0.650
   0.270
  +4.712
   6.532

EXAMPLE 4 ▪

66.96 + 32 = 66.96
       + 32.00
         98.96

QUICK REVIEW

▪ To add or subtract decimals, align the decimal points and add zeros at the end of the decimal fraction, making all decimals of equal length. Eliminate unnecessary zeros at the end in the final answer.

EXAMPLES ■

$1.5 + 0.05 = 1.5\underline{0}$

$$\begin{array}{r} 1.50 \\ + \; 0.05 \\ \hline 1.55 \end{array}$$

$7.8 + 1.12 = 7.8\underline{0}$

$$\begin{array}{r} 7.80 \\ + \; 1.12 \\ \hline 8.92 \end{array}$$

$0.725 - 0.5 = 0.725$

$$\begin{array}{r} 0.725 \\ - \; 0.5\underline{00} \\ \hline 0.225 \end{array}$$

$12.5 - 1.5 = 12.5$

$$\begin{array}{r} 12.5 \\ - \; 1.5 \\ \hline 11.0 = 11 \end{array}$$

Review Set 5

Find the results of the following problems.

1. $0.16 + 5.375 + 1.05 + 16 =$ _____

2. $7.517 + 3.2 + 0.16 + 33.3 =$ _____

3. $13.009 - 0.7 =$ _____

4. $5.125 + 6.025 + 0.15 =$ _____

5. $175.1 + 0.099 =$ _____

6. $25.2 - 0.193 =$ _____

7. $0.58 - 0.062 =$ _____

8. $\$10.10 - \$0.62 =$ _____

9. $\$19 - \$0.09 =$ _____

10. $\$5.05 + \$0.17 + \$17.49 =$ _____

11. $4 + 1.98 + 0.42 + 0.003 =$ _____

12. $0.3 - 0.03 =$ _____

13. $16.3 - 12.15 =$ _____

14. $2.5 - 0.99 =$ _____

15. $5 + 2.5 + 0.05 + 0.15 + 2.55 =$ _____

16. $0.03 + 0.16 + 2.327 =$ _____

17. $700 - 325.65 =$ _____

18. $645.32 - 40.9 =$ _____

19. $18 + 2.35 + 7.006 + 0.093 =$ _____

20. $13.529 + 10.09 =$ _____

21. A dietitian calculates the sodium in a patient's breakfast: raisin bran cereal = 0.1 gram, 1 cup 2% milk = 0.125 gram, 6 ounces orange juice = 0.001 gram, 1 corn muffin = 0.35 gram, and butter = 0.121 gram. How many grams of sodium did the patient consume? _____

22. In a 24-hour period, a premature infant drank 7.5 milliliters, 15 milliliters, 10 milliliters, 15 milliliters, 6.25 milliliters, and 12.5 milliliters of formula. How many milliliters did the infant drink in 24 hours?

_____

23. A patient has a hospital bill for $16,709.43. Her insurance company pays $14,651.37. What is her balance due? _____

24. A patient's hemoglobin was 14.8 grams before surgery. During surgery, the hemoglobin dropped 4.5 grams. What was the hemoglobin value after it dropped? _____

25. A home health nurse accounts for her day of work. If she spent 3 hours and 20 minutes at the office, 40 minutes traveling, $3\frac{1}{2}$ hours caring for patients, 24 minutes for lunch, and 12 minutes on break, what is her total number of hours including all of her activities? Express your answer as a decimal. (Hint: First convert each time to hours and minutes.) _____

After completing these problems, see page 590 to check your answers.

Multiplying Decimals

The procedure for multiplication of decimals is similar to that used for whole numbers. The only difference is the decimal point, which must be properly placed in the product or answer. Use the following simple rule.

RULE
To multiply decimals:

1. Multiply the decimals without concern for decimal point placement.

2. Count off the total number of decimal places in both of the decimals multiplied.

3. Move the decimal point in the product by moving it to the left the number of places counted.

EXAMPLE 1 ■

$1.5 \times 0.5 =$

$$
\begin{array}{r}
1.5 \\
\times\ 0.5 \\
\hline
0.75
\end{array}
$$

(1 decimal place)
(1 decimal place)
(The decimal point is located 2 places to the left, because a total of 2 decimal places are counted in the numbers that are multiplied.)

EXAMPLE 2 ■

$1.72 \times 0.9 =$

$$
\begin{array}{r}
1.72 \\
\times\ 0.9 \\
\hline
1.548
\end{array}
$$

(2 decimal places)
(1 decimal place)
(The decimal point is located 3 places to the left, because a total of 3 decimal places are counted.)

EXAMPLE 3 ■

$5.06 \times 1.3 =$

$$
\begin{array}{r}
5.06 \\
\times\ 1.3 \\
\hline
1518 \\
506 \\
\hline
6.578
\end{array}
$$

(2 decimal places)
(1 decimal place)

(The decimal point is located 3 places to the left, because a total of 3 decimal places are counted.)

EXAMPLE 4 ■

$1.8 \times 0.05 =$

$$
\begin{array}{r}
1.8 \\
\times\ 0.05 \\
\hline
0.090
\end{array}
$$

(1 decimal place)
(2 decimal places)
(The decimal point is located 3 places to the left. Notice that a zero has to be inserted between the decimal point and the 9 to allow for enough decimal places.)

$0.090 = 0.09$ (Eliminate unnecessary zero.)

RULE
When multiplying a decimal by a power of 10, move the decimal point as many places to the right as there are zeros in the multiplier.

EXAMPLE 1 ▪

1.25×10

The multiplier 10 has 1 zero; move the decimal point 1 place to the right.

$1.25 \times 10 = 1.2\underset{\smile}{5} = 12.5$

EXAMPLE 2 ▪

2.3×100

The multiplier 100 has 2 zeros; move the decimal point 2 places to the right. (Note: Add zeros as necessary to complete the operation.)

$2.3 \times 100 = 2.\underset{\smile}{30.} = 230$

EXAMPLE 3 ▪

$0.001 \times 1,000$

The multiplier 1,000 has 3 zeros; move the decimal point 3 places to the right.

$0.001 \times 1,000 = 0.\underset{\smile}{001.} = 1$

Dividing Decimals

When dividing decimals, set up the problem the same as for the division of whole numbers. Follow the same procedure for dividing whole numbers after you apply the following rule.

RULE
To divide decimals:

1. Move the decimal point in the *divisor* (number divided by) and the *dividend* (number divided) the number of places needed to make the *divisor* a *whole number*.

2. Place the decimal point in the *quotient* (answer) above the *new* decimal point place in the *dividend*.

EXAMPLE 1 ▪   EXAMPLE 2 ▪

$$100.75 \div 2.5 = 2.5\overline{)100.7\,5} = 40.3$$

$$
\begin{array}{r}
40.3 \text{ (quotient)} \\
2.5\,)\overline{100.7\,5} \\
\underline{100} \\
07 \\
\underline{00} \\
75 \\
\underline{75} \\
\end{array}
$$

(dividend) (divisor)

$$56.5 \div 0.02 = 0.02\overline{)56.50} = 2,825$$

$$
\begin{array}{r}
2,825. \\
0.02\,)\overline{56.50} \\
\underline{4} \\
16 \\
\underline{16} \\
5 \\
\underline{4} \\
10 \\
\underline{10} \\
\end{array}
$$

MATH TIP
Recall that adding a zero at the end of a decimal number does not change its value (56.5 = 56.50). Adding a zero was necessary in the last example to complete the operation.

RULE
When dividing a decimal by a power of 10, move the decimal point to the left as many places as there are zeros in the divisor.

EXAMPLE 1 ▪

$0.65 \div 10$

The divisor 10 has 1 zero; move the decimal point 1 place to the left.

$0.65 \div 10 = .0.65 = 0.065$

(Note: Place a zero to the left of the decimal point to avoid confusion and to emphasize that this is a decimal.)

EXAMPLE 2 ▪

$7.3 \div 100$

The divisor 100 has 2 zeros; move the decimal point 2 places to the left.

$7.3 \div 100 = .07.3 = 0.073$

(Note: Add zeros as necessary to complete the operation.)

EXAMPLE 3 ▪

$0.5 \div 1,000$

The divisor 1,000 has 3 zeros; move the decimal point 3 places to the left.

$0.5 \div 1,000 = .000.5 = 0.0005$

Rounding Decimals

For many dosage calculations, it will be necessary to compute decimal calculations to *thousandths* (*three* decimal places) and round back to *hundredths* (*two* places) for the final answer. For example, pediatric care and critical care require this degree of accuracy. At other times, you will need to round to *tenths* (*one* place). Let's look closely at this important math skill.

RULE
To round a decimal to hundredths, drop the number in thousandths place, and

1. Do not change the number in hundredths place if the number in thousandths place was 4 or less.

2. Increase the number in hundredths place by 1 if the number in thousandths place was 5 or more.

When rounding for dosage calculations, unnecessary zeros can be dropped. For example, 5.20 rounded to hundredths place should be written as 5.2, because the 0 is not needed to clarify the number.

EXAMPLES ■

Tenths Hundredths Thousandths	All rounded to hundredths (2 places)

0 . 1 2 3   = 0.12

1 . 7 4 4   = 1.74

5 . 3 2 5   = 5.33

0 . 6 6 6   = 0.67

0 . 3 0   = 0.3   (When this is rounded to hundredths, the final zero should be dropped. It is not needed to clarify the number and is potentially confusing.)

RULE

To round a decimal to tenths, drop the number in hundredths place, and

1. Do not change the number in tenths place if the number in hundredths place was 4 or less.

2. Increase the number in tenths place by 1 if the number in hundredths place was 5 or more.

EXAMPLES ■

Tenths Hundredths   All rounded to tenths (1 place)

0 . 1 3   = 0.1

5 . 6 4   = 5.6

0 . 7 5   = 0.8

1 . 6 6   = 1.7

0 . 9 5   = 1.0 = 1   (The zero at the end of this decimal number is dropped, because it is unnecessary and potentially confusing.)

QUICK REVIEW

■ To multiply decimals, place the decimal point in the product to the left as many total decimal places as there are in the two decimals multiplied.

Example:
$0.25 \times 0.2 = 0.050 = 0.05$ (Zero at the end of the decimal is unnecessary.)

■ To divide decimals, move the decimal point in the divisor and dividend the number of decimal places that will make the divisor a whole number and align it in the quotient.

Example: $24 \div 1.2$

$$\begin{array}{r} 2\,0. \\ 1.2\,\overline{)\,24.0} \end{array}$$

■ To multiply or divide decimals by a power of 10, move the decimal point to the right (to multiply) or to the left (to divide) the same number of decimal places as there are zeros in the power of 10.

Examples:
5.06 × 10 = 5.0̣6 = 50.6
2.1 ÷ 100 = .02̣1 = 0.021

■ When rounding decimals, add 1 to the place value considered if the next decimal place is 5 or greater.

Examples:
Rounded to hundredths: 3.054 = 3.05; 0.566 = 0.57

Rounded to tenths: 3.05 = 3.1; 0.54 = 0.5

Review Set 6

Multiply, and round your answers to two decimal places.

1. 1.16 × 5.03 = _____
2. 0.314 × 7 = _____
3. 1.71 × 25 = _____
4. 3.002 × 0.05 = _____
5. 16.1 × 25.04 = _____

6. 75.1 × 1,000.01 = _____
7. 16.03 × 2.05 = _____
8. 55.5 × 0.05 = _____
9. 23.2 × 15.025 = _____
10. 1.14 × 0.014 = _____

Divide, and round your answers to two decimal places.

11. 16 ÷ 0.04 = _____
12. 25.3 ÷ 6.76 = _____
13. 0.02 ÷ 0.004 = _____
14. 45.5 ÷ 15.25 = _____
15. 515 ÷ 0.125 = _____

16. 73 ÷ 13.40 = _____
17. 16.36 ÷ 0.06 = _____
18. 0.375 ÷ 0.25 = _____
19. 100.04 ÷ 0.002 = _____
20. 45 ÷ 0.15 = _____

Multiply or divide by the power of 10 indicated. Draw an arrow to demonstrate movement of the decimal point. Do not round answers.

21. 562.5 × 100 = _____
22. 16 × 10 = _____
23. 25 ÷ 1,000 = _____
24. 32.005 ÷ 1,000 = _____
25. 0.125 ÷ 100 = _____

26. 23.25 × 10 = _____
27. 717.717 ÷ 10 = _____
28. 83.16 × 10 = _____
29. 0.33 × 100 = _____
30. 14.106 × 1,000 = _____

After completing these problems, see page 590 to check your answers.

PRACTICE PROBLEMS—CHAPTER 1

1. Convert 0.35 to a fraction in lowest terms. __7/20__

2. Convert $\frac{3}{8}$ to a decimal. __.375__

Find the least common denominator for the following pairs of fractions.

3. $\frac{5}{7}$; $\frac{2}{3}$ _____

5. $\frac{4}{9}$; $\frac{5}{6}$ _____

4. $\frac{1}{5}$; $\frac{4}{11}$ _____

6. $\frac{1}{3}$; $\frac{3}{5}$ _____

Perform the indicated operation, and reduce fractions to lowest terms.

7. $1\frac{2}{3} + \frac{9}{5} =$ _____

15. $8\frac{4}{11} \div 1\frac{2}{3} =$ _____

8. $4\frac{5}{12} + 3\frac{1}{15} =$ _____

16. $\dfrac{9\frac{1}{2}}{1\frac{4}{5}} =$ _____

9. $\frac{7}{9} - \frac{5}{18} =$ _____

17. $\dfrac{13\frac{1}{3}}{4\frac{6}{13}} =$ _____

10. $5\frac{1}{6} - 2\frac{7}{8} =$ _____

18. $\dfrac{\frac{1}{10}}{\frac{2}{3}} =$ _____

11. $\frac{4}{9} \times \frac{7}{12} =$ _____

19. $\frac{1}{125} \times \frac{1}{25} =$ _____

12. $1\frac{1}{2} \times 6\frac{3}{4} =$ _____

20. $\dfrac{\frac{7}{8}}{\frac{1}{3}} \div \dfrac{3\frac{1}{2}}{\frac{1}{3}} =$ _____

13. $7\frac{1}{5} \div 1\frac{7}{10} =$ _____

21. $\frac{20}{35} \times 3 =$ _____

14. $\frac{3}{16} + \frac{3}{10} =$ _____

22. $2\frac{1}{4} \times 7\frac{1}{8} =$ _____

Perform the indicated operations, and round the answers to two decimal places.

23. $11.33 + 29.16 + 19.78 =$ _____

30. $5 + 2.5 + 0.05 + 0.15 =$ _____

24. $93.712 - 26.97 =$ _____

31. $1.71 \times 25 =$ _____

25. $43.69 - 0.7083 =$ _____

32. $45 \div 0.15 =$ _____

26. $66.4 \times 72.8 =$ _____

33. $2,974 \div 0.23 =$ _____

27. $360 \times 0.53 =$ _____

34. $51.21 \div 0.016 =$ _____

28. $268.4 \div 14 =$ _____

35. $0.74 \div 0.37 =$ _____

29. $10.10 - 0.62 =$ _____

36. $1.5 + 146.73 + 1.9 + 0.832 =$ _____

Multiply or divide by the power of 10 indicated. Draw an arrow to demonstrate movement of the decimal point. Do not round answers.

37. $9.716 \times 1,000 =$ _____

40. $5.75 \times 1,000 =$ _____

38. $50.25 \div 100 =$ _____

41. $0.25 \div 10 =$ _____

39. $0.25 \times 100 =$ _____

42. $11.525 \times 10 =$ _____

43. A 1-month-old infant drinks $3\frac{1}{2}$ fluid ounces of formula every 4 hours day and night. How many fluid ounces will the infant drink in 1 week on this schedule? _____

44. There are 368 people employed at Riverview Clinic. If $\frac{3}{8}$ of the employees are nurses, $\frac{1}{8}$ are maintenance personnel/cleaners, $\frac{1}{4}$ are technicians, and $\frac{1}{4}$ are all other employees, calculate the number of employees that each fraction represents. _____

45. True or false? A specific gravity of urine of $1\frac{2}{32}$ falls within the normal range of 1.01 to 1.025 for an adult patient. _____

46. Last week, a nurse earning $20.43 per hour gross pay worked 40 hours plus 6.5 hours overtime, which is paid at twice the hourly rate. What is the total regular and overtime gross pay for last week? _____

47. The instructional assistant is ordering supplies for the nursing skills laboratory. A single box of 12 urinary catheters costs $98.76. A case of 12 boxes of these catheters costs $975. Calculate the savings per catheter when a case is purchased. _____

48. If each ounce of a liquid laxative contains 0.065 gram of a drug, how many grams of the drug would be contained in 4.75 ounces? (Round answer to the nearest hundredth.) _____

49. A patient is to receive 1,200 milliliters of fluid in a 24-hour period. How many milliliters should the patient drink between the hours of 7:00 AM and 7:00 PM if he is to receive $\frac{2}{3}$ of the total amount during that time? _____

50. A baby weighed 3.7 kilograms at birth. The baby now weighs 6.65 kilograms. How many kilograms did the baby gain? _____

After completing these problems, see pages 590–591 to check your answers.

For additional practice, visit the online practice software at www.CengageBrain.com, using the Premium Website access code found in the front of your text.

REFERENCE

The Joint Commission. (2010). Facts about the Official "Do Not Use" List. Retrieved April 28, 2011 from http://www.jointcommission.org/assets/1/18/Official_Do%20Not%20Use_List_%206_10.pdf

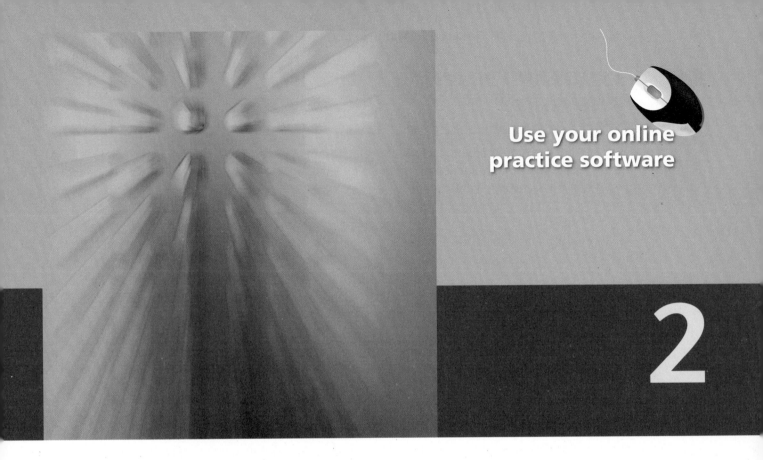

2

Ratios, Percents, Simple Equations, and Ratio-Proportion

OBJECTIVES

Upon mastery of Chapter 2, you will be able to perform basic mathematical computations that involve ratios, percents, simple equations, and proportions. Specifically, you will be able to:

- Interpret values expressed in ratios.
- Convert among fractions, decimals, ratios, and percents.
- Compare the size of fractions, decimals, ratios, and percents.
- Determine the value of X in simple equations.
- Set up proportions for solving problems.
- Cross-multiply to find the value of X in a proportion.
- Calculate the percentage of a quantity.

Health care professionals need to understand ratios and percents to be able to accurately interpret, prepare, and administer a variety of medications and treatments. Let's take a look at each of these important ways of expressing ratios and percents and how they are related to fractions and decimals. It is important for you to be able to convert equivalent ratios, percents, decimals, and fractions quickly and accurately.

RATIOS AND PERCENTS

Ratios

Like a fraction, a *ratio* is used to indicate the relationship of one part of a quantity to the whole. The two quantities are written as a fraction or separated by a colon (:). The use of the colon is a traditional way to write the division sign within a ratio.

EXAMPLE ▪

On an evening shift, if there are 5 nurses and 35 patients, what is the ratio of nurses to patients? 5 nurses to 35 patients = 5 nurses per 35 patients = $\frac{5}{35} = \frac{1}{7}$. This is the same as a ratio of 5:35 or 1:7.

> **MATH TIP**
> The terms of a ratio are the numerator (always to the left of the colon) and the denominator (always to the right of the colon) of a fraction. Like fractions, ratios should be stated in lowest terms.

If you think back to the discussion of fractions and parts of a whole, it is easy to see that a ratio is actually the same as a fraction and its equivalent decimal. It is just a different way of expressing the same quantity. Recall from Chapter 1 that to convert a fraction to a decimal, you simply divide the numerator by the denominator.

EXAMPLE ▪

Adrenalin 1:1,000 for injection = 1 part Adrenalin to 1,000 total parts of solution. It is a fact that 1:1,000 is the same as $\frac{1}{1,000}$.

In some drug solutions, such as Adrenalin 1:1,000, the ratio is used to indicate the drug's concentration. This will be covered in more detail later.

Percents

A percent is a type of ratio. *Percent* comes from the Latin phrase *per centum*, translated *per hundred*. This means per hundred parts or hundredth part.

> **MATH TIP**
> To remember the value of a given percent, replace the % symbol with "/" for *per* and "100" for *cent*. THINK: Percent (%) means "/100" or "*per hundred*."

EXAMPLE ▪

$3\% = 3$ percent $= 3/100 = \frac{3}{100} = 0.03$

Converting Among Ratios, Percents, Fractions, and Decimals

When you understand the relationship of ratios, percents, fractions, and decimals, you can readily convert from one to the other. Let's begin by converting a percent to a fraction.

RULE

To convert a percent to a fraction:

1. Delete the % sign.

2. Write the remaining number as the numerator.

3. Write 100 as the denominator.

4. Reduce the result to lowest terms.

EXAMPLE ■

$5\% = \frac{5}{100} = \frac{1}{20}$

It is also easy to express a percent as a ratio.

RULE

To convert a percent to a ratio:

1. Delete the % sign.

2. Write the remaining number as the numerator.

3. Write 100 as the denominator.

4. Reduce the result to lowest terms.

5. Express the fraction as a ratio.

EXAMPLE ■

$25\% = \frac{25}{100} = \frac{1}{4} = 1{:}4$

Because the denominator of a percent is always 100, it is easy to find the equivalent decimal. Recall that to divide by 100, you move the decimal point two places to the left, the number of places equal to the number of zeros in the denominator.

RULE

To convert a percent to a decimal:

1. Delete the % sign.

2. Divide the remaining number by 100, which is the same as moving the decimal point two places to the left.

EXAMPLE ■

$25\% = \frac{25}{100} = 25 \div 100 = .25. = 0.25$

Conversely, it is easy to change a decimal to a percent.

RULE

To convert a decimal to a percent:

1. Multiply the decimal number by 100, which is the same as moving the decimal point two places to the right.

2. Add the % sign.

EXAMPLE ▪

$0.25 \times 100 = 0.\underset{\smile}{25}. = 25\%$

MATH TIP

When converting a decimal to a percent, always move the decimal point two places so that the resulting percent is the larger number.

Now you know all the steps to change a ratio to the equivalent percent.

RULE

To convert a ratio to a percent:

1. Convert the ratio to a fraction.
2. Convert the fraction to a decimal.
3. Convert the decimal to a percent.

EXAMPLE ▪

Convert 1:1,000 Adrenalin solution to the equivalent concentration expressed as a percent.

1. $1:1,000 = \dfrac{1}{1,000}$ (ratio converted to fraction)

2. $\dfrac{1}{1,000} = .\underset{\smile}{001}. = 0.001$ (fraction converted to decimal)

3. $0.001 = 0.\underset{\smile}{00}1 = 0.1\%$ (decimal converted to percent)

Thus, 1:1,000 Adrenalin solution = 0.1% Adrenalin solution.

Review the preceding example again slowly until it is clear. Ask your instructor for assistance as needed. If you go over this one step at a time, you can master these important calculations. You need never fear fractions, decimals, ratios, and percents again.

Comparing Percents and Ratios

Nurses and other health care professionals frequently administer solutions with the concentration expressed as a percent or ratio. Consider two intravenous (which means given directly into a person's vein) solutions: one that is 0.9%, the other 5%. It is important to be clear that 0.9% is *less* than 5%. A 0.9% solution means that there are 0.9 parts of the solid per 100 total parts (0.9 parts is less than one whole part, so it is less than 1%). Compare this to the 5% solution, with 5 parts of the solid (or more than five times 0.9 parts) per 100 total parts. Therefore, the 5% solution is much more concentrated, or stronger, than the 0.9% solution. A misunderstanding of these numbers and the quantities they represent can have dire consequences.

Likewise, you may see a solution concentration expressed as $\frac{1}{3}\%$ and another expressed as 0.45%. Convert these amounts to equivalent decimals to clarify values and compare concentrations.

EXAMPLE 1 ▪

$$\frac{1}{3}\% = \frac{\frac{1}{3}}{100} = \frac{1}{3} \div \frac{100}{1} = \frac{1}{3} \times \frac{1}{100} = \frac{1}{300} = 0.00\overline{33}$$

EXAMPLE 2 ▪

$$0.45\% = \frac{0.45}{100} = 0.0045 \text{ (greater value, stronger concentration)}$$

MATH TIP

In the last set of examples, the line over the last 3 in the decimal fraction $0.003\overline{3}$ indicates that the number 3 repeats itself indefinitely.

Compare solution concentrations expressed as a ratio, such as 1:1,000 and 1:100.

EXAMPLE 1 ■

$1:1,000 = \dfrac{1}{1,000} = 0.001$

EXAMPLE 2 ■

$1:100 = \dfrac{1}{100} = 0.01$ or 0.010 (add zero for comparison); 1:100 is a stronger concentration

QUICK REVIEW

- Fractions, decimals, ratios, and percents are related equivalents.
  Example: $1:2 = \dfrac{1}{2} = 0.5 = 50\%$
- Like fractions, ratios should be reduced to lowest terms.
  Example: $2:4 = 1:2$
- To express a ratio as a fraction, the number to the left of the colon becomes the numerator and the number to the right of the colon becomes the denominator. The colon in a ratio is equivalent to the division sign in a fraction.
  Example: $2:3 = \dfrac{2}{3}$
- To change a ratio to a decimal, convert the ratio to a fraction and divide the numerator by the denominator.
  Example: $1:4 = \dfrac{1}{4} = 1 \div 4 = 0.25$
- To change a percent to a fraction, drop the % sign and place the remaining number as the numerator over the denominator 100. Reduce the fraction to lowest terms. THINK: per (/) cent (100).
  Example: $75\% = \dfrac{75}{100} = \dfrac{3}{4}$
- To change a percent to a ratio, first convert the percent to a fraction in lowest terms. Then, place the numerator to the left of a colon and the denominator to the right of that colon.
  Example: $35\% = \dfrac{35}{100} = \dfrac{7}{20} = 7:20$
- To change a percent to a decimal, drop the % sign and divide by 100.
  Example: $4\% = .04. = 0.04$
- To change a decimal to a percent, multiply by 100 and add the % sign.
  Example: $0.5 = 0.50. = 50\%$
- To change a ratio to a percent, first convert the ratio to a fraction. Convert the resulting fraction to a decimal and then to a percent.
  Example: $1:2 = \dfrac{1}{2} = 1 \div 2 = 0.5 = 0.50. = 50\%$

Review Set 7

Change the following ratios to fractions that are reduced to lowest terms.

1. $3:150 =$ _____

2. $6:10 =$ _____

3. $0.05:0.15 =$ _____

4. $4:7 =$ _____

5. $6:8 =$ _____

Change the following ratios to decimals; round to two decimal places, if needed.

6. $20:40 =$ _____   9. $0.3:4.5 =$ _____

7. $\frac{1}{1,000}:\frac{1}{150} =$ _____   10. $1\frac{1}{2}:6\frac{2}{9} =$ _____

8. $0.12:0.88 =$ _____

Change the following ratios to percents; round to two decimal places, if needed.

11. $12:48 =$ _____   14. $7:10 =$ _____

12. $2:5 =$ _____   15. $50:100 =$ _____

13. $0.08:0.64 =$ _____

Change the following percents to fractions that are reduced to lowest terms.

16. $45\% =$ _____   19. $1\% =$ _____

17. $60\% =$ _____   20. $66\frac{2}{3}\% =$ _____

18. $0.5\% =$ _____

Change the following percents to decimals; round to two decimal places, if needed.

21. $2.94\% =$ _____   24. $33\% =$ _____

22. $4.5\% =$ _____   25. $0.9\% =$ _____

23. $6.32\% =$ _____

Change the following percents to ratios that are reduced to lowest terms.

26. $16\% =$ _____   29. $45\% =$ _____

27. $25\% =$ _____   30. $6\% =$ _____

28. $50\% =$ _____

Which of the following is largest? Circle your answer.

31. 0.9% 0.9 $1:9$ $\frac{1}{90}$ 34. $\frac{1}{150}$ $\frac{1}{300}$ 0.5 $\frac{2}{3}\%$

32. 0.05 $\frac{1}{5}$ 0.025 $1:25$ 35. $1:1,000$ 0.0001 $\frac{1}{100}$ 0.1%

33. 0.0125% 0.25% 0.1% 0.02%

After completing these problems, see page 591 to check your answers.

SOLVING SIMPLE EQUATIONS FOR X

You can set up and solve dosage calculations in different ways. One way is to use a simple equation form. The following examples demonstrate the various forms of this equation. Learn to express your answers in decimal form, because decimals will be used most often in dosage calculations and administration.

MATH TIP
Round decimals to hundredths or to two places. For most dosage calculations, you will round to no more than two decimal places.

MATH TIP
The unknown quantity is represented by X.

EXAMPLE 1 ▪

$$\frac{100}{200} \times 1 = X$$

MATH TIP

You can drop the 1, because a number multiplied by 1 is the same number.

$\frac{100}{200} \times 1 = X$ is the same as $\frac{100}{200} = X$.

1. Reduce to lowest terms: $\frac{100}{200} = \frac{\overset{1}{\cancel{100}}}{\underset{2}{\cancel{200}}} = \frac{1}{2} = X$

2. Convert to decimal form: $\frac{1}{2} = 0.5 = X$

3. You have your answer. $X = 0.5$

EXAMPLE 2 ▪

$$\frac{3}{5} \times 2 = X$$

MATH TIP

Dividing a number by 1 does not change its value.

1. Convert: Express 2 as a fraction: $\frac{3}{5} \times \frac{2}{1} = X$

2. Multiply fractions: $\frac{3}{5} \times \frac{2}{1} = \frac{6}{5} = X$

3. Convert to a mixed number: $\frac{6}{5} = 1\frac{1}{5} = X$

4. Convert to decimal form: $1\frac{1}{5} = 1.2 = X$

5. You have your answer. $X = 1.2$

EXAMPLE 3 ▪

$$\frac{\frac{1}{6}}{\frac{1}{4}} \times 5 = X$$

1. Convert: Express 5 as a fraction: $\frac{\frac{1}{6}}{\frac{1}{4}} \times \frac{5}{1} = X$

2. Divide fractions: $\frac{1}{6} \div \frac{1}{4} \times \frac{5}{1} = X$

3. Invert the divisor, and multiply: $\frac{1}{6} \times \frac{4}{1} \times \frac{5}{1} = X$

4. Cancel terms: $\frac{1}{\underset{3}{\cancel{6}}} \times \frac{\overset{2}{\cancel{4}}}{1} \times \frac{5}{1} = \frac{1}{3} \times \frac{2}{1} \times \frac{5}{1} = \frac{10}{3} = X$

5. Convert to a mixed number: $\frac{10}{3} = 3\frac{1}{3} = X$

6. Convert to decimal form: $3\frac{1}{3} = 3.33\overline{3} = X$

7. Round to hundredths place: $3.33\overline{3} = 3.33 = X$

8. It is easy, when you take it one step at a time. $X = 3.33$

EXAMPLE 4 ▪

$$\frac{\frac{1}{10}}{\frac{1}{15}} \times 2.2 = X$$

1. Convert: Express 2.2 in fraction form: $\dfrac{\frac{1}{10}}{\frac{1}{15}} \times \dfrac{2.2}{1} = X$

2. Divide fractions: $\dfrac{1}{10} \div \dfrac{1}{15} \times \dfrac{2.2}{1} = X$

3. Invert the divisor, and multiply: $\dfrac{1}{10} \times \dfrac{15}{1} \times \dfrac{2.2}{1} = X$

4. Cancel terms: $\dfrac{1}{\cancel{10}_2} \times \dfrac{\cancel{15}^3}{1} \times \dfrac{2.2}{1} = \dfrac{1}{\cancel{2}_1} \times \dfrac{3}{1} \times \dfrac{\cancel{2.2}^{1.1}}{1} = \dfrac{1}{1} \times \dfrac{3}{1} \times \dfrac{1.1}{1} = X$

5. Multiply: $\dfrac{1}{1} \times \dfrac{3}{1} \times \dfrac{1.1}{1} = \dfrac{3.3}{1} = 3.3 = X$

6. That's it! $X = 3.3$

EXAMPLE 5 ▪

$$\frac{0.125}{0.25} \times 1.5 = X$$

1. Convert: Express 1.5 in fraction form: $\dfrac{0.125}{0.25} \times \dfrac{1.5}{1} = X$

2. Convert: For easier comparison, add a zero to thousandths place for 0.25: $\dfrac{0.125}{0.250} \times \dfrac{1.5}{1} = X$

3. Cancel terms: $\dfrac{\cancel{0.125}^1}{\cancel{0.250}_2} \times \dfrac{1.5}{1} = \dfrac{1}{2} \times \dfrac{1.5}{1} = X$

4. Multiply: $\dfrac{1}{2} \times \dfrac{1.5}{1} = \dfrac{1.5}{2} = X$

5. Divide: $\dfrac{1.5}{2} = 0.75 = X$

6. You've got it! $X = 0.75$

MATH TIP

It may be easier to work with whole numbers than decimals. If you had difficulty with Step 3, try multiplying the numerator and denominator by 1,000 to eliminate the decimal fractions.

$$\frac{0.125}{0.250} \times \frac{1,000}{1,000} = \frac{125}{250} = \frac{1}{2}$$

Example 5 can also be solved by computing with fractions instead of decimals.

Try this: $\dfrac{0.125}{0.25} \times 1.5 = X$

1. Convert: Express 1.5 in fraction form: $\dfrac{0.125}{0.25} \times \dfrac{1.5}{1} = X$

2. Convert: Add zeros for easier comparison, making *both* decimals of equal length:
$\dfrac{0.125}{0.250} \times \dfrac{1.5}{1.0} = X$

3. Cancel terms: $\dfrac{\overset{1}{\cancel{0.125}}}{\underset{2}{\cancel{0.250}}} \times \dfrac{\overset{3}{\cancel{1.5}}}{\underset{2}{\cancel{1.0}}} = \dfrac{1}{2} \times \dfrac{3}{2} = X$ (It is easier to work with whole numbers.)

4. Multiply: $\dfrac{1}{2} \times \dfrac{3}{2} = \dfrac{3}{4} = X$

5. Convert: $\dfrac{3}{4} = 0.75 = X$

6. You've got it again! $X = 0.75$

Which way do you find easier?

EXAMPLE 6 ■

$\dfrac{3}{4} \times 45\% = X$

1. Convert: Express 45% as a fraction reduced to lowest terms: $45\% = \dfrac{45}{100} = \dfrac{9}{20}$

2. Multiply fractions: $\dfrac{3}{4} \times \dfrac{9}{20} = X$

   $\dfrac{27}{80} = X$

3. Divide: $\dfrac{27}{80} = 0.337 = X$

4. Round to hundredths place: $0.34 = X$

5. You have your answer. $X = 0.34$

QUICK REVIEW

- To solve simple equations, perform the mathematical operations indicated to find the value of the unknown X.

- Express the result (value of X) in decimal form.

Review Set 8

Solve the following problems for X. Express answers as decimals rounded to two places.

1. $\dfrac{75}{125} \times 5 = X$ _____

2. $\dfrac{\frac{3}{4}}{\frac{1}{2}} \times 2.2 = X$ _____

3. $\dfrac{150}{300} \times 2.5 = X$ _____

4. $\dfrac{40\%}{60\%} \times 8 = X$ _____

5. $\dfrac{0.35}{2.5} \times 4 = X$ _____

6. $\dfrac{0.15}{0.1} \times 1.2 = X$ _____

7. $\dfrac{0.4}{2.5} \times 4 = X$ _____

8. $\dfrac{1,200,000}{400,000} \times 4.2 = X$ _____

9. $\dfrac{\frac{2}{3}}{\frac{1}{6}} \times 10 = X$ _____

10. $\dfrac{30}{50} \times 0.8 = X$ _____

11. $\dfrac{200,000}{300,000} \times 1.5 = X$ _____

12. $\dfrac{0.08}{0.1} \times 1.2 = X$ _____

13. $\dfrac{7.5}{5} \times 3 = X$ _____

14. $\dfrac{250,000}{2,000,000} \times 7.5 = X$ _____

15. $\dfrac{600}{150} \times 2.5 = X$ _____

16. $\dfrac{600,000}{750,000} \times 0.5 = X$ _____

17. $\dfrac{75\%}{60\%} \times 1.2 = X$ _____

18. $\dfrac{0.25}{0.125} \times 5 = X$ _____

19. $\dfrac{1,000,000}{250,000} \times 5 = X$ _____

20. $\dfrac{\frac{1}{100}}{\frac{1}{150}} \times 1.2 = X$ _____

After completing these problems, see pages 591–592 to check your answers.

RATIO-PROPORTION: CROSS-MULTIPLYING TO SOLVE FOR X

A *proportion* is two ratios that are equal or an equation between two equal ratios.

MATH TIP

A proportion is written as two ratios separated by an equal sign, such as 5:10 = 10:20. The two ratios in a proportion may also be separated by a double colon sign, such as 5:10 ::10:20.

Some of the calculations you will perform will have the unknown X as a different term in the equation. To determine the value of the unknown X, you must apply the rule for cross-multiplying used in a proportion.

RULE

In a proportion, the product of the means (the two inside numbers) equals the product of the extremes (the two outside numbers). Finding the product of the means and the extremes is called cross-multiplying.

EXAMPLE ■

Extremes

$5{:}10 \;=\; 10{:}20$

Means

$5 \times 20 = 10 \times 10$

$100 = 100$

Because ratios are the same as fractions, the same proportion can be expressed like this: $\dfrac{5}{10} = \dfrac{10}{20}$. The fractions are *equivalent,* or equal. The numerator of the first fraction and the denominator of the second fraction are the *extremes,* and the denominator of the first fraction and the numerator of the second fraction are the *means*.

EXAMPLE ■

Extreme Mean
Mean $\dfrac{5}{10} \diagdown \dfrac{10}{20}$ Extreme

Cross-multiply to find the equal products of the means and extremes.

RULE

If two fractions are equivalent, or equal, their cross-products are also equal.

EXAMPLE ■

$$\frac{5}{10} \times \frac{10}{20}$$

$5 \times 20 = 10 \times 10$

$100 = 100$

When one of the quantities in a proportion is unknown, a letter, such as X, may be substituted for this unknown quantity. You would solve the equation to find the value of X. In addition to cross-multiplying, there is one more rule you need to know to solve for X in a proportion.

RULE

Dividing or multiplying each side (member) of an equation by the same nonzero number produces an equivalent equation.

MATH TIP

Dividing each side of an equation by the same nonzero whole number is the same as reducing or simplifying the equation. Multiplying each side by the same nonzero whole number enlarges the equation.

Let's examine how to simplify an equation.

EXAMPLE ■

$25X = 100$ (25X means $25 \times X$)

Simplify the equation to find X. Divide both sides by 25, the number before X. Reduce to lowest terms.

$$\frac{\overset{1}{\cancel{25}}X}{\underset{1}{\cancel{25}}} = \frac{\overset{4}{\cancel{100}}}{\underset{1}{\cancel{25}}}$$

$\frac{1X}{1} = \frac{4}{1}$ (Dividing or multiplying a number by 1 does not change its value. 1X is understood to be simply X.)

$X = 4$

Replace X with 4 in the same equation, and you can prove that the calculations are correct.

$25 \times 4 = 100$

Now you are ready to apply the concepts of cross-multiplying and simplifying an equation to solve for X in a proportion.

EXAMPLE 1 ■

$$\frac{90}{2} = \frac{45}{X}$$

You have a proportion with an unknown quantity X in the denominator of the second fraction. Find the value of X.

1. Cross-multiply: $\frac{90}{2} \diagup\kern-1.2em\diagdown \frac{45}{X}$

2. Multiply terms: $90 \times X = 2 \times 45$

$$90X = 90 \ (90X \text{ means } 90 \times X)$$

3. Simplify the equation: Divide both sides of the equation by the number before the unknown X. You are equally reducing the terms on both sides of the equation.

$$\frac{\overset{1}{\cancel{90}}X}{\underset{1}{\cancel{90}}} = \frac{\overset{1}{\cancel{90}}}{\underset{1}{\cancel{90}}}$$

$$X = 1$$

Try another one. You will use a proportion to solve this equation.

EXAMPLE 2 ■

$$\frac{80}{X} \times 60 = 20$$

1. Convert: Express 60 as a fraction.

$$\frac{80}{X} \times \frac{60}{1} = 20$$

2. Multiply fractions: $\frac{80}{X} \times \frac{60}{1} = 20$

$$\frac{4,800}{X} = 20$$

3. Convert: Express 20 as a fraction.

$$\frac{4,800}{X} = \frac{20}{1}$$

You now have a proportion.

4. Cross-multiply: $\frac{4,800}{X} \diagup\kern-1.2em\diagdown \frac{20}{1}$

$$20X = 4,800$$

5. Simplify: Divide both sides of the equation by the number before the unknown X.

$$\frac{\overset{1}{\cancel{20}}X}{\underset{1}{\cancel{20}}} = \frac{\overset{240}{\cancel{4,800}}}{\underset{1}{\cancel{20}}}$$

$$X = 240$$

EXAMPLE 3 ■

$$\frac{X}{160} = \frac{2.5}{80}$$

1. Cross-multiply: $\frac{X}{160} \diagup\kern-1.2em\diagdown \frac{2.5}{80}$

$$80 \times X = 2.5 \times 160$$

$$80X = 400$$

2. Simplify: $\dfrac{\overset{1}{\cancel{80}}X}{\underset{1}{\cancel{80}}} = \dfrac{\overset{5}{\cancel{400}}}{\underset{1}{\cancel{80}}}$

   X = 5

EXAMPLE 4 ■

$\dfrac{40}{100} = \dfrac{X}{2}$

1. Cross-multiply: $\dfrac{40}{100} \diagdown\kern-1.1em\diagup \dfrac{X}{2}$

2. Multiply terms: $100 \times X = 40 \times 2$

   $100X = 80$

3. Simplify the equation: $\dfrac{\overset{1}{\cancel{100}}X}{\underset{1}{\cancel{100}}} = \dfrac{\overset{}{\cancel{80}}}{100}$

   X = 0.8

Calculations that result in an amount less than 1 should be expressed as a decimal. Most medications are ordered and supplied in metric measure. Metric measure is a decimal-based system.

QUICK REVIEW

■ A *proportion* is an equation of two equal ratios. The ratios may be expressed as fractions.

■ Example: $1:4 = X:8$ or $\dfrac{1}{4} = \dfrac{X}{8}$

■ In a proportion, the product of the means equals the product of the extremes.

   Extremes

■ Example: $1{:}4 \quad = \quad X{:}8$ Therefore, $4 \times X = 1 \times 8$

   Means

■ If two fractions are equal, their cross-products are equal. This operation is referred to as cross-multiplying.

■ Example: $\dfrac{1}{4} \diagdown\kern-1.1em\diagup \dfrac{X}{8}$ Therefore, $4 \times X = 1 \times 8$, or $4X = 8$

■ Dividing each side of an equation by the same number produces an equivalent equation. This operation is referred to as *simplifying the equation*.

■ Example: If $4X = 8$, then $\dfrac{4X}{4} = \dfrac{8}{4}$, and $X = 2$

Review Set 9

Find the value of X. Express answers as decimals rounded to two places.

1. $\dfrac{1,000}{2} = \dfrac{125}{X}$ _____

2. $\dfrac{500}{2} = \dfrac{250}{X}$ _____

3. $\dfrac{500}{1} = \dfrac{280}{X}$ _____

4. $\dfrac{0.5}{2} = \dfrac{250}{X}$ _____

5. $\dfrac{75}{1.5} = \dfrac{35}{X}$ _____

6. $\dfrac{40}{X} \times 12 = 60$ _____

7. $\dfrac{10}{X} \times 60 = 28$ _____

8. $\dfrac{2}{2,000} \times X = 0.5$ _____

9. $\frac{15}{500} \times X = 6$ _____

10. $\frac{5}{X} = \frac{10}{21}$ _____

11. $\frac{250}{1} = \frac{750}{X}$ _____

12. $\frac{80}{5} = \frac{10}{X}$ _____

13. $\frac{5}{20} = \frac{X}{40}$ _____

14. $\frac{\frac{1}{100}}{1} = \frac{\frac{1}{150}}{X}$ _____

15. $\frac{2.2}{X} = \frac{8.8}{5}$ _____

16. $\frac{60}{15} = \frac{125}{X}$ _____

17. $\frac{60}{10} = \frac{100}{X}$ _____

18. $\frac{80}{X} \times 60 = 20$ _____

19. $\frac{X}{0.5} = \frac{6}{4}$ _____

20. $\frac{5}{2.2} = \frac{X}{1}$ _____

21. $\frac{\frac{1}{4}}{15} = \frac{X}{60}$ _____

22. $\frac{25\%}{30\%} = \frac{5}{X}$ _____

23. In any group of 100 nurses, you would expect to find 45 nurses who will specialize in a particular field of nursing. In a class of 240 graduating nurses, how many would you expect to specialize? _____

24. Low-fat cheese has 48 calories per ounce. A client who is having his caloric intake measured has eaten $1\frac{1}{2}$ ounces of low-fat cheese. How many calories has he eaten? _____

25. If a patient receives 450 milligrams of a medication given evenly over 5.5 hours, how many milligrams does the patient receive per hour? _____

After completing these problems, see page 592 to check your answers.

FINDING THE PERCENTAGE OF A QUANTITY

An important computation that health care professionals use for dosage calculations is to find a given percentage or part of a quantity. *Percentage* is a term that describes a *part* of a whole quantity. A *known percent* determines the part in question. Said another way, the percentage (or part in question) is equal to some known percent multiplied by the whole quantity.

RULE

Percentage (Part) = Percent × Whole Quantity
To find a percentage or part of a whole quantity:

1. Change the percent to a decimal.

2. Multiply the decimal by the whole quantity.

EXAMPLE ▪

A patient reports that he drank 75% of his 8 fluid ounce cup of coffee for breakfast. To record in his chart the amount he actually drank, you must determine what amount is 75% of 8 fluid ounces.

MATH TIP

In a mathematical expression, the word "*of*" means "*times*" and indicates that you should multiply.

To continue with the example:

Percentage (Part) = Percent × Whole Quantity

Let X represent the unknown.

1. Change 75% to a decimal: $75\% = \frac{75}{100} = .75. = 0.75$

2. Multiply 0.75 × 8 fluid ounces: X = 0.75 × 8 fluid ounces = 6 fluid ounces

Therefore, 75% of 8 fluid ounces is 6 fluid ounces.

QUICK REVIEW

■ Percentage (Part) = Percent × Whole Quantity

   Example: What is 12% of 48? X = 12% × 48 = 0.12 × 48 = 5.76

Review Set 10

Perform the indicated operation; round decimals to hundredths place.

1. What is 0.25% of 520? _____   6. What is 20% of 75? _____

2. What is 5% of 95? _____   7. What is 4% of 20? _____

3. What is 40% of 140? _____   8. What is 7% of 34? _____

4. What is 0.7% of 62? _____   9. What is 15% of 250? _____

5. What is 3% of 889? _____   10. What is 75% of 150? _____

11. A patient has an order for an anti-infective in the amount of 500 milligrams by mouth twice a day for 10 days to treat pneumonia. He received a bottle of 20 pills. How many pills has this patient taken if he has used 40% of the 20 pills? _____

12. The patient is on oral fluid restrictions of 1,200 milliliters for a 24-hour period. For breakfast and lunch he has consumed 60% of the total fluid allowance. How many milliliters has he had? _____

13. A patient's hospital bill for surgery is $17,651.07. Her insurance company pays 80%. How much will the patient owe? _____

14. Table salt (sodium chloride) is 40% sodium by weight. If a box of salt weighs 18 ounces, how many ounces of sodium is in the box of salt? _____

15. A patient has an average daily intake of 3,500 calories. At breakfast she eats 20% of the total daily caloric allowance. How many calories did she ingest? _____

After completing these problems, see pages 592–593 to check your answers.

PRACTICE PROBLEMS—CHAPTER 2

Find the equivalent decimal, fraction, percent, and ratio forms. Reduce fractions and ratios to lowest terms; round decimals to hundredths and percents to the nearest whole number.

	Decimal	Fraction	Percent	Ratio
1.	_____	$\frac{2}{5}$	_____	_____
2.	0.05	_____	_____	_____
3.	_____	_____	17%	_____
4.	_____	_____		1:4
5.	_____	_____	6%	_____
6.	_____	$\frac{1}{6}$	_____	_____
7.	_____	_____	50%	_____
8.	_____	_____	_____	1:100
9.	0.09	_____	_____	_____
10.	_____	$\frac{3}{8}$	_____	_____
11.	_____	_____	_____	2:3
12.	_____	$\frac{1}{3}$	_____	_____
13.	0.52	_____	_____	_____
14.	_____	_____	_____	9:20
15.	_____	$\frac{6}{7}$	_____	_____
16.	_____	_____	_____	3:10
17.	_____	$\frac{1}{50}$	_____	_____
18.	0.6	_____	_____	_____
19.	0.04	_____	_____	_____
20.	_____	_____	10%	_____

Convert as indicated.

21. 1:25 to a decimal _____

22. $\frac{10}{400}$ to a ratio _____

23. 0.075 to a percent _____

24. 17:34 to a fraction _____

25. 75% to a ratio _____

Perform the indicated operation. Round decimals to hundredths.

26. What is 35% of 750? _____

27. What is 7% of 52? _____

28. What is 8.2% of 24? _____

Identify the strongest solution in each of the following groups:

29. 1:40   1:400   1:4   _____

30. 1:10   1:200   1:50   _____

Find the value of X in the following equations. Express your answers as decimals rounded to the nearest hundredth.

31. $\frac{20}{400} = \frac{X}{1,680}$ = _____

32. $\frac{75}{X} = \frac{\frac{1}{300}}{4}$ _____

33. $\frac{X}{5} = \frac{3}{15}$ _____

34. $\frac{500}{250} = \frac{2.2}{X}$ _____

35. $\frac{0.6}{1.2} = \frac{X}{200}$ _____

36. $\frac{3}{9} = \frac{X}{117}$ _____

37. $\frac{\frac{1}{8}}{\frac{1}{3}} \times 2 = X$ _____

38. $\frac{X}{7} = \frac{12}{4}$ _____

39. $\frac{X}{8} = \frac{9}{0.6}$ _____

40. $\frac{0.4}{0.1} \times 22.5 = X$ _____

41. A portion of meat totaling 125 grams contains 20% protein and 5% fat. How many grams each of protein and fat does the meat contain? _____ protein _____ fat

42. The total points for a course in a nursing program is 308. A nursing student needs to achieve 75% of the total points to pass the semester. How many points are required to pass? _____

43. To work off 90 calories, Angie must walk for 27 minutes. How many minutes would she need to walk to work off 200 calories? _____

44. The doctor orders a record of the patient's fluid intake and output. The patient drinks 25% of a bowl of broth. How many milliliters of intake will be recorded if the bowl holds 200 milliliters?

_____

45. The recommended daily allowance (RDA) of a particular vitamin is 60 milligrams. If a multivitamin tablet claims to provide 45% of the RDA, how many milligrams of the particular vitamin would a patient receive from the multivitamin tablet? _____

46. A label on a dinner roll wrapper reads, "2.7 grams of fiber per $\frac{3}{4}$ ounce serving." If you eat $1\frac{1}{2}$ ounces of dinner rolls, how many grams of fiber will you consume? _____

47. A patient received an intravenous medication at a rate of 6.75 milligrams per minute. After 42 minutes, how much medication had she received? _____

48. A person weighed 130 pounds at his last doctor's office visit. At this visit the patient has lost 5% of his weight. How many pounds has the patient lost? _____

49. The cost of a certain medication is expected to decrease by 17% next year. If the cost is $12.56 now, how much would you expect it to cost at this time next year? _____

50. A patient is to be started on 150 milligrams of a medication that is then decreased by 10% of the original dose for each dose until he is receiving 75 milligrams. When he takes his 75 milligram dose, how many total doses will he have taken? HINT: Be sure to count his first (150 milligrams) and last (75 milligrams) doses. _____

After completing these problems, see page 593 to check your answers.

🔧 For additional practice, visit the online practice software at www.CengageBrain.com, using the Premium Website access code found in the front of your text.

SECTION 1 SELF-EVALUATION

Directions

1. Round decimals to two places, as needed.

2. Express fractions in lowest terms.

Section 1 Mathematics Review for Dosage Calculations

Multiply or divide by the power of 10 indicated. Draw an arrow to demonstrate movement of the decimal point.

1. $30.5 \div 10 =$ _____

2. $40.025 \times 100 =$ _____

3. $63 \div 100 =$ _____

4. $72.327 \times 10 =$ _____

Identify the least common denominator for the following sets of numbers.

5. $\frac{1}{6}, \frac{2}{3}, \frac{3}{4}$ _____

6. $\frac{2}{5}, \frac{3}{10}, \frac{3}{11}$ _____

Complete the operations indicated.

7. $\frac{1}{4} + \frac{2}{3} =$ _____

8. $\frac{6}{7} - \frac{1}{9} =$ _____

9. $1\frac{3}{5} \times \frac{5}{8} =$ _____

10. $\frac{3}{8} \div \frac{3}{4} =$ _____

11. $13.2 + 32.55 + 0.029 =$ _____

12. 20% of $0.09 =$ _____

13. $80.3 - 21.06 =$ _____

14. $0.3 \times 0.3 =$ _____

15. $1.5 \div 0.125 =$ _____

16. $\frac{1}{150} \div \frac{1}{100} =$ _____

Arrange in order from smallest to largest.

17. $\frac{1}{3}$ $\frac{1}{2}$ $\frac{1}{6}$ $\frac{1}{10}$ $\frac{1}{5}$ _____

18. $\frac{3}{4}$ $\frac{7}{8}$ $\frac{5}{6}$ $\frac{2}{3}$ $\frac{9}{10}$ _____

19. 0.25 0.125 0.3 0.009 0.1909 _____

20. 0.9% $\frac{1}{2}\%$ 50% 500% 100% _____

21. Identify the strongest solution of the following: $1:3$, $1:60$, $1:6$ _____

22. Identify the weakest solution of the following: $1:75$, $1:600$, $1:60$ _____

Convert as indicated.

23. $1:100$ to a decimal _____

24. 0.009 to a percent _____

25. $33\frac{1}{3}\%$ to a fraction _____

26. $\frac{5}{9}$ to a ratio _____

27. 0.05 to a fraction _____

28. $\frac{1}{2}\%$ to a ratio _____

29. $2:3$ to a fraction _____

30. $3:4$ to a percent _____

31. $\frac{2}{5}$ to a percent _____

32. $\frac{1}{6}$ to a decimal _____

Find the value of X in the following equations. Express your answers as decimals; round to the nearest hundredth.

33. $\frac{0.35}{1.3} \times 4.5 = X$ _____

34. $\frac{0.3}{2.6} = \frac{0.15}{X}$ _____

35. $\frac{1,500,000}{500,000} \times X = 7.5$ _____

36. $\frac{1:100}{1:4} \times 2,500 = X$ _____

37. $\frac{0.25}{0.125} \times 2 = X$ _____

38. $\frac{1,000,000}{600,000} \times 5 = X$ _____

39. In a drug study, it was determined that 4% of the participants developed the headache side effect. If there were 600 participants in the study, how many developed headaches? _____

40. You are employed in a health care clinic where each employee must work 25% of 8 major holidays. How many holidays will you expect to work? _____

41. If the cost of 1 roll of gauze is $0.69, what is the cost of $3\frac{1}{2}$ rolls? _____

42. To prepare a nutritional formula from frozen concentrate, you mix 3 cans of water to every 1 can of concentrate. How many cans of water will you need to prepare formula from 4 cans of concentrate? _____

43. If 1 centimeter equals $\frac{3}{8}$ inch, how many centimeters is a laceration that measures 3 inches? _____

Section 1 Board Examination Practice

To obtain licensure, you will be required to pass a board examination. The following problems represent a simulated version of the various types of computerized items on the NCLEX-RN (National Council Licensure Examination for Registered Nurses) and NCLEX-PN (National Council Licensure Examination for Practical Nurses) computerized exams. Whether you will be taking one of these board examinations or one from another licensure board, alternate test items such as these are good practice. The board examination may not utilize every alternate format question to evaluate dosage calculation skills, but items such as these help you to prepare for other content areas too. For additional practice, go to the online practice software that accompanies this text to respond to more interactive test items, including those using the calculator tool.

44. NCLEX *Fill-in-the-Blank* Item

You are recording Intake and Output for your patient who is on fluid restrictions of 1,000 milliliters per day. During the last 24 hours, the patient has consumed $3\frac{1}{2}$ fluid ounces milk, 725 milliliters intravenous fluid, and 4 fluid ounces of juice with the potassium supplement. If 1 fluid ounce is equivalent to 30 milliliters, how many milliliters of liquids did the patient consume in 24 hours?

Answer: _____

45. NCLEX *Multiple-Choice One-Response* Item

An infant requires 3.5 fluid ounces of formula per day for each kilogram of body weight. The infant weighs 6.6 kilograms. How much formula does the infant need? (Express the answer rounded to one decimal place. Place a check mark beside the correct answer.)

Answer:

a. 23 fluid ounces _____

b. 23.1 fluid ounces _____

c. 26.4 fluid ounces _____

d. 35 fluid ounces _____

e. 42 fluid ounces _____

46. NCLEX *Fill-in-the-Blank* Item

A child weighs 39 pounds. If each kilogram is equivalent to 2.2 pounds, what is the child's weight in kilograms? (Express the answer rounded to one decimal place.)

Answer: _____ kilograms

47. NCLEX *Exhibit* Item

Use the information in the table to determine which is the largest amount of fluid. (Place a check mark beside the correct answer.)

Answer:

a. Strawberry gelatin   _____

b. Orange juice   _____

c. Intravenous fluid   _____

d. Milk   _____

Fluid	Milliliters
Orange juice	25.25
Strawberry gelatin	30
Milk	120
Intravenous fluid	25.5

48. NCLEX *Drag-and-Drop / Ordered-Response* Item

Simulate the drag-and-drop computer response by copying the amounts from the box onto the list in ascending order from smallest to largest.

Answer:

0.05   _____
5   _____
2.5   _____
2.25   _____
5.075   _____
0.175   _____
0.049   _____

49. NCLEX *Multiple-Response* Item

Which of the following amounts are greater than 2.05? (Place a check mark beside all that apply.)

a. 0.26   _____   d. 2.06   _____

b. 2.104   _____   e. 2.4   _____

c. 2.006   _____

50. NCLEX *Hot Box* Item

Place an X in the box that contains the amount that is written using safe decimal notation.

.913	0.913
0.9130	9.130

After completing these problems, see page 594 to check your answers. Give yourself 2 points for each correct answer.

Perfect score = 100   My score = _____

Minimum mastery score = 86 (43 correct)

For more practice, go back to the beginning of this section and repeat the Mathematics Diagnostic Evaluation.

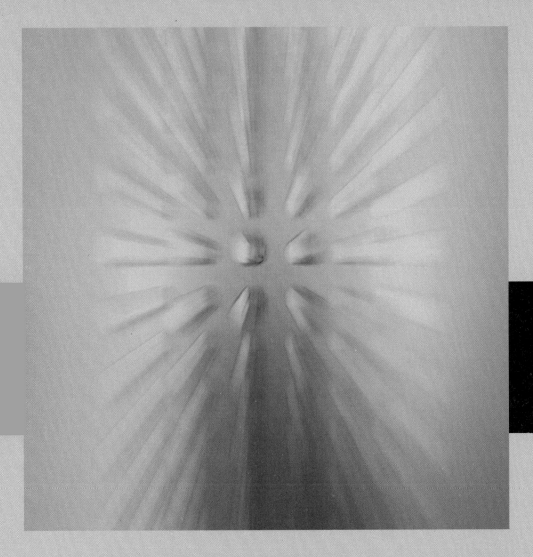

Measurement Systems, Drug Orders, and Drug Labels

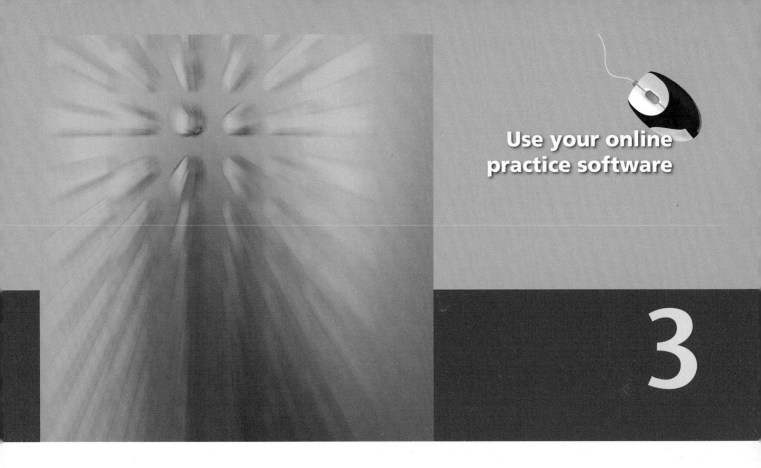

3

Systems of Measurement

OBJECTIVES

Upon mastery of Chapter 3, you will be able to recognize and express the basic systems of measurement used to calculate dosages. To accomplish this, you will also be able to:

- Differentiate metric, apothecary, and household systems of measurement.
- Recall metric and household notation and equivalents.
- Explain the use of milliequivalent (mEq), international unit, unit, and milliunit in dosage calculation.

To administer the correct amount of the prescribed medication to the patient, you must have a thorough knowledge of the measurement systems used to prescribe, measure, and administer medications. Metric is the preferred system of measurement in health care. The household system is still in use in home care. As metric measure is the universal and international system, let's first concentrate on the metric system.

METRIC SYSTEM

All prescriptions should be written in the metric system, and all U.S. Food and Drug Administration (FDA) approved prescription drug labels provide metric dosage. The metric system was first adopted in 1799 in France. It is the most widely used system of measurement in the world. It is preferred for prescribing, measuring, and recording the administration of medications because, as a decimal system, it is the most precise. It is based on powers of 10 with three base units: gram, liter, and meter.

Three essential parameters of measurement are associated with the prescription and administration of medications: weight, volume, and length. Weight is the most utilized parameter. It is important as a dosage unit. The metric base unit of weight is the *gram* (g).

Think of capacity or how much a container holds as you contemplate volume, which is the next most important parameter. Volume usually refers to liquids. Volume also adds two additional parameters to dosage calculations: quantity and concentration. Quantity defines the amount, and concentration describes the strength, of a solution. The *liter* (L) is the metric base unit for volume, and the *milliliter* (mL) is the most common metric volume unit for dosage calculations.

Length is the least utilized parameter for dosage calculations, but linear measurement is still important in health care. A person's height, the circumference of an infant's head, body surface area, length of an amount of ointment, and the size of lacerations and tumors are examples of important length measurements. The metric length base unit is the *meter* (m). Most length measurements in health care are *millimeters* (mm) and *centimeters* (cm).

In the metric system, prefixes are used to show which portion of the base unit is being considered. It is important that you learn the most commonly used prefixes for health care.

REMEMBER
Metric Prefixes

micro	=	one millionth or 0.000001 or $\frac{1}{1,000,000}$ of the base unit
milli	=	one thousandth or 0.001 or $\frac{1}{1,000}$ of the base unit
centi	=	one hundredth or 0.01 or $\frac{1}{100}$ of the base unit
deci	=	one tenth or 0.1 or $\frac{1}{10}$ of the base unit
kilo	=	one thousand or 1,000 times the base unit

Figure 3-1 demonstrates the relationship of metric units. Notice that the values of most of the common prefixes used in health care and the ones applied in this text are highlighted in red: **kilo-, base, milli-,** and **micro-.** These units are three places away from the next place. Often you can either multiply or divide by 1,000 to calculate an equivalent quantity. The only exception is **centi-,** which is also highlighted. Centi- is easy to remember, though, if you think of the relationship between one cent and one U.S. dollar as a clue to the relationship of centi- to the base, $\frac{1}{100}$. **Deci-** is one-tenth ($\frac{1}{10}$) of the base. See Chapter 1 to review the rules of multiplying and dividing decimals by a power of 10.

MATH TIP
Try this to remember the order of six of the metric units—<u>k</u>ilo-, <u>h</u>ecto-, <u>d</u>eca-, (BASE), <u>d</u>eci-, <u>c</u>enti-, and <u>m</u>illi-: "King Henry Died from a Disease Called Mumps."

			gram			
			liter			
			meter			
kilo	hecto	deca	BASE	deci	centi	milli
K	**H**	**D**	**Δ**	**D**	**C**	**M**
"King	Henry	Died	from a	Disease	Called	Mumps."

The international standardization of metric units was adopted throughout much of the world in 1960 with the International System of Units, or SI (from the French *Système International*). The abbreviations of this system of metric notation are the most widely accepted. The metric units of measurement and the SI abbreviations most often used for dosage calculations and measurements of health status are given in the following units of weight, volume, and length. This text uses SI standardized abbreviations throughout. Learn and practice these notations.

FIGURE 3-1   Relationship and value of metric units, with comparison of common metric units used in health care

Prefix	Kilo-	Hecto-	Deca-	BASE	Deci-	Centi-	Milli-	Decimilli-	Centimilli-	Micro-
Weight	kilogram			gram			milligram			microgram
Volume				liter	deciliter		milliliter			
Length				meter		centimeter	millimeter			
Value to Base	1,000	100	10	1	0.1	0.01	0.001	0.0001	0.00001	0.000001

© Cengage Learning 2013

REMEMBER

SI METRIC SYSTEM

	Unit	Abbreviation	Equivalents
Weight	**gram** (base unit)	g	**1 g** = 1,000 mg = 1,000,000 mcg
	milligram	mg	0.001 g = **1 mg** = 1,000 mcg
	microgram	mcg	0.000001 g = 0.001 mg = **1 mcg**
	kilogram	kg	**1 kg** = 1,000 g
Volume	**liter** (base unit)	L	**1 L** = 1,000 mL
	deciliter	dL	0.1 L = **1 dL**
	milliliter	mL	0.001 L = **1 mL**
Length	**meter** (base unit)	m	**1 m** = 100 cm = 1,000 mm
	centimeter	cm	0.01 m = **1 cm** = 10 mm
	millimeter	mm	0.001 m = 0.1 cm = **1 mm**

CAUTION

You may see gram abbreviated as Gm or gm, liter as lowercase l, milliliter as ml, or microgram as μg. These abbreviations are considered obsolete or too easily misinterpreted, and should be avoided. You should only use the standardized SI abbreviations. Use g for gram, L for liter, and mL for milliliter. Further, the unit of measurement *cubic centimeter,* abbreviated cc, has been used interchangeably with mL. The use of cc for mL is now prohibited by many health care organizations because cc can be mistaken for zeros (00) or units (U). The abbreviation U is also now prohibited and must be spelled out (unit).

CAUTION

The SI abbreviations for milligram (mg) and milliliter (mL) appear to be somewhat similar, but in fact mg is a weight unit and mL is a volume unit. Confusing these two units can have dire consequences in dosage calculations. Learn now to clearly differentiate them.

In addition to learning the metric units, their equivalent values, and their abbreviations, it is important to use the following rules of metric notation.

RULES

The following 10 critical rules will help to ensure that you accurately write and interpret metric notation.

1. The unit or abbreviation always follows the amount. Example: *5 g* NOT *g 5*

2. Do not put a period after the unit abbreviation, because it may be mistaken for the number 1 if poorly written. Example: *20 mg* NOT *20 mg.*

3. Do not add an s to make the unit plural, because it may be misread for another unit. Example: *5 mL* NOT *5 mLs*

4. Separate the amount from the unit so the number and unit of measure do not run together, because the unit can be mistaken as zero or zeros, risking a 10-fold to 100-fold overdose. Example: *20 mg* NOT *20mg*

5. Place commas for amounts at or above 1,000. Example: *10,000 mcg* NOT *10000 mcg*

6. Decimals are used to designate fractional amounts. Example: *1.5 mL* NOT *1½ mL*

7. Use a leading zero to emphasize the decimal point for fractional amounts less than 1. Without the zero, the amount may be interpreted as a whole number, resulting in serious overdosing. Example: *0.5 mg* NOT *.5 mg*

8. Omit unnecessary or trailing zeros that can be misread as part of the amount if the decimal point is not seen. Example: *1.5 mg* NOT *1.50 mg*

9. Do not use the abbreviation μg for microgram, because it might be mistaken for mg, which is 1,000 times the intended amount. Example: *150 mcg* NOT *150 μg*

10. Do not use the abbreviation cc for mL, because the unit can be mistaken for zeros. Example: *500 mL* NOT *500 cc*

Always ask the writer to clarify if you are not sure of the abbreviation or notation used. Never guess!

The metric system is the most common and the only standardized system of measurement in health care. Take a few minutes to review the following essential points.

QUICK REVIEW

■ The metric base units are gram (g), liter (L), and meter (m).

■ Subunits are designated by the appropriate prefix and the base unit (such as milligram) and standard abbreviations (such as mg).

■ There are 10 critical rules for ensuring that units and amounts are accurately interpreted. Review them again now, and learn to rigorously adhere to them.

■ Never guess as to the meaning of metric notation. When in doubt about the exact amount or the abbreviation used, ask the writer to clarify.

Review Set 11

1. The system of measurement most commonly used for prescribing and administering medications is the _____ system.

2. Liter and milliliter are metric units that measure _____.

3. Gram and milligram are metric units that measure _____.

4. Meter and millimeter are metric units that measure _____.

5. 1 mg is _____ of a g.

6. There are _____ mL in a liter.

7. Which is smaller—milligram or microgram? _____

8. Which is the largest—kilogram, gram, or milligram? _____

9. Which is the smallest—kilogram, gram, or milligram? _____

10. 1 liter = _____ mL

11. 1,000 mcg = _____ mg

12. 1 kg = _____ g

13. 1 cm = _____ mm

Select the correctly written metric notation.

14. .3 g, 0.3 Gm, 0.3 g, .3 Gm, 0.30 g _____

15. $1\frac{1}{3}$ ml, 1.33 mL, 1.33 ML, $1\frac{1}{3}$ ML, 1.330 mL _____

16. 5 Kg, 5.0 kg, kg 05, 5 kg, 5 kG _____

17. 1.5 mm, $1\frac{1}{2}$ mm, 1.5 Mm, 1.50 MM, $1\frac{1}{2}$ MM _____

18. mg 10, 10 mG, 10.0 mg, 10 mg, 10 MG _____

Interpret these metric abbreviations.

19. mcg _____   23. mm _____

20. mL _____   24. kg _____

21. mg _____   25. cm _____

22. g _____

After completing these problems, see page 594 to check your answers.

APOTHECARY AND HOUSEHOLD SYSTEMS

Apothecary and household measures are most prevalent in home care settings but began to disappear from hospitals and other health care organizations in the 1950s. The historic interconnection between these systems is interesting. The ancient apothecary system was the first system of medication measurement used by apothecaries (pharmacists) and physicians. It originated in Greece and made its way to Europe. The English used it during the late 1600s, and the colonists brought it to America. A modified system of measurement for everyday use evolved; it is now recognized as the household system. Large liquid volumes were based on familiar trading measurements—such as pints, quarts, and gallons—which originated as apothecary measurements. Vessels to accommodate each measurement were made by craftspersons and widely circulated in colonial America. Likewise, units of weight (such as grain, ounce, and pound) are rooted in apothecary. The grain originated as the standard weight of a single grain of wheat.

As the accrediting body for health care organizations, The Joint Commission discourages the use of apothecary units and symbols, such as minims (♏), drams (ʒ), ounces (℥), and grains (gr). But remnants of this system are still evident in health care. After more than 100 years as the world's most popular pill, 5 grains of aspirin is now labeled in the metric equivalent of 325 milligrams. Drams and ounces still appear on some disposable medicine cups along with the metric equivalent, and some 3 mL syringes still show minims (see Chapter 6). Further, it was customary to express apothecary amounts using lowercase Roman numerals and to write the amount after the unit of measure. Oddly, the lowercase Roman numeral also had a horizontal line over it. Some physicians continue to write amounts using apothecary notation, as in the following examples.

EXAMPLES

give iii tablets   Meaning: "Give 3 tablets"

give grains v̄ aspirin   Meaning: "Give a 5-grain aspirin tablet"

While measurement in grains is disappearing from medication labels and physician orders, some medication labels may still include both apothecary and metric measure. Let's compare an older label for morphine sulfate (Figure 3-2) that includes both the apothecary measure in *grains* and metric measure in *milligrams* with a current label for the same drug measured in *milligrams* only (Figure 3-3).

FIGURE 3-2 Morphine sulfate 10 mg/mL (1/8 gr/mL)

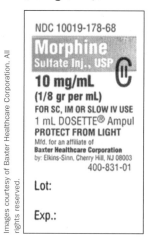

FIGURE 3-3 Morphine sulfate 10 mg/mL

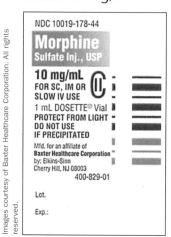

FIGURE 3-4 Nitrostat 0.4 mg (1/150 gr)

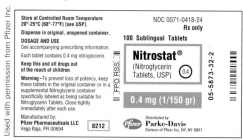

And notice the apothecary measure on the Nitrostat (nitroglycerin) label (Figure 3-4). The information on the label also tells you that $\frac{1}{150}$ *gr* is equivalent to *0.4 mg*. You can see how the grain abbreviation can easily be misread and confused with gram. It is apparent why The Joint Commission (2010) strongly discourages the use of apothecary measure, to prevent medication errors. It is the metric measurement on these labels that you will need to identify for dosage calculations.

CAUTION

The following apothecary units and symbols may appear on some labels, syringes, and medicine cups, or may be written as shorthand by older practitioners. Because they are considered obsolete, do not use these symbols, and be careful to differentiate them from acceptable units of measure. They are provided here for recognition purposes only, but they can easily be misinterpreted and lead to a medication error. **If you receive a written order using one of these symbols or abbreviations, be safe and ask for clarification.**

DO NOT USE THESE SYMBOLS OR ABBREVIATIONS:

gr   **grains:** apothecary unit of weight, approximately 60 mg; easily confused with metric *gram*

ɱ   **minim:** apothecary drop, approximately 16 minims per mL

ℨ   **dram:** apothecary symbol for amount that is slightly less than a teaspoon, approximately 4 mL

ℨ   **ounce:** apothecary symbol for fluid ounce, approximately 30 mL

ss   **one-half:** apothecary symbol for $\frac{1}{2}$

See Appendix B for a comparison of apothecary units and their metric equivalents.

The following household units are likely to be used by the patient at home where metric measuring devices may not be available. They are important for discharge teaching when advising patients and their families about take-home prescriptions. We will consider the metric equivalents of these units in Chapter 4. Unlike the more precise metric system, fractional amounts in the household system are expressed as common fractions (rather than decimals), such as $\frac{1}{2}$ or $\frac{3}{4}$.

REMEMBER

Household		
Unit	Abbreviation	Equivalents
teaspoon	t (or tsp)	
tablespoon	T (or tbs)	1 T = 3 t
ounce (fluid)	fl oz	1 fl oz = 2 T
cup	cup	1 cup = 8 fl oz
pint	pt	1 pt = 2 cups = 16 fl oz
quart	qt	1 qt = 2 pt = 4 cups = 32 fl oz
ounce (weight)	oz	16 oz = 1 lb
pound	lb	

MATH TIP

When comparing the tablespoon and the teaspoon, the tablespoon is the larger unit, and its abbreviation is expressed with a capital, or "large," T. The teaspoon is the smaller unit, and its abbreviation is expressed with a lowercase, or "small," t.

CAUTION

Although some households may use metric measure, many do not, especially in the United States. There can be a wide variation in household measuring devices, such as in tableware teaspoons, which can constitute a safety risk. Talking to your patients and their families about administering medications at home is an excellent teaching opportunity. Determine their familiarity with metric units, such as milliliters, and ask what kind of medicine measuring devices they use at home. It is best to advise your patients and their families to use the measuring devices packaged with the medication or provided by the pharmacy.

OTHER COMMON DRUG MEASUREMENTS: UNITS AND MILLIEQUIVALENTS

Four other measurements may be used to indicate the quantity of medicine prescribed: international unit, unit, milliunit, and milliequivalent (mEq). The quantity is expressed in Arabic numbers with the unit of measure following. The *international unit* represents a unit of potency used to measure such things as vitamins and chemicals. The *unit* is a standardized amount needed to produce a desired effect. Medications such as penicillin, heparin, and insulin have their own meaning and numeric value related to the type of unit. One thousandth ($\frac{1}{1,000}$) of a unit is a *milliunit*. The equivalent of 1 unit is 1,000 milliunits. Oxytocin is a drug measured in milliunits. The *milliequivalent* (mEq) is one thousandth ($\frac{1}{1,000}$) of an equivalent weight of a chemical. The mEq is the unit used when referring to the concentration of serum electrolytes, such as calcium, magnesium, potassium, and sodium.

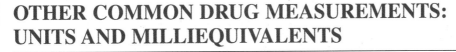

CAUTION

The abbreviations *U* and *IU* are included on the *Official "Do Not Use" List* published by The Joint Commission (2010). The written words *unit* and *international unit* should be used instead, because the abbreviations are considered obsolete and too easily misinterpreted for safe practice. See Chapter 9 for the full "Do Not Use" list.

It is not necessary to learn conversions for the international unit, unit, or milliequivalent, because medications prescribed in these measurements are also prepared and administered in the same system.

EXAMPLE 1 ■

Heparin 800 units is ordered, and *heparin 1,000 units per 1 mL* is the stock drug.

Because there is no standard metric equivalent for units, when a medication is ordered in units (such as heparin), the stock drug should be supplied in units.

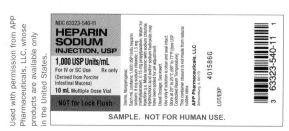

EXAMPLE 2 ■

Potassium chloride 10 mEq is ordered, and *potassium chloride 20 mEq per 15 mL* is the stock drug.

Because there is no standard metric equivalent for mEq, when a medication is ordered in mEq (such as potassium chloride), the stock drug should be supplied in mEq.

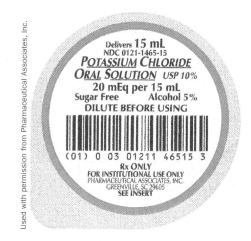

EXAMPLE 3 ■

Oxytocin 2 milliunits (0.002 usp units) intravenous per minute is ordered, and *oxytocin 10 usp units per 1 mL* to be added to 1,000 mL intravenous solution is available. Very small doses of a medication (such as oxytocin), may be ordered in milliunits. Remember, the prefix milli- means one thousandth. Sometimes converting from units to milliunits is necessary.

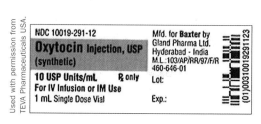

QUICK REVIEW

- Some symbols and abbreviations are obsolete or can lead to medication errors. If you come across these symbols, ask the writer to clarify. Do not use: gr, ɱ, ʒ, ℥, l, ml, cc, U, or IU.

- Household measurement developed from the ancient apothecary system. Household units are most frequently used in home care: t, T, fl oz, cup, pt, qt, and lb.

- Fractional amounts in the household system are expressed as common fractions.

- No conversion is necessary for unit, international unit, and mEq, because the ordered dosage and supply dosage are in the same system.

- 1 unit = 1,000 milliunits

Review Set 12

Interpret the following notations.

1. 3 qt _____   4. $2\frac{1}{2}$ lb _____
2. 10 lb _____   5. 10 T _____
3. 10 mEq _____

Express the following using medical notation.

6. seventy-five pounds   _____

7. thirty milliequivalents   _____

8. five tablespoons   _____

9. one and one-half teaspoons   _____

10. fourteen units   _____

11. True or False? The household system of measurement is commonly used in hospital dosage calculations. _____

12. True or False? 1,000 mcg = 1 g _____

13. True or False? 1 kg = 1,000 g _____

14. Drugs such as heparin and insulin are commonly measured in _____.

15. 1 T = _____ t   18. 2 pt = _____ qt

16. 1 fl oz = _____ T   19. 8 fl oz = _____ cup

17. 16 oz = _____ lb

20. The unit used to measure the concentration of serum electrolytes (such as calcium, magnesium, potassium, and sodium) is the _____ and is abbreviated _____.

After completing these problems, see page 594 to check your answers.

CLINICAL REASONING SKILLS

The importance of the placement of the decimal point cannot be overemphasized. Let's look at some examples of potential medication errors related to placement of the decimal point.

ERROR

Not placing a zero before a decimal point in medication orders.

Possible Scenario

An emergency room physician wrote an order for the bronchodilator terbutaline for a patient with asthma. The order was written as follows.

Incorrectly Written

Terbutaline .5 mg subcutaneously now, repeat dose in 30 minutes if no improvement

Suppose the nurse, not noticing the faint decimal point, administered 5 mg of terbutaline subcutaneously instead of 0.5 mg. The patient would receive ten times the dose intended by the physician.

Potential Outcome

Within minutes of receiving the injection, the patient would likely complain of headache and develop tachycardia, nausea, and vomiting. The patient's hospital stay would be lengthened because of the need to recover from the overdose.

Prevention

This type of medication error is avoided by remembering the rule to place a 0 in front of a decimal to avoid confusion regarding the dosage: 0.5 mg. Further, remember to question orders that are unclear or seem unsafe or impractical.

Correctly Written
Terbutaline 0.5 mg subcutaneously now, repeat dose in 30 minutes if no improvement

CLINICAL REASONING SKILLS

Many medication errors occur by confusing mg and mL. Remember that mg is the weight of the medication and mL is the volume of the medication preparation.

ERROR

Confusing mg and mL.

Possible Scenario

Suppose a physician ordered the steroid prednisolone syrup 15 mg by mouth twice a day for a patient with cancer. Prednisolone syrup is supplied in a concentration of 15 mg in 5 mL. The pharmacist supplied a bottle of prednisolone containing a total volume of 240 mL with 15 mg of prednisolone in every 5 mL. The nurse, in a rush to give her medications on time, misread the order as 15 mL and gave the patient 15 mL of prednisolone instead of 5 mL. Therefore, the patient received 45 mg of prednisolone, or three times the correct dosage.

Potential Outcome

The patient could develop a number of complications related to a high dosage of steroids: gastrointestinal bleeding, hyperglycemia, hypertension, agitation, and severe mood disturbances, to name a few.

Prevention

The mg is the weight of a medication, and mL is the volume you prepare. Do not allow yourself to get rushed or distracted so that you confuse milligrams with milliliters. When you know you are distracted or stressed, have another nurse double-check the calculation of the dose.

PRACTICE PROBLEMS—CHAPTER 3

Give the metric prefix for the following parts of the base units.

1. 0.001 _____

3. 0.01 _____

2. 0.000001 _____

4. 1,000 _____

Identify the equivalent unit with a value of 1 that is indicated by the following amounts (such as 1 unit = 1,000 milliunits).

5. 0.001 gram _____

7. 0.001 milligram _____

6. 1,000 grams _____

8. 0.01 meter _____

Identify the metric base unit for the following.

9. length _____

10. weight _____

11. volume _____

Interpret the following notations.

12. fl oz _____

13. oz _____

14. mg _____

15. mcg _____

16. lb _____

17. mEq _____

18. t _____

19. qt _____

20. mL _____

21. pt _____

22. T _____

23. mm _____

24. g _____

25. cm _____

26. L _____

27. m _____

28. kg _____

29. lb _____

Express the following amounts in proper notation.

30. three hundred and twenty-five micrograms _____

31. one-half teaspoon _____

32. two teaspoons _____

33. one-third fluid ounce _____

34. five million units _____

35. one-half liter _____

36. five hundredths of a milligram _____

37. six hundred milliliters _____

38. two and five tenths centimeters _____

39. eight hundredths of a milliliter _____

40. five and five tenths kilograms _____

Express the following numeric amounts in words.

41. $8\frac{1}{4}$ fl oz _____

42. 375 g _____

43. 0.5 kg _____

44. 2.6 mL _____

45. 20 mEq _____

46. 0.4 L _____

47. 3.05 mcg _____

48. 0.17 mg _____

49. $14\frac{1}{2}$ lb _____

50. Describe the clinical reasoning that you would use to prevent the medication error.

Possible Scenario

Suppose a physician ordered oral Coumadin (warfarin), an anticoagulant, for a patient with a history of deep vein thrombosis. The physician wrote an order for 10 mg but while writing the order placed a decimal point after the 10 and added a 0:

Incorrectly Written

Coumadin 10.0 mg orally once per day

Coumadin 10.0 mg was transcribed on the medication record as Coumadin 100 mg. The patient received ten times the correct dosage.

Potential Outcome

The patient would likely begin hemorrhaging. An antidote, such as vitamin K, would be necessary to reverse the effects of the overdose. However, it is important to remember that not all drugs have antidotes.

Prevention

_____

_____

51. **BONUS:** Describe the strategy that would prevent this medication error.

Possible Scenario

Suppose a physician ordered oral codeine, a narcotic analgesic, for an adult patient recovering from nasal surgery. The physician wrote the following order for one grain of codeine (approximately equivalent to 60 mg). The gr smeared, and the abbreviation of i gr is now unclear. Is it *grains* or *grams*?

Physician's Apothecary Order

Codeine i gr orally every 4 hours as needed for pain

Codeine 1 gram was transcribed on the medication record. Because 1 gram is equivalent to 1,000 mg or about 15 grains, this erroneous dosage is about 15 times more than the intended amount.

Potential Outcome

The maximum dosage of codeine is 60 mg every 4 to 6 hours, not to exceed 360 mg per day. If the nurse had administered the transcribed dosage, the patient could have experienced acute intoxication resulting in violent GI tract symptoms, abdominal pain, burning of the throat, rapid and weak pulse, CNS depression, respiratory paralysis, and even death, depending on the fragility of the patient's prior status.

Prevention

_____

_____

_____

After completing these problems, see pages 594–596 to check your answers.

For additional practice, visit the online practice software at www.CengageBrain.com, using the Premium Website access code found in the front of your text.

REFERENCE

The Joint Commission. (2010). Facts about the Official "Do Not Use" List. Retrieved April 28, 2011, from http://www.jointcommission.org/assets/1/18/Official_Do%20Not%20Use_List_%206_10.pdf

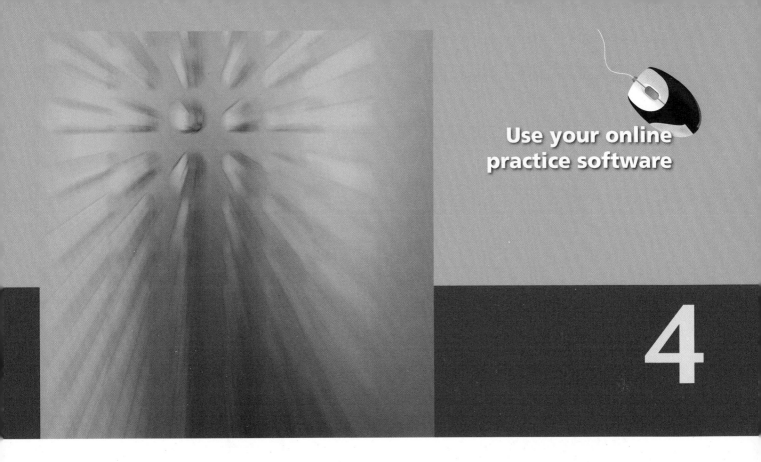

4

Conversions: Metric and Household Systems

OBJECTIVES

Upon mastery of Chapter 4, you will be able to complete Step 1, Conversion, in the Three-Step Approach to dosage calculations. To accomplish this, you will also be able to:

- Recall from memory the metric and household approximate equivalents.
- Convert among units of measurement within the same system.
- Convert units of measurement from one system to another.

Medications are usually prescribed or ordered in a unit of weight measurement such as grams or milligrams. The nurse must interpret this order and administer the correct number of tablets, capsules, teaspoons, milliliters, or some other unit of volume or capacity measurement to deliver the prescribed amount of medication.

EXAMPLE 1 ■

A prescription notation may read:

> Aldactone 100 mg to be given orally twice a day

The nurse has on hand a 100 tablet bottle of *Aldactone labeled 50 mg in each tablet.* To administer the correct amount of the drug, the nurse must calculate the prescribed weight of 100 mg to the correct number of tablets. In this case, the nurse gives the patient two of the 50 mg tablets, which equals *100 mg of Aldactone.* To give the prescribed dosage, the nurse must be able to calculate the order in weight to the correct number of tablets of the drug on hand or in stock. THINK: If one tablet equals 50 mg, then two tablets equal 100 mg.

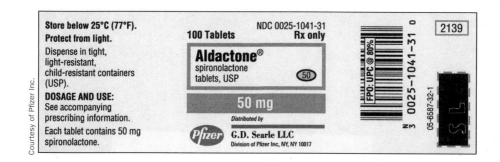

EXAMPLE 2 ■

A prescription notation may read:

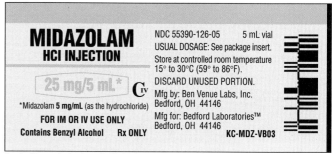

midazolam HCl 2.5 mg by intravenous
injection immediately

The nurse has on hand a vial of *midazolam HCl* labeled *25 mg per 5 mL* or *5 mg/mL*. To administer the correct amount of the drug, the nurse must be able to fill the injection syringe with the correct number of milliliters. As the nurse, how many milliliters would you give? THINK: If 5 mg = 1 mL, then 2.5 mg = 0.5 mL. Therefore, 0.5 mL should be administered.

IDENTIFYING NEED FOR UNIT CONVERSION

Sometimes a drug order may be written in a unit of measurement that is different from the supply of drugs the nurse has on hand. Usually this will be an order for a medicine that is written in one size of metric unit (such as milligrams) but where the medicine is supplied in another metric unit (such as grams). You will occasionally encounter a medicine ordered in household or apothecary measure (such as fluid ounces). However, the drug will be supplied in metric measure (such as milliliters). The Joint Commission (2010) discourages the use of apothecary measure; but until it is prohibited, you may still see it in use. Therefore, we will consider examples of conversion within the metric system and between other systems. Converting a unit of measure does not change the amount of the ordered dosage of medication, but provides an equal but alternate expression of the dosage. Let's look at examples of medicines ordered and supplied in both different size units and different systems of measurement.

EXAMPLE 1 ■

Medication order: triazolam 250 mcg orally at bedtime

Supply on hand: Halcion 0.25 mg tablets

The drug order is written in micrograms, but the drug is supplied in milligrams.

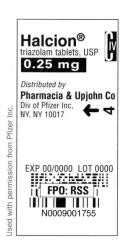

EXAMPLE 2 ■

Medication order: Antacid Plus $\frac{1}{2}$ fl oz after meals

Supply on hand: Antacid Plus 1 fl oz (30 mL)

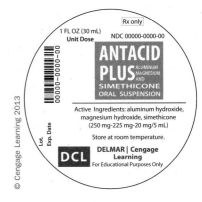

The drug order is written in fluid ounces (household measure), but the drug is supplied in a form that measures both milliliters (metric measure) and fluid ounces (household measure).

In the first example, the prescribed quantity must be converted into the unit of measure as supplied. The nurse or other health care professional can then calculate the correct dosage to prepare and administer to the patient. But in this second example, the nurse must take care to select the correct unit of measure from the two options provided on the label before calculating the ordered dose. Thus, determining the need for and calculating unit conversions are the first steps in dosage calculations.

CONVERTING FROM ONE UNIT TO ANOTHER USING THE CONVERSION FACTOR METHOD

After learning the systems of measurement common for dosage calculations and their equivalents (Chapter 3), the next step is to learn how to use them. First, you must be able to convert or change from one unit to another within the same measurement system. To accomplish this simple operation, you need to:

- Recall the equivalents

- Multiply or divide

The following information will help you remember when to multiply and when to divide.

The *conversion factor* is a number used with either multiplication or division to change a measurement from one unit of measurement to its equivalent in another unit of measurement.

RULE

To convert from a larger to a smaller unit of measurement, multiply by the conversion factor.
THINK: "*Larger* is going down to *smaller*, so you will multiply." Larger ↓ Smaller → Multiply (×)

Stop and think about this. You know this is true because it takes *more* parts of a *smaller* unit to make an equivalent amount of a larger unit. To get *more* parts, *multiply*. Let's look at how this works with units already familiar to you.

EXAMPLE 1 ■

How many cups are in 3 quarts? You know that 1 quart = 4 cups. It takes 4 of the cup units to equal 1 of the quart units. Cups are *smaller* than quarts. THINK: Larger ↓ Smaller → Multiply (×). The conversion factor for the cup and quart units is 4 cups/qt.

Multiply by the conversion factor:

quarts (larger unit) × cups/qt (conversion factor) = cups (smaller unit)

3 qt × 4 cups/qt = 12 cups

MATH TIP

Notice that the original unit (qt) cancels out, leaving the desired unit (cups) in the answer.

$\frac{3 \text{ qt}}{1} \times \frac{4 \text{ cups}}{1 \text{ qt}} = 12$ cups; or, written more simply, 3 qt × 4 cups/qt = 12 cups

EXAMPLE 2 ■

Now consider two metric units of measurement: gram (g) and kilogram (kg). How many grams are in 4.5 kilograms? In metric units of measurement, 1 kg = 1,000 g. It takes 1,000 of the gram units to equal 1 of the kilogram units. Grams are smaller than kilograms; therefore, more are needed to make an equivalent amount. THINK: Larger ↓ Smaller → Multiply (×). The conversion factor for kilograms to grams is 1,000 g/kg. Multiply by the conversion factor.

kilograms (larger unit) × g/kg (conversion factor) = grams (smaller unit)

4.5 k̶g̶ × 1,000 mg/k̶g̶ = 4,500 g

Therefore, 4.5 kg = 4,500 g

RULE

To convert from a smaller to a larger unit of measurement, divide by the conversion factor. THINK: "*Smaller* is going up to *larger*, so you will divide." Smaller ↑ Larger → Divide (÷)

You know this is true because it takes *fewer* parts of the *larger* unit to make an equivalent amount of a smaller unit. To get *fewer* parts, *divide*. Again, let's first convert units already familiar to you.

EXAMPLE 1 ■

How many tablespoons are in 6 teaspoons? You know that 1 T = 3 t. The conversion factor is 3t/T. Tablespoons are larger units than teaspoons. Divide by the conversion factor because it takes fewer of the tablespoon units to equal the equivalent amount in teaspoon units. THINK: Smaller ↑ Larger → Divide (÷)

teaspoons (smaller unit) ÷ t/T (conversion factor) = tablespoons (larger unit)

6 t ÷ 3 t/T = 6 t × 1 T/3 t = 2 T

MATH TIP

Recall that dividing by a fraction involves inverting the divisor and multiplying.

$6\,t \div 3\,t/T = \frac{6\,t}{1} \div \frac{3\,t}{1\,T} = \frac{6\,t̶}{1} \times \frac{1\,T}{3\,t̶} = \frac{6}{3}\,T = 2\,T$

Or, more simply: $6\,t \div 3\,t/T = 6\,t̶ \times 1\,T/3\,t̶ = 2\,T$

Now let's examine conversion of units used for health care.

EXAMPLE 2 ■

How many grams are equal to 500 milligrams? Recall that 1 g = 1,000 mg. Grams are larger than milligrams; therefore, fewer are needed to make an equivalent amount. THINK: Smaller ↑ Larger → Divide (÷). The conversion factor for milligrams to grams is 1,000 mg/g. Divide by the conversion factor.

milligrams (smaller unit) ÷ mg/g (conversion factor) = grams (larger unit)

500 mg ÷ 1,000 mg/g = 500 m̶g̶ × 1 g/1,000 m̶g̶ = 0.5 g

Therefore, 500 mg = 0.5 g

CONVERTING WITHIN THE METRIC SYSTEM

The most common conversions in dosage calculations and health care are within the metric system. As you recall from Chapter 3, most metric conversions are simply derived by multiplying or dividing by 1,000. Recall from Chapter 1 that multiplying by 1,000 is the same as moving the decimal point three places to the right. Notice that in the following examples you are asked to find the equivalent amount of the smaller unit. It makes sense that the resulting number of smaller units would be greater than the original number of larger units. In this first example, you are converting grams to milligrams, so you multiply.

EXAMPLE 1 ▪

Convert 2 grams to the equivalent number of milligrams.

1. Recall the known equivalent: 1 g = 1,000 mg; conversion factor is 1,000 mg/g

2. THINK: To convert 2 grams to the equivalent number of milligrams, you would first determine that the gram is the larger unit. Larger ↓ Smaller → Multiply (×). Therefore, you would multiply to convert to milligrams, the smaller unit.

3. Multiply by 1,000 mg/g: 2 g̶ × 1,000 mg/g̶ = 2,000 mg

   or

   2 g = 2.000. = 2,000 mg (moving decimal 3 places to the right; add 3 zeros to complete the operation)

   Thus, you know that a medicine container labeled 2 grams per tablet means the same as 2,000 milligrams per tablet.

MATH TIP

Notice that to multiply 2 by 1,000, you are moving the decimal three places to the right. This is a shortcut. Sometimes to complete this operation, you add zeros to hold the places equal to the number of zeros in the equivalent. In this case, 1 g = 1,000 mg, so you add three zeros: 2 × 1,000 = 2.000. = 2,000

EXAMPLE 2 ▪

Convert: 0.3 mg to mcg

Equivalent: 1 mg = 1,000 mcg; therefore, conversion factor is 1,000 mcg/mg

THINK: Larger ↓ Smaller → Multiply (×)

Multiply by 1,000 mcg/mg: 0.3 m̶g̶ × 1,000 mcg/m̶g̶ = 300 mcg
or move decimal point 3 places to the right
0.3 mg = 0.300. = 300 mcg (2 zeros are added to complete the operation)

EXAMPLE 3 ▪

Convert: 2.5 g to mg

Equivalent: 1 g = 1,000 mg; therefore, conversion factor is 1,000 mg/g

THINK: Larger ↓ Smaller → Multiply (×)

Multiply by 1,000 mg/g: 2.5 g̶ × 1,000 mg/g̶ = 2,500 mg
or move decimal point 3 places to the right
2.5 g = 2.500. = 2,500 mg (2 zeros are added to complete the operation)

EXAMPLE 4 ▪

Convert: 0.15 kg to g

Equivalent: 1 kg = 1,000 g; therefore, conversion factor is 1,000 g/kg

THINK: Larger ↓ Smaller → Multiply (×)

Multiply by 1,000 g/kg: 0.15 k̶g̶ × 1,000 g/k̶g̶ = 150 g
or move decimal point 3 places to the right
0.15 kg = 0.150. = 150 g (1 zero is added to complete the operation)

EXAMPLE 5 ▪

Convert: 0.04 L to mL

Equivalent: 1 L = 1,000 mL; therefore, conversion factor is 1,000 mL/L

THINK: Larger ↓ Smaller → Multiply (×)

Multiply by 1,000 mL/L: 0.04 L̶ × 1,000 mL/L̶ = 40 mL
or move decimal point 3 places to the right
0.04 L = 0.040. = 40 mL (1 zero is added to complete the operation)

EXAMPLE 6 ▪

Knowing how to do unit conversions is also helpful when conducting physical assessment. An infant's head circumference is 40.5 cm. How many millimeters does that equal?

Convert: 40.5 cm to mm

Equivalent: 1 cm = 10 mm; therefore, conversion factor is 10 mm/cm (not 1,000 this time), so you move the decimal point 1 place to the right.

THINK: Larger ↓ Smaller → Multiply (×)

Multiply by 10 mm/cm: 40.5 c̶m̶ × 10 mm/c̶m̶ = 405 mm
or move decimal point 1 place to the right
40.5 cm = 40.5. = 405 mm

Now let's consider conversions that go the opposite way—from a smaller unit (such as mL) to a larger unit (such as L). It makes sense that the resulting number of larger units will now be less than the original number of smaller units.

Remember that to convert a smaller unit to its equivalent larger unit, such as milliliters to liters, you divide. THINK: Smaller ↑ Larger → Divide (÷). Recall the equivalent of 1 L = 1,000 mL and then divide the number of milliliters by 1,000 mL/L. Thus, if you have a bottle that contains 5,000 milliliters of boric acid solution, you know that this is the same as 5 liters of solution. Dividing by 1,000 is the same as moving the decimal point three places to the left.

EXAMPLE 1 ▪

Convert: 5,000 mL to L

Equivalent: 1 L = 1,000 mL; therefore, conversion factor is 1,000 mL/L

THINK: Smaller ↑ Larger → Divide (÷)

Divide by 1,000 mL/L: 5,000 mL ÷ 1,000 mL/L = 5,000 m̶L̶ × 1 L/1,000 m̶L̶ = 5 L
or move decimal point 3 places to the left
5,000 mL = 5.000. = 5 L (eliminate unnecessary zeros)

MATH TIP
Let's look again at the shortcut for dividing 5,000 by 1,000. Now you are moving the decimal three places to the left, and then eliminating unnecessary zeros. 5,000 ÷ 1,000 = 5.000. = 5

CAUTION
Leaving unnecessary zeros may lead to confusion and misinterpretation. For safety, the unnecessary zeros must be eliminated. Likewise, use a leading zero for emphasis of a decimal point when a decimal number is less than 1. Both of these cautions are demonstrated in the next example.

EXAMPLE 2 ▪

Convert: 500 mcg to mg

Equivalent: 1 mg = 1,000 mcg; therefore, conversion factor is 1,000 mcg/mg

THINK: Smaller ↑ Larger → Divide (÷)

Divide by 1,000 mcg/mg: 500 mcg ÷ 1,000 mcg/mg = 500 ~~mcg~~ × 1 mg/1,000 ~~mcg~~ = 0.5 mg
or move decimal point 3 places to the left
500 mcg = .500. = 0.5 mg (Eliminate unnecessary zeros. As the amount is less than 1, use a leading zero for emphasis of the decimal point.)

MATH TIP
Sometimes, to complete the operation, you must add zeros equal to the number of zeros in the equivalent to hold the places, as shown in Examples 3 and 4.

EXAMPLE 3 ▪

Convert: 20 mg to g

Equivalent: 1 g = 1,000 mg; therefore, conversion factor is 1,000 mg/g

THINK: Smaller ↑ Larger → Divide (÷)

Divide by 1,000 mg/g: 20 mg ÷ 1,000 mg/g = 20 ~~mg~~ × 1 g/1,000 ~~mg~~ = 0.02 g
or move decimal point 3 places to the left
20 mg = .020. = 0.02 g (First you must add a zero to complete the operation. Then eliminate the unnecessary zero and use a leading zero for emphasis in your final answer.)

EXAMPLE 4 ▪

Convert: 5 g to kg

Equivalent: 1 g = 1,000 kg; therefore, conversion factor is 1,000 g/kg

THINK: Smaller ↑ Larger → Divide (÷)

Divide by 1,000 g/kg: 5 g ÷ 1,000 g/kg = 5 ~~g~~ × 1 kg/1,000 ~~g~~ = 0.005 kg
or move decimal point 3 places to the left
5 g = 0.005. = 0.005 kg (Add zeros to complete the operation. Use a leading zero for emphasis.)

EXAMPLE 5 ▪

A patient's wound measures 31 millimeters. How many centimeters does that equal?

Convert: 31 mm to cm

Equivalent: 1 cm = 10 mm; therefore, conversion factor is 10 mm/cm (not 1,000 this time)

THINK: Smaller ↑ Larger → Divide (÷) Notice that you are dividing by 10, so you will move the decimal 1 place to the left.

Divide by 10 mm/cm: 31 mm ÷ 10 mm/cm = 31 ~~mm~~ × 1 cm/10 ~~mm~~ = 3.1 cm
or move decimal point 1 place to the left
31 mm = 3.1. = 3.1 cm

REMEMBER
When converting from a larger to a smaller unit of measure, the resulting number of smaller units should be greater than the original number of larger units. Conversely, when converting from a smaller to a larger unit of measure, the resulting number of larger units should be less than the original number of smaller units. After all calculations, ask yourself, "Does this answer make sense?" If it does not, stop and check for your mistake.

MATH TIP

Remember this diagram when converting within the metric system.

Move decimal point three places to the left for each step.

◄───

kg   g   mg   mcg

───►

Move decimal point three places to the right for each step.

EXAMPLES ▪

1 mcg = 0.001 mg (moved decimal point to the left 3 places)

2 g = 2,000 mg (moved decimal point to the right 3 places)

2 g = 2,000,000 mcg (moved decimal point to the right 6 places, as the conversion required two steps)

　　　In time, you will probably do these calculations in your head with little difficulty. If you feel you do not understand the concept of conversions within the metric system, review again the decimal section in Chapter 1 and the metric section in Chapter 3. Also get help from your instructor before proceeding further.

QUICK REVIEW

Use the conversion factor method to convert from one unit of measurement to another.

■ Recall the equivalents.

■ Identify the conversion factor.

■ MULTIPLY by the conversion factor to convert to a smaller unit.
　THINK: Larger ↓ Smaller → Multiply (×)

■ DIVIDE by the conversion factor to convert to a larger unit.
　THINK: Smaller ↑ Larger → Divide (÷)

Review Set 13

Convert each of the following to the equivalent unit indicated.

1. 500 mL = _____ L		16. 0.75 L = _____ mL	
2. 0.015 g = _____ mg		17. 5,000 mL = _____ L	
3. 8 mg = _____ g		18. 1 L = _____ mL	
4. 10 mg = _____ g		19. 1 g = _____ mg	
5. 60 mg = _____ g		20. 3,000 mL = _____ L	
6. 300 mg = _____ g		21. 23 mcg = _____ mg	
7. 0.2 g = _____ mg		22. 1.05 g = _____ kg	
8. 1.2 g = _____ mg		23. 18 mcg = _____ mg	
9. 0.0025 kg = _____ g		24. 0.4 mg = _____ mcg	
10. 0.065 g = _____ mg		25. 2,625 g = _____ kg	
11. 0.005 L = _____ mL		26. 50 cm = _____ m	
12. 1.5 L = _____ mL		27. 10 L = _____ mL	
13. 100 mcg = _____ mg		28. 450 mL = _____ L	
14. 250 mL = _____ L		29. 5 mL = _____ L	
15. 2 kg = _____ g		30. 30 mg = _____ mcg	

After completing these problems, see page 595 to check your answers.

APPROXIMATE EQUIVALENTS

Fortunately, the use of the apothecary and household systems is infrequent and may soon become completely obsolete in health care, to prevent medication errors. These systems are most often still used in the home care setting. Conversions between the apothecary and household units still in use are based on approximate equivalents. More exact equivalents are not practical and, therefore, rarely used by health care workers. For example, a more exact equivalent of 1 U.S. fluid ounce as measured in milliliters is 29.5735296875 milliliters, or approximately 30 milliliters; but in the U.K. 1 fluid ounce is 28.4130625 milliliters. There are 32 fluid ounces per 1 U.S. quart, and this is generally accepted to be approximately 1 liter; but the more exact conversion is 946.35295 milliliters. This is further complicated by the relationship of pints, quarts, and fluid ounces, all of which explains why these systems are discouraged by The Joint Commission (2010) and are becoming obsolete in traditional health care settings.

The approximate equivalents in the following Remember Box are the ones you need to learn so that you can convert from one system to another. Other obsolete approximate equivalents are included in Appendix B: *drams* (volume measure which is still evident on some disposable medicine cups along with teaspoons, tablespoons, fluid ounces, and milliliters), *minims* (volume measure which is still evident on some hypodermic syringes along with the metric equivalent), and *grains* (weight measure, still evident on labels of some older medications along with the metric equivalent). Memorize these approximate equivalents.

REMEMBER
Approximate Equivalents

$$1\ t = 5\ mL$$
$$1\ T = 3\ t = 15\ mL = \frac{1}{2}\ fl\ oz$$
$$1\ fl\ oz = 30\ mL = 6\ t$$
$$1\ L = 1\ qt = 32\ fl\ oz = 2\ pt = 4\ cups$$
$$1\ pt = 16\ fl\ oz = 2\ cups$$
$$1\ cup = 8\ fl\ oz = 240\ mL$$
$$1\ kg = 2.2\ lb$$
$$1\ in = 2.5\ cm$$

CONVERTING BETWEEN SYSTEMS OF MEASUREMENT USING THE CONVERSION FACTOR METHOD

Now let's convert units between systems of measurement using approximate equivalents and the conversion factor method. Recall that to convert from a larger to a smaller unit of measure, you must multiply by the conversion factor. THINK: Larger ↓ Smaller → Multiply (×)

EXAMPLE 1 ▪

Convert: 2 fl oz to mL

Approximate equivalent: 1 fl oz = 30 mL. Conversion factor is 30 mL/fl oz.

THINK: Larger ↓ Smaller → Multiply (×)

2 f̶l̶ o̶z̶ × 30 mL/f̶l̶ o̶z̶ = 60 mL

EXAMPLE 2

Convert: 75 in to cm

Approximate equivalent: 1 in = 2.5 cm. Conversion factor is 2.5 cm/in.

THINK: Larger ↓ Smaller → Multiply (×)

75 i̶n̶ × 2.5 cm/i̶n̶ = 187.5 cm

EXAMPLE 3 ■

The hospital scale weighs a child at 40 kg. The mother wants to know her child's weight in pounds.

Convert: 40 kg to lb

Approximate equivalent: 1 kg = 2.2 lb. Conversion factor is 2.2 lb/kg.

THINK: Larger ↓ Smaller → Multiply (×)

40 k̶g̶ × 2.2 lb/k̶g̶ = 88 lb

   Recall that to convert from a smaller to a larger unit of measure, you must divide by the conversion factor. THINK: Smaller ↑ Larger → Divide (÷). Now the resulting number of larger units will be less than the original number of smaller units.

EXAMPLE 1 ■

Convert: 45 mL to t

Approximate equivalent: 1 t = 5 mL. Conversion factor is 5 mL/t.

THINK: Smaller ↑ Larger → Divide (÷)

45 mL ÷ 5 mL/t = 45 m̶L̶ × 1 t/5 m̶L̶ = 9 t

EXAMPLE 2 ■

Convert: 66 lb to kg

Approximate equivalent: 1 kg = 2.2 lb. Conversion factor is 2.2 lb/kg.

THINK: Smaller ↑ Larger → Divide (÷)

66 lb ÷ 2.2 lb/kg = 66 l̶b̶ × 1 kg/2.2 l̶b̶ = 30 kg

EXAMPLE 3 ■

Convert: 40 cm to in

Approximate equivalent: 1 in = 2.5 cm. Conversion factor is 2.5 cm/in.

THINK: Smaller ↑ Larger → Divide (÷)

40 cm ÷ 2.5 cm/in = 40 c̶m̶ × 1 in/2.5 c̶m̶ = 16 in

MATH TIP

A clue for remembering the approximate equivalent 1 kg = 2.2 lb is to realize that there are about 2 pounds for every kilogram, so the number of kilograms you weigh is about half the number of pounds you weigh. (This could almost make getting on a metric scale pleasant.)

   Try this: Convert your weight in pounds to kilograms rounded to hundredths, or two decimal places. Now check your answer. Is your weight in kilograms approximately $\frac{1}{2}$ your weight in pounds? Then you are correct!

   By using the approximate equivalents that you know, you can determine an unknown equivalent using the common equivalent between them. For example, we know that 1 teaspoon = 5 milliliters, and we know that 1 fluid ounce = 30 milliliters. Therefore, we can convert fluid ounces to teaspoons. The common equivalent is milliliters. Notice that in this example you will multiply *and* divide.

EXAMPLE

Convert: $1\frac{1}{2}$ fl oz to t

Approximate equivalents: 1 t = 5 mL

                             1 fl oz = 30 mL

THINK: Larger ↓ Smaller → Multiply (×)

Smaller ↑ Larger → Divide (÷)

$1\frac{1}{2}$ fl oz × 30 mL/fl oz = 1.5 f̶l̶ o̶z̶ × 30 mL/f̶l̶ o̶z̶ = 45 mL

45 mL ÷ 5 mL/t = 45 m̶L̶ × 1 t/5 m̶L̶ = 9 t

QUICK REVIEW

To perform dosage calculations, you must be able to convert between systems of measurement. To use the *conversion factor method*, recall the approximate equivalent, identify the conversion factor, and

- MULTIPLY by the conversion factor to convert to a SMALLER unit.
  THINK: Larger ↓ Smaller → Multiply (×)

- DIVIDE by the conversion factor to convert to a LARGER unit.
  THINK: Smaller ↑ Larger → Divide (÷)

Review Set 14

Convert each of the following amounts to the unit indicated. Indicate the approximate equivalent(s) used in the conversion. If rounding is necessary, round decimals to two places (hundredths).

Approximate Equivalent

1. 3 g = _____ kg   _____

2. 13 t = _____ mL   _____

3. 15 mL = _____ fl oz   _____

4. $2\frac{1}{2}$ fl oz = _____ mL   _____

5. 750 mL = _____ qt   _____

6. 20 mL = _____ t   _____

7. 4 T = _____ mL   _____

8. 9 kg = _____ lb   _____

9. 250 lb = _____ kg   _____

10. 3 L = _____ qt   _____

11. 55 kg = _____ lb   _____

12. 12 in = _____ cm   _____

13. 2 qt = _____ L   _____

14. 3 t = _____ mL   _____

15. 99 lb = _____ kg   _____

16. 1 pt = _____ mL   _____

17. $1\frac{1}{2}$ cups = _____ mL   _____

18. 1.5 m = _____ ft   _____

19. 30 cm = _____ in   _____

20. 60 mL = _____ fl oz   _____

21. 32 in = _____ cm   _____

22. 350 mm = _____ in   _____

23. 7.5 cm = _____ in   _____

24. 2 in = _____ mm   _____

25. 40 kg = _____ lb   _____

26. 7.16 kg = _____ lb   _____

27. 110 lb = _____ kg   _____

28. 3.5 kg = _____ lb   _____

29. 63 lb = _____ kg   _____

30. A newborn infant is $21\frac{1}{2}$ inches long. Her length is _____ cm.

31. The label for a granular medicine recommends mixing it with at least 120 mL of water or juice. At the time of discharge, the nurse should advise the patient to mix the medicine with _____ fluid ounce(s) or _____ cup(s) of water or juice.

32. A patient who weighs 250 lb starts a weight-loss program with a goal of losing 10 lb before the next doctor's appointment. At the next office visit, the patient is weighed at 108 kg. Has the patient met the weight-loss goal? _____

33. Calculate the total fluid intake in mL for 24 hours.

Breakfast	8 fl oz milk	
	6 fl oz orange juice	
	4 fl oz water with medication	
Lunch	8 fl oz iced tea	
Snack	10 fl oz coffee	
	4 fl oz gelatin dessert	
Dinner	8 fl oz water	
	6 fl oz tomato juice	
	6 fl oz beef broth	
Snack	5 fl oz pudding	
	12 fl oz diet soda	
	4 fl oz water with medication	Total = _____ mL

34. A child who weighs 55 lb is to receive 0.05 mg of a drug per kg of body weight per dose. How much of the drug should the child receive for each dose? _____ mg

35. A child is taking 12 mL of a medication 4 times per day. If the full bottle contains 16 fluid ounces of the medication, how many days will the bottle last? _____ day(s)

36. The doctor prescribes 10 mL of Betadine concentrate in 480 mL of warm water as a soak for a finger infection. Using measures commonly found in the home, how would you instruct the patient to prepare the solution?

_____

37. The patient is to receive 10 mL of a drug. How many teaspoonsful should the patient take?

_____ t

38. An infant is taking a ready-to-feed formula. The formula comes in quart containers. If the infant usually takes 4 fluid ounces of formula every 3 hours during the day and night, how many quarts of formula should the mother buy for a 3-day supply? _____ qt

39. An infant's head circumference is 40 cm. The parents ask for the equivalent in inches. You tell the parents their infant's head circumference is _____ in.

40. The patient tells you he was weighed in the physician's office and was told he is 206 pounds. What is his weight in kilograms? _____ kg

After completing these problems, see pages 595–596 to check your answers.

SUMMARY

At this point, you should be quite familiar with the equivalents for converting within the metric and household systems and from one system to another. From memory, you should be able to recall quickly and accurately the equivalents for conversions. If you are having difficulty understanding the concept of converting from one unit of measurement to another, review this chapter and seek additional help from your instructor.

Consider the two Clinical Reasoning Skills scenarios, and work the Practice Problems for Chapter 4. Concentrate on accuracy. One error can be a serious mistake when calculating the dosages of medicines or performing critical measurements of health status.

CLINICAL REASONING SKILLS

ERROR

Incorrectly interpreting an apothecary symbol.

Possible Scenario

To prevent hypokalemia (lowered potassium), a physician ordered $\frac{1}{2}$℥ *potassium gluconate 20 mEq elixir three times a day*, for a hospitalized patient who was also receiving digitalis and diuretic therapy. The nursing student did not recognize the fluid ounce symbol and interpreted the order as $\frac{1}{2}$ of the 20 mEq amount. The potassium gluconate was supplied as 20 mEq per 15 mL, and the physician intended for the patient to receive 15 mL three times a day; instead, the student nurse prepared 7.5 mL or $1\frac{1}{2}$ t of the elixir in a medicine cup. The nursing instructor asked the student nurse to explain how she determined the amount to give, and the student explained that the order is for $\frac{1}{2}$ of the 20 mEq per 15 mL amount, so $\frac{1}{2}$ of 15 mL is 7.5 mL, or $1\frac{1}{2}$ t. The instructor pointed to the ℥ symbol and suggested that the physician likely intended $\frac{1}{2}$ fl oz, which is the same as 15 mL.

Potential Outcome

If the student nurse had given over several days the dose amount she prepared, the patient would have received only 50% of the intended dosage of the potassium gluconate and could potentially have developed digitalis toxicity leading to confusion, vomiting, diarrhea, blurred vision, irregular pulse, and palpitations.

Prevention

This type of medication error is avoided by clarifying all drug orders that are confusing or that include unfamiliar symbols. If you are not sure: stop, think, and ask. In this case, the physician should have been contacted to clarify the order. Ideally, the hospital would follow The Joint Commission (2010) recommendations regarding unsafe use of abbreviations, acronyms, and symbols and put apothecary symbols on its "Do Not Use" List.

CLINICAL REASONING SKILLS	ERROR

ERROR

Not moving the correct number of decimal spaces when using the shortcut method to multiply by a power of 10.

Possible Scenario

A physician ordered **125 mcg of digoxin once each day** for a patient treated for congestive heart failure. Supplied were scored tablets in individual packages labeled 0.25 mg per tablet. The conversion needed was mg to mcg, a larger unit to a smaller unit. The nurse remembered that to convert from a larger unit to a smaller unit you multiply by the conversion factor. The nurse also knew that 1,000 mcg = 1 mg and that the conversion factor was 1,000 mcg/mg. But, in a hurry, the nurse forgot to add a zero to create the correct number of decimal spaces and incorrectly figured the problem this way:

$$0.25 \times 1,000 = 0.25. = 25 \text{ mcg} \qquad \textbf{INCORRECT}$$

The nurse then reasoned, "If the physician's order was 125 mcg, then with 25 mcg tablets on hand, the patient must need 5 tablets because 5 tablets of 25 mcg each equal 125 mcg." The nurse started to administer the 5 tablets but hesitated because it seemed like a large number of tablets. The nurse asked a fellow nurse to double-check the calculations. The second nurse found the error. The **correct** conversion is:

$$0.25 \text{ mg} \times 1,000 \text{ mcg/mg} = 0.250. = 250 \text{ mcg} \qquad \textbf{CORRECT}$$

The tablets are 250 mcg each, not 25 mcg each. The patient should receive $\frac{1}{2}$ tablet, not 5 tablets.

Potential Outcome

Digoxin is a high-alert cardiac medication that may lead to serious adverse reactions at toxic levels. If the nurse had proceeded with the incorrect amount, the patient would have received 10 times the normal dose and very likely would have had serious complications, such as severe bradycardia or cardiac arrhythmias.

Prevention

Fortunately, the error was caught and the patient was given the correct amount, which was $\frac{1}{2}$ tablet. A medication administration error was prevented because the nurse stopped to consider, "Does this make sense?" After every dosage calculation, ask if the answer makes sense. If still in doubt, especially with high-alert medications, ask another nurse to double-check your thinking and the calculation.

PRACTICE PROBLEMS–CHAPTER 4

Give the following equivalents without consulting conversion tables. If rounding is necessary, round decimals to two places (hundredths).

1. 0.5 g = _500_ mg		7. 250 mL = _.5_ pt
2. 0.01 g = _10_ mg		8. 300 g = _.3_ kg
3. 7.5 mL = _.0075_ L		9. 28 in = _61_ cm
4. 3 qt = _1.08_ L		10. 68 kg = _149.6_ lb
5. 4 mg = _4000_ mcg		11. 2,025 g = _4.46_ lb
6. 500 mL = _.5_ L		12. $3\frac{1}{2}$ fl oz = _105_ mL

13. 5 lb 4 oz = _____ kg   30. 90 mL = _____ fl oz

14. 16 cm = _____ in   31. 375 mcg = _____ mg

15. 4 T = _____ fl oz   32. 2 T = _____ mL

16. 65 in = _____ m   33. 2.2 lb = _____ kg

17. $70\frac{1}{2}$ lb = _____ kg   34. 5 mL = _____ t

18. 3,634 g = _____ lb   35. 1,000 mL = _____ L

19. 8 mL = _____ L   36. 1.5 g = _____ mg

20. 450 mg = _____ g   37. $1\frac{1}{2}$ fl oz = _____ mL

21. 237.5 cm = _____ in   38. 1,500 mL = _____ qt

22. 0.5 g = _____ mg   39. 2 kg = _____ lb

23. 0.6 mg = _____ mcg   40. 25 mg = _____ .025 g

24. 4,050 mL = _____ L   41. 4.3 kg = _____ 4300 g

25. 150 lb = _____ kg   42. 60 mg = _____ .06 g

26. 7.5 L = _____ qt   43. 0.015 g = _____ 15.0 mg

27. 22 lb = _____ kg   44. 45 mL = _____ 3 T

28. 2 cups = _____ mL   45. 0.25 mg = _____ 250 mcg

29. 6 t = _____ T

46. As a camp nurse for 9- to 12-year-old children, you are administering $2\frac{1}{2}$ teaspoons of oral liquid Children's Tylenol to 6 feverish campers every 4 hours for oral temperatures above 100°F. You have on hand a 4 fluid ounce bottle of liquid Children's Tylenol. How many complete, or full, doses are available from this bottle? _____ full doses

47. At this same camp, the standard dosage of Pepto-Bismol for 9- to 12-year-old children is 1 tablespoon. How many full doses are available in a 120 mL bottle? _____ full doses

48. Calculate the total fluid intake in mL of this clear liquid lunch:

    apple juice   4 fluid ounces   120

    chicken broth   8 fluid ounces   240

    gelatin dessert   6 fluid ounces   180

    hot tea   10 fluid ounces   300

    TOTAL =   _____ 840 mL   840

49. A newborn weighs 5,250 g. Her weight is approximately equivalent to _____ 11½ lb.

50. Describe the strategy to prevent this medication error.

Possible Scenario

2000 mg

An attending physician ordered **cefotaxime 2 g intravenously immediately** for a patient with a leg abscess. The supply dosage available is *1,000 mg per 10 mL*. The nurse was in a rush to give the medication and calculated the dose this way:

(20)

    If: 1 g = 1,000 mg

    then: 2 g = 1,000 ÷ 2 = 500 mg per 5 mL

Then the nurse administered 5 mL of the available cefotaxime.

Potential Outcome

The patient received only $\frac{1}{4}$, or 25%, of the dosage ordered. The patient should have received 2,000 mg, or 20 mL, of cefotaxime. The leg abscess could progress to osteomyelitis (a severe bone infection) or septicemia (a blood infection) because of underdosage.

Prevention

_____

_____

After completing these problems, see page 596 to check your answers.

For additional practice, visit the online practice software at www.CengageBrain.com, using the Premium Website access code found in the front of your text.

REFERENCES

The Joint Commission. (2010). Facts about the Official "Do Not Use" List. Retrieved April 28, 2011, from http://www.jointcommission.org/assets/1/18/Official_Do%20Not%20Use_List_%206_10.pdf

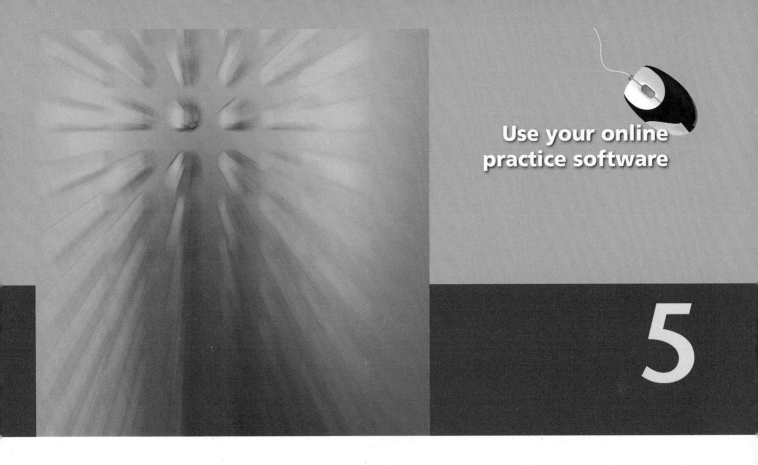

5

Conversions for Other Clinical Applications: Time and Temperature

OBJECTIVES

Upon mastery of Chapter 5, you will be able to:

- Convert between traditional and international time.
- Convert between Celsius and Fahrenheit temperature.

This chapter focuses on two other conversions applied in health care. *Time* is an essential part of the drug order. *Temperature* is an important measurement of health status.

CONVERTING BETWEEN TRADITIONAL AND INTERNATIONAL TIME

It is becoming increasingly popular in health care settings to keep time with a system more straightforward than traditional time, using the 24-hour clock. In use around the world and in the U.S. military for many years, this system is known as *international time* or *military time.*

Look at the 24-hour clock (Figure 5-1). Each time designation is comprised of a unique four-digit number. Notice that there are two circles of numbers (an inner and an outer circle) that identify the hours from 0100 to 2400. The inside numbers correlate to traditional AM time (midnight to 11:59 AM)—time periods that are ante meridian, or before noon. The outside numbers correlate to traditional PM time (noon to 11:59 PM)—time periods that are post meridian, or after noon.

113

FIGURE 5-1   24-hour clock depicting 0015 (12:15 AM)
and 1215 (12:15 PM)
© Cengage Learning 2013

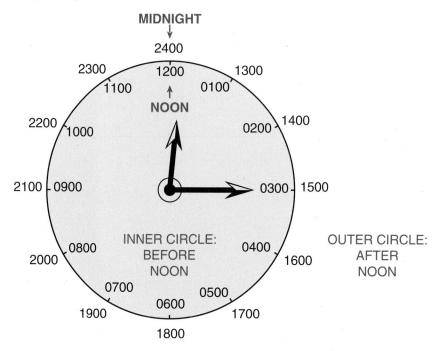

Hours on the 24-hour clock after 0059 minutes (zero-zero fifty-nine) are stated in hundreds, and the word **zero** precedes hours under ten hundred (single-digit hours in traditional time).

EXAMPLE 1 ▪

0400 is stated as *zero four hundred.*

EXAMPLE 2 ▪

1600 is stated as *sixteen hundred.*

Between each hour, the time is read simply as the hour and the number of minutes, preceded by *zero* as needed.

EXAMPLE 1 ▪

0421 is stated as *zero four twenty-one.*

EXAMPLE 2 ▪

1659 is stated as *sixteen fifty-nine.*

The minutes between 2400 (midnight) and 0100 (1:00 AM) are written as 0001, 0002, 0003 . . . 0058, 0059. Each zero is stated before the number of minutes.

EXAMPLE 1 ▪

0009 is stated as *zero-zero-zero nine.*

EXAMPLE 2 ▪

0014 is stated as *zero-zero fourteen.*

Midnight can be written two different ways in international time:

- 2400 and read as *twenty-four hundred,* or

- 0000 (used by the military) and read as *zero hundred.*

Use of the 24-hour clock decreases the possibility for error in administering medications and documenting time, because no two times are expressed by the same number. There is less chance for misinterpreting time using the 24-hour clock.

EXAMPLE 1 ▪

13 minutes after 1 AM is written *0113.*

EXAMPLE 2 ▪

13 minutes after 1 PM is written *1313.*

The same cannot be said for traditional time. The AM or PM notations are the only things that differentiate traditional times.

EXAMPLE 1 ■

13 minutes after 1 AM is written *1:13 AM*

EXAMPLE 2 ■

13 minutes after 1 PM is written *1:13 PM*

Careless notation in a medical order or in patient records can create misinterpretation about when a therapy is due or actually occurred. Figure 5-2 shows the comparison of traditional and international time. Notice that international time is less ambiguous.

FIGURE 5-2 Comparison of traditional and international time

AM	Int'l Time	PM	Int'l Time
12:00 midnight	2400	12:00 noon	1200
1:00	0100	1:00	1300
2:00	0200	2:00	1400
3:00	0300	3:00	1500
4:00	0400	4:00	1600
5:00	0500	5:00	1700
6:00	0600	6:00	1800
7:00	0700	7:00	1900
8:00	0800	8:00	2000
9:00	0900	9:00	2100
10:00	1000	10:00	2200
11:00	1100	11:00	2300

© Cengage Learning 2013

RULES

1. Traditional time and international time have similar numbering from 1:00 AM (0100) through 12:59 PM (1259).

2. Minutes after 12:00 AM (midnight) and before 1:00 AM are 0001 through 0059 in international time.

3. Hours from 1:00 PM through 12:00 AM (midnight) are 1200 hours greater in international time (1300 through 2400).

4. International time is designated by a unique four-digit number.

5. The hour(s) and minute(s) are separated by a colon in traditional time, but no colon is typically used in international time. However, you may see international time represented with a colon, such as 14:00 for 1400 (for 2:00 PM) and so forth.

MATH TIP

For the hours between 1:00 PM (1300) and 12:00 AM (2400), add 1200 to traditional time to find equivalent international time; subtract 1200 from international time to convert to equivalent traditional time.

Let's apply these rules to convert between the two time systems.

EXAMPLE 1 ■

3:00 PM = 300 + 1200 = 1500

EXAMPLE 2 ■

2212 = 2212 − 1200 = 10:12 PM

EXAMPLE 3 ■

12:45 AM = 0045

EXAMPLE 4 ■

0004 = 12:04 AM

EXAMPLE 5 ▪
0130 = 1:30 AM

EXAMPLE 6 ▪
11:00 AM = 1100

QUICK REVIEW

■ International time is designated by 0001 through 1259 for 12:01 AM through 12:59 PM and 1300 through 2400 for 1:00 PM through 12:00 midnight.

■ The hours from 1:00 PM through 12:00 midnight in traditional time are 1200 hours greater in international time (1300 through 2400).

Review Set 15

Convert international time to traditional AM/PM time.

1. 0032 =	_____	6. 1215 =		_____
2. 0730 =	_____	7. 0220 =		_____
3. 1640 =	_____	8. 1010 =		_____
4. 2121 =	_____	9. 1315 =		_____
5. 2359 =	_____	10. 1825 =		_____

Convert traditional to international time.

11. 1:30 PM =	_____	16. 3:45 AM =		_____
12. 12:04 AM =	_____	17. 12:00 midnight =		_____
13. 9:45 PM =	_____	18. 3:30 PM =		_____
14. 12:00 noon =	_____	19. 6:20 AM =		_____
15. 11:15 PM =	_____	20. 5:45 PM =		_____

Fill in the blanks by writing out in words the times indicated.

21. In 24-hour time, 0623 is stated _____.

22. In 24-hour time, 0041 is stated _____.

23. In 24-hour time, 1903 is stated _____.

24. In 24-hour time, 2311 is stated _____.

25. In 24-hour time, 0300 is stated _____.

After completing these problems, see page 597 to check your answers.

CONVERTING BETWEEN CELSIUS AND FAHRENHEIT TEMPERATURE

Another important conversion in health care involves Celsius and Fahrenheit temperatures. Simple formulas are used for converting between the two temperature scales. It is easier to remember the formulas when you understand how they are related. The Fahrenheit (F) scale establishes the freezing point of pure water at 32° and the boiling point of pure water at 212°. The Celsius (C) scale establishes the freezing point of pure water at 0° and the boiling point of pure water at 100°.

FIGURE 5-3 Comparison of Celsius and Fahrenheit temperature scales
© Cengage Learning 2013

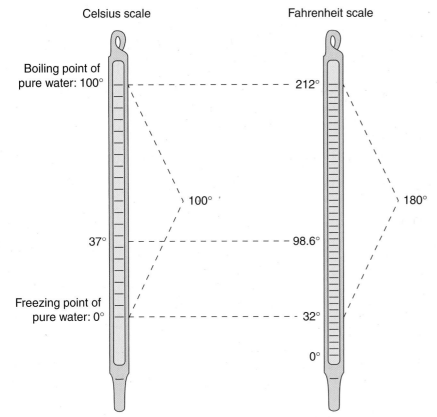

FIGURE 5-4 Comparison of Celsius and Fahrenheit body temperature scales. Bold type indicates normal body temperature.
© Cengage Learning 2013

°C	°F
40.6	105.1
40.4	104.7
40.2	104.4
40.0	104.0
39.8	103.6
39.6	103.3
39.4	102.9
39.2	102.6
39.0	102.2
38.8	101.8
38.6	101.5
38.4	101.1
38.2	100.8
38.0	100.4
37.8	100.0
37.6	99.7
37.4	99.3
37.2	99.0
37.0	**98.6**
36.0	96.8
35.0	95.0
34.0	93.2
33.0	91.4

Look at Figure 5-3. Note that there is 180° difference between the boiling and freezing points on the Fahrenheit thermometer and 100° between the boiling and freezing points on the Celsius thermometer. The ratio of the difference between the Fahrenheit and Celsius scales can be expressed as 180:100 or $\frac{180}{100}$. When reduced, this ratio is equivalent to 1.8. You will use this constant in temperature conversions.

The glass thermometers pictured in Figure 5-3 are for demonstration purposes. Electronic digital temperature devices are more commonly used in health care settings. Most electronic devices can instantly convert between the two scales, freeing the health care provider from doing the actual calculations. However, the health care provider's ability to understand the difference between Celsius and Fahrenheit remains important.

The range of body temperatures seen in health care situations is usually limited to those that are compatible with life, so it is practical to keep a chart handy that lists potential equivalent temperatures (Figure 5-4). You will find it helpful to memorize Celsius and Fahrenheit normal body temperature and some other commonly reported ones (as highlighted on the body temperature chart) for quick conversions.

To convert between Fahrenheit and Celsius temperature, formulas have been developed based on the differences between the freezing and boiling points on each scale.

RULE

To convert a given Fahrenheit temperature to Celsius, first subtract 32 and then divide the result by 1.8.

$$°C = \frac{°F - 32}{1.8}$$

EXAMPLE ■

Convert 98.6°F to °C

$$°C = \frac{98.6 - 32}{1.8}$$

$$°C = \frac{66.6}{1.8}$$

$$°C = 37°$$

RULE

To convert Celsius temperature to Fahrenheit, multiply by 1.8 and add 32.

$$°F = 1.8°C + 32$$

EXAMPLE ■

Convert 35°C to °F

$$°F = 1.8 \times 35 + 32$$

$$°F = 63 + 32$$

$$°F = 95°$$

QUICK REVIEW

Use these formulas to convert between Fahrenheit and Celsius temperatures:

■ $°C = \frac{°F - 32}{1.8}$

■ $°F = 1.8°C + 32$

Review Set 16

Convert these temperatures as indicated. Round your answers to tenths.

1. 100.4°F = _____ °C   3. 36.2°C = _____ °F

2. 38.4°C = _____ °F   4. 32°C = _____ °F

5. 98.6°F = _____ °C   11. 100°F = _____ °C

6. 99°F = _____ °C   12. 39°C = _____ °F

7. 103.6°F = _____ °C   13. 37.4°C = _____ °F

8. 40°C = _____ °F   14. 94.2°F = _____ °C

9. 38.9°C = _____ °F   15. 102.8°F = _____ °C

10. 36.4°C = _____ °F

For each of the following statements, convert the given temperature in °F or °C to its corresponding equivalent in °C or °F.

16. An infant has a body temperature of 95.5°F.   _____ °C

17. Store the vaccine serum at 7°C.   _____ °F

18. Do not expose medication to temperatures greater than 88°F.   _____ °C

19. Normal body temperature is 37°C.   _____ °F

20. If Mr. Rose's temperature is greater than 103.5°F, call MD.   _____ °C

After completing these problems, see page 597 to check your answers.

CLINICAL REASONING SKILLS

ERROR

Incorrect interpretation of an order because of a misunderstanding of traditional time.

Possible Scenario

A physician ordered a mild sedative for an anxious patient who is scheduled for a sigmoidoscopy in the morning. The order read *Valium 5 mg orally at 6:00 × 1 dose.* The evening nurse interpreted that single-dose order to be scheduled for 6 o'clock PM along with the enema and other preparations to be given to the patient. The doctor meant for the Valium to be given at 6 o'clock AM to help the patient relax prior to the test.

Potential Outcome

Valium would help the patient relax during the enema and make the patient sleepy. But it is not desirable for the patient to be drowsy or sedated during the evening preparations. Because of the omission of the AM designation, the patient would not benefit from this mild sedative at the intended time, just before the test. The patient would have likely experienced unnecessary anxiety both before and during the test.

Prevention

This scenario emphasizes the benefit of the 24-hour clock. If international time had been in use at this facility, the order would have been written as *Valium 5 mg orally at 0600 × 1 dose,* clearly indicating the exact time of administration. *Be careful to verify AM and PM times if your facility uses traditional time.*

PRACTICE PROBLEMS—CHAPTER 5

Give the following time equivalents as indicated.

AM/PM Clock	24-Hour Clock	AM/PM Clock	24-Hour Clock
1. _2:57 AM_	0257	11. 7:31 PM	_____
2. 3:10 AM	_0310_	12. 12:00 midnight	_____
3. 4:22 PM	_1622_	13. 6:45 AM	_____
4. _08:01 pm_	2001	14. _____	0915
5. _11:02 am_	1102	15. _____	2107
6. 12:33 AM	_0033_	16. _____	1823
7. 2:16 AM	_0216_	17. _____	0540
8. _4:42 p_	1642	18. 11:55 AM	_____
9. _11:56_	2356	19. 10:12 PM	_____
10. 4:20 AM	_____	20. 9:06 PM	_____

Find the length of each time interval in hours and minutes for questions 21 through 30.

21. 0200 to 0600	_4 hr_	26. 2316 to 0328	_____
22. 1100 to 1800	_7 hr_	27. 8:22 AM to 1:10 PM	_____
23. 1500 to 2330	_8 hr 30 mn_	28. 4:35 PM to 8:16 PM	_____
24. 0935 to 2150	_____	29. 1:00 AM to 7:30 AM	_____
25. 0003 to 1453	_____		

30. 10:05 AM Friday to 2:43 AM Saturday _16h 38m_   _12_

31. True or False? The 24-hour clock is imprecise and not suited to health care.   _F_ _____

32. Indicate whether these international times would be AM or PM when converted to traditional time.

    a. 1030 _____   c. 0158 _____

    b. 1920 _____   d. 1230 _____

_(F-32 ÷ 1.8_

_C × 1.8C+32_

Give the following temperature equivalents as indicated.

33. 99.6°F	_____ °C	41. 97.8°F	_____ °C
34. 36.5°C	_____ °F	42. 35.4°C	_____ °F
35. 39.2°C	_____ °F	43. 103.5°F	_____ °C
36. 100.2°F	_____ °C	44. 39°C	_____ °F
37. 98°F	_____ °C	45. 36.9°C	_____ °F
38. 37.4°C	_____ °F	46. 101.4°F	_____ °C
39. 38.2°C	_____ °F	47. 97.2°F	_____ °C
40. 104°F	_____ °C		

48. Four temperature readings in °C for Mrs. Baskin are 37.6, 35.5, 38.1, and 37.6. Find her average (or mean) °C temperature and convert it to °F. Average: _____ °C = _____ °F

49. True or False? The freezing and boiling points of pure water on the Fahrenheit and Celsius temperature scales were used to develop the conversion formulas. _____

50. Describe the clinical reasoning you would use to prevent this conversion error.

Possible Scenario

A student nurse takes a child's temperature and finds that it is 38.2°C. The child's mother asks what that equates to in Fahrenheit temperature. The student nurse does a quick calculation in her head and multiplies 38° by 2 and adds 32, because she recalls that the conversion constant is 1.8 and thinks 2 is close enough. The student nurse tells the mother, "Well, about 108°." The mother replies, "I hope not" and smiles.

Potential Outcome

The student nurse immediately recognizes that she has made an error and feels embarrassed. The mother could have become alarmed and experienced undue anxiety and a loss of confidence in the student nurse. The correct temperature measurement is 100.8°F. Fever-reducing medical orders often vary the dosage depending on the severity of the elevated temperature. An incorrect conversion could result in over- or undermedication of the child.

Prevention

_____

_____

After completing these problems, see page 597 to check your answers.

For additional practice, visit the online practice software at www.CengageBrain.com, using the Premium Website access code found in the front of your text.

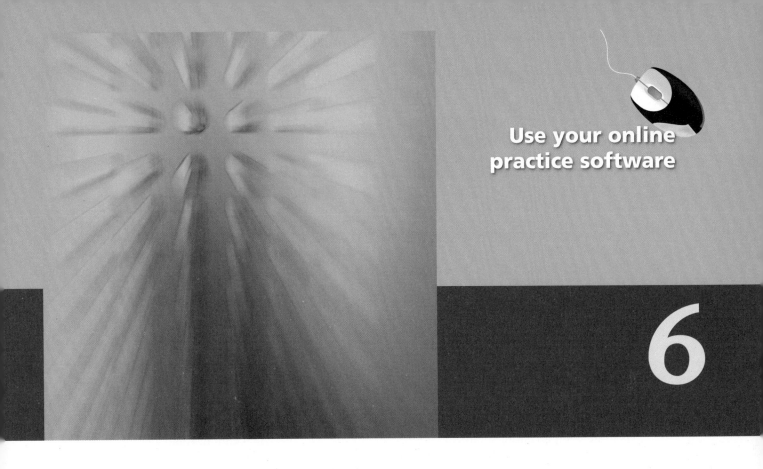

6

Equipment Used in Dosage Measurement

OBJECTIVES

Upon mastery of Chapter 6, you will be able to correctly measure the prescribed dosages that you calculate. To accomplish this, you will also be able to:

- Recognize and select the appropriate equipment for the medication, dosage, and method of administration ordered.
- Read and interpret the calibrations of each utensil presented.

Now that you are familiar with the systems of measurement used in the calculation of dosages, let's take a look at the common measuring utensils. In this chapter, you will learn to recognize and read the calibrations of devices used in both oral and parenteral (other than gastrointestinal) administration. The oral utensils include the medicine cup, pediatric oral devices, and calibrated droppers. The parenteral devices include the 3 mL syringe, the prefilled syringe, a variety of insulin syringes, the 1 mL syringe, and special safety and intravenous syringes.

ORAL ADMINISTRATION

Medicine Cup

Figure 6-1 shows three side views of the 30-milliliter 1-fluid-ounce medicine cup that is used to measure most liquids for oral administration. Three views are presented to show all of the scales. Notice that the approximate equivalents of the metric, apothecary, and household systems of measurement are indicated

FIGURE 6-1 Medicine cup (three views) with approximate equivalent measures

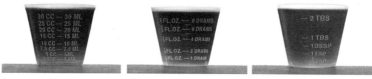

© Cengage Learning 2013

on the cup. The medicine cup can serve as a great study aid to help you learn the volume equivalents of the three systems of measurement. Look at the calibrations for milliliters, teaspoons, tablespoons, fluid ounces, and drams. As you fill the cup, you can see that 30 milliliters equal 1 fluid ounce, 5 milliliters equal 1 teaspoon, and so forth. Dram, a unit of measurement in the apothecary system, is no longer used but may still appear on medicine cups. Cubic centimeters (cc), formerly used interchangeably with milliliters (mL) in clinical situations, may still be noted on measuring devices. The correct unit to use is milliliter (mL). For volumes less than 2.5 mL, a smaller, more accurate device should be used (see Figures 6-2, 6-3, and 6-4).

Calibrated Dropper

Figure 6-2 shows the calibrated dropper, which is used to administer some small quantities. A dropper is used when giving medicine to children and the elderly and when adding small amounts of liquid to water or juice. Eye and ear medications are also dispensed from a medicine dropper or squeeze drop bottle.

The amount of the drop, abbreviated gtt, varies according to the diameter of the hole at the tip of the dropper. For this reason, a properly calibrated dropper usually accompanies the medicine (Figure 6-3). It is calibrated according to the way in which that drug is prescribed. The calibrations are usually given in milliliters or drops.

FIGURE 6-2 Calibrated dropper

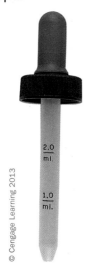

© Cengage Learning 2013

FIGURE 6-3 Furosemide Oral Solution label

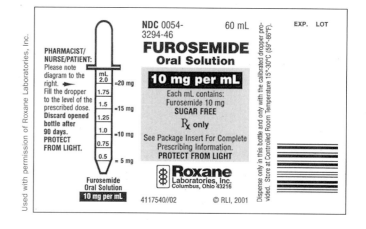

Used with permission of Roxane Laboratories, Inc.

CAUTION

To be safe, never exchange packaged droppers between medications, because drop size varies from one dropper to another.

Pediatric Oral Devices

Various types of calibrated equipment are available to administer oral medications to children. Two devices intended only for oral use are shown in Figure 6-4. Parents and child caregivers should be taught to always use calibrated devices when administering medications to children. Household spoons vary in size and are not reliable for accurate dosing.

FIGURE 6-4 Devices for administering oral medications

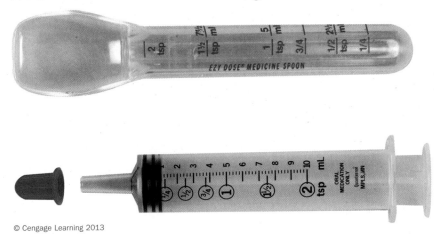

© Cengage Learning 2013

CAUTION
To be safe, do not use syringes intended for injections in the administration of oral medications. Confusion about the route of administration may occur.

You can distinguish oral from parenteral syringes in two ways. Syringes intended for oral use typically do not have a luerlock hub (see Figures 6-5 and 6-6). They also usually have a cap on the tip which must be removed before administering the medication. Syringes intended for parenteral use have a luerlock hub that allows a needle to be secured tightly.

PARENTERAL ADMINISTRATION

The term *parenteral* interpreted literally designates routes of administration other than gastrointestinal. However, in this text, as well as most clinical settings, parenteral means injection routes.

3 mL Syringe

Figure 6-5 shows a 3 mL syringe assembled with needle unit. The parts of the syringe are identified in Figure 6-6. Notice that the black rubber tip of the suction plunger is visible. The nurse pulls back on the plunger to withdraw the medicine from the storage container. *The calibrations are read from the top (needle end) black ring, NOT the raised middle section and NOT the bottom (plunger end) ring.* Look closely at the metric scale in Figure 6-5, which is calibrated in milliliters (mL) for each tenth (0.1) of a milliliter. Each 0.5 (or $\frac{1}{2}$) milliliter is marked up to the maximum volume of 3 milliliters.

Standardized to the syringe calibrations, standard drug dosages of 1 mL or greater can be rounded to the nearest tenth (0.1) of a mL and measured on the mL scale. Refer to Chapter 1 to review the rules of decimal rounding. For example, 1.45 mL is rounded to 1.5 mL. Notice that the volume of the colored liquid in Figure 6-5 is 1.5 mL, which is also illustrated in Figure 6-6.

FIGURE 6-5   3 mL syringe with needle unit measuring 1.5 mL

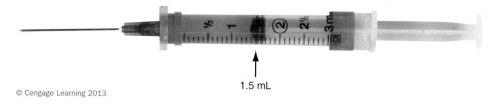

1.5 mL

© Cengage Learning 2013

FIGURE 6-6   Illustration of 3 mL syringe with needle unit measuring 1.5 mL

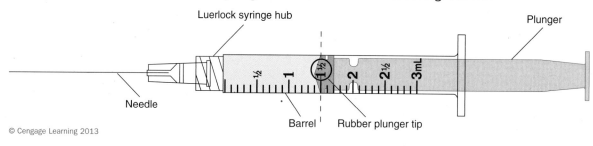

© Cengage Learning 2013

Prefilled Single-Dose Syringe

Figure 6-7 is an example of a *prefilled single-dose syringe.* Such syringes contain the usual single dose of a medication and are to be used only once. The syringe is discarded after the single use.

If you are to give *less* than the full single dose of a drug provided in a prefilled single-dose syringe, you should discard the extra amount *before* injecting the patient.

EXAMPLE ■

The drug order prescribes 100 mg of medroxyprogesterone acetate to be administered to a patient. You have a prefilled single-dose syringe containing 150 mg per mL of solution (as in Figure 6-7). You would discard 50 mg of the drug solution; then 100 mg would remain in the syringe. You will learn more about calculating drug dosages beginning in Chapter 10. (Some medications, such as controlled substances, require another nurse to observe the discarding of the unused portion.)

FIGURE 6-7   Prefilled single-dose syringe

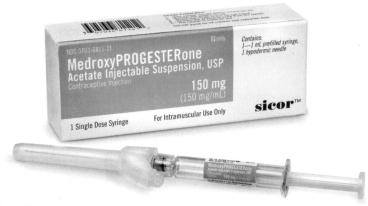

Used with permission from TEVA Pharmaceuticals USA.

Insulin Syringe

Figure 6-8(a) shows both sides of a standard U-100 insulin syringe. This syringe is to be used for the measurement and administration of U-100 insulin *only*. It must not be used to measure other medications that are measured in units.

CAUTION

U-100 insulin should only be measured in a U-100 insulin syringe. U-100 insulin concentration is 100 units of insulin per mL.

Notice that Figure 6-8(a) pictures one side of the insulin syringe calibrated in odd-number two-unit increments and the other side calibrated in even-number two-unit increments. The plunger in Figure 6-9(a) simulates the measurement of 70 units of U-100 insulin. It is important to note that for U-100 insulin, 100 units equal 1 mL.

Figure 6-8(b) shows two Lo-Dose U-100 insulin syringes. The enlarged scale is easier to read and is calibrated for each 1 unit up to 50 units per 0.5 mL, or 30 units per 0.3 mL. Every unit is marked, with the scale designating corresponding numbers by fives. The 30 unit syringe is commonly used for pediatric administration of insulin. The plunger in Figure 6-9(b) simulates the measurement of 19 units of U-100 insulin.

FIGURE 6-8   Insulin syringes with safety covers removed for easy viewing of calibrations: (a) Front and back of a standard U-100 insulin syringe; (b) Lo-Dose U-100 insulin syringes, 50 and 30 units

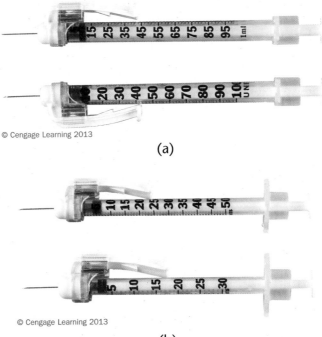

© Cengage Learning 2013

(a)

© Cengage Learning 2013

(b)

FIGURE 6-9   (a) Standard U-100 insulin syringe measuring 70 units of U-100 insulin; (b) Lo-Dose U-100 insulin syringe measuring 19 units of U-100 insulin; all with safety covers removed for easy viewing of calibrations

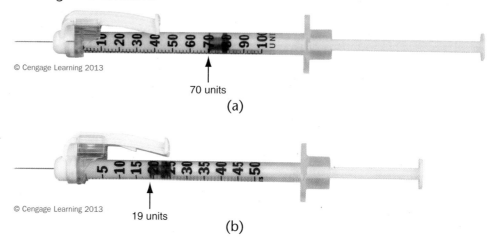

70 units

(a)

19 units

(b)

 CAUTION
Be careful to measure the insulin dose by reading the units at the top of the black rubber stopper at the end of the plunger, not the bottom. A common error is to incorrectly read the dose by looking at the bottom of the stopper. Look again at Figure 6-9 to see that the insulin syringes demonstrate doses of 70 and 19 units, respectively.
   All insulin doses should be double-checked by another nurse before administration to the patient.

1 mL Syringe

Figure 6-10 shows the 1 mL syringe. This syringe is also referred to as the *tuberculin*, or *TB, syringe*. It is used when a small dose of a drug must be measured, such as an allergen extract, vaccine, or child's medication. Notice that the 1 mL syringe is calibrated in hundredths (0.01) of a milliliter, with each one tenth (0.1) milliliter labeled on the metric scale. Pediatric and critical care doses of less than 1 mL can be rounded to hundredths and measured in the 1 mL syringe. It is preferable to measure all amounts less than 0.5 mL in a 1 mL syringe.

EXAMPLE ■

The amount 0.366 mL would be rounded to 0.37 mL and measured in the 1 mL syringe (Figure 6-10).

FIGURE 6-10   1 mL syringe

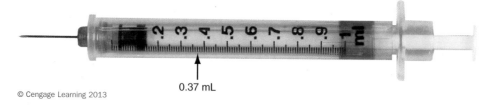

0.37 mL

Safety Syringe

Figures 6-10 and 6-11 show 3 mL, 1 mL, and insulin safety syringes. Notice that the needles may be protected by shields after administration of an injectable medication, to prevent accidental needlestick injury to the nurse.

FIGURE 6-11 Safety syringes: (a) 3 mL; (b) 1 mL; (c) Lo-Dose U-100 insulin; (d) Standard U-100 insulin

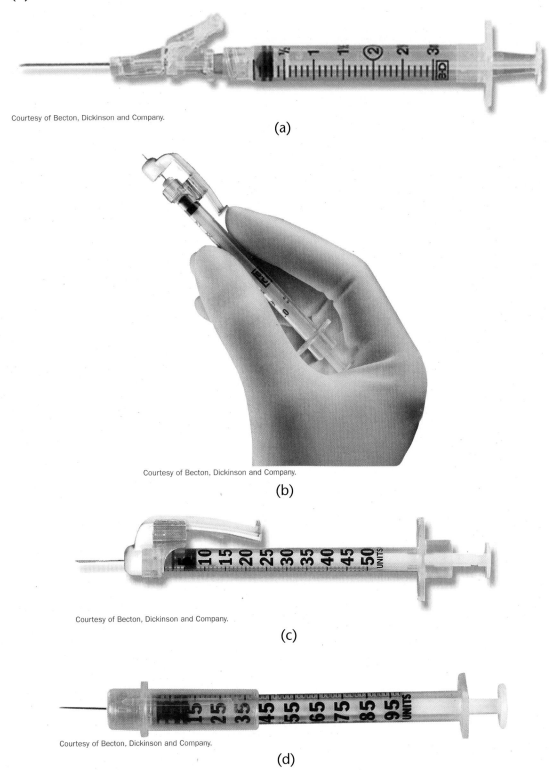

Courtesy of Becton, Dickinson and Company.

(a)

Courtesy of Becton, Dickinson and Company.

(b)

Courtesy of Becton, Dickinson and Company.

(c)

Courtesy of Becton, Dickinson and Company.

(d)

Intravenous Syringe

Figure 6-12 shows large syringes commonly used to prepare medications for intravenous administration. The volume and calibration of these syringes vary. To be safe, examine the calibrations of the syringes, and select the one best suited for the volume to be administered.

FIGURE 6-12   Intravenous syringes: (a) 5 mL; (b) 10 mL ; (c) 30 mL ; (d) 60 mL

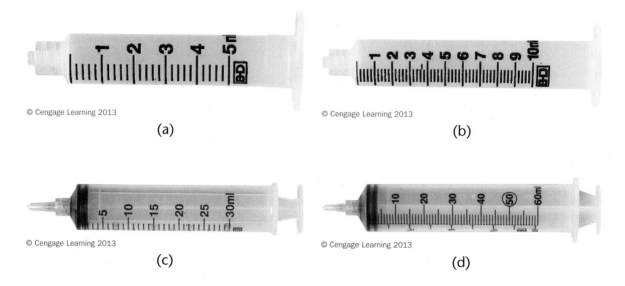

© Cengage Learning 2013

(a)

© Cengage Learning 2013

(b)

© Cengage Learning 2013

(c)

© Cengage Learning 2013

(d)

Needleless Syringe

Figure 6-13 pictures a needleless syringe system designed to prevent accidental needlesticks during intravenous administration.

FIGURE 6-13   Example of a needleless syringe system

Courtesy of Becton, Dickinson and Company.

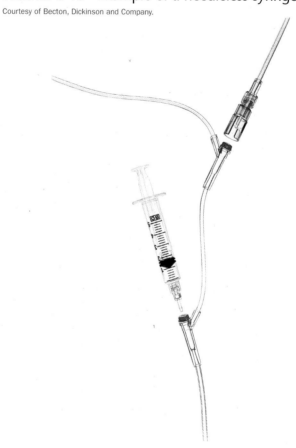

QUICK REVIEW

- The medicine cup has a 1 fluid ounce, or 30 milliliter, capacity for oral liquids. It is also calibrated to measure teaspoons, tablespoons, and drams. The apothecary measurement dram is no longer used. Amounts less than 2.5 milliliters should be measured in a smaller device, such as an oral syringe.

- The calibrated dropper measures small amounts of oral liquids. The size of the drop varies according to the diameter of the tip of the dropper. Drop is abbreviated as gtt.

- The standard 3 mL syringe is used to measure most injectable drugs. It is calibrated in tenths of a mL.

- The prefilled single-dose syringe cartridge is to be used once and then discarded.

- The Standard U-100 insulin syringe is only used to measure U-100 insulin. It is calibrated for a total of 100 units per 1 mL.

- The Lo-Dose U-100 insulin syringe is used for measuring small amounts of U-100 insulin. It is calibrated for a total of 50 units per 0.5 mL or 30 units per 0.3 mL. The smaller syringe is commonly used for administering small amounts of insulin.

- The 1 mL syringe is used to measure small or critical amounts of injectable drugs. It is calibrated in hundredths of a mL.

- Safety and needleless syringes prevent needlestick injuries.

- Syringes intended for injections should never be used to measure or administer oral medications.

Review Set 17

1. In which syringe should 0.25 mL of a drug solution be measured? _____

2. How can 1.25 mL be measured in the regular 3 mL syringe? _____

_____

3. Should insulin be measured in a 1 mL syringe? _____

4. Fifty (50) units of U-100 insulin equal how many milliliters? _____

5. a. True or False? The gtt is considered a consistent quantity for comparisons between different droppers. _____

   b. Why? _____

6. Can you measure 3 mL in a medicine cup? _____

7. How would you measure 3 mL of oral liquid to be administered to a child? _____

_____

8. The medicine cup indicates that each teaspoon is the equivalent of _____ mL.

9. Describe your action if you are to administer less than the full amount of a drug supplied in a prefilled single-dose syringe. _____

10. What is the primary purpose of the safety and needleless syringes? _____

_____

Draw an arrow to point to the calibration that corresponds to the dose to be administered.

11. Administer 0.75 mL.

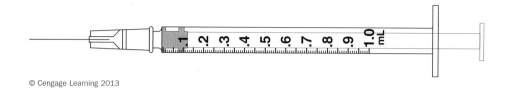

© Cengage Learning 2013

12. Administer 1.33 mL.

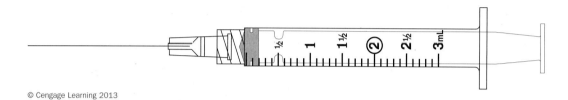

© Cengage Learning 2013

13. Administer 2.2 mL.

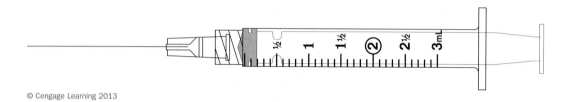

© Cengage Learning 2013

14. Administer 1.3 mL.

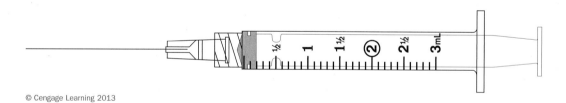

© Cengage Learning 2013

15. Administer 0.33 mL.

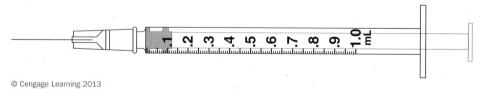

© Cengage Learning 2013

16. Administer 65 units of U-100 insulin.

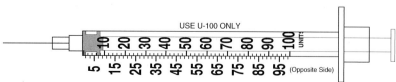

© Cengage Learning 2013

17. Administer 27 units of U-100 insulin.

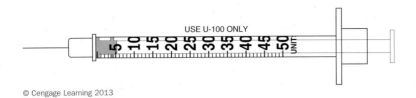

© Cengage Learning 2013

18. Administer 75 units of U-100 insulin.

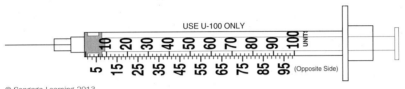

© Cengage Learning 2013

19. Administer 4.4 mL.

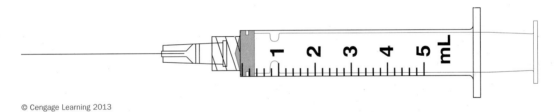

© Cengage Learning 2013

20. Administer 16 mL.

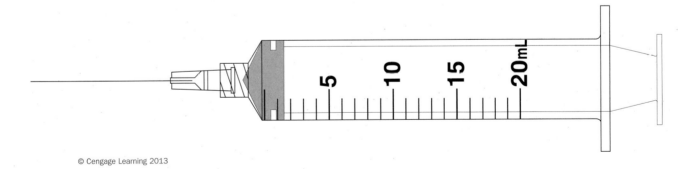

© Cengage Learning 2013

21. On the 5 mL syringe, each calibration is equal to _____. (Express the answer as a decimal.)

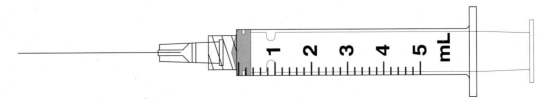

© Cengage Learning 2013

22. On the 20 mL syringe, each calibration is equal to _____.

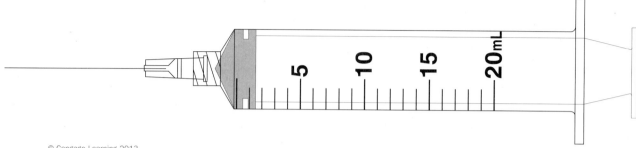

© Cengage Learning 2013

23. On the 10 mL syringe, each calibration is equal to _____. (Express the answer as a decimal.)

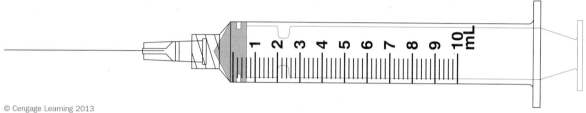

© Cengage Learning 2013

After completing these problems, see pages 597–599 to check your answers.

CLINICAL REASONING SKILLS

Select correct equipment to prepare medications. In the following situation, the correct dosage was not given, because an incorrect measuring device was used.

ERROR

Using an inaccurate measuring device for oral medications.

Possible Scenario

Suppose a pediatrician ordered Amoxil suspension (250 mg per 5 mL) 1 teaspoon every 8 hours to be given to a child. The child should receive the medication for 10 days for otitis media, an ear infection. The pharmacy dispensed the medication in a bottle containing 150 mL, or a 10-day supply. The nurse did not clarify for the mother how to measure and administer the medication. The child returned to the clinic in 10 days for routine follow-up. The nurse asked whether the child had taken all the prescribed Amoxil. The child's mother stated, "No, we have almost half of the bottle left." When the nurse asked how the medication had been given, the mother described small plastic disposable teaspoons she had obtained from the grocery store. The nurse measured the spoon's capacity and found it to be less than 3 mL (remember, 1 t = 5 mL). The child would have received only $\frac{3}{5}$, or 60%, of the correct dose.

Potential Outcome

The child did not receive a therapeutic dosage of the medication and was actually underdosed. The child could develop a resistant infection, which could lead to a more severe illness such as meningitis.

Prevention

Teach family members (and patients, as appropriate) to use calibrated measuring spoons or specially designed oral syringes to measure the correct dosage of medication. The volumes of serving spoons can vary considerably, as this situation illustrates.

CLINICAL REASONING SKILLS

Recognize variations in syringes used to measure insulin. In the following situation, the nurse administered the incorrect dose of insulin because the nurse did not understand the design of the insulin syringe and the relationship of the rubber stopper at the end of the plunger as the measuring device for the insulin dose.

ERROR

Incorrectly reading the dose of insulin in an insulin syringe.

Possible Scenario

The physician ordered **25 units of U-100 Regular Humulin insulin** for a patient with diabetes. In a hurry, the nurse prepared and administered the incorrect insulin dose as shown.

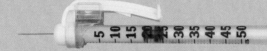

INCORRECT DOSE

© Cengage Learning 2013

Potential Outcome

The patient received only 19 units of insulin, which is a significant underdosage of almost 25 percent less than the prescribed dosage. The patient would likely develop symptoms of hyperglycemia. If the nurse continued to incorrectly measure each insulin dose, the patient could progress into a diabetic coma.

Prevention

The nurse needs to review the proper measurement of injectable medications in syringes. Inaccurate measurement of insulin is a common and extremely serious medication error with dire consequences. The insulin syringe above showing the incorrect dose measures 19 units of insulin. The top of the rubber stopper is the correct part of the syringe for determining the amount of insulin and the proper dose. Notice the difference between the correct and incorrect dose as shown. Further, each insulin dose should be double-checked by another nurse before administration.

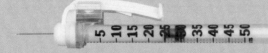

CORRECT DOSE

© Cengage Learning 2013

CLINICAL REASONING SKILLS

Precisely measure doses in 1 mL and 3 mL syringes. In the following situation, an incorrect dose was administered because the computed volume was not rounded properly.

ERROR

Rounding more decimal places than are necessary and selecting the wrong-size syringe.

Possible Scenario

A newborn infant was ordered to receive **gentamicin sulfate 7.5 mg intravenously every 24 hours.** Using the 2 mL vial supplied with 10 mg/mL of gentamicin, the nurse calculated the volume needed as 0.75 mL. This volume may be administered precisely using a 1 mL syringe. No rounding is needed. In this case, the nurse rounded 0.75 to the whole number 1 and administered 1 mL of medication using a 3 mL syringe. The infant was given 0.25 mL, or 2.5 mg, additional medication. If the nurse continued to care for this infant on subsequent days, the error might continue, with serious overdosage implications.

Potential Outcome

Gentamicin sulfate, an aminoglycoside, is a high-alert drug with serious potential adverse effects. One adverse effect associated with high doses is ototoxicity, leading to irreversible hearing loss. Blood levels are monitored during therapy to ensure that safe doses are ordered. By administering this higher dose, the nurse may have placed this infant at an increased risk for ototoxicity.

Prevention

It is important to know the correct size of syringe to use and the number of decimal places to round for computed dose volumes. Syringes with a total volume of 1 mL are calibrated in hundredths (2 decimal places), and 3 mL syringes are calibrated in tenths (1 decimal place). Volumes of less than 1 mL should be measured as precisely as possible in a 1 mL syringe, especially when administering high-alert medications.

PRACTICE PROBLEMS—CHAPTER 6

1. In the U-100 insulin syringe, 100 units = _____ mL.

2. The 1 mL syringe is calibrated in _____ of a mL.

3. Can you measure 1.25 mL in a single tuberculin syringe? _____ Explain. _____
   _____
   _____

4. How would you measure 1.33 mL in a 3 mL syringe? _____

5. The medicine cup has a _____ mL, or _____ fl oz, capacity.

6. To administer exactly 0.52 mL to a child, select a _____ syringe.

7. Seventy-five (75) units of U-100 insulin equals _____ mL.

8. True or False? All droppers are calibrated to deliver standardized drops of equal amounts regardless of the dropper used. _____

9. True or False? The prefilled syringe is a multiple-dose system. _____

10. True or False? Insulin should only be measured in an insulin syringe. _____

11. The purpose of needleless syringes is _____

12. Medications are measured in syringes by aligning the calibrations with the _____ of the black rubber tip of the plunger (top ring, raised middle, or bottom ring).

13. The medicine cup calibrations indicate that 2 teaspoons are approximately _____ milliliters.

14. True or False? Safety syringes are designed to protect the patient. _____

15. The _____ syringe(s) is (are) intended to measure parenteral doses of medications. (3 mL, 1 mL, or insulin)

Draw an arrow to indicate the calibration that corresponds to the dose to be administered.

16. Administer 0.45 mL.

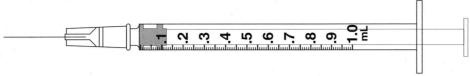

© Cengage Learning 2013

17. Administer 80 units of U-100 insulin.

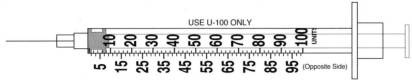

© Cengage Learning 2013

18. Administer $\frac{1}{2}$ fluid ounce.

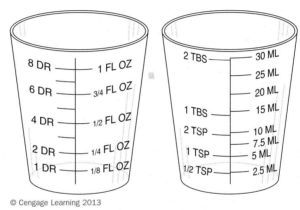

© Cengage Learning 2013

19. Administer 2.4 mL.

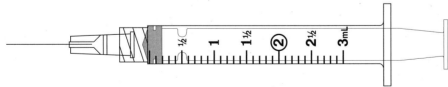

© Cengage Learning 2013

20. Administer 1.1 mL.

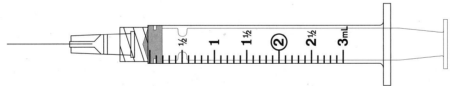

© Cengage Learning 2013

21. Administer 6.2 mL.

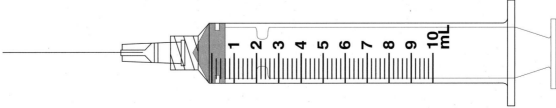

© Cengage Learning 2013

22. Administer 3.6 mL.

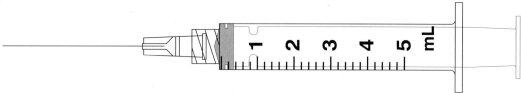

© Cengage Learning 2013

23. Administer 4.8 mL.

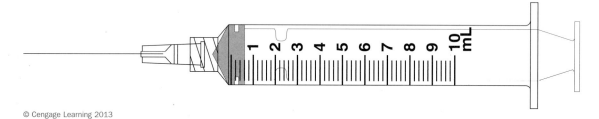

© Cengage Learning 2013

24. Administer 12 mL.

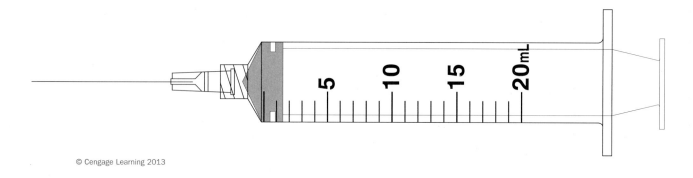

© Cengage Learning 2013

25. Describe the clinical reasoning you would use to prevent this medication error.

Possible Scenario

Suppose a patient with cancer has oral Compazine (prochlorperazine) liquid ordered for nausea. Because the patient has had difficulty taking the medication, the nurse decided to draw up the Compazine in a syringe without a needle to facilitate giving the medication. The nurse found this to be quite helpful and prepared several doses in syringes without the needles. A nurse from another unit covered for the nurse during lunch, and when the patient complained of nausea, the nurse assumed that the Compazine prepared in an injection syringe was to be given via injection. The nurse attached a needle and injected the oral medication.

Potential Outcome

The oral preparation may not be sterile and, if absorbed systemically, could lead to a bloodstream infection. Also, oral preparations have different preparative agents that likely should not be injected (such as glucose, which is traumatic to veins).

Prevention

_____

_____

26. Describe the strategy that would prevent this medication administration error.

   Possible Scenario

   A child with ear infections is to receive cefaclor oral liquid as an anti-infective. The medication is received in oral syringes for administration. The nurse fails to remove the cap on the tip of the syringe and attempts to administer the medication.

   Potential Outcome

   The nurse would exert enough pressure on the syringe plunger that the protective cap could pop off in the child's mouth and possibly cause the child to choke.

   Prevention

   _____

   _____

After completing these problems, see pages 599–601 to check your answers.

   For additional practice, visit the online practice software at www.CengageBrain.com, using the Premium Website access code found in the front of your text.

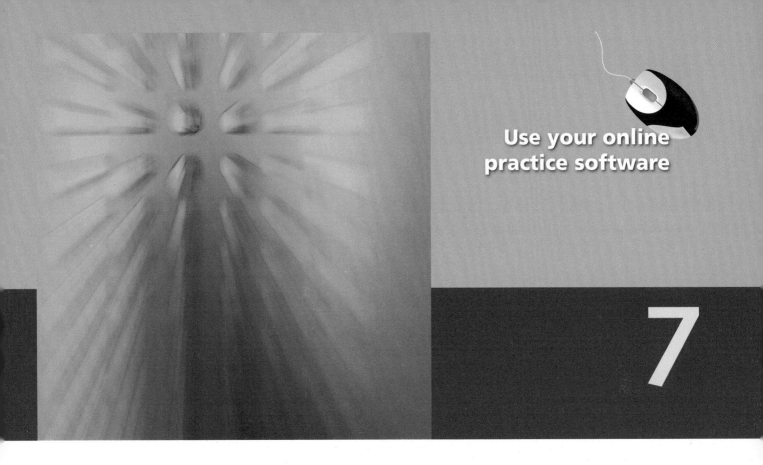

Interpreting Drug Orders

OBJECTIVES

Upon mastery of Chapter 7, you will be able to interpret drug orders. To accomplish this, you will also be able to:

- Read and write correct medical notation.
- Write the standard medical abbreviation from a list of common terminology.
- Interpret medicine orders of physicians and other prescribing practitioners.
- Interpret medication administration records.

The prescription, or medication order, conveys the therapeutic drug plan for the patient. It is the responsibility of the nurse to:

- Interpret the order.
- Gather information about the drug.
- Select and prepare the exact dosage of the prescribed drug.
- Identify the patient.
- Administer the proper dosage by the prescribed route, at the prescribed time intervals.
- Educate the patient regarding the medication.
- Record the administration of the prescribed drug.
- Monitor the patient's response for desired (therapeutic) and adverse effects.

Before you can prepare the correct dosage of the prescribed drug, you must learn to interpret, or read, the written drug order. For brevity and speed, the health care professions have adopted certain standards and common abbreviations for use in notation. You should learn to recognize and interpret the abbreviations from memory. As you practice reading drug orders, you will find that this skill becomes second nature to you.

An example of a typical written drug order is:

9/4/XX 0730 Amoxil 500 mg p.o. q.i.d. p.c. et bedtime
J. Physician, M.D.

This order means that the patient should receive 500 milligrams of an antibiotic named Amoxil (or amoxicillin) orally 4 times a day after meals and at bedtime. You can see that the medical notation shortens the written-out order considerably.

▬▬▬ MEDICAL ABBREVIATIONS

The following table lists common medical abbreviations used in writing drug orders. The abbreviations are grouped according to the route (or method) of administration, the frequency (time interval), and other general terms. Commit these to memory, along with the other abbreviations related to systems of measurement presented in Chapter 3.

REMEMBER

Common Medical Abbreviations

Abbreviation	Interpretation	Abbreviation	Interpretation
Route:		**Frequency:**	
IM	intramuscular	h	hour
IV	intravenous	q.h	every hour
IV PB	intravenous piggyback	q.2h	every 2 hours
subcut	subcutaneous	q.3h	every 3 hours
SL	sublingual, under the tongue	q.4h	every 4 hours
ID	intradermal	q.6h	every 6 hours
GT	gastrostomy tube	q.8h	every 8 hours
NG	nasogastric tube	q.12h	every 12 hours
NJ	nasojejunal tube	**General:**	
p.o.	by mouth, orally	$\bar{a}$	before
p.r.	per rectum, rectally	$\bar{p}$	after
Frequency:		$\bar{c}$	with
a.c.	before meals	$\bar{s}$	without
p.c.	after meals	q	every
ad. lib.	as desired, freely	qs	quantity sufficient
p.r.n.	when necessary	aq	water
stat	immediately, at once	NPO	nothing by mouth
asap	as soon as possible	gtt	drop
b.i.d.	twice a day	tab	tablet
t.i.d.	3 times a day	cap	capsule
q.i.d.	4 times a day	et	and
min	minute	noct	night

THE DRUG ORDER

The drug order consists of seven parts:

1. Name of the *patient*.

2. Name of the *drug* to be administered.

3. *Dosage* of the drug.

4. *Route* by which the drug is to be administered.

5. *Frequency*, time, and special instructions related to administration.

6. *Date and time* when the order was written.

7. *Signature and licensure* of the person writing the order.

CAUTION

If any of the seven parts is missing or unclear, the order is considered incomplete and is therefore not a legal drug order.

Parts one through five of the drug order are known as the original Five Rights of safe medication administration. They are essential, and each one must be faithfully checked every time a medication is prepared and administered. After safe administration of the medication, the nurse or health care practitioner must accurately document the drug administration. Combining accurate documentation with the original Five Rights, the patient is entitled to *Six Rights* of safe and accurate medication administration and documentation with each and every dose.

REMEMBER

The Six Rights of safe and accurate medication administration are as follows:

The *right patient* must receive the *right drug* in the *right amount* by the *right route* at the *right time*, followed by the *right documentation*.

Each drug order should follow a specific sequence. The name of the drug is written first, followed by the dosage, route, and frequency. When correctly written, the brand (or trade) name of the drug begins with a capital, or uppercase, letter. The generic name begins with a lowercase letter.

EXAMPLE ■

Procanbid 500 mg p.o. b.i.d.

1. **Procanbid** is the brand name of the drug.

2. **500 mg** is the dosage.

3. **p.o.** is the route.

4. **b.i.d.** is the frequency.

This order means: *Give 500 milligrams of Procanbid orally twice a day.*

CAUTION

If the nurse has difficulty understanding and interpreting the drug order, the nurse must clarify the order with the writer. Usually this person is the physician or another authorized practitioner, such as an advanced registered nurse practitioner.

Let's practice reading and interpreting drug orders.

EXAMPLE 1 ■

phenytoin 100 mg p.o. t.i.d.

This order means: *Give 100 milligrams of phenytoin orally 3 times a day.*

EXAMPLE 2 ■

procaine penicillin G 400,000 units IV q.6h

This order means: *Give 400,000 units of procaine penicillin G intravenously every 6 hours.*

EXAMPLE 3 ■

hydromorphone 2 mg IM q.4h p.r.n., moderate to severe pain

This order means: *Give 2 milligrams of hydromorphone intramuscularly every 4 hours when necessary for moderate to severe pain.*

CAUTION

The p.r.n. frequency designates the minimum time allowed between doses. There is no maximum time other than automatic stops as defined by hospital or agency policy.

EXAMPLE 4 ■

Humulin R regular U-100 insulin 5 units subcut stat

This order means: *Give 5 units of Humulin R regular U-100 insulin subcutaneously immediately.*

EXAMPLE 5 ■

cefazolin 1 g IV PB q.6h

This order means: *Give 1 gram of cefazolin by intravenous piggyback every 6 hours.*

The administration times are designated by hospital policy. For example, t.i.d. administration times may be 0900 or 9 AM, 1300 or 1 PM, and 1700 or 5 PM. This is different than q.8h administration times, which may be 0600, 1400, and 2200. Administration times for b.i.d., t.i.d., and q.i.d. are typically during waking hours.

QUICK REVIEW

- The *right patient* must receive the *right drug* in the *right amount* by the *right route* at the *right time* followed by the *right documentation*.
- Understanding drug orders requires interpreting common medical abbreviations.
- The drug order must contain (in this sequence): drug name, dosage, route, and frequency.
- All parts of the drug order must be stated clearly for accurate, exact interpretation.
- If you are ever in doubt as to the meaning of any part of a drug order, ask the writer to clarify before proceeding.

Review Set 18

Interpret the following medication (drug) orders:

1. naproxen 250 mg p.o. b.i.d. _____

_____

2. Humulin N NPH insulin 30 units subcut daily 30 min ā breakfast _____

_____

3. cefaclor 500 mg p.o. stat, then 250 mg q.8h _____

_____

4. Synthroid 25 mcg p.o. daily _____

_____

5. Ativan 10 mg IM q.4h p.r.n., agitation _____

_____

6. furosemide 20 mg slow IV stat _____

_____

7. Mylanta 10 mL p.o. p.c. et bedtime _____

_____

8. atropine sulfate ophthalmic 1% 2 gtt right eye q.15 min × 4 _____

_____

9. morphine sulfate 15 mg IM q.3h p.r.n., pain _____

_____

10. digoxin 0.25 mg p.o. daily _____

_____

11. tetracycline 250 mg p.o. q.i.d. _____

_____

12. nitroglycerin 150 mcg SL stat _____

_____

13. Cortisporin otic suspension 2 gtt each ear t.i.d. et bedtime _____

_____

14. Compare and contrast *t.i.d.* and *q.8h* administration times. Include sample administration times for each in your explanation. _____

_____

15. Describe your action if no method of administration is written. _____

_____

16. Do q.i.d. and q.4h have the same meaning? _____ Explain. _____

_____

17. Who determines the medication administration times? _____

_____

18. Name the seven parts of a written medication prescription. _____

_____

19. Which parts of the written medication prescription/order are included in the original Five Rights of medication administration? _____

_____

20. State the Six Rights of safe and accurate medication administration. _____

_____

After completing these problems, see page 601 to check your answers.

MEDICATION ORDER AND ADMINISTRATION FORMS

Hospitals have a special form for recording drug orders. As hospitals transition to electronic medical records, handwritten forms will be replaced by electronic order entry. Figure 7-1 shows a sample written physician's order form. Find and name each of the seven parts of the drug orders listed. Notice that the nurse or other health care professional must verify and initial each order, ensuring that each of the seven parts is accurate. In some facilities, the pharmacist may be responsible for verifying the order as part of the computerized record.

FIGURE 7-1 Paper-based physician's order form

① Patient
② Drug
③ Dosage
④ Route
⑤ Frequency and special instructions
⑥ Date and time
⑦ Signature

		ENTERED	FILLED	CHECKED	VERIFIED

NOTE: A NON-PROPRIETARY DRUG OF EQUAL QUALITY MAY BE DISPENSED - IF THIS COLUMN IS NOT CHECKED!

DATE	TIME WRITTEN	PLEASE USE BALL POINT - PRESS FIRMLY	✓	TIME NOTED	NURSES SIGNATURE
⑥ 11/3/xx	0815	② cephalexin ③ 250 mg ④ p.o. ⑤ q.6h	✓	0830	G. Pickar, R.N.
		Humulin N NPH Insulin 40 units subcut ā breakfast	✓		
		hydromorphone 2 mg IV q. 3h p.r.n., severe pain	✓		
		codeine 30 mg p.o. q.4h p.r.n., mild–mod pain ⑤	✓		
		Tylenol 650 mg p.o. q.4h p.r.n., fever greater than 101° F	✓		
		furosemide 40 mg p.o. daily	✓		
		K-Dur 10 mEq p.o. b.i.d.	✓		
		⑦ J. Physician, M.D.			
11/3/xx	2200	furosemide 80 mg IV stat	✓		
		J. Physician, M.D.		2210	M. Smith, R.N.

AUTO STOP ORDERS: UNLESS REORDERED, FOLLOWING WILL BE D/C^D AT 0800 ON:

DATE	ORDER		PHYSICIAN SIGNATURE
		☐ CONT ☐ D/C	
		☐ CONT ☐ D/C	
		☐ CONT ☐ D/C	

CHECK WHEN ANTIBIOTICS ORDERED   ☐ Prophylactic   ☐ Empiric   ☐ Therapeutic

Allergies:
None Known

PATIENT DIAGNOSIS
Diabetes

HEIGHT 5' 5"   WEIGHT 130 lb

FORM 959-708 (8-XX)   **PHYSICIANS ORDER**   Reynolds • Reynolds   LITHO IN U.S.A. K41814 (7 X X) D339380

① *Patient, Mary Q.*
#3-11316-7

①

If traditional handwritten records are still in use, the drug orders from the physician's order form are transcribed to a medication administration record (MAR) and the administration times are scheduled (Figure 7-2). The nurse or other health care professional uses this record as a guide to:

- Check the drug order.
- Prepare the correct dosage.
- Record the drug administered and time.

These three checkpoints help to ensure accurate medication administration.

FIGURE 7-2 Paper-based medication administration record

MEDICATION ADMINISTRATION RECORD — PAGE 1 of 1

ORIGINAL ORDER DATE	DATE STARTED/RENEWED	MEDICATION - DOSAGE	ROUTE	SCHEDULE 11-7	7-3	3-11	DATE 11/3/xx 11-7	7-3	3-11	DATE 11/4/xx 11-7	7-3	3-11	DATE 11/5/xx 11-7	7-3	3-11	DATE 11/6/xx 11-7	7-3	3-11
11/3/xx	11/3/xx	cephalexin 250 mg q. 6 h	PO	12 6	12	6		GP 12	MS 6	12JJ 6JJ	GP 12	MS 6						
11/4/xx	11/4/xx	Humulin N NPH U-100 insulin 40 units ā breakfast	subcut		7³⁰						GP 7³⁰ Ⓑ							
11/3/xx	11/3/xx	furosemide 40 mg daily	PO		9			GP 9			GP 9							
11/3/xx	11/3/xx	K-Dur 10 mEq b.i.d.	PO		9	9			MS 9		GP 9	MS 9						

PRN

11/3/xx	11/3/xx	hydromorphone 2 mg q.3h	IV	severe pain			GP 12 Ⓛ	MS 6 Ⓜ	JJ 11 Ⓙ									
11/3/xx	11/4/xx	codeine 30 mg q. 4 h	PO	mild-mod pain						JJ 6	GP 2							
11/3/xx	11/3/xx	Tylenol 650 mg q.4h	PO	fever greater than 101°F			GP 12	MS 4-8	MS JJ 12-4	JJ GP 8-12	GP							

INJECTION SITES

B - RIGHT ARM   C - RIGHT ABDOMEN   D - RIGHT ANTERIOR THIGH   G - LEFT ARM   H - LEFT ABDOMEN   J - LEFT ANTERIOR THIGH   L - LEFT BUTTOCKS   M - RIGHT BUTTOCKS

DATE GIVEN	TIME	INT.	ONE - TIME MEDICATION - DOSAGE	R.T.	SCHEDULE 11-7	7-3	3-11	DATE			DATE			DATE			DATE		
11/3/xx	2200	ms	furosemide 80 mg stat	IV															

SIGNATURE OF NURSE ADMINISTERING MEDICATIONS

11-7: JJ J. Jones, LPN
7-3: GP G. Pickar, RN   GP G. Pickar, RN
3-11: MS M. Smith, RN   MS M. Smith, RN

| DATE GIVEN | TIME | INT. | MEDICATION-DOSAGE-CONT. | RT. |

RECOPIED BY:
CHECKED BY:

Patient, Mary Q.
#3-11316-7

ALLERGIES: None Known

① ORIGINAL COPY

© Cengage Learning 2013

COMPUTERIZED MEDICATION ADMINISTRATION SYSTEMS

Many health care facilities now use or will soon use computers for processing drug orders. The Health Information Technology for Economic and Clinical Health Act (HITECH) of 2009 calls for electronic medical records for all patients by 2014. To earn stimulus incentives, physicians and hospitals must demonstrate meaningful use of a certified electronic health record (EHR) solution. Drug orders are either electronically transmitted or manually entered into the computer from an order form, such as Figure 7-3.

FIGURE 7-3 Paper-based physician's order form

		ENTERED	FILLED	CHECKED	VERIFIED

NOTE: A NON-PROPRIETARY DRUG OF EQUAL QUALITY MAY BE DISPENSED - IF THIS COLUMN IS NOT CHECKED!

DATE	TIME WRITTEN	PLEASE USE BALL POINT - PRESS FIRMLY	✓	TIME NOTED	NURSES SIGNATURE
8/31/XX	1500	Procanbid 500 mg p.o. b.i.d.	✓		
		J. Physician, M.D.		1515	M. Smith, R.N.
9/3/XX	0715	digoxin 0.125 mg p.o. every other day	✓		
		Lasix 40 mg p.o. daily	✓		
		Reglan 10 mg p.o. stat a.c. et bedtime	✓		
		Micro-K 16 mEq p.o. b.i.d.—start 9/4/xx	✓	0730	G. Pickar, R.N.
		nitroglycerin gr 0.4 mg SL p.r.n., mild to moderate chest pain	✓		
		Darvocet-N 100 tab. 1 p.o. q.4h p.r.n., mild to moderate pain	✓		
		ketorolac 30 mg IM q.6h p.r.n., severe pain	✓		
		J. Physician, M.D.			

AUTO STOP ORDERS: UNLESS REORDERED, FOLLOWING WILL BE D/C'D AT 0800 ON:

DATE	ORDER		
		☐ CONT	PHYSICIAN SIGNATURE
		☐ D/C	
		☐ CONT	PHYSICIAN SIGNATURE
		☐ D/C	
		☐ CONT	PHYSICIAN SIGNATURE
		☐ D/C	

CHECK WHEN ANTIBIOTICS ORDERED ☐ Prophylactic ☐ Empiric ☐ Therapeutic

Allergies:
No known allergies

Patient, John D.
#3-81512-3

PATIENT DIAGNOSIS
congestive heart failure

HEIGHT 5' 10"   WEIGHT 165 lb

FORM 959-708 (8-XX) **PHYSICIANS ORDER** Reynolds + Reynolds LITHO IN U.S.A. K41814 (7-xx) D326060

①

Through the computer, the nurse or other health care professional can transmit the order within seconds to the pharmacy for filling. The computer can keep track of drug stock and usage patterns and even notify the business office to post charges to the patient's account. Most importantly, it can scan for information previously entered, such as drug incompatibilities, drug allergies, safe dosage ranges, doses already given, or recommended administration times. The health care staff can be readily alerted to potential problems or inconsistencies. The corresponding medication administration record may also be printed directly from the computer as in Figure 7-4. Such computerized records reduce the risk of misinterpreting handwriting.

FIGURE 7-4 Printed computerized medication administration record

PHARMACY MAR

START	STOP	MEDICATION	SCHEDULED TIMES	OK'D BY	0001 HRS. TO 1200 HRS.	1201 HRS. TO 2400 HRS.
08/31/xx 1800 SCH		PROCAINAMIDE LONG ACTING (PROCANBID) 500 MG TAB-SR [500 MG] b.i.d. [PO]	0900 2100	JD	0900 GP	2100 MS
09/03/xx 0900 SCH		DIGOXIN (LANOXIN) 0.125 MG TAB [1 TAB] EVERY [PO] OTHER DAY ODD DAYS-SEPT	0900	JD	0900 GP	
09/03/xx 0900 SCH		FUROSEMIDE (LASIX) 40 MG TAB [1 TAB] DAILY [PO]	0900	JD	0900 GP	
09/03/xx 0730 SCH		METOCLOPRAMIDE (REGLAN) 10 MG TAB [10 MG] AC AND HS [PO] GIVE ONE NOW!!	0730 1130 1630 2100	JD	0730 GP 1130 GP	1630 MS 2100 MS
09/04/xx 0900 SCH		POTASSIUM CHLORIDE EXTENDED RELEASE (MICRO-K) 16 MEQ CAP [16 mEq] BID [PO] START 09/04/XX	0900 2100	JD	0900 GP	2100 MS
09/03/xx 1507 PRN		NITROGLYCERIN 0.4 mg 0.4 MG TAB-SL [1 TABLET] PRN* [SL] PRN CHEST PAIN		JD		
09/03/xx 1700 PRN		PROPOXYPHENE NAPSYLATE/ACETAMINOPHEN (DARVOCET-N 100*) CAP [1 TAB] Q4H [PO] PRN MILD–MODERATE PAIN		JD		
09/03/xx 2100 PRN		KETOROLAC (TORADOL) INJ [30 MG] Q6H [IM] PRN SEVERE PAIN		JD		2200 Ⓗ MS
		[ ] [ ]				

Gluteus A. Right B. Left **Ventro Gluteal** C. Right J. Right D. Left K. Left E. Abdomen 1｜2 3｜4 730-13 (12/xx)	**Thigh** H. Right I. Left	NURSE'S SIGNATURE INITIAL 7–3 G. Pickar, R.N. GP 3–11 M. Smith, R.N. MS 11–7 J. Doe, R.N. JD	ALLERGIES: **NKA** DIAGNOSIS: **CHF** FROM: 09/05/xx 0701	Patient: Patient, John D. Patient #: 3-81512-3 Admitted: 08/31/xx Physician: J. Physician, MD Room: PCU-14 PCU TO: 09/06/xx 0700

The computerized MAR may be viewed from a printed copy or at the computer. The nurse may be able to look back at the patient's cumulative medication administration record, document administration times and comments at the computer terminal, and then keep a printed copy of the information obtained and entered. The data analysis, storage, and retrieval abilities of computers are making them essential tools for safe and accurate medication administration.

QUICK REVIEW

■ Drug orders are prescribed on the physician's order form.

■ The person who administers a drug records it on the medication administration record (MAR). This record may be handwritten or computerized.

■ All parts of the drug order must be stated clearly for accurate, exact interpretation. If you are ever in doubt as to the meaning of any part of a drug order, ask the writer to clarify.

Review Set 19

Refer to the computerized MAR, Figure 7-4 on page 149, to answer questions 1 through 10. Convert the scheduled international time to traditional AM/PM time.

1. Scheduled times for administering Procanbid. _____

2. Scheduled times for administering Lanoxin and Lasix. _____

3. Scheduled times for administering Reglan. _____

4. Scheduled times for administering Micro-K. _____

5. How often can the Toradol be given? _____

6. If the Lanoxin was last given on 9/5/xx at 0900, when is the next date and time it will be given?

   _____

7. What is the ordered route of administration for the nitroglycerin? _____

8. How many times a day is furosemide ordered? _____

9. The equivalent dosage of digoxin is _____ mcg.

10. Which drugs are ordered to be administered "as necessary"? _____

Refer to the paper-based MAR (Figure 7-2) on page 147 to answer questions 11 through 20.

11. What is the route of administration for the insulin? _____

12. How many times in a 24-hour period will furosemide be administered? _____

13. What is the only medication ordered to be given routinely at noon? _____

14. At what time of day is the insulin to be administered? _____

15. A dosage of 10 mEq of K-Dur is ordered. What does mEq mean? _____

16. You work 3 PM to 11 PM on November 5. Which routine medications will you administer to Mary Q. Patient during your shift? _____

17. Mary Q. Patient has a fever of 101.4°F. What medication should you administer? _____

18. How many times in a 24-hour period will K-Dur be administered? _____

19. What is the equivalent of the scheduled administration time(s) for the K-Dur as converted to international time?

_____

20. What is the equivalent of the scheduled administration time(s) for the cephalexin as converted to international time? _____

21. Identify the place on the MAR where the stat IV furosemide was charted. _____

After completing these problems, see page 601 to check your answers.

CLINICAL REASONING SKILLS

It is the responsibility of the nurse to clarify any drug order that is incomplete—that is, an order that does not contain the essential seven parts discussed in this chapter. Let's look at an example in which an error resulted from not clarifying an incomplete order.

ERROR

Failing to clarify incomplete orders.

Possible Scenario

Suppose a physician ordered *omeprazole capsules p.o. ā bedtime* for a patient with an active duodenal ulcer. You will note that there is no dosage listed. The nurse thought the medication came in only one dosage strength, added 20 mg to the order, and sent it to the pharmacy. The pharmacist prepared the dosage written on the physician's order sheet. Two days later, during rounds, the physician noted that the patient had not responded well to the medication. When asked about this, the nurse explained that the patient had received 20 mg at bedtime. The physician informed the nurse that the patient should have received the 40 mg dosage for high acid suppression.

Potential Outcome

Potentially, the delay in correct dosage could result in gastrointestinal bleeding or delayed healing of the ulcer.

Prevention

This medication error could have been avoided simply by the physician writing the strength of the medication. Because it was omitted, the nurse should have checked the dosage before sending the order to the pharmacy. When you add to an incomplete order, you are essentially practicing medicine without a license, which is illegal and potentially dangerous.

CLINICAL REASONING SKILLS

Read the entire medication record to ensure that the planned administration times are scheduled correctly according to the medication order. In the following situation, two doses of a medication were omitted each day until an observant nurse picked up on the transcription error.

ERROR

Omitting medication due to incorrect scheduling of doses.

Possible Scenario

An order was written for **ampicillin 500 mg IV PB q.4h**, which was handwritten on the medication administration record (MAR). The registered nurse was distracted while verifying the order and writing in the scheduled times of administration. The nurse saw the number 4 and instead of scheduling the medication every 4 hours, scheduled the medication to be given 4 times a day—at 0600, 1200, 1800, and 2400. For 2 days, the shift nurses each checked to see what medications needed to be given on their scheduled shifts but did not take the time to compare the ordered frequency to the scheduled times. Eventually, a nurse did look over the entire medication record and noticed the error. The medication times were corrected and the doctor was notified. A medication variance form was completed, documenting the error, and it was submitted to the hospital risk management department.

Potential Outcome

Over the course of 2 days the patient missed 4 doses, for a total of 2 grams of ampicillin. This could have led to a prolonged illness as a result of the persistent infection, increased patient discomfort, and a prolonged hospitalization.

Prevention

At the beginning of each shift, read the entire medication administration record. Verify that the times scheduled for medications to be administered on your shift comply with the ordered frequency. Also review medications scheduled for other shifts, to consider any potential drug interactions or inconsistencies. This practice might also prevent others from making a medication error.

PRACTICE PROBLEMS—CHAPTER 7

Interpret the following abbreviations and symbols without consulting another source.

1. b.i.d. _____

2. p.r. _____

3. a.c. _____

4. $\bar{p}$ _____

5. t.i.d. _____

6. q.4h _____

7. p.r.n. _____

8. p.o. _____

9. IV _____

10. q.i.d. _____

11. stat _____

12. ad.lib. _____

13. p.c. _____

14. IM _____

15. $\bar{s}$ _____

Give the abbreviations for the following terms without consulting another source.

16. night _____

17. drop _____

18. milliliter _____

19. under the tongue _____

20. gram _____

21. 4 times a day _____

22. with _____

23. subcutaneous _____

24. teaspoon _____

25. twice daily _____

26. every 3 hours _____

27. after meals _____

28. before _____

29. kilogram _____

Interpret the following physician's drug orders without consulting another source.

30. Toradol 60 mg IV stat et q.6h p.r.n., pain _____

31. procaine penicillin G 300,000 units IV q.i.d. _____

32. Mylanta 5 mL p.o. 1 h a.c., 1 h p.c., bedtime, et q.2h p.r.n. at noct, gastric upset _____

_____

33. Librium 25 mg p.o. q.6h p.r.n., agitation _____

34. heparin 5,000 units subcut stat _____

35. morphine sulfate 5 mg IV q.4h p.r.n., moderate to severe pain _____

36. digoxin 0.25 mg p.o. daily _____

37. Neo-Synephrine ophthalmic 10% 2 gtt left eye q.30 min × 2 _____

_____

38. Lasix 40 mg IM stat _____

39. Decadron 4 mg IV b.i.d. _____

Refer to the paper-based MAR in Figure 7-2 on page 147 to answer questions 40 through 44.

40. Convert the scheduled times for isosorbide SR to traditional AM/PM times.

_____   _____   _____

41. How many units of heparin will be used to flush the central line at 2200? _____

42. What route is ordered for the Humulin R regular U-100 insulin? _____

43. Interpret the order for Cipro. _____

44. If the administration times for the sliding scale insulin are accurate (30 minutes before meals), at what times will meals be served? (Use traditional AM/PM time.) _____

Refer to the computerized pharmacy MAR in Figure 7-4 on page 149 to answer questions 45 through 49.

45. The physician visited about 5:00 PM on 8/8/xx. What order did the physician write? _____

_____

46. Using the time as a clue, interpret the symbol "w/" in the Zantac order and give the proper medical abbreviation. _____

_____

47. Interpret the order for ranitidine. _____

FIGURE 7-5 Paper-based MAR for Chapter 7 Practice Problems (questions 40–44)

PAGE _1_ of _1_

MEDICATION ADMINISTRATION RECORD

ORIGINAL ORDER DATE	DATE STARTED / RENEWED	MEDICATION - DOSAGE	ROUTE	SCHEDULE 11-7	7-3	3-11	DATE 11/3/xx 11-7	7-3	3-11	DATE 11/4/xx 11-7	7-3	3-11	DATE 11/5/xx 11-7	7-3	3-11	DATE 11/6/xx 11-7	7-3	3-11
11/3/xx	11/3/xx	heparin lock central line flush (10 units per mL solution) 2 mL	IV b.i.d.		1000	2200												
11/3/xx	11/3/xx	isosorbide SR 40 mg q.8h	PO	2400	0800	1600												
11/3/xx	11/3/xx	Cipro 500 mg q.12h	PO		1000	2200												
11/3/xx	11/3/xx	Humulin N NPH U-100 insulin 15 units q.am	subcut	0700														
11/3/xx	11/3/xx	Humulin R regular U-100 insulin 30 min. ac and bedtime per sliding scale Blood glucose 0-150 3 units 151-250 8 units 251-350 13 units 351-400 18 units greater than 400 call Dr.	subcut	0730 1130	1730 2200													
11/3/xx	11/3/xx	PRN Tylenol 1,000 mg q.4h p.r.n., headache	PO															

PRN

INJECTION SITES

B - RIGHT ARM C - RIGHT ABDOMEN
D - RIGHT ANTERIOR THIGH G - LEFT ARM
H - LEFT ABDOMEN J - LEFT ANTERIOR THIGH
L - LEFT BUTTOCKS M - RIGHT BUTTOCKS

DATE GIVEN	TIME	INT.	ONE - TIME MEDICATION - DOSAGE	RT.	11-7	7-3	3-11	11-7	7-3	3-11	11-7	7-3	3-11	11-7	7-3	3-11
					SCHEDULE			DATE			DATE			DATE		DATE

SIGNATURE OF NURSE ADMINISTERING MEDICATIONS

11-7

7-3

3-11

DATE GIVEN	TIME	INT.	MEDICATION-DOSAGE-CONT.	RT.

RECOPIED BY:

CHECKED BY:

Patient, Pat H.
#6-33725-4

ALLERGIES:
None Known

(1)

ORIGINAL COPY

48. Which of the routine medications is (are) ordered for 6:00 PM? _____

49. How many hours are between the scheduled administration times for Megace? _____

FIGURE 7-6   Computerized pharmacy MAR for Chapter 7 Practice Problems
(questions 45–49)

PHARMACY MAR

START	STOP	MEDICATION	SCHEDULED TIMES	OK'D BY	0701 TO 1500	1501 TO 2300	2301 TO 0700
21:00 8/17/xx SCH		MEGESTROL ACETATE (MEGACE) 40 MG TAB 2 TABS PO BID	0900 2100				
12:00 8/17/xx SCH		VANCOMYCIN 250 MG CAP 1 CAPSULE PO QID	0800 1200 1800 2200				
9:00 8/13/xx SCH		FLUCONAZOLE (DIFLUCAN) 100 MG TAB 100 MG PO DAILY	0900				
21:00 8/11/xx SCH		PERIDEX ORAL RINSE 480 ML 30 ML ORAL RINSE BID SWISH AND SPIT	0900 2100				
17:00 8/10/xx SCH		RANITIDINE (ZANTAC) 150 MG TAB 1 TABLET PO BID W/BREAKFAST AND SUPPER	0800 1700				
17:00 8/08/xx SCH		DIGOXIN (LANOXIN) 0.125 MG TAB 1 TAB PO daily at 1700 CHECK PULSE RATE	1700				
0:01 8/27/xx PRN		LIDOCAINE 5% OINT 35 GM TUBE APPLY TOPICAL PRN TO RECTAL AREA					
14:00 8/22/xx PRN		SODIUM CHLORIDE INJ 10 ML AS DIR IV TID DILUENT FOR ATIVAN IV					
14:00 8/22/xx PRN		LORAZEPAM (ATIVAN) 2 MG INJ 1 MG IV TID PRN ANXIETY					
9:30 8/21/xx PRN		TUCKS 40 PADS APPLY APPLY TOPICAL Q4H TO RECTUM PRN					
9:30 8/21/xx PRN		ANUSOL SUPP 1 SUPP 1 SUPP PR Q4H					
16:00 8/18/xx PRN		OXYCODONE 5 MG TAB 5 MG PO Q4H PRN PAIN					

Gluteus	Thigh
A. Right	H. Right
B. Left	I. Left
Ventro Gluteal	Deltoid
C. Right	J. Right
D. Left	K. Left
E. Abdomen	1 | 2
	3 | 4
Page **1** of **2**	DAILY

STANDARD TIMES
DAILY = 0900
BID = Q12H = 0900 & 2100
TID = 0800, 1400, 2200
Q8H = 0800, 1600, 2400
QID = 0800, 1200, 1800, 2200
Q6H = 0600, 1200, 1800, 2400
Q4H = 0400, 0800, 1200. . .
DAILY DIGOXIN = 1700
DAILY WARFARIN = 1600

NURSE'S SIGNATURE   INITIAL
0701- _____
1500 _____
1501- _____
2300 _____
2301- _____
0700 _____
Ok'd
by _____

ALLERGIES: NAFCILLIN
             BACTRIM
             SULFA
             TRIMETHOPRIM
             CIPROFLOXACIN HCL

Patient   Smith, John
Patient #   3-90301-4

Physician: J. Physician, M.D.
Room: 407-4 South

FROM: 08/30/xx   0701   TO: 08/31/xx   0700

50. Describe the clinical reasoning you would use to prevent this medication error.

Possible Scenario

Suppose a physician wrote an order for *gentamicin 100 mg IV q.8h* for a patient hospitalized with meningitis. The unit secretary transcribed the order as:

gentamicin 100 mg IV q.8h

(12 AM–6 AM–12 PM–6 PM)

The medication nurse checked the order without noticing the discrepancy in the administration times. Suppose the patient received the medication every 6 hours for 3 days before the error was noticed.

Potential Outcome

The patient would have received one extra dose each day, which is equivalent to one third more medication daily than prescribed. Most likely, the physician would be notified of the error, the medication discontinued, and the serum gentamicin levels drawn. The levels would likely be in the toxic range, and the patient's gentamicin levels would be monitored until the levels returned to normal. This patient would be at risk of developing ototoxicity or nephrotoxicity from the overdose of gentamicin.

Prevention

_____

_____

After completing these problems, see page 602 to check your answers.

For additional practice, visit the online practice software at www.CengageBrain.com, using the Premium Website access code found in the front of your text.

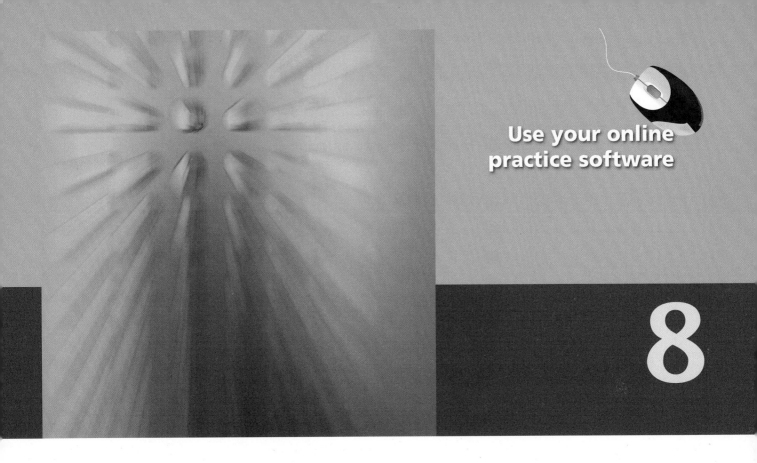

8

Understanding Drug Labels

OBJECTIVES

Upon mastery of Chapter 8, you will be able to read and understand the labels of the medications you have available. To accomplish this, you will also be able to:

- Recognize pertinent information on drug labels including:

  - Drug form
  - Dosage strength
  - Supply dosage or concentration
  - Total volume of drug container
  - Administration route
  - Expiration date

as well as

- Differentiate the brand and generic names of drugs.
- Find the directions for mixing or preparing the supply dosage of drugs, as needed.
- Recognize and follow drug alerts.
- Locate the lot or control number, National Drug Code, barcode symbols, and controlled substance classifications.
- Determine if containers are for single-dose or multidose use.
- Identify combination drugs.
- Describe supply dosage expressed as a ratio or percent.

Throe drug order prescribes how much of a drug the patient is to receive. The nurse must prepare the order from the drugs on hand. The drug label tells how the available drug is supplied. Examine the various preparations, labels, and dosage strengths of Valium injection, Figure 8-1.

Look at the following common drug labels to learn to recognize pertinent information about the drugs supplied.

FIGURE 8-1   Various Valium preparations

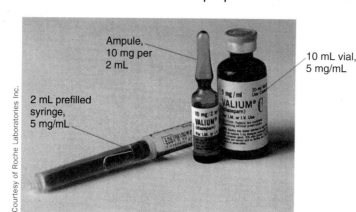

BRAND AND GENERIC NAMES

The brand, trade, or proprietary name is the manufacturer's name for a drug. Notice that the brand name is usually the most prominent word on the drug label—set in large type and boldly visible to easily identify and promote the product. It is often followed by the registered sign (®), meaning that both the name and formulation are so designated. The generic, or established, nonproprietary name appears directly under the brand name. Sometimes the generic name is placed inside parentheses. By law, the generic name must be identified on all drug labels.

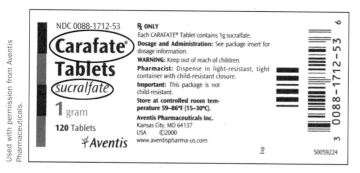

Brand name (Carafate) and generic name (sucralfate)   Generic drug (famotidine)

Generic equivalents of many brand-name drugs are ordered as substitutes or allowed by the prescribing practitioner. Because only the generic name appears on these labels, nurses need to carefully cross-check all medications. Failure to do so could cause inaccurate drug identification.

DOSAGE STRENGTH

The dosage strength refers to the dosage *weight* or amount of drug provided in a specific unit of measurement. The dosage strength of Lopid tablets is 600 milligrams (the weight and specific unit of measurement) per tablet. Some drugs, such as penicillin V potassium, have two different but equivalent dosage strengths. Penicillin V potassium has a dosage strength of 250 milligrams (per tablet), or 400,000 units (per tablet). This allows prescribers to order the drug using either unit of measurement.

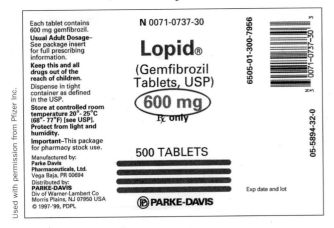

600 milligrams (per tablet)

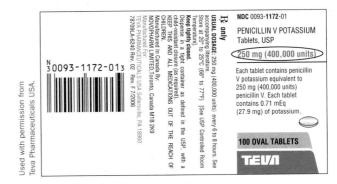

250 milligrams (400,000 units) (per tablet)

▨▨▨▨ FORM

The form identifies the *structure* and *composition* of the drug. Solid dosage forms for oral use include tablets and capsules. Some powdered or granular medications that are not manufactured in tablet or capsule form can be directly combined with food or beverages and administered. Others must be reconstituted (liquefied) and measured in a precise liquid volume, such as milliliters, drops, or ounces. They may be a crystalloid (clear solution) or a suspension (solid particles in liquid that separate when held in a container).

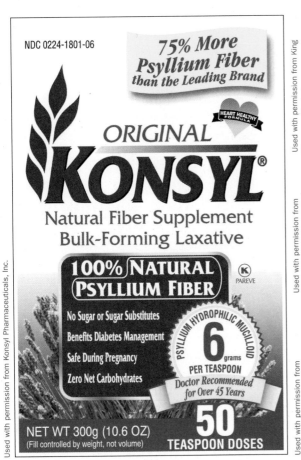

Fiber granular drug added to beverage

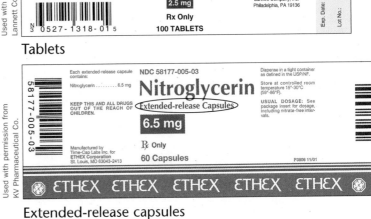

Oral solution

Tablets

Extended-release capsules

Injectable medications may be supplied in solution or dry powdered form to be reconstituted. Once reconstituted, they are measured in milliliters.

Medications are also supplied in a variety of other forms, such as suppositories, creams, and patches.

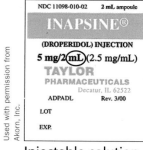

Injectable solution

SUPPLY DOSAGE

The supply dosage refers to both *dosage strength* and *form*. It is read *X measured units per some quantity*. For solid-form medications, such as tablets, the supply dosage is X measured units per tablet. For liquid medications, the supply dosage is the same as the medication's concentration, such as X measured units per milliliter. Take a minute to read the supply dosage printed on the following labels.

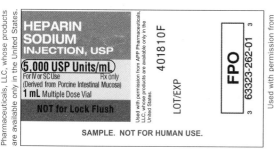

5,000 USP units per milliliter

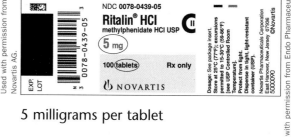

5 milligrams per tablet

20 milligrams per milliliter

TOTAL VOLUME

The total volume refers to the *full quantity* contained in a package, bottle, or vial. For tablets and other solid medications, it is the total number of individual items. For liquids, it is the total fluid volume.

All too frequently, dosage strength and total volume are misinterpreted, resulting in medication errors. Beginning February 1, 2009, a new Food and Drug Administration (FDA) requirement became official that calls for the strength per total volume to be the prominent expression on single- and multidose injectable product labels, followed in close proximity by the strength per mL enclosed in parentheses (Cohen, 2008). Notice the Inapsine (droperidol injection) label on this page, which complies with the new rule: 2 mL ampule size, **5 mg/2 mL** (2.5 mg/mL). Clearly providing all of this information lowers the risk of misinterpretation and medication error.

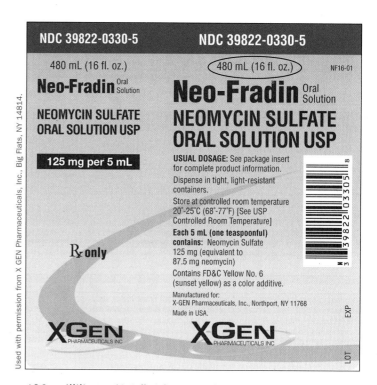

480 milliliters (16 fluid ounces)

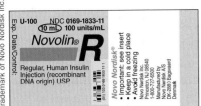

10 milliliters

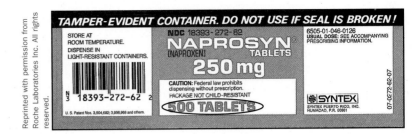

500 tablets

ADMINISTRATION ROUTE

The administration route refers to the *site* (of the body) or the *method of drug delivery* into the patient. Examples of routes of administration include oral, enteral (into the gastrointestinal tract through a tube), sublingual, injection (IV, IM, subcut), otic, optic, topical, rectal, vaginal, and others. Unless specified otherwise, tablets, capsules, and caplets are intended for oral use.

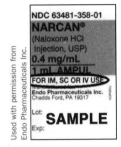

Intramuscular (IM), subcutaneous (subcut), or intravenous (IV)

Sublingual

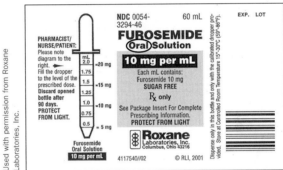

Oral

DIRECTIONS FOR MIXING OR RECONSTITUTING

Some drugs are dispensed in *powder* form and must be *reconstituted for use*. (Reconstitution is discussed further in Chapters 10 and 12.)

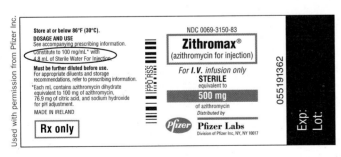

See directions

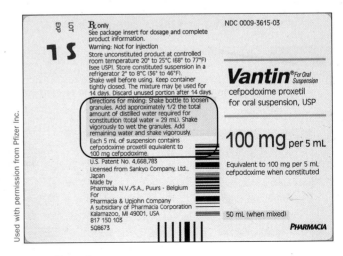

See directions

LABEL ALERTS

Manufacturers may print warnings on the packaging, or special alerts may be added by the pharmacy before dispensing. Look for special storage alerts such as "refrigerate at all times," "keep in a dry place," "replace cap and close tightly before storing," or "protect from light." Reconstituted suspensions may be dispensed already prepared for use, and directions may instruct the health care professional to "shake well before using," as a reminder to remix the components. Read and follow all label instructions carefully.

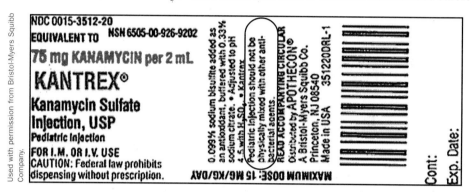

See alert

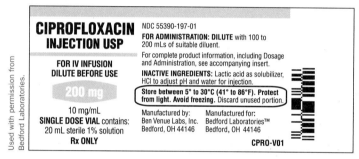

See alert

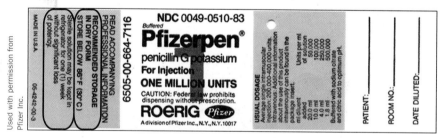

See alerts

NAME OF THE MANUFACTURER

The name of the manufacturer is circled on the following labels.

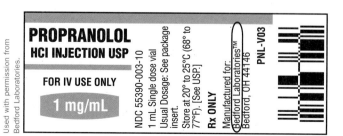

Bedford Laboratories

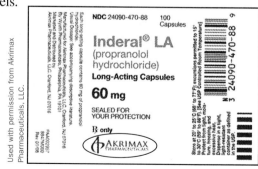

Akrimax Pharmaceuticals, Inc.

EXPIRATION DATE

The medication should be used, discarded, or returned to the pharmacy by the expiration date. Further, note the special expiration instructions given on labels for reconstituted medications. Refer to the discard instructions on the Vantin label on page 161.

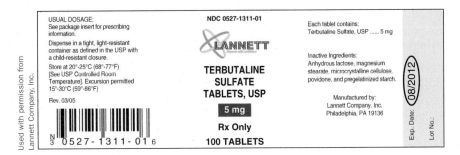

Expiration date: 08/2012

LOT OR CONTROL NUMBERS

Federal law requires all medication packages to be identified with a lot or control number. If a drug is recalled for reasons such as damage or tampering, the lot number quickly identifies the particular group of medication packages to be removed from shelves. This number has been invaluable for vaccine and over-the-counter medication recalls.

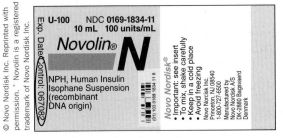

Control number: 067082

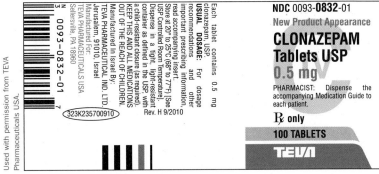

Lot number: 323K235700910

NATIONAL DRUG CODE (NDC)

Federal law requires every prescription medication to have a unique identifying number, much like every U.S. citizen has a unique Social Security number. This number must appear on every manufacturer's label and is printed with the letters "NDC" followed by three discrete groups of numbers.

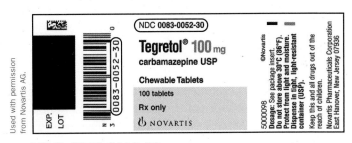

NDC: 0083-0052-30

CONTROLLED SUBSTANCE SCHEDULE

The Controlled Substances Act was passed in May 1971. One of its purposes was to improve the administration and regulation of the production, distribution, and dispensing of controlled substances. Drugs considered controlled substances are classified according to their potential for use and abuse. Drugs are classified into numbered levels, or schedules, from Schedule I to Schedule V. Drugs that have the highest potential for abuse are Schedule I drugs, and those with the lowest potential for abuse are Schedule V drugs. The schedule number of controlled substances is indicated on the drug label.

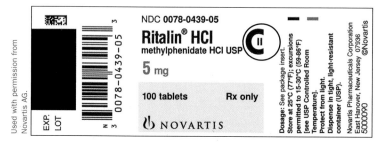

Schedule II

BARCODE SYMBOLS

Barcode symbols are commonly used in retail sales. They also document drug dosing for recordkeeping and stock reordering and can automate medication documentation right at the patient's bedside.

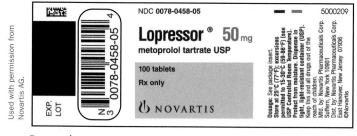

Barcode

UNITED STATES PHARMACOPEIA (USP) AND NATIONAL FORMULARY (NF)

These codes are found on many manufacturer-printed medication labels, and they are placed after the generic drug name. The USP and NF are the two official national lists of approved drugs. Each manufacturer follows special guidelines that determine when to include these initials on a label. Be careful not to mistake these abbreviations for other initials that designate specific characteristics of a drug, such as *SR*, which means *sustained release.*

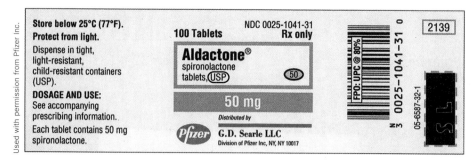

USP

UNIT- OR SINGLE-DOSE LABELS

Most oral medications administered in the hospital setting are available in unit dosage, such as a single capsule or tablet packaged separately in a typical blister pack. The pharmacy provides a 24-hour supply of each drug for the patient. The only major difference in this form of labeling is that the total volume of the container is usually omitted because the volume is 1 tablet or capsule. Likewise, the dosage strength is understood as *per one*. Further, injectable medicines may be packaged in single-dose preparations.

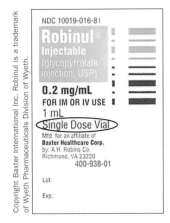

Unit dose
single-use vial

COMBINATION DRUGS

Some medications are a combination of two or more drugs in one form. Read the labels for Percocet and Lortab and notice the different substances that are combined in each tablet. Combination drugs are sometimes prescribed by the number of tablets, capsules, or milliliters to be given rather than by the dosage strength.

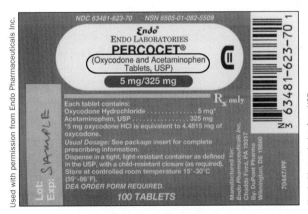

oxycodone and acetaminophen

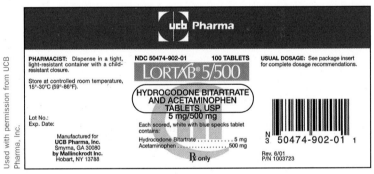

hydrocodone bitartrate and acetaminophen

SUPPLY DOSAGE EXPRESSED AS A RATIO OR PERCENT

Occasionally, solutions will be ordered and/or manufactured in a supply dosage expressed as a ratio or percent.

RULE

Ratio solutions express the number of grams of the drug per total milliliters of solution.

EXAMPLE ■

Epinephrine 1:1,000 contains 1 g pure drug per
1,000 mL solution;
1 g:1,000 mL = 1,000 mg:1,000 mL = 1 mg:1 mL.

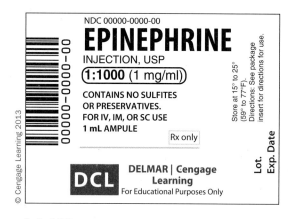

1:1,000

RULE

Percentage (%) solutions express the number of grams of the drug per 100 milliliters of solution.

EXAMPLE ■

Lidocaine 2% contains 2 g pure drug
per 100 mL solution; 2 g per
100 mL = 2,000 mg per 100 mL =
20 mg/mL.

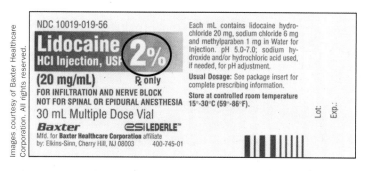

2%

Although these labels look different from many of the other labels, it is important to recognize that the supply dosage can still be determined. Many times the label will have a more commonly identified supply dosage and not just the ratio or percent. Look at the epinephrine and lidocaine labels. On the epinephrine label, the ratio is 1:1,000; the supply dosage can also be identified as 1 mg/mL. On the lidocaine label, the percentage is 2%; the supply dosage can also be identified as 20 mg/mL.

CHECKING LABELS

Recall the Six Rights of medication administration: The *right patient* must receive the *right drug* in the *right amount* by the *right route* at the *right time* followed by the *right documentation*. To be absolutely sure the patient receives the right drug, check the label three times.

CAUTION

Before administering a medication to a patient, check the drug label three times:

1. Against the medication order or MAR.

2. Before preparing the medication.

3. After preparing the medication and before administering it.

QUICK REVIEW

Read labels carefully to:

- Identify the drug and the manufacturer.

- Differentiate between brand and generic names, dosage strength, form, supply dosage, total container volume, and administration route.

- Recognize that the drug's supply dosage similarly refers to a drug's weight per unit of measure or concentration.

- Find the directions for reconstitution, as needed.

- Note expiration date and alerts.

- Describe lot or control number, NDC number, and schedule (if controlled substance).

- Identify supply dosage on labels with ratios and percents.

- Be sure that you administer the right drug.

Review Set 20

Used with permission from Novartis AG.

NDC 0083-0052-30

Tegretol® 100 mg

carbamazepine USP

Chewable Tablets

100 tablets

Rx only

◊ NOVARTIS

5000098
Dosage: See package insert.
Do not store above 30°C (86°F).
Protect from light and moisture.
Dispense in tight, light-resistant container (USP).

Keep this and all drugs out of the reach of children.

Novartis Pharmaceuticals Corporation
East Hanover, New Jersey 07936

©Novartis

EXP.
LOT
0083-0052-30

A

Used with permission from Bedford Laboratories.

TERBUTALINE
SULFATE INJECTION USP

FOR SC INJECTION ONLY.

1 mg/mL

Rx ONLY

NDC 55390-101-10

1 mL Sterile Vial

Protect from light.

Manufactured for:
Bedford Laboratories™
Bedford, OH 44146

TBT-V01

B

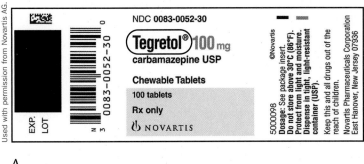

Used with permission from Abbott Laboratories.

SPECIMEN

©Abbott

Exp.
Lot 03-2127-3/R4

0074336860

Store tablets at 15° to 30°C (59° to 86°F).

NDC 0074-3368-60
60 Tablets

BIAXIN®
FILMTAB®

clarithromycin tablets

250 mg

Caution: Federal (U.S.A.) law prohibits dispensing without prescription.

6505-01-354-8582
Do not accept if break-away ring on cap is broken or missing.
Dispense in a USP tight, light-resistant container.
Each tablet contains:
250 mg clarithromycin.
Each yellow tablet bears the Ⓐ and Abbo-Code KT for product identification.
Usual Adult Dose: One or two tablets every twelve hours. See enclosure for full prescribing information.
Filmtab – Film-sealed tablets, Abbott.
Abbott Laboratories
North Chicago, IL60064, U.S.A.

C

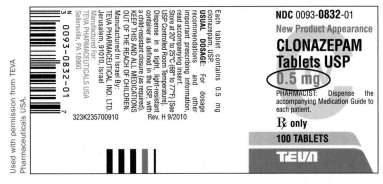

Used with permission from TEVA Pharmaceuticals USA.

0093-0832-01

323K235700910

Each tablet contains 0.5 mg clonazepam, USP.
USUAL DOSAGE: For dosage recommendations and other important prescribing information, read accompanying insert.
Store at 20° to 25°C (68° to 77°F) [See USP Controlled Room Temperature].
Dispense in a tight, light-resistant container as defined in the USP with a child-resistant closure (as required).
KEEP THIS AND ALL MEDICATIONS OUT OF THE REACH OF CHILDREN.
Manufactured in Israel By:
TEVA PHARMACEUTICAL IND. LTD.
Jerusalem, 91010, Israel
Manufactured For:
TEVA PHARMACEUTICALS USA
Sellersville, PA 18960
Rev. H 9/2010

NDC 0093-**0832**-01

New Product Appearance

CLONAZEPAM
Tablets USP

0.5 mg

PHARMACIST: Dispense the accompanying Medication Guide to each patient.

℞ only

100 TABLETS

TEVA

D

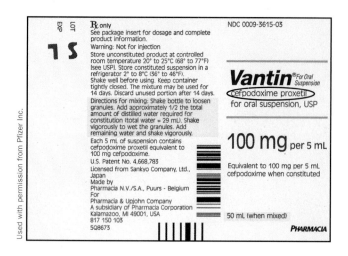

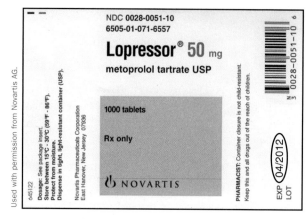

E

F

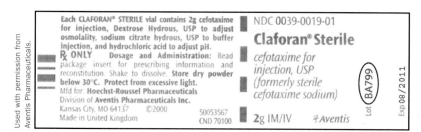

G

Use labels A through G to find the information requested in questions 1 through 15. Indicate your answer by letter (A through G).

1. The total volume of the liquid container is circled.   _____

2. The dosage strength is circled.   _____

3. The form of the drug is circled.   _____

4. The brand name of the drug is circled.   _____

5. The generic name of the drug is circled.   _____

6. The expiration date is circled.   _____

7. The lot number is circled.   _____

8. Look at label E and determine how much of the supply drug you will administer
   to the patient per dose for the order *cefpodoxime 100 mg p.o. q.12h.*   _____

9. Look at label A and determine the route of administration.   _____

10. Indicate which labels have a visible imprinted barcode symbol.   _____

11. Look at label C. What does the word *Filmtab* mean on this label?   _____

12. Look at label B and determine the supply dosage.   _____

13. Look at label F, and determine how much of the supply drug you will administer
    to the patient per dose for the order *metoprolol 100 mg p.o. daily.*   _____

14. Which drug label(s) represent controlled substance(s)?   _____

15. Evaluate the potential for abuse of the controlled substance drug(s) identified in question 14.

Refer to the following label to identify the specific drug information described in questions 16 through 21.

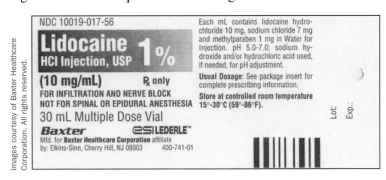

16. Generic name _____

17. Brand name _____

18. Dosage strength _____

19. Route of administration _____

20. National Drug Code _____

21. Manufacturer _____

Refer to the following label to answer questions 22 through 24.

22. The supply dosage of the drug is _____ %.

23. The supply dosage of the drug is _____ g per 100 mL.

24. The supply dosage of the drug is _____ mg per mL.

After completing these problems, see page 602 to check your answers.

CLINICAL REASONING SKILLS

Reading the labels of medications is critical. Make sure that the drug you want is what you have on hand before you prepare it. Let's look at an example of a medication error related to reading the label incorrectly.

ERROR

Not checking the label for correct dosage.

Possible Scenario

A nurse flushed a triple central venous catheter (an IV with three ports). According to hospital policy, the nurse was to flush each port with 10 mL of normal saline followed by 2 mL of heparin flush solution in the concentration of 100 units/mL. The nurse mistakenly picked up a vial of heparin containing heparin 10,000 units/mL. Without checking the label, she prepared the solution for all three ports. The patient received 60,000 units of heparin instead of 600 units.

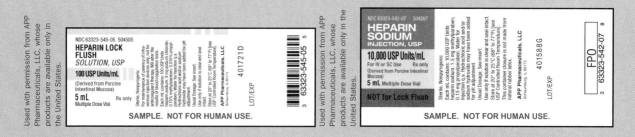

Potential Outcome

The patient in this case would be at great risk for hemorrhage, leading to shock and death. Protamine sulfate would likely be ordered to counteract the action of the heparin, but a successful outcome is questionable.

Prevention

There is no substitute for checking the label before administering a medication. The nurse in this case, having drawn three different syringes of medication for the three ports, had three opportunities to catch the error.

CLINICAL REASONING SKILLS

Many drugs have brand names or generic names that look alike or sound alike (LASA). Inattention to detail while preparing medications may lead to administration of the wrong drug, which can have serious consequences. Let's consider the safety risk of two look-alike/sound-alike medications.

ERROR

Mixing up two medications with similar names.

Possible Scenario

A patient who was receiving hydromorphone, an opioid analgesic for postoperative pain, complained of nausea. The physician had written an order for *hydroxyzine 50 mg IM q.3–4h p.r.n., nausea*. Instead of retrieving the ordered antiemetic medication, the nurse selected a vial of hydralazine 20 mg/mL, an antihypertensive, from the automated dispensing cabinet. After calculating the dose to be 2.5 mL, the nurse administered the medication by the intramuscular route. Although he still felt nauseous an hour later, the patient tried to amubulate for the first time since surgery with the assistance of the nurse technician but experienced severe dizziness and could not stand at the side of the bed. His blood pressure was taken and noted to have dropped to 92/48 mm/Hg. The nurse called the physician, who ordered vital signs to be taken q.2h and for the patient to remain on bed rest until his blood pressure returned to normal. Eight hours later the patient's blood pressure returned to normal and he was able to get out of bed to a chair. Neither the nurse nor the physician was able to determine the reason for the blood pressure drop.

Potential Outcome

The patient needed an antiemetic medication but received an antihypertensive medication. Besides continuing to suffer from nausea, the patient was inconvenienced and lost needed rest by having vital signs taken more frequently than otherwise would have been required. He was also at risk for a serious injury from a fall due to orthostatic hypotension when attempting to ambulate the first time following surgery.

Prevention

Administering the antihypertensive agent (hydralazine) instead of the antiemetic (hydroxyzine) could lead to a serious adverse drug event. Observe that the first four letters in the drug names are identical. Pharmacies are likely to stock these drugs next to each other on pharmacy shelves or in automated dispensing cabinets. Nurses may also locate these drugs alphabetically on computer screens. Additionally, their similar dosage strengths may not indicate a potential problem to the nurse. The nurse and the physician not recognizing the error is an all too common occurrence. According to the Institute of Medicine (IOM, 2000), most errors and safety issues go undetected and unreported. Nurses should comply with the National Safety Goals of The Joint Commission (2008) and "identify and, at a minimum, annually review a list of look-alike/sound-alike drugs used in the organization, and take action to prevent errors involving the interchange of these drugs."

PRACTICE PROBLEMS—CHAPTER 8

Look at labels A through G and identify the information requested.

Label A:

1. The supply dosage of the drug in milliequivalents is _____.

2. The total volume of the vial is _____.

3. The supply dosage of the drug in milligrams is _____.

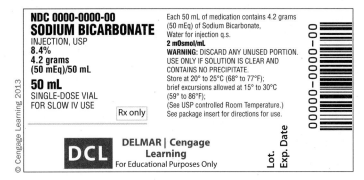

A

Label B:

4. The generic name of the drug is _____.

5. The reconstitution instruction to mix a supply dosage of 100 mg per 5 mL for oral suspension is

_____.

6. The manufacturer of the drug is _____.

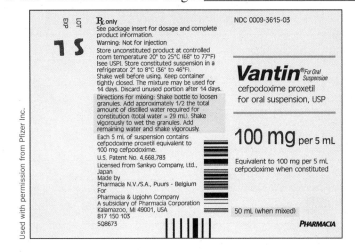

B

Label C:

7. The total volume of the medication container is _____.

8. The supply dosage is _____.

9. How much will you administer to the patient per dose for the order **methotrexate 25 mg IV stat?**

_____.

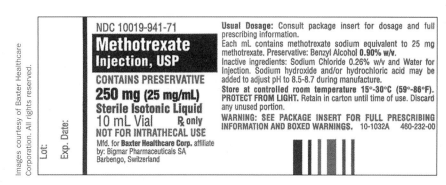

NDC 10019-941-71

Methotrexate Injection, USP

CONTAINS PRESERVATIVE

250 mg (25 mg/mL)

Sterile Isotonic Liquid

10 mL Vial   ℞ only

NOT FOR INTRATHECAL USE

Mfd. for **Baxter Healthcare Corp.** affiliate by: Bigmar Pharmaceuticals SA Barbengo, Switzerland

Lot: Exp. Date:

Usual Dosage: Consult package insert for dosage and full prescribing information.
Each mL contains methotrexate sodium equivalent to 25 mg methotrexate. Preservative: Benzyl Alcohol **0.90% w/v.**
Inactive ingredients: Sodium Chloride 0.26% w/v and Water for Injection. Sodium hydroxide and/or hydrochloric acid may be added to adjust pH to 8.5-8.7 during manufacture.
Store at controlled room temperature 15°-30°C (59°-86°F).
PROTECT FROM LIGHT. Retain in carton until time of use. Discard any unused portion.
WARNING: SEE PACKAGE INSERT FOR FULL PRESCRIBING INFORMATION AND BOXED WARNINGS. 10-1032A   460-232-00

C

Label D:

10. The brand name of the drug is _____.

11. The generic name is _____.

12. The National Drug Code of the drug is _____.

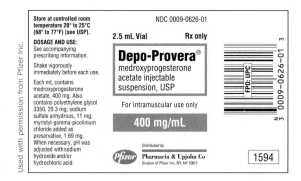

Store at controlled room temperature 20° to 25°C (68° to 77°F) [see USP].

DOSAGE AND USE: See accompanying prescribing information.

Shake vigorously immediately before each use.

Each mL contains medroxyprogesterone acetate, 400 mg. Also contains polyethylene glycol 3350, 20.3 mg; sodium sulfate anhydrous, 11 mg; myristyl-gamma-picolinium chloride added as preservative, 1.69 mg. When necessary, pH was adjusted with sodium hydroxide and/or hydrochloric acid.

NDC 0009-0626-01

2.5 mL Vial   Rx only

Depo-Provera®
medroxyprogesterone acetate injectable suspension, USP

For intramuscular use only

400 mg/mL

Distributed by
Pfizer **Pharmacia & Upjohn Co**
Division of Pfizer Inc, NY, NY 10017

1594

D

Label E:

13. The form of the drug is _____.

14. The total volume of the drug container is _____.

15. The administration route is _____.

FOR INTRAMUSCULAR USE ONLY.

USUAL ADULT DOSE: Intramuscularly: 25 - 100 mg stat; repeat every 4 to 6 hours, as needed.

See accompanying prescribing information.

Each mL contains **50 mg** of hydroxyzine hydrochloride, 0.9% benzyl alcohol and sodium hydroxide to adjust to optimum pH.

To avoid discoloration, protect from prolonged exposure to light.

Rx only

10 mL   NDC 0049-5460-74

Vistaril®
(hydroxyzine hydrochloride)

Intramuscular Solution

50 mg/mL

Pfizer **Roerig**
Division of Pfizer Inc, NY, NY 10017

Store below 86°F (30°C).

PROTECT FROM FREEZING.

PATIENT: _____

ROOM NO.: _____

05-1111-32-4 9249
MADE IN USA

E

Label F:

16. The name of the drug manufacturer is _____.

17. The form of the drug is _____.

18. The appropriate temperature for storage of this drug is _____.

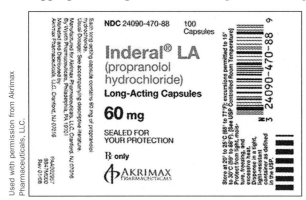

F

Label G:

19. The supply dosage of the drug is _____.

20. The dosage strength of the drug container is _____.

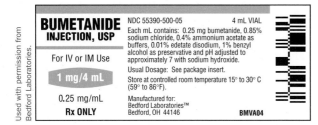

G

Match label H or I with the correct descriptive statement.

21. This label represents a unit- or single-dose drug.   _____

22. This label represents a combination drug.   _____

23. This label represents a drug that may be ordered by the number of tablets or capsules to be administered rather than the dosage strength.   _____

24. The administration route for the drug labeled H is _____.

25. The label represents a brand name drug. _____.

26. The controlled substance schedule for the drug labeled H is _____.

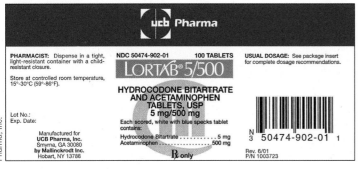

H

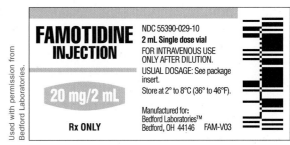

I

Label J:

27. Expressed as a percentage, the supply dosage of the drug is _____.

28. The supply dosage is equivalent to _____ g per 100 mL, or _____ mg per mL.

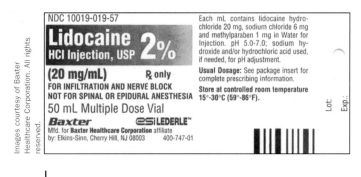

NDC 10019-019-57

Lidocaine **2**%
HCl Injection, USP

(20 mg/mL)   ℞ only
FOR INFILTRATION AND NERVE BLOCK
NOT FOR SPINAL OR EPIDURAL ANESTHESIA
50 mL Multiple Dose Vial

Baxter   **℮S**i**LEDERLE**™
Mfd. for **Baxter Healthcare Corporation** affiliate
by: Elkins-Sinn, Cherry Hill, NJ 08003   400-747-01

Each mL contains lidocaine hydrochloride 20 mg, sodium chloride 6 mg
and methylparaben 1 mg in Water for
Injection. pH 5.0-7.0; sodium hydroxide and/or hydrochloric acid used,
if needed, for pH adjustment.

Usual Dosage: See package insert for
complete prescribing information.

Store at controlled room temperature
15°-30°C (59°-86°F).

Lot: Exp.:

J

29. Describe the clinical reasoning you would use to prevent this medication error.

Possible Scenario

Suppose a physician ordered the antibiotic **Principen .5 g p.o. q.6h.** The writing was not clear on the order, and Prinivil (an antihypertensive medication) 5 mg was sent up by the pharmacy. However, the order was correctly transcribed to the MAR. In preparing the medication, the nurse did not read the MAR or label carefully and administered Prinivil, the wrong medication.

Potential Outcome

A medication error occurred because the wrong medication was given. The patient's infection treatment would be delayed. Furthermore, the erroneous blood pressure drug could have harmful effects.

Prevention

_____

_____

30. Describe the strategy you would implement to prevent this medication error.

Possible Scenario

Suppose a physician wrote the order **Celebrex 100 mg p.o. q.12h** (anti-inflammatory to treat rheumatoid arthritis pain), but the order was difficult to read. The unit secretary and pharmacy interpreted the order as *Celexa* (antidepressant), a medication with a similar spelling. Celexa was written on the MAR.

Potential Outcome

The nurse administered the Celexa for several days, and the patient began complaining of severe knee and hip pain from rheumatoid arthritis. Also, the patient experienced side effects of Celexa, including drowsiness and tremors. A medication error occurred because several health care professionals misinterpreted the order.

Prevention

a) What should have alerted the nurse that something was wrong?

_____

b) What should have been considered to prevent this error?

_____

After completing these problems, see page 602 to check your answers.

For additional practice, visit the online practice software at www.CengageBrain.com, using the Premium Website access code found in the front of your text.

REFERENCES

Cohen, Michael R. (2008). ISMP medication error report analysis: Strength misread as total dose [Electronic version]. *Hospital Pharmacy, 43,* 7. Retrieved November 23, 2008, from http://www.factsandcomparisons.com/assets/hpdatenamed/20080701_July2008_ismp.pdf

Institute of Medicine (2000). Committee on the Quality of Health Care in America. Kohn, Linda T., Corrigan, Janet M., and Donaldson, Molla S., Editors. To err is human: Building a safer health system. National Academy Press, Washington, DC, page 43.

The Joint Commission (2008). *Patient safety goals 2006–2008.* Retrieved November 28, 2010, from http://www.jointcommission.org/nr/rdonlyres/c92aab3f-a9bd-431c-8628-11dd2d1d53cc/0/lasa.pdf

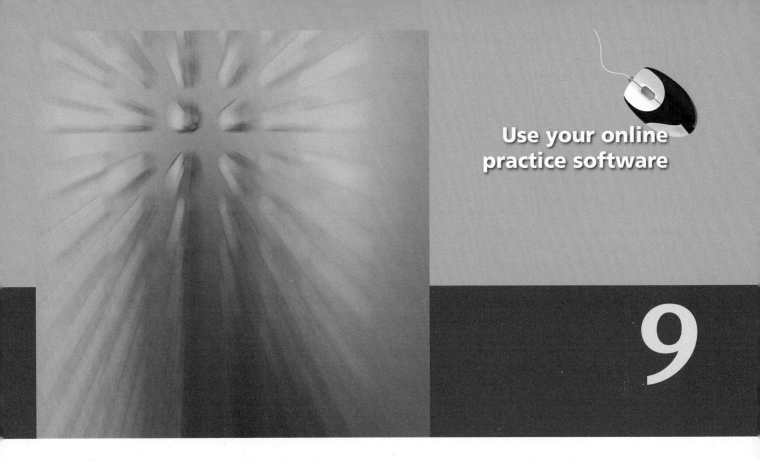

Preventing Medication Errors

OBJECTIVES

Upon mastery of Chapter 9, you will be able to identify and prevent the common situations that lead to medication administration errors. To accomplish this, you will also be able to:

- Describe the consequences and costs of medication errors.
- Cite the incidence of hospital injuries and deaths attributable to medication errors.
- Explore evidence and rationale for the underreporting of medication errors.
- Name the steps involved in medication administration.
- Identify six common causes of medication errors.
- Identify the role of the nurse in preventing medication errors.
- Describe the role of technology and health care administration in medication error prevention.
- Recognize examples of prescription, transcription, and recording notation errors.
- Correct medical notation errors.
- Describe the requirements of The Joint Commission to prevent medication errors.
- Provide a sound rationale for the critical nature of medication administration and the importance of accurate and safe dosage calculations and medication administration.

Medication administration is one of the primary functions of the nurse and the other health care practitioners in most health care settings. Unfortunately, medication administration errors are common. Any health care practitioner is potentially at risk for making an error. Several studies addressing the problem indicate that there is no relationship between the incidence of medication errors and the characteristics of the nurses who usually make them (that is, years of practice and education).

The frequency of medication errors made by nurses and the consequences of these errors affect not only the health of the patient but also the overall cost of health care. These medication errors and the reactions that result from them cause increased length of stay, increased cost, patient disability, and death. There are additional indirect consequences as well. These include harm to the nurse involved, in regard to his or her personal and professional status, confidence, and practice (Mayo & Duncan, 2004).

Although prescription and administration mistakes are the most commonly reported, the incidence of medication errors by nurses is difficult to accurately determine. The Institute of Medicine (IOM, 2006) reported that medication errors may occur during any step of the medication process, from procuring the drug, prescribing it, dispensing it, administering it, and monitoring the effects. IOM estimates that when all steps of the medication administration process are taken into account, hospitalized patients are subjected to an average of one medication error per day.

Studies addressing nurses' perception of medication errors support the existence of underreporting by nurses (Mayo & Duncan, 2004; Stetina, Groves, & Pafford, 2005; Wolf & Serembus, 2004). Other research indicates confusion among nurses about what constitutes a drug error. Failure to administer a medication and administering a medication late are the most underreported errors, because some nurses erroneously perceive that the patients will not be harmed in these situations (Mayo & Duncan, 2004; Stetina et al., 2005).

Statistics indicate that 10% to 18% of all hospital injuries are attributable to medication errors (Mayo & Duncan, 2004). The Institute of Medicine (2006) estimated that at least 400,000 medication errors a year resulting in $3.5 billion in annual costs, occur in U.S. hospitals and could have been prevented.

Medications that have been designated as high-alert drugs have the highest risk of causing injuries when errors are made. The Joint Commission (1999) identified insulin, opiates and narcotics, injectable potassium chloride, and intravenous anticoagulants as the high-alert medications with the greatest safety risk. A complete list of high-alert medications may be obtained on the Institute for Safe Medication Practices Website, www.ismp.org (see Figure 9-1).

The medication delivery process is complex and involves many individuals and departments. This chapter will focus on the critical role of the nurse in this process and the importance of legible medication orders, correct transcription and interpretation, safe medication administration, and accurate recording.

▆▆▆▆ PRESCRIPTION

The steps involved in safe medication administration begin with the *prescription,* followed by *transcription* and then *administration.* Only those licensed health care providers who have authority by their state to write prescriptions are permitted to do so, such as a medical doctor (MD), an osteopathic doctor (DO), a podiatrist (DPM), a dentist (DDS), a physician's assistant (PA), or an advanced registered nurse practitioner (ARNP).

Although nurses are not the originators of drug prescriptions, they play an important role in preventing errors in the *prescription* step. Refer back to Chapter 7 to review the seven parts of drug orders: patient's name, date and time of the order, name of the drug, amount of the drug (including the unit of measure), route, frequency or specific administration schedule, and the prescriber's name and licensure. It is important to always remember that the practitioner who administers a drug shares the liability for patient injury, even if the medical order was incorrect. The wise nurse always verifies the safety of the drug order by consulting a reputable drug reference, such as the American Hospital Formulary Service *AHFS Drug Information,* published annually by the American Society of Health-System Pharmacists, *Delmar's Nurse's Drug Handbook* published annually by Delmar Cengage Learning, and the *Physicians' Desk Reference* published annually by Thomson Reuters. Most hospitals and health care systems have access to electronic drug guides available online, with many accessed directly from the electronic medication administration record (MAR) by clicking on the drug name, such as the Thomson Reuters Micromedex system for point-of-care decision support.

FIGURE 9-1 ISMP's list of high-alert medications

 Institute for Safe Medication Practices

ISMP's List of *High-Alert Medications*

High-alert medications are drugs that bear a heightened risk of causing significant patient harm when they are used in error. Although mistakes may or may not be more common with these drugs, the consequences of an error are clearly more devastating to patients. We hope you will use this list to determine which medications require special safeguards to reduce the risk of errors. This may include strategies like improving access to information about these drugs; limiting access to high-alert medications; using auxiliary labels and automated alerts; standardizing the ordering, storage, preparation, and administration of these products; and employing redundancies such as automated or independent double-checks when necessary. (Note: manual independent double-checks are not always the optimal error-reduction strategy and may not be practical for all of the medications on the list).

Classes/Categories of Medications
adrenergic agonists, IV (e.g., epinephrine, phenylephrine, norepinephrine)
adrenergic antagonists, IV (e.g., propranolol, metoprolol, labetalol)
anesthetic agents, general, inhaled and IV (e.g., propofol, ketamine)
antiarrhythmics, IV (e.g., lidocaine, amiodarone)
antithrombotic agents (anticoagulants), including warfarin, low-molecular-weight heparin, IV unfractionated heparin, Factor Xa inhibitors (fondaparinux), direct thrombin inhibitors (e.g., argatroban, lepirudin, bivalirudin), thrombolytics (e.g., alteplase, reteplase, tenecteplase), and glycoprotein IIb/IIIa inhibitors (e.g., eptifibatide)
cardioplegic solutions
chemotherapeutic agents, parenteral and oral
dextrose, hypertonic, 20% or greater
dialysis solutions, peritoneal and hemodialysis
epidural or intrathecal medications
hypoglycemics, oral
inotropic medications, IV (e.g., digoxin, milrinone)
liposomal forms of drugs (e.g., liposomal amphotericin B)
moderate sedation agents, IV (e.g., midazolam)
moderate sedation agents, oral, for children (e.g., chloral hydrate)
narcotics/opiates, IV, transdermal, and oral (including liquid concentrates, immediate and sustained-release formulations)
neuromuscular blocking agents (e.g., succinylcholine, rocuronium, vecuronium)
radiocontrast agents, IV
total parenteral nutrition solutions

Specific Medications
colchicine injection***
epoprostenol (Flolan), IV
insulin, subcutaneous and IV
magnesium sulfate injection
methotrexate, oral, non-oncologic use
opium tincture
oxytocin, IV
nitroprusside sodium for injection
potassium chloride for injection concentrate
potassium phosphates injection
promethazine, IV
sodium chloride for injection, hypertonic (greater than 0.9% concentration)
sterile water for injection, inhalation, and irrigation (excluding pour bottles) in containers of 100 mL or more

***Although colchicine injection should no longer be used, it will remain on the list until shipments of unapproved colchicine injection cease in August 2008. For details, please visit: www.fda.gov/bbs/topics/NEWS/2008/NEW01791.html.

Background
Based on error reports submitted to the USP-ISMP Medication Errors Reporting Program, reports of harmful errors in the literature, and input from practitioners and safety experts, ISMP created and periodically updates a list of potential high-alert medications. During February-April 2007, 770 practitioners responded to an ISMP survey designed to identify which medications were most frequently considered high-alert drugs by individuals and organizations. Further, to assure relevance and completeness, the clinical staff at ISMP, members of our advisory board, and safety experts throughout the US were asked to review the potential list. This list of drugs and drug categories reflects the collective thinking of all who provided input.

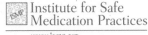 Institute for Safe Medication Practices

www.ismp.org

Verbal Orders

In most health care institutions, the nurse (or other authorized individual, such as a transcriptionist) can receive verbal orders either in person or by phone from licensed physicians or other practitioners who are licensed to prescribe. As the accrediting body for health care organizations and agencies, The Joint Commission (2011) annually publishes Patient Safety Goals. Goal 2 is designed to improve the effectiveness of communication among caregivers. It requires that the authorized individual receiving a verbal or telephone order first **write it down** in the patient's chart or enter it into the computer record; second, **read it back** to the prescriber; and third, **get confirmation** from the prescriber that it is correct. For the nurse to only repeat back the order as heard or repeat it while writing it down is not sufficient to regularly prevent errors, and this is not allowed by The Joint Commission. The order must first be **written** and then it must be **read back** after it is written to ensure that the order is clear to the recipient and in turn **confirmed** by the prescriber giving the order. As with written orders, the nurse must also verify that all seven parts of the verbal order have been included and are accurate. If the nurse has any question or concern about the order, it should be clarified during the conversation. Of course, The Joint Commission advises that in emergency situations, such as a code in the ER, doing a formal read-back would not be feasible and would compromise patient safety. In such cases, a repeat-back is acceptable.

CAUTION

Accepting verbal orders is a major responsibility and a situation that can readily lead to medication errors. Most health care institutions have policies concerning telephone or verbal orders, and the nurse or other authorized staff member should be informed of his or her responsibility in this regard.

▬▬▬▬ TRANSCRIPTION

One of the main causes of medication errors is incorrect *transcription* of the original prescriber's order. Many studies addressing the causes of medication errors identify one of the main sources to be illegible physician handwriting (Stetina et al., 2005). During the transcription process, the transcriber must ensure that the drug order includes all seven parts. If any of the components are absent or illegible, the nurse must obtain or clarify that information prior to signing off and implementing the order.

Further, The Joint Commission and the Institute for Safe Medication Practices have published lists of abbreviations, acronyms, and symbols to avoid in prescriptions and patient records because they have been common sources of errors and can be easily misinterpreted. The Joint Commission first published the Official "Do Not Use" List (Figure 9-2) in 2004 and required that health care organizations publish their own lists of abbreviations not to use. It suggested that there may be other abbreviations, acronyms, and symbols added to its list in the future (Figure 9-3) and referred health care organizations to the ISMP list of dangerous abbreviations relating to medication use. The ISMP recommends that these abbreviations, symbols, and dose designations be strictly prohibited when communicating medical information (Figure 9-4).

CAUTION

Stay alert to the guidelines and restrictions of The Joint Commission, the ISMP, and your own health care facility regarding abbreviations and medical notation. Acceptable medical communication is subject to abrupt change. Check the Websites listed at the end of this chapter often to stay up to date.

FIGURE 9-2   The Joint Commission's Official "Do Not Use" List of medical abbreviations, acronyms, and symbols

Official "Do Not Use" List[1]

Do Not Use	Potential Problem	Use Instead
U (unit)	Mistaken for "0" (zero), the number "4" (four) or "cc"	Write "unit"
IU (International Unit)	Mistaken for IV (intravenous) or the number 10 (ten)	Write "International Unit"
Q.D., QD, q.d., qd (daily)	Mistaken for each other	Write "daily"
Q.O.D., QOD, q.o.d, qod (every other day)	Period after the Q mistaken for "I" and the "O" mistaken for "I"	Write "every other day"
Trailing zero (X.0 mg)* Lack of leading zero (.X mg)	Decimal point is missed	Write X mg Write 0.X mg
MS	Can mean morphine sulfate or magnesium sulfate	Write "morphine sulfate" Write "magnesium sulfate"
MSO_4 and $MgSO_4$	Confused for one another	

[1] Applies to all orders and all medication-related documentation that is handwritten (including free-text computer entry) or on pre-printed forms.

*Exception: A "trailing zero" may be used only where required to demonstrate the level of precision of the value being reported, such as for laboratory results, imaging studies that report size of lesions, or catheter/tube sizes. It may not be used in medication orders or other medication-related documentation.

FIGURE 9-3   The Joint Commission's list of additional abbreviations, acronyms, and symbols

Additional Abbreviations, Acronyms and Symbols
(For possible future inclusion in the Official "Do Not Use" List)

Do Not Use	Potential Problem	Use Instead
> (greater than) < (less than)	Misinterpreted as the number "7" (seven) or the letter "L" Confused for one another	Write "greater than" Write "less than"
Abbreviations for drug names	Misinterpreted due to similar abbreviations for multiple drugs	Write drug names in full
Apothecary units	Unfamiliar to many practitioners Confused with metric units	Use metric units
@	Mistaken for the number "2" (two)	Write "at"
cc	Mistaken for U (units) when poorly written	Write "mL" or "ml" or "milliliters" ("mL" is preferred)
µg	Mistaken for mg (milligrams) resulting in one thousand-fold overdose	Write "mcg" or "micrograms"

FIGURE 9-4 ISMP's list of error-prone abbreviations, symbols, and dose designations

Institute for Safe Medication Practices

ISMP's List of *Error-Prone Abbreviations*, Symbols, and *Dose Designations*

The abbreviations, symbols, and dose designations found in this table have been reported to ISMP through the ISMP National Medication Errors Reporting Program (ISMP MERP) as being frequently misinterpreted and involved in harmful medication errors. They should **NEVER** be used when commu- nicating medical information. This includes internal communica- tions, telephone/verbal prescriptions, computer-generated labels, labels for drug storage bins, medication administration records, as well as pharmacy and prescriber computer order entry screens.

Abbreviations	Intended Meaning	Misinterpretation	Correction
μg	Microgram	Mistaken as "mg"	Use "mcg"
AD, AS, AU	Right ear, left ear, each ear	Mistaken as OD, OS, OU (right eye, left eye, each eye)	Use "right ear," "left ear," or "each ear"
OD, OS, OU	Right eye, left eye, each eye	Mistaken as AD, AS, AU (right ear, left ear, each ear)	Use "right eye," "left eye," or "each eye"
BT	Bedtime	Mistaken as "BID" (twice daily)	Use "bedtime"
cc	Cubic centimeters	Mistaken as "u" (units)	Use "mL"
D/C	Discharge or discontinue	Premature discontinuation of medications if D/C (intended to mean "discharge") has been misinterpreted as "discontinued" when followed by a list of discharge medications	Use "discharge" and "discontinue"
IJ	Injection	Mistaken as "IV" or "intrajugular"	Use "injection"
IN	Intranasal	Mistaken as "IM" or "IV"	Use "intranasal" or "NAS"
HS	Half-strength	Mistaken as bedtime	Use "half-strength" or "bedtime"
hs	At bedtime, hours of sleep	Mistaken as half-strength	
IU**	International unit	Mistaken as IV (intravenous) or 10 (ten)	Use "units"
o.d. or OD	Once daily	Mistaken as "right eye" (OD-oculus dexter), leading to oral liquid medications administered in the eye	Use "daily"
OJ	Orange juice	Mistaken as OD or OS (right or left eye); drugs meant to be diluted in orange juice may be given in the eye	Use "orange juice"
Per os	By mouth, orally	The "os" can be mistaken as "left eye" (OS-oculus sinister)	Use "PO," "by mouth," or "orally"
q.d. or QD**	Every day	Mistaken as q.i.d., especially if the period after the "q" or the tail of the "q" is misunderstood as an "i"	Use "daily"
qhs	Nightly at bedtime	Mistaken as "qhr" or every hour	Use "nightly"
qn	Nightly or at bedtime	Mistaken as "qh" (every hour)	Use "nightly" or "at bedtime"
q.o.d. or QOD**	Every other day	Mistaken as "q.d." (daily) or "q.i.d. (four times daily) if the "o" is poorly written	Use "every other day"
q1d	Daily	Mistaken as q.i.d. (four times daily)	Use "daily"
q6PM, etc.	Every evening at 6 PM	Mistaken as every 6 hours	Use "daily at 6 PM" or "6 PM daily"
SC, SQ, sub q	Subcutaneous	SC mistaken as SL (sublingual); SQ mistaken as "5 every;" the "q" in "sub q" has been mistaken as "every" (e.g., a heparin dose ordered "sub q 2 hours before surgery" misunderstood as every 2 hours before surgery)	Use "subcut" or "subcutaneously"
ss	Sliding scale (insulin) or ½ (apothecary)	Mistaken as "55"	Spell out "sliding scale;" use "one-half" or "½"
SSRI	Sliding scale regular insulin	Mistaken as selective-serotonin reuptake inhibitor	Spell out "sliding scale (insulin)"
SSI	Sliding scale insulin	Mistaken as Strong Solution of Iodine (Lugol's)	
i/d	One daily	Mistaken as "tid"	Use "1 daily"
TIW or tiw	3 times a week	Mistaken as "3 times a day" or "twice in a week"	Use "3 times weekly"
U or u**	Unit	Mistaken as the number 0 or 4, causing a 10-fold overdose or greater (e.g., 4U seen as "40" or 4u seen as "44"); mistaken as "cc" so dose given in volume instead of units (e.g., 4u seen as 4cc)	Use "unit"
UD	As directed ("ut dictum")	Mistaken as unit dose (e.g., diltiazem 125 mg IV infusion "UD" misin- terpreted as meaning to give the entire infusion as a unit [bolus] dose)	Use "as directed"
Dose Designations and Other Information	**Intended Meaning**	**Misinterpretation**	**Correction**
Trailing zero after decimal point (e.g., 1.0 mg)**	1 mg	Mistaken as 10 mg if the decimal point is not seen	Do not use trailing zeros for doses expressed in whole numbers
"Naked" decimal point (e.g., .5 mg)**	0.5 mg	Mistaken as 5 mg if the decimal point is not seen	Use zero before a decimal point when the dose is less than a whole unit
Abbreviations such as mg. or mL. with a period following the abbreviation	mg mL	The period is unnecessary and could be mistaken as the number 1 if written poorly	Use mg, mL, etc. without a terminal period

FIGURE 9-4 Continued

Institute for Safe Medication Practices

ISMP's List of *Error-Prone Abbreviations*, *Symbols*, and *Dose Designations* (continued)

Dose Designations and Other Information	Intended Meaning	Misinterpretation	Correction
Drug name and dose run together (especially problematic for drug names that end in "l" such as Inderal40 mg; Tegretol300 mg)	Inderal 40 mg Tegretol 300 mg	Mistaken as Inderal 140 mg Mistaken as Tegretol 1300 mg	Place adequate space between the drug name, dose, and unit of measure
Numerical dose and unit of measure run together (e.g., 10mg, 100mL)	10 mg 100 mL	The "m" is sometimes mistaken as a zero or two zeros, risking a 10- to 100-fold overdose	Place adequate space between the dose and unit of measure
Large doses without properly placed commas (e.g., 100000 units; 1000000 units)	100,000 units 1,000,000 units	100000 has been mistaken as 10,000 or 1,000,000; 1000000 has been mistaken as 100,000	Use commas for dosing units at or above 1,000, or use words such as 100 "thousand" or 1 "million" to improve readability

Drug Name Abbreviations	Intended Meaning	Misinterpretation	Correction
To avoid confusion, do not abbreviate drug names when communicating medical information. Examples of drug name abbreviations involved in medication errors include:			
ARA A	vidarabine	Mistaken as cytarabine (ARA C)	Use complete drug name
AZT	zidovudine (Retrovir)	Mistaken as azathioprine or aztreonam	Use complete drug name
CPZ	Compazine (prochlorperazine)	Mistaken as chlorpromazine	Use complete drug name
DPT	Demerol-Phenergan-Thorazine	Mistaken as diphtheria-pertussis-tetanus (vaccine)	Use complete drug name
DTO	Diluted tincture of opium, or deodorized tincture of opium (Paregoric)	Mistaken as tincture of opium	Use complete drug name
HCl	hydrochloric acid or hydrochloride	Mistaken as potassium chloride (The "H" is misinterpreted as "K")	Use complete drug name unless expressed as a salt of a drug
HCT	hydrocortisone	Mistaken as hydrochlorothiazide	Use complete drug name
HCTZ	hydrochlorothiazide	Mistaken as hydrocortisone (seen as HCT250 mg)	Use complete drug name
MgSO4**	magnesium sulfate	Mistaken as morphine sulfate	Use complete drug name
MS, MSO4**	morphine sulfate	Mistaken as magnesium sulfate	Use complete drug name
MTX	methotrexate	Mistaken as mitoxantrone	Use complete drug name
PCA	procainamide	Mistaken as patient controlled analgesia	Use complete drug name
PTU	propylthiouracil	Mistaken as mercaptopurine	Use complete drug name
T3	Tylenol with codeine No. 3	Mistaken as liothyronine	Use complete drug name
TAC	triamcinolone	Mistaken as tetracaine, Adrenalin, cocaine	Use complete drug name
TNK	TNKase	Mistaken as "TPA"	Use complete drug name
ZnSO4	zinc sulfate	Mistaken as morphine sulfate	Use complete drug name

Stemmed Drug Names	Intended Meaning	Misinterpretation	Correction
"Nitro" drip	nitroglycerin infusion	Mistaken as sodium nitroprusside infusion	Use complete drug name
"Norflox"	norfloxacin	Mistaken as Norflex	Use complete drug name
"IV Vanc"	intravenous vancomycin	Mistaken as Invanz	Use complete drug name

Symbols	Intended Meaning	Misinterpretation	Correction
℥	Dram	Symbol for dram mistaken as "3"	Use the metric system
♏	Minim	Symbol for minim mistaken as "mL"	
x3d	For three days	Mistaken as "3 doses"	Use "for three days"
> and <	Greater than and less than	Mistaken as opposite of intended; mistakenly use incorrect symbol; "< 10" mistaken as "40"	Use "greater than" or "less than"
/ (slash mark)	Separates two doses or indicates "per"	Mistaken as the number 1 (e.g., "25 units/10 units" misread as "25 units and 110" units)	Use "per" rather than a slash mark to separate doses
@	At	Mistaken as "2"	Use "at"
&	And	Mistaken as "2"	Use "and"
+	Plus or and	Mistaken as "4"	Use "and"
°	Hour	Mistaken as a zero (e.g., q2° seen as q 20)	Use "hr," "h," or "hour"

**These abbreviations are included on The Joint Commission's "minimum list" of dangerous abbreviations, acronyms, and symbols that must be included on an organization's "Do Not Use" list, effective January 1, 2004. Visit www.jointcommission.org for more information about this Joint Commission requirement.

© ISMP 2011. Permission is granted to reproduce material with proper attribution for internal use within healthcare organizations. Other reproduction is prohibited without written permission from ISMP. Report actual and potential medication errors to the ISMP National Medication Errors Reporting Program (ISMP MERP) via the Web at www.ismp.org or by calling 1-800-FAIL-SAF(E).

INSTITUTE FOR SAFE MEDICATION PRACTICES

www.ismp.org

Many health care institutions are utilizing a computerized physician/prescriber order entry (CPOE) system to help eliminate transcription sources of error. Physicians choose drug orders from a menu screen (Figure 9-5) and then choose the route and dosage strength offered on the following screen (Figure 9-6). These systems can also be implemented with clinical decision support systems (CDSS). The CDSS may include suggestions or default values for drug dosages, routes, and frequencies. The chance still exists that the order may be entered incorrectly, but the computer system does remove the variable of illegible handwriting and is known to foster a *safety culture*.

FIGURE 9-5 A CPOE menu screen allows the user to select a drug

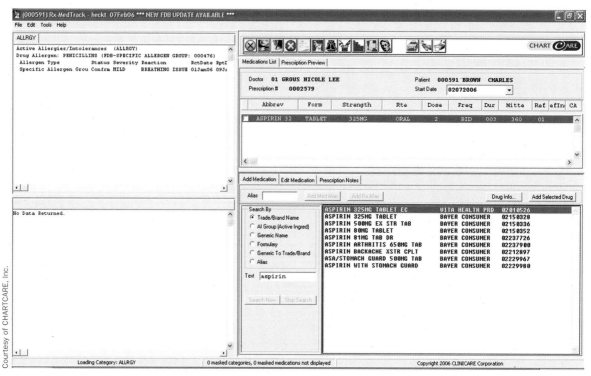

FIGURE 9-6 A CPOE offers options for route and dose of the drug chosen

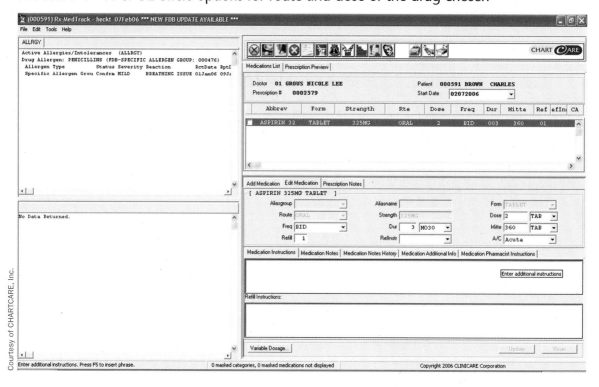

SAFE MEDICATION ADMINISTRATION

The Five Rights of medication administration *(right patient, right drug, right amount, right route, and right time)* have been the cornerstones for safe and effective nursing practice in the area of medication administration. A sixth right, *right documentation,* is often added to the list. These Six Rights were introduced in Chapter 7. Thoroughly and consistently following these rights can ensure that nurses administer medications safely.

> **REMEMBER**
> Nurses should refer to reputable drug reference resources to validate the safety of the medication as ordered and transcribed. Whoever administers a medication is legally responsible for patient safety. Any medication errors that result also fall under the responsibility of the person who administered the drug, regardless of the primary source of the error.

Right Patient

The administration of a medication to a patient other than the one for whom it was ordered is clearly an error. It is also one that should be easily prevented. Yet the literature shows this to be one of the three most common causes of medication errors. The failure of the nurse to accurately identify a patient is the most common cause for the error. The Joint Commission (2011) has a Patient Safety Goal to improve the accuracy of patient identification when administering medications. The Joint Commission requires that patients be identified with at least two unique person-specific identifiers (neither of which can be the patient's room number), such as name and date of birth or name and patient ID number. Electronic identification technology coding, such as barcoding, that includes two or more person-specific identifiers (not room number) will also comply. Basic nursing education emphasizes the importance of correctly identifying a patient prior to administering a medication, by comparing the two person-specific identifiers with the patient's arm band, medication administration record (MAR), or chart and by asking the patient to state his or her name (as a third identifier). Both steps should be consistently implemented regardless of the nurse's familiarity with the patient or the practice arena.

It is also wise to tell the patient at the time of administration what medication and dosage strength of the drug the nurse is administering. This extra step can often prevent errors, because patients who are familiar with their medications may spot an error or question a drug dosage. This is also an opportunity to engage the patient in medication teaching and learning. However, the nurse should never rely on this practice as the primary means to prevent errors. Instead, this is an extra precaution.

Technological advances in medication administration and documentation have included mechanisms to help prevent errors in this area. Computers installed at the patient's bedside and/or handheld devices that enable the nurse to scan the barcodes on the patient's identification band and on the medications serve as reinforcement to visual checks by the nurse. Few studies have been published in regard to the effectiveness of these systems in preventing errors. However, this additional mechanism to ensure correct patient identification increases efficiency, ensuring that the right patient receives the right drug. The health care industry has invested heavily in technology to help prevent costly medication errors caused by carelessness and distraction.

Right Drug

Nurses can ensure that the right drug criterion is maintained by checking the medication label against the order or MAR at three points during the administration process:

1. On first contact with the drug (removing it from the medication cart, drawer, or shelf).

2. Prior to measuring the drug (pouring, counting, or withdrawing the drug).

3. After preparing the drug, just prior to administration.

Distraction in the workplace has been identified as a key reason for error in obtaining the right drug (Pape, Guerra, Muzquiz, & Bryant, 2005). Nurses should take measures to ensure that they are not distracted during this phase of medication administration. Optimally, the physical workplace should provide for the nurse to move to an area without distractions. However, if this is not available, the nurse should be conscious of the need to focus solely on the task at hand and avoid the temptation to multi-task while dispensing medications.

In February 2004, the U.S. Food and Drug Administration (FDA) issued a regulation that requires all new pharmaceuticals to be barcoded upon launch into the market (FDA, 2006). Studies by U.S. Pharmacopeia in 2003 indicated that insulin products have the highest rates of error (Information Technology, 2005). Projections by the FDA indicate that barcoding on prescription drugs will reduce errors in the United States by 500,000 instances over the next 20 years, with estimated savings of $93 billion in additional health care costs, patient pain, and lost wages (FDA, 2004). This represents a 50% reduction in the medication errors that would otherwise occur without the use of barcoding (FDA, 2004).

Barcodes on drugs are used with a barcode-scanning system and computerized database. At a minimum, the code must contain the drug's National Drug Code. This number uniquely identifies the drug. The process starts as a patient enters the hospital and is given a barcoded patient identification band. The hospital has barcode scanners that are linked to the hospital's electronic medical records system. Before a health care worker administers a medication, he or she scans the patient's barcode, which allows the computer to access the patient's medical records. The health care worker then scans each drug prior to administration. This notifies the computer of each medication to be administered. The information is compared to the patient's database to ensure a match. If there is a problem, the health care worker receives an error message and investigates the problem.

Nurses are responsible for being knowledgeable about the actions, indications, and contraindications of the medications they administer. The constant changes that are occurring in health care delivery and the steady influx of new medications being released into the market have challenged the individual nurse's ability to meet this responsibility. A valid and current drug-reference system should be available in every practice setting. The nurse should not hesitate to seek information about any medication that is unfamiliar. The prescribing clinician should be contacted for clarification or confirmation for any medication order that appears inappropriate or incorrect.

Automated dispensing cabinets (ADCs) (Figure 9-7) have been utilized in many health care settings since the 1980s and are now used in the majority of hospitals. There are many safety measures in place with the use of this technology, but the possibility still exists that the patient may receive the wrong medication. It is important that the correct medication be stocked by the pharmacy in the correct location within the ADC to avoid mistakes in drug selection (ISMP, 2008a). In a survey conducted by the ISMP (2008b), nurses reported that at least half of the ADCs were not located in areas free from distractions. Nurses also reported that they always or frequently wait in line to access the ADC, and one-third of the respondents indicated that they often remove multiple patients' medications at a time. This identified "workaround" is known to lead to drug administration errors. Recognizing that few resources exist to guide health care organizations in the safest use of this technology, the ISMP has developed and posted guidelines that include 12 interdisciplinary core processes for safe use of automated dispensing cabinets.

CAUTION

When medications are distributed with automated dispensing cabinets, follow the ISMP *Core Processes* for safe ADC use (ISMP, 2008a).

1. Provide ideal environmental conditions for the use of ADCs

2. Ensure ADC system security

3. Use pharmacy-profiled ADCs

4. Identify and include information that should appear on the ADC screen

5. Select and maintain proper ADC inventory

6. Select appropriate ADC configuration (e.g., lidded compartments are preferred to matrix drawers)

7. Define and implement safe ADC restocking processes

8. Develop procedures to ensure the accurate withdrawal of medications from the ADC

9. Establish strict criteria for ADC system overrides

10. Standardize processes for transporting medications from the ADC to the patient's bedside

11. Eliminate the process for returning medications directly to their original ADC location

12. Provide staff education and competency validation

FIGURE 9-7 The Pyxis MedStation® is an example of an automated dispensing cabinet (ADC) system

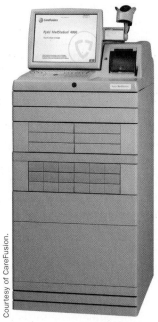

Courtesy of CareFusion.

(a) Pyxis MedStation System®

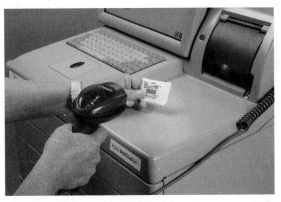

(b) Pyxis Barcode Scanner®

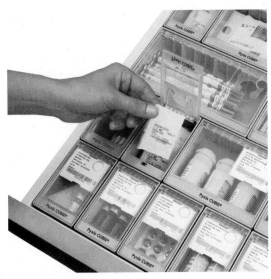

(c) Pyxis CUBIE System®

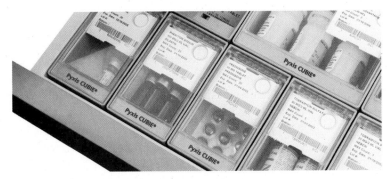

(d) Pyxis CUBIE System®

In addition, nurses who practice in a setting utilizing this technology should continue to implement the three checks described at the beginning of this section to avoid administering the wrong drug: during retrieval, preparation, and administration. Review the information about reading drug labels in Chapter 8 to ensure that all of the important information is confirmed.

A common preventable medication error is interchanging look-alike/sound-alike (LASA) medication pairs—prescribing and administering one for the other. The Joint Commission (2011) Patient Safety Goal 3 addresses this issue and posts online an extensive list of LASA medications that pose the greatest risk for medication errors, including drugs such as ephedrine and epinephrine, hydromorphone injection and morphine injection, hydroxyzine and hydralazine, OxyContin (controlled release) and oxycodone (immediate release). Hospitals are independently required to list at least 10 look-alike/sound-alike drug pairs commonly prescribed and administered in their institution for their caregivers to monitor. A survey conducted by the Institute for Safe Medication Practices (ISMP, 2009a) indicated that compliance with The Joint Commission National Patient Safety Goal 3 for LASA drugs has been high, with rates of at least 95% for hospitals. Yet 27% of staff nurses responding were still uncertain whether their organization maintained a list of LASA drug name pairs. To reduce the risk of errors, all clinical staff, but especially nurses administering medications, must know the hospital's list of LASA drugs and its importance to patient safety.

The ISMP and the Food and Drug Administration (FDA) also suggest the use of "Tall Man" lettering to differentiate drugs with look-alike names (ISMP, 2010b). Using this method, the drug name is highlighted by various means such as uppercase letters, colors, bolding, and italics to call attention to the dissimilarities between look-alike drug names; the FDA-approved Tall Man list is shown in Figure 9-8. Tall Man lettering is being used in many hospitals on computerized physician/prescriber order entry (CPOE) screens, automated dispensing cabinet (ADC) screens, computer-generated medication administration records (MARs), computer-generated pharmacy labels, preprinted standard orders, and medication shelf labels.

The Joint Commission (2011) National Patient Safety Goal 8 addresses the practice of reconciling the right medications across the continuum of care, beginning with admission and following the patient through transfers within the health care facility (such as from a hospital intensive care unit to a medical floor) and back home or to a long-term care facility. A complete list of current medications the patient is taking at home (including dosage, route, and frequency) is created and documented upon admission, ideally before prescribing any new medications. The medications ordered for the patient while under care are compared to this list and discrepancies are reconciled and documented. Likewise, when the patient is transferred to another unit within the hospital or to another facility, or discharged to home, the up-to-date, reconciled medication list is communicated and documented. Strict adherence to these standards will prevent many medication errors of transcription, omission, duplication, and drug interactions.

Right Amount

Illegible prescriber's handwriting, transcription error, miscalculation of the amount, or misreading of the label can result in errors involving the administration of an incorrect dose of a medication. The need for each nurse to carefully read and clarify drug orders and recheck drug labels has been previously discussed. Two nurses must check some potent high-alert drugs, such as insulin or heparin, which are common sources of errors. Transcription errors involving dosage can be avoided if nurses consult drug references to confirm the dosage of medications when they are in doubt. The Joint Commission's Official "Do Not Use" List (Figure 9-2) will also help eliminate dosage problems for those medications ordered daily, ordered every other day, or measured in units.

While medication errors are known to be the most common type of medical error in general, the risk of harm from dosage errors is a significant risk in the pediatric population. Increased caution must be taken when administering medication to children because of the greater frequency of weight-based dosage calculations, fractional dosage, and the need for decimal points in calculations (The Joint Commission, 2008b).

FIGURE 9-8 FDA-approved list of generic drug names with Tall Man letters

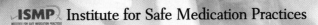

ISMP Institute for Safe Medication Practices

FDA and ISMP Lists of
Look-Alike Drug Names with Recommended Tall Man Letters

FDA-Approved List of Generic Drug Names with Tall Man Letters	
Drug Name with Tall Man Letters	**Confused with**
acetaZOLAMIDE	acetoHEXAMIDE
acetoHEXAMIDE	acetaZOLAMIDE
buPROPion	busPIRone
busPIRone	buPROPion
chlorproMAZINE	chlorproPAMIDE
chlorproPAMIDE	chlorproMAZINE
clomiPHENE	clomiPRAMINE
clomiPRAMINE	clomiPHENE
cycloSERINE	cycloSPORINE
cycloSPORINE	cycloSERINE
DAUNOrubicin	DOXOrubicin
dimenhyDRINATE	diphenhydrAMINE
diphenhydrAMINE	dimenhyDRINATE
DOBUTamine	DOPamine
DOPamine	DOBUTamine
DOXOrubicin	DAUNOrubicin
glipiZIDE	glyBURIDE
glyBURIDE	glipiZIDE
hydrALAZINE	hydrOXYzine
hydrOXYzine	hydrALAZINE
medroxyPROGESTERone	methylPREDNISolone - methylTESTOSTERone
methylPREDNISolone	medroxyPROGESTERone - methylTESTOSTERone
methylTESTOSTERone	medroxyPROGESTERone - methylPREDNISolone
niCARdipine	NIFEdipine
NIFEdipine	niCARdipine
prednisoLONE	predniSONE
predniSONE	prednisoLONE
sulfADIAZINE	sulfiSOXAZOLE
sulfiSOXAZOLE	sulfADIAZINE
TOLAZamide	TOLBUTamide
TOLBUTamide	TOLAZamide
vinBLAStine	vinCRIStine
vinCRIStine	vinBLAStine

Ensuring that the patient receives the right amount when administering parenteral fluids is equally important. Electronic infusion pumps have enabled nurses to have greater control over the rate of infusion of intravenous solutions and medications, thereby reducing medication errors. The newest innovation with infusion pumps is the Smart Pump, which is equipped with computer software that includes a library of medications and dosage guidelines (ISMP, 2009b). Other infusion pumps, such as the patient-controlled analgesia (PCA) pump and the insulin pump, have enabled patients to be active participants in their own care (FDA, 2010a). Although infusion pump technology has increased administration safety, one cannot rely fully on these devices. Because electronic infusion pumps are primarily used for patients who require a precise delivery of fluids or critical medications, errors can result in serious consequences to the patient. Recently, the Food and Drug Administration (FDA) has become greatly concerned with the number of adverse events associated with the use of infusion pumps. Some of these events are attributed to user error, while others have been associated with pump malfunction. The FDA Infusion Pump Improvement Initiative (2010b) addresses infusion pump safety problems. Along with establishing additional safety requirements for infusion pump manufacturers, the FDA is increasing user awareness with a new infusion pump Website (http://www.fda.gov/MedicalDevices/ProductsandMedicalProcedures/GeneralHospitalDevicesandSupplies/InfusionPumps/default.htm). It is the responsibility of the nurse to be trained on the proper use of infusion pumps and to be watchful for potential problems associated with emerging technologies.

Teaching effective dosage calculation methods is the main purpose of this text. The need for each nurse to estimate the correct dosage prior to calculating the exact amount is stressed throughout the book. The inclusion of this commonsense approach to calculating dosages is crucial in preventing errors in dosage calculation. Calculating, preparing, and administering the wrong dose of a drug are preventable medication errors. Full attention to accurate dosage calculations will ensure that you avoid such liabilities.

Right Route

Errors involving the route of medication administration can occur for several reasons. One of the most common problems has already been addressed: that of illegible prescriber's handwriting. Another common error relates to the nurse's knowledge of medications and their dosage forms. Nurses are usually familiar with medications commonly ordered and administered in their area of practice, but the nurse should consult a drug information source to confirm that the correct route is ordered for an unfamiliar medication, particularly in regard to injectable forms of medications.

Nurses should also be alert to the need to change or clarify administration forms or routes for the patient receiving medication through a feeding tube, such as a nasogastric or surgically inserted gastric tube. Medication errors related to this route of administration may occur due to administering multiple medications that are incompatible, preparing the medications improperly, or using improper administration techniques (ISMP, 2010d). Sometimes the patient may not be allowed any oral intake (NPO status) or may have a nasogastric tube but the medications are ordered for oral administration. Prescribers may order time-released or enteric-coated medications to be administered via a feeding tube but not realize that medications must be crushed or dissolved to be administered. The Institute for Safe Medication Practices (2010e) provides a comprehensive drug list of oral dosage forms that should not be crushed, including the rationale for the restriction. Such situations require the nurse to contact the prescriber for a change in the medication form or route or to seek clarification for the drug to be administered safely and correctly. Enteral infusion pumps are often used to administer liquid nutrients and medications by the gastrointestinal route. These pumps may be used with patients who also have intravenous infusion pumps or other pumps in place. Serious adverse events as a result of misconnections of tubing have been reported due to a mix-up with electronic infusion devices as well as tubing regulated by manual devices (The Joint Commission, 2006). To ensure that the patient receives the ordered medication by the right route, it is recommended that the tube or catheter from the patient be traced to the point of origin before connecting any new device or infusion. Additionally, a "line reconciliation" should be conducted to recheck connections and trace all patient tubes and catheters to their sources upon a patient's arrival at a new setting as part of the handoff process (The Joint Commission, 2006). It is the nurse's responsibility to be alert to potential errors of all kinds that may interfere with patient safety and rights.

Right Time

Medication orders should include the frequency with which a drug is to be administered or the specific administration schedule. Computerized hospital drug administration systems automatically indicate these times on the medication administration record. The nurse is responsible for checking these records to be sure they are accurate. For example, a physician writes an order for an antibiotic to be given q.i.d., or 4 times a day. The computer system might transcribe these times to 9:00 AM, 1:00 PM, 5:00 PM, and 9:00 PM. The nurse should recognize that an antibiotic should be administered at regular intervals around the clock so that the 4 doses would be 6 hours apart. The right time for the order should have been q.6h or *every 6 hours*. The nurse should contact the physician to clarify the order.

The Joint Commission has recognized the problem of misinterpretation of time and frequency in medication orders. It has taken steps to prevent common errors in regard to the time a drug is to be administered, by prohibiting the use of some abbreviations related to dosing frequency (Figure 9-2). For example, the notation to give a drug q.d. has frequently been transcribed as q.i.d., with the period being mistaken for an *i*, resulting in a daily medication being administered four times a day instead of once daily.

Right Documentation

The last step in medication administration is correct documentation. The policy in most institutions directs nurses to administer a medication prior to documentation. Numerous studies indicate that fatigue and lack of time are factors that contribute to medication errors. Nurses who prioritize their time may find that they give medications correctly but fail to document that they have done so. This omission can result in unintentional overmedication of the patient when the follow-on nurse responds as though the drug was not given. Many of the new ADCs document drug administration at the time the drug is removed from the machine. This ensures that administration is documented, but an error occurs if the patient does not take the medication. In that situation, the nurse must follow the institution's policy for clarifying or deleting the initial documentation. Often, this is a time-consuming process, but if omitted, it can result in undermedication of the patient.

THE NURSE'S CRITICAL ROLE IN MEDICATION ERROR PREVENTION

As the largest segment of the health care workforce, nurses are essential to reducing medication errors and improving patient outcomes. In the Institute of Medicine (2006) landmark report, *Preventing Medication Errors*, the most effective way to reduce errors was identified as a partnership between patients and their health care providers. Communication between nurses and patients should be open, with nurses not only talking to patients, but listening to them as well. To this end, The Joint Commission (2002) launched a Speak Up™ campaign to urge patients to take a larger role in preventing errors by becoming more active participants in their care. When administering medications, nurses should be prepared for and encourage patients' questions. By way of brochures, buttons, and posters displayed in health care facilities, patients are instructed to use six strategies to avoid medication mistakes at the hospital or clinic (Figure 9-9).

FIGURE 9-9   The Joint Commission Speak Up™ Program—Tips for patients to reduce medication errors

Speak UP™

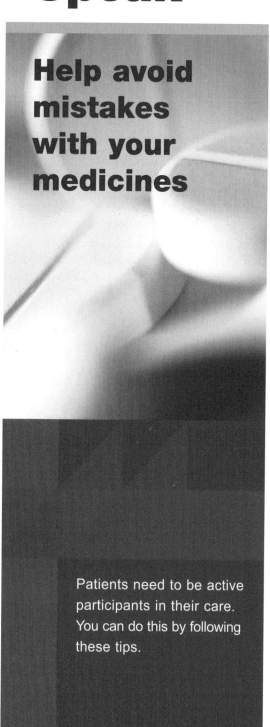

Help avoid mistakes with your medicines

Patients need to be active participants in their care. You can do this by following these tips.

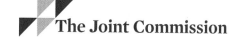
The Joint Commission

A lot of people are responsible for your medicine—including you!

☐ Check all of your medicines with your doctor to make sure they are OK to take together.

☐ Check with your pharmacist to see if there are other medicines, foods or drinks you should not take with your new medicines. This helps to avoid a bad reaction.

☐ Give your doctors, pharmacists and other caregivers a list of all your medicines. This list should have your

    prescription medicines
    over-the-counter medicines (for example, aspirin)
    vitamins
    herbs
    diet supplements
    natural remedies
    recreational drugs
    amount of alcohol you drink each day or week

Check your medicines and ask questions

☐ Make sure you can read the handwriting on the prescription. If you can't read it, the pharmacist may not be able to read it. Ask to have the prescription printed.

☐ Read the label. Make sure it has your name on it and the right medicine name.

☐ Understand all of the instructions for your medicines.

☐ If you have doubts about a medicine, ask your doctor, pharmacist or caregiver about it.

☐ Call your doctor or pharmacist if you forget the instructions for taking a medicine.

☐ Don't be afraid to ask questions about any of your medicines.

How to avoid medicine mistakes at the hospital or clinic

☐ Make sure your doctors, nurses and other caregivers check your wristband and ask your name before giving you medicine. Sometimes patients get a medicine that was supposed to go to another patient.

☐ Don't be afraid to tell a caregiver if you think you are about to get the wrong medicine.

☐ Know what time you should get a medicine. If you don't get it then, speak up.

☐ Tell your caregiver if you don't feel well after taking a medicine. Ask for help immediately if you think you are having a bad reaction.

☐ You may be given IV (intravenous) fluids. Read the bag to find out what is in it. Ask the caregiver how long it should take for the liquid to run out. Tell the caregiver if it's dripping too fast or too slow.

☐ Get a list of your medicines—including your new ones. Read the list carefully. Make sure it lists everything you are taking. If you're not well enough to do this, ask a friend or relative to help.

The goal of the Speak Up™ program is to help patients become more informed and involved in their health care.

Additionally, the number of medication errors may be reduced by making greater use of information technologies when prescribing and administering medications. Nurses cannot be expected to keep up with all the relevant information on all the medications they administer. Using point-of-care reference information provided with the electronic medical record or by automated dispensing units, the Internet, or downloaded content on personal digital assistants (PDAs) will enhance the nurse's ability to apply critical reasoning when making judgments related to medication administration. Yet, while technological interventions such as smart infusion pumps, patient-controlled analgesia, computerized physician/provider order entry (CPOE), automated dispensing cabinets (ADCs), automated medication dispensing machines (AMDMs), electronic medical records (EMRs), and barcoding identification have contributed to improved patient care, there is considerable data on incidences of adverse events while using these tools (The Joint Commission, 2008a). As health technologies are increasingly adopted by health care organizations, nurses must be mindful of the safety risks and preventable adverse events that these new innovations may bring about. Still, some nurses will be involved in medication errors and they must be aware of the appropriate response. Whenever a medication error is identified, the nurse must follow the health organization's procedure for reporting. This enables organizations to track errors and implement improvement processes aimed at preventing repeat errors. Organizations have also been encouraged to have specific plans in place in order to guide health providers in the appropriate manner to disclose harmful errors to patients and family members (ISMP, 2006). Many organizations have participated in the Medication Errors Reporting Program (MERP), a confidential national voluntary reporting program. The ISMP publishes *Medication Safety Alerts* that provide vital information about medication and device errors and adverse drug reactions (ISMP, 2010a). Nurses may also receive a monthly safety newsletter, *ISMP Medication Safety Alert! Nurse Advise-ERR*, specifically designed to meet the needs of frontline nurses who are actively involved with medication administration (ISMP, 2010c). Another source for error-prevention advice, provided on the Website of The Joint Commission (2008b), is the *Sentinel Event Alert*, which includes reduction strategies for sentinel events that occur with significant frequency.

Throughout this text there are **Clinical Reasoning Skills** that require critical thinking. They are designed to alert you to common medication errors and to practice how to prevent them. Combating errors requires diligent adherence to safety standards prescribed by organizations such as The Joint Commission, the Institute of Medicine, the Institute for Safe Medication Practices, and your health care agency. Stay alert by practicing the *Six Rights of Safe Medication Administration*, regularly reading prevention publications, and spotting and reporting medication errors.

SUMMARY

In conclusion, medication administration is a critical nursing skill that can lead to costly errors, morbidity, and death if not carried out correctly. It is the nurse's responsibility to ensure that the right patient receives the right drug, in the right amount, by the right route, at the right time, and with the right documentation. The nurse who administers a medication is legally liable for medication errors whether the primary cause was an unsafe order, an incorrect transcription, a wrong drug, an inaccurate dosage calculation, an improper preparation, or an administration error.

Review Set 21

1. What are the six patient rights of safe medication administration?

_____

2. Using The Joint Commission's Official "Do Not Use" List, correct the notations in the following medication order: NPH insulin 20.0 U SC qd

_____

3. Safe medication administration requires that you check the drug against the order three times:

   1) when you first make contact with the drug (such as removing it from the medication drawer),

   2) when you measure it, and 3) _____.

4. Give two examples of acceptable patient identification according to The Joint Commission, using two unique person-specific identifiers.

_____.

5. True or False? The nurse who administers a drug based on an incorrect or unsafe medication order shares legal liability for patient injury that results from that drug. _____.

6. According to the Institute of Medicine landmark report, *Preventing Medication Errors,* what strategy is the most effective way to reduce errors?

   a. partnership between the patient and health care providers

   b. double-checking insulin dosage

   c. checking medications three times

   d. safe use of prescribing, dispensing, and recording technologies

   e. strict adherence to "Do Not Use" lists of abbreviations, symbols, and acronyms

7. Identify one common "workaround" known to lead to drug administration errors during the use of an automated dispensing cabinet (ADC). _____.

8. Where are the two barcodes located that are scanned during medication administration? _____

_____.

9. Name four drugs or drug categories that have the highest risk of causing injuries when errors are made. How are these drugs designated? _____

_____.

10. To ensure the accuracy of the order, what nursing actions should you implement following the receipt of a verbal or telephone order from a licensed prescribing practitioner?

_____.

After completing these problems, see page 603 to check your answers.

CLINICAL REASONING SKILLS

It is important for the nurse to check the label on each medication administered, regardless of the medication dispensing mechanism.

ERROR

Failing to check the medication label.

Possible Scenario

Suppose a physician orders 40 mg of Lasix (a diuretic) for an adult with congestive heart failure. The Lasix is supplied in 20 mg tablets. The nurse plans to administer 2 tablets and use an automated medication dispensing machine. The nurse chooses the correct medication from the computer screen. The medication drawer, which should contain the medication, opens. The nurse removes 2 tablets without reading the label, goes to the patient's room, and administers the medication. The medication the nurse removed was Lanoxin 0.25 mg tablets (a cardiac glycoside). The pharmacy technician incorrectly stocked the medication drawer.

Potential Outcome

Although the patient has an order for Lanoxin 0.25 mg daily, he had already received his dose for the day. At this point, he has received three times the correct amount. He becomes nauseated, and when the nurse checks his pulse, it is 40 beats per minute. The nurse notifies the doctor of the change in the patient's condition. As the one who administered the incorrect medication, the nurse clearly shares responsibility for the medication error.

Prevention

The nurse should read the label on each medication and compare it to the order or MAR three times before administering the drug. If the nurse had checked the label as the drug was removed from the medication drawer, the error could have been prevented. And the nurse had two more opportunities to prevent this error: prior to calculating the dose (the amount should have been 40 mg, not 0.25 mg) and prior to administering the medication.

CLINICAL REASONING SKILLS

The nurse should ensure that the medication ordered can be administered by the right route.

ERROR

Opening a time-released capsule and administering it through a nasogastric tube.

Possible Scenario

Suppose a patient is hospitalized to treat a stroke. The physician's orders state to continue all of the patient's home medications. One of the medications is theophylline 100 mg, to be administered daily as a 24-hour extended-release capsule (Theo-24) for the treatment of asthma. The patient is unable to swallow as a result of the stroke, and all of his medications must be given through his nasogastric tube. The nurse opens the capsule and dissolves the contents in water and administers it via the nasogastric tube. The patient begins complaining of palpitations, and his pulse increases to 180 beats per minute. The nurse evaluates the changes in the patient's condition and realizes the error.

Potential Outcome

The physician would be notified of the error, and a peak level of theophylline would be ordered. If the patient had a history of cardiac problems, the sympathetic stimulation caused by the theophylline could result in anginal pain or an acute myocardial infarction. The patient would be treated symptomatically until his theophylline blood levels returned to therapeutic range.

Prevention

The nurse should have recognized that a time-released medication could not safely be administered through a nasogastric tube. The physician should have been contacted to obtain orders for a different dosage form of the medication.

PRACTICE PROBLEMS—CHAPTER 9

1. Which of the following statements is/are true?

   a) Statistics show that 5% of all hospital injuries are attributable to medication errors.

   b) According to the Institute of Medicine, most medication errors occur during the administration step of the medication process.

c) A nurse with more experience and education is less likely to make medication errors.

d) The medication delivery process involves many individuals and departments.

e) c and d

2. True or False? Studies indicate that nurses' education and years of practice are closely correlated to the incidence of medication errors. _____

3. True or False? Ten percent (10%) to 18% of patient injuries are attributable to preventable medication errors. _____

4. True or False? Administering a drug late is a frequently underreported medication error. _____

5. True or False? Illegible prescriber's handwriting is a major contributor to transcription errors. _____

6. Fill in the blanks of the following statement. "The right _____ must receive the right _____ in the right _____ by the right _____ at the right _____, followed by the right _____."

7. What are the three steps of medication administration?

_____

8. The nurse can ensure that the patient receives the right drug by checking the drug label three times. When should the nurse perform these label checks?

_____

9. Which of the following medical notations is (are) written in the recommended format?
0.75 mg .2 cm q.d. _____

10. Describe a nursing action to prevent medication errors when receiving verbal drug orders.

_____

11. Cite four of the direct and/or indirect costs of medication errors.

_____

12. Describe the strategy or strategies you would implement to prevent this potential medication error.

Possible Scenario

Suppose the physician writes the following order: Dilacor XR 240 mg p.o. q.d.

The order is transcribed as *Dilacor XR 240 mg p.o. q.i.d.,* and the medication is scheduled for administration at 0600, 1200, 1800, and 2400 on the medication administration record.

The nurse reviews the order prior to obtaining the medication for administration. The nurse notices the XR following the name of the medication and recognizes that the letters usually indicate a sustained-release form of medication. The nurse consults the current *AHFS Drug Information* resource and finds that the drug is a sustained-release formula and is only to be given once daily. The nurse reviews the original orders and notes that there was a transcription error. The medication administration record is corrected, and the patient receives the correct amount of medication at the correct time.

Potential Outcome

Had the nurse administered the medication at each of the times indicated on the medication administration record, the patient would have received four times the intended dosage. The drug's therapeutic effect is a decrease in the cardiac output and decrease in blood pressure. However, the toxic effects caused by overdosing could have resulted in congestive heart failure. The patient's life would have been jeopardized.

Prevention

_____

_____

After completing these questions, see page 603 to check your answers.

For additional practice, visit the online practice software at www.CengageBrain.com, using the Premium Website access code found in the front of your text.

REFERENCES

Information Technology: Drug company announces individual bar coding on all insulin vials [Electronic version]. *Medical Letter on the CDC & FDA*, March 13, 2005.

Institute for Safe Medication Practices. (2006). Medication safety alert. Harmful errors: How will your facility respond? Retrieved December 4, 2010, from http://www.ismp.org/Newsletters/acutecare/articles/20061005.asp

Institute for Safe Medication Practices. (2008a). Guidance on the interdisciplinary safe use of automated dispensing cabinets. Retrieved December 14, 2010, from http://www.ismp.org/Tools/guidelines/ADC_Guidelines_Final.pdf

Institute for Safe Medication Practices. (2008b). Medication safety alert. ADC survey shows some improvements, but unnecessary risks still exist. Retrieved December 14, 2010, from http://www.ismp.org/Newsletters/acutecare/articles/20080117.asp

Institute for Safe Medication Practices. (2009a). Medication safety alert. Survey on LASA drug name pairs. Retrieved December 14, 2010, from http://www.ismp.org/Newsletters/acutecare/articles/20090521.asp

Institute for Safe Medication Practices. (2009b). Proceedings from the ISMP summit on the use of smart infusion pumps: Guidelines for safe implementation and use. Retrieved December 12, 2010, from http://www.ismp.org/tools/guidelines/smartpumps/printerVersion.pdf

Institute for Safe Medication Practices. (2010a). Medication safety alerts. Retrieved December 4, 2010, from http://www.ismp.org/Newsletters/acutecare/default.asp

Institute for Safe Medication Practices. (2010b). Medication safety alert. ISMP updates its list of drug name pairs with TALL Man Letters. Retrieved December 14, 2010, from http://www.ismp.org/Newsletters/acutecare/articles/20101118.asp

Institute for Safe Medication Practices. (2010c). Medication safety alert. Nurse Advise-ERR. Retrieved December 4, 2010, from http://www.ismp.org/Newsletters/nursing/default.asp

Institute for Safe Medication Practices. (2010d). Medication safety alert. Preventing errors when administering drugs via an enteral feeding tube. Retrieved December 12, 2010, from http://www.ismp.org/Newsletters/acutecare/articles/20100506.asp

Institute for Safe Medication Practices. (2010e). J. F. Mitchell, PharmD. ISMP Tool, Oral forms that should not be crushed. Retrieved December 12, 2010, from http://www.ismp.org/Tools/DoNotCrush.pdf

Institute of Medicine. (2006). Report Brief—Preventing medication errors. Retrieved December 4, 2010, from http://www.iom.edu/~/media/Files/Report%20Files/2006/Preventing-Medication-Errors-Quality-Chasm-Series/medicationerrorsnew.pdf

The Joint Commission. (1999). Sentinel event alert, Issue 11. High-alert medications and patient safety. Retrieved December 14, 2010, from http://www.jointcommission.org/assets/1/18/SEA_11.pdf

The Joint Commission. (2002). Facts about Speak Up initiatives. Retrieved December 4, 2010, from http://www.jointcommission.org/assets/1/6/Speak%20Up_initiatives_11_%2009.pdf

The Joint Commission. (2006). Sentinel event alert, Issue 36. Tubing misconnections—A persistent and potentially deadly occurrence. Retrieved December 12, 2010, from http://www.jointcommission.org/assets/1/18/SEA_36.PDF

The Joint Commission. (2008a). Sentinel event alert, Issue 42. Safely implementing health information and converging technologies. Retrieved December 4, 2010, from http://www.jointcommission.org/assets/1/18/SEA_42.PDF

The Joint Commission. (2008b). Sentinel event alert, Issue 39. Preventing pediatric medication errors. Retrieved December 14, 2010, from http://www.jointcommission.org/assets/1/18/SEA_39.PDF

The Joint Commission. (2011). National patient safety goals. Retrieved January 11, 2011, from http://www.jointcommission.org/standards_information/npsgs.aspx

Mayo, A. M., & Duncan, D. (2004). Nurse perceptions of medication errors: What we need to know for patient safety [Electronic version]. *Journal of Nursing Quality Care, 19*, 3.

Pape, T. M., Guerra, D. M., Muzquiz, M., & Bryant, J. B. (2005). Innovative approaches to reducing nurses' distractions during medication administration. *Journal of Continuing Nursing Education, 36*, 3.

Stetina, P., Groves, M., & Pafford, L. (2005). Managing medication errors—A qualitative study. *Medsurg Nursing, 14*, 3.

U.S. Food and Drug Administration (FDA). (2004). FDA issues bar code regulation. Retrieved May 6, 2006, from http://www.fda.gov/oc/initiates/barcode-sadr/fs-barcode.html

U.S. Food and Drug Administration (FDA). (2006). Guidance for industry: Bar code label requirements. Retrieved December 16, 2010, from http://www.fda.gov/downloads/Drugs/GuidanceCompliance RegulatoryInformation/Guidances/ucm070259.pdf

U.S. Food and Drug Administration (FDA). (2010a). Infusion pumps. Retrieved December 12, 2010, from http://www.fda.gov/MedicalDevices/ProductsandMedicalProcedures/GeneralHospitalDevices andSupplies/InfusionPumps/default.htm

U.S. Food and Drug Administration (FDA). (2010b). Infusion pump improvement initiative. Retrieved December 12, 2010, from http://www.fda.gov/downloads/MedicalDevices/ProductsandMedical Procedures/GeneralHospitalDevicesandSupplies/InfusionPumps/UCM206189.pdf

Wolf, Z. R., & Serembus, J. F. (2004). Medication errors: Ending the blame game. *Nursing Management, 35*, 8.

SECTION 2 SELF-EVALUATION

Directions

1. Round decimals to two places. Round temperatures to one decimal place.

2. Reduce fractions to lowest terms.

Chapter 3—Systems of Measurement

Express the following amounts in proper medical notation.

1. six-tenths gram   _____

2. four teaspoons   _____

3. two hundred fifty thousand units   _____

4. one-half milliliter   _____

5. one-half fluid ounce   _____

Interpret the following notations.

6. 4 gtt   _____

7. 0.25 mg   _____

8. 125 mcg   _____

9. 2 T   _____

10. 0.25 L   _____

Chapters 4 and 5—Conversions

Convert each of the following to the equivalent units indicated.

11. 350 mcg   =   _____ mg   =   _____ g

12. 1.2 g   =   _____ mg   =   _____ mcg

13. 4 T   =   _____ t   =   _____ mL

14. 5 fl oz   =   _____ mL   =   _____ L

15. 56 oz   =   _____ lb   =   _____ kg

16. 56.2 mm   =   _____ cm   =   _____ in

17. 198 lb   =   _____ kg   =   _____ g

18. 11.59 kg   =   _____ g   =   _____ lb

19. A patient is told to take $\frac{1}{2}$ t of a medication. What is the equivalent dose amount in milliliters? _____ mL

20. A patient is being treated for an infection with two 250 mg tablets of cephalexin four times daily for 10 days. How many grams will he receive in the total dose amount over 10 days? _____ g

21. A full-term infant that weighs less than 2,500 g at birth is considered small for gestational age (SGA). Would a full-term infant with a birth weight of 6 lb 4 oz be SGA? _____

22. Your patient drinks the following for breakfast: 3 fl oz orange juice, 8 fl oz coffee with 1 fl oz cream, and 4 fl oz water. Your patient's total fluid intake is _____ mL.

Convert the following times as indicated. Designate AM or PM where needed.

Traditional Time	International Time
23. 11:35 PM	_____
24. _____	1844
25. 8:03 AM	_____

Convert the following temperatures as indicated.

26. 38°C   _____ °F

27. _____ °C   101.5°F

28. 37.2°C   _____ °F

Chapter 6—Equipment Used in Dosage Measurement

Draw an arrow to demonstrate the correct measurement of the doses given.

29. 1.5 mL

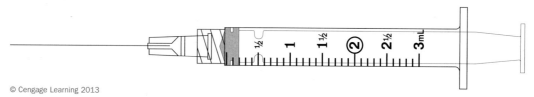

© Cengage Learning 2013

30. 0.33 mL

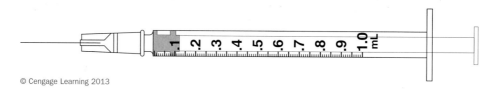

© Cengage Learning 2013

31. 44 units U-100 insulin

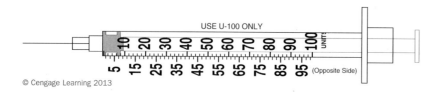

© Cengage Learning 2013

32. 37 units U-100 insulin

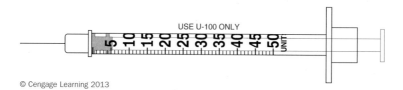

© Cengage Learning 2013

33. $1\frac{1}{2}$ t

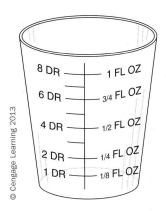 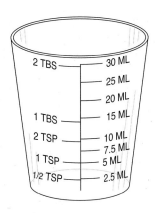

Chapters 7 and 8—Interpreting Drug Orders and Understanding Drug Labels

Use label A to identify the information requested for questions 34 through 36.

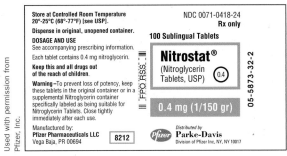

A

34. The generic name is _____.

35. The route of administration intended for this tablet is _____.

36. Interpret this order: **nitroglycerin 400 mcg SL stat.** _____

_____

Use label B to identify the information requested for questions 37 through 39.

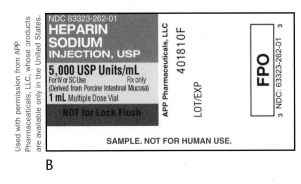

B

37. The supply dosage is _____

38. The National Drug Code is _____.

39. Interpret: **heparin 3,750 units subcut q.8h.** _____

_____

Use label C to identify the information requested for questions 40 and 41.

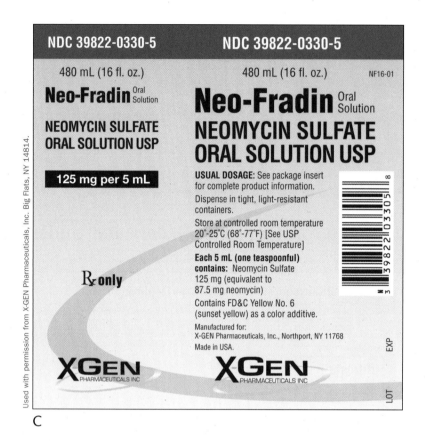

C

40. The generic name is _____.

41. The supply dosage is _____.

Chapter 9—Preventing Medication Errors

42. Using abbreviations from both The Joint Commission and Institute for Safe Medication Practices (ISMP) sources, correct the medical notation of the following order.

    Heparin 5000 U SC qd _____

43. Complete the following statement that defines the six rights of safe medication administration.

    "The right patient must receive the right . . . _____

    _____."

Section 2 Board Examination Practice

To obtain licensure, you will be required to pass a board examination. The following problems represent the various types of items on the NCLEX-RN (National Council Licensure Examination for Registered Nurses) and NCLEX-PN (National Council Licensure Examination for Practical Nurses) exams. Whether you will be taking one of these board examinations or one from another licensure board, alternate test items such as these are good practice. For additional practice, go to the online practice software that accompanies this text to respond to more interactive test items, including those using the calculator tool.

44. NCLEX *Fill-in-the-Blank* Item

A medication order is written for 0.25 mg of medication. The supplied dosage is expressed in mcg. What would be an equivalent ordered dosage expressed in the supplied unit of measure?

Answer: _____

45. NCLEX *Multiple-Choice One-Response* Item

A hospital nursing unit is preparing signs for the medication room, to alert the staff to look-alike/sound-alike (LASA) drugs that have been associated with medication errors. Which of the following would be an example of the recommended use of Tall Man letters? (Place a check mark beside the correct answer.)

Answer:

    a. CHLORPROmazine – CHLORPROpamide   _____

    b. **PREDNISONE – PREDNISOLONE**   _____

    c. DOBUTamine – DOPamine   _____

    d. VINBLASTINE – VINCRISTINE   _____

46. NCLEX *Fill-in-the-Blank* Item

If a patient who has an order for **hydromorphone (Dilaudid) 2 mg IV q.4h p.r.n., *severe pain*** received the medication at 5:00 PM, when is the earliest time the medication may be administered again if requested? Write your answer using the 24-hour clock.

Answer: _____

47. NCLEX *Exhibit* Item

Look at the syringe pictured. What is the amount of medication contained in the syringe? (Place a check mark beside the correct answer.)

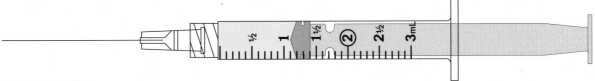

© Cengage Learning 2013

Answer:

    a. 0.12 mL   _____

    b. $1\frac{1}{2}$ mL   _____

    c. 1.2 mL   _____

    d. 1.4 mL   _____

48. NCLEX *Drag-and-Drop / Ordered-Response* Item

Copy the parts of a medication order from the box onto the list in the proper sequence.

Answer:

| 650 mg |
| acetaminophen (Tylenol) |
| fever greater than 101°F |
| p.o. |
| p.r.n. |
| q.4h |

_____

_____

_____

_____

_____

_____

49. NCLEX *Multiple-Response* Item

A medication is ordered to be administered q.i.d. Which of the following possible administration times would be appropriate? (Place a check mark beside all that apply.)

a. 0400, 0800, 1200, 1600, 2000, 2400 _____

b. 0730, 1330, 1830, 2230 _____

c. 2:00 AM, 6:00 AM, 10:00 AM, 2:00 PM, 6:00 PM, 10:00 PM _____

d. 0800, 1200, 2000, 2400 _____

e. 7:00 AM, 12:00 PM, 5:00 PM, 10:00 PM _____

50. NCLEX *Hot Box* Item

Place an X on the circled section of the label that identifies the supply dosage of the medication.

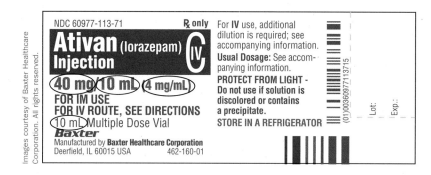

After completing these problems, see pages 603–605 to check your answers. Give yourself 2 points for each correct answer.

Perfect score = 100   My score = _____

Minimum mastery score = 86 (43 correct)

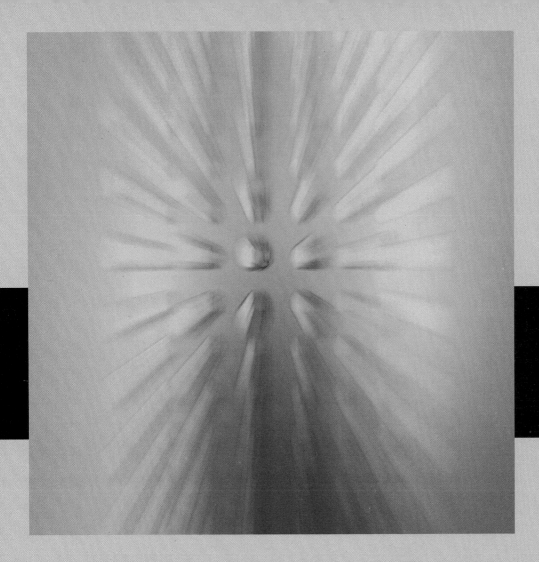

Drug Dosage Calculations

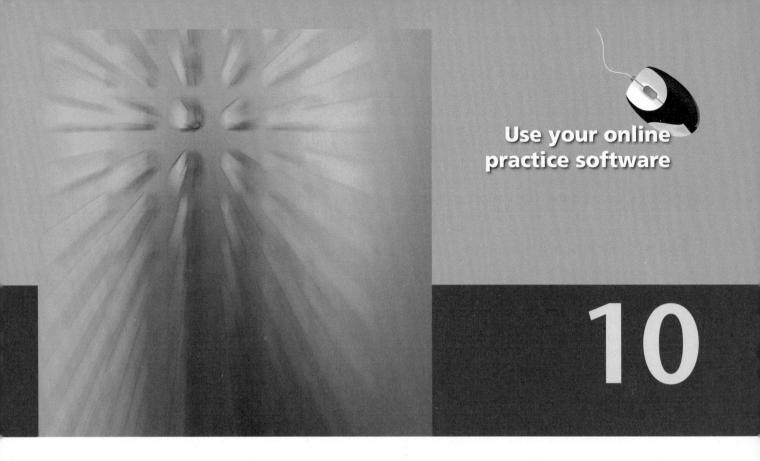

Oral Dosage of Drugs

OBJECTIVES

Upon mastery of Chapter 10, you will be able to apply clinical reasoning skills to prepare safe and accurate oral dosages of drugs. To accomplish this, you will also be able to:

- Gather current information about the drug.
- Retrieve the right drug in the correct supply dosage strength.
- Convert all units of measurement to the same system and same size units.
- Estimate the reasonable amount of the drug to be administered.
- Use the formula $\frac{D}{H} \times Q = X$ to calculate drug dosage.
- Calculate the dose amount (number) of tablets or capsules required to administer oral prescribed dosages.
- Calculate the volume of liquid per dose when the prescribed dosage is in solution form.
- Measure oral dose amounts.

Medications for oral administration are supplied in a variety of forms, such as tablets, capsules, and liquids. They are usually ordered to be administered by mouth, or *p.o.,* which is an abbreviation for the Latin phrase *per os.* To reduce errors in dosage calculations, safety organizations have recommended that all medications supplied to hospital patient care areas be provided in unit-dose packaging, preferably in the original package from the manufacturer (Cohen, 2007). This is not always possible, as hospital pharmacies are frequently supplied with large bulk containers of tablets, capsules, and drugs for injection. Whenever possible, hospital pharmacists should repackage medication into unit doses for distribution to inpatient areas.

When a liquid form of a drug is unavailable, children and many elderly patients may need to have a tablet crushed or a capsule opened and mixed with a small amount of food or fluid to enable them to swallow the medication. Many of these crushed medications and oral liquids also may be ordered to be given enterally or into the gastrointestinal tract via a specially placed tube. Such tubes and their associated enteral routes include the *nasogastric* (NG) tube from nares to stomach, the *nasojejunal* (NJ) tube from nares to jejunum, the *gastrostomy tube* (GT) inserted directly through the abdomen into the stomach, the *jejunum tube* (J-tube) that goes directly into the jejunum of the small intestines, and the *percutaneous endoscopic gastrostomy* (PEG) tube which is placed directly into a patient's stomach through the abdominal wall.

It is important to recognize that some solid-form medications are intended to be given whole to achieve a specific effect in the body. For example, enteric-coated medications protect the stomach by dissolving in the duodenum. Sustained-release capsules allow for gradual release of medication over time and should be swallowed whole. Consult a drug reference or the pharmacist if you are in doubt about the safety of crushing tablets or opening capsules.

Accurate and safe medication preparation requires that the nurse understand the medication order, gather information about the drug, retrieve the right drug in the correct supply dosage strength, accurately calculate the dose amount, and select the proper equipment for accurate measurement of the dose. An error can be made at any point in this process. To help you to avoid costly errors, the examples and problems in this chapter and the next will lead you through the process of critically thinking about the medication and supply dosage before performing dosage calculations, as all are related. A knowledgeable and safety-minded nurse is the best defense against calculation errors.

To foster clinical reasoning skills, extra clinical information will be provided in this and the next chapters to detail how the dosage calculation skill is an integral step in the safe preparation and administration of medication. Simple illustrations will be used in examples to simulate medications supplied either by floor stock in medication cabinets or refrigerators (Figure 10-1a), by individual patient drawers in a unit-dose cart (Figure 10-1b), or by cubbies in an automated dispensing cabinet (Figure 10-1c).

FIGURE 10-1(a)   Stock medication cabinet and refrigerator with sample stock drug labels

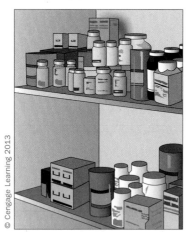

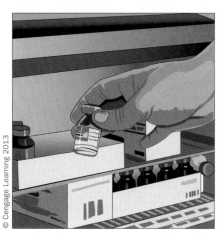

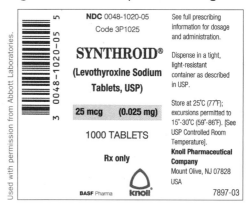

NDC 0048-1020-05
Code 3P1025

SYNTHROID®
(Levothyroxine Sodium Tablets, USP)

25 mcg   (0.025 mg)

1000 TABLETS

Rx only

See full prescribing information for dosage and administration.

Dispense in a tight, light-resistant container as described in USP.

Store at 25°C (77°F); excursions permitted to 15°-30°C (59°-86°F). [See USP Controlled Room Temperature].
Knoll Pharmaceutical Company
Mount Olive, NJ 07828 USA

BASF Pharma   knoll   7897-03

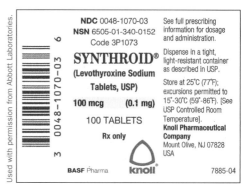

NDC 0048-1070-03
NSN 6505-01-340-0152
Code 3P1073

SYNTHROID®
(Levothyroxine Sodium Tablets, USP)

100 mcg   (0.1 mg)

100 TABLETS

Rx only

See full prescribing information for dosage and administration.

Dispense in a tight, light-resistant container as described in USP.

Store at 25°C (77°F); excursions permitted to 15°-30°C (59°-86°F). [See USP Controlled Room Temperature].
Knoll Pharmaceutical Company
Mount Olive, NJ 07828 USA

BASF Pharma   knoll   7885-04

FIGURE 10-1(b) Medication cart with individual patient drawers stocked with 24-hour supply of sample unit-dose drug labels and example of images that will be used in text to illustrate this supply system

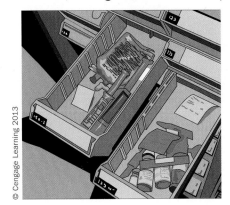

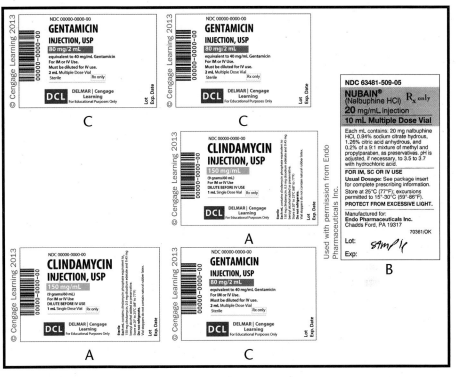

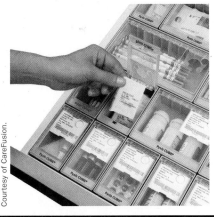

FIGURE 10-1(c) Automated Dispensing Cabinet (ADC) cubbies, and example of image that will be used in text to illustrate this supply system, stocked with supply of sample unit-dose drug labels depicting look-alike/sound-alike (LASA) drugs

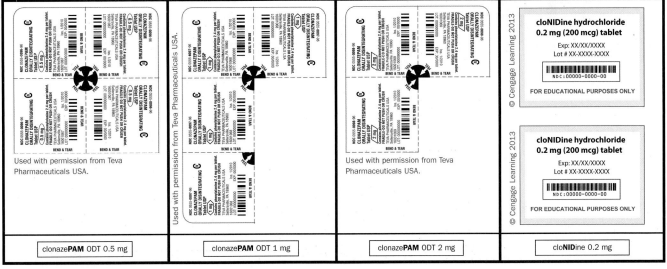

clonazePAM ODT 0.5 mg	clonazePAM ODT 1 mg	clonazePAM ODT 2 mg	cloNIDine 0.2 mg
A	B	C	D

Used with permission from Teva Pharmaceuticals USA.

Used with permission from Teva Pharmaceuticals USA.

TABLETS AND CAPSULES

Complicated calculations are rarely necessary when preparing tablets or capsules for administration. Usually, the amount required for the ordered dose is one or two pills. Medications with a limited recommended dosage range are often only manufactured in one dosage strength per tablet or capsule. Medications with a wide range of recommended dosages are supplied in capsules or tablets with a variety of strengths, or in scored tablets that are specially prepared for accurate splitting into half or quarter tablets. Only tablets that have scored lines should be split. Splitting tablets that are not scored may result in uneven parts and an inaccurate dosage.

CAUTION

It is safest and most accurate to give the fewest number of whole, undivided tablets possible. Do not split tablets unless they are scored.

EXAMPLE 1 ■

The doctor's order reads: **sucralfate 1 g p.o. q.i.d. a.c. and at bedtime**

As a safety-minded nurse, you gather information about the medication and your patient before determining the amount to give. You consult your drug reference and find that sucralfate, an antiulcer agent, is supplied in 1 g tablets and 500 mg per 5 mL oral suspension. The recommended adult dosage is 1 g q.i.d. 1 hour before meals and at bedtime or 2 g b.i.d. upon waking and at bedtime. The recommended children's dosage is 500 mg q.i.d. 1 hour before meals and at bedtime. Administration guidelines state that tablets should be administered on an empty stomach 1 hour before meals and at bedtime. Guidelines also state that tablets should not be crushed, broken, or chewed. Before selecting the form of the drug to use, the nurse will need to assess whether the patient is able to swallow medication. For this example, we will assume that the patient is an adult who is able to swallow tablets without difficulty.

FIGURE 10-2(a) Label for stock bottle of sucralfate (Carafate) 1 g tablets; **(b)** Example of hospital pharmacy-repackaged sucralfate in unit-dose package

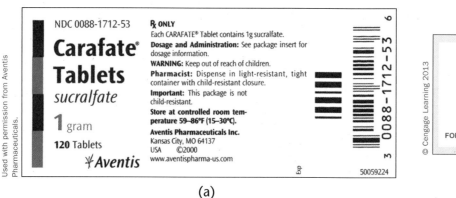
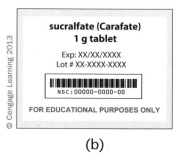

(a)   (b)

The label pictured in Figure 10-2a is from a stock bottle containing 120 tablets of sucralfate (Carafate) in 1 g tablets. It should be obvious to the nurse that, for the ordered dosage, no calculation is necessary and 1 tablet should be administered to the patient at the scheduled time. While this task seems simple, caution must be taken to ensure the right medication in the right amount is given. In a study reported by the Institute of Medicine (IOM, 2006) of the adverse drug events in U.S. hospitals attributed to administration errors, 10% resulted from faulty drug-identity checking and 10% from faulty dose verification.

There are several options for supplying this medication to the patient unit. Less commonly, the nurse might locate and select the correct stock-supply bottle with the pictured label among many stock medication bottles in a medication supply cabinet. The nurse would remove exactly one tablet from the bottle and return the bottle to the supply cabinet in the correct spot before proceeding to the patient's room. More commonly, the one tablet would be supplied individually in a unit-dose package supplied directly from the manufacturer or in a unit-dose package prepared by the hospital pharmacist, with the drug name and dosage typed on the label as shown in Figure 10-2b. If the hospital uses the unit-dose supply system, the medication will be retrieved from individually labeled patient drawers stocked by the pharmacy daily. It is becoming more common for nurses to find ordered medications in labeled cubicles or cubbies in automated dispensing cabinets (ADC). While unit-dose distribution systems have been credited with a decrease in medication errors, mistakes still do happen (Cohen, 2007). To avoid errors, the nurse must take the time to select the correct drug in the correct amount from the correct patient unit-dose drawer (such as in Figure 10-1b) or the correctly labeled ADC cubby (such as in Figure 10-1c). The nurse must verify that the medication found in the cubby was stocked correctly by the pharmacy. As you can see, even with the simplest calculation, errors may be made if the nurse omits any steps of the medication administration process.

Let's consider another order with a simple calculation.

EXAMPLE 2 ■

The doctor's order reads: clarithromycin 500 mg p.o. q.12h

Clarithromycin, an anti-infective indicated for a variety of infections, is supplied in 250 mg and 500 mg tablets, 500 mg extended-release tablets, and 125 mg per 5 mL and 250 mg per 5 mL oral suspension. Before proceeding with the dosage calculation, the nurse will need to determine which of the available supplied dosage forms are most appropriate for the patient. For this example, we will again assume that the patient is an adult who is able to swallow tablets without difficulty. Depending on the indication, the usual adult dosage is 250 to 500 mg q.12h or 1,000 mg once daily as XL (extended-release) tablets. The nurse should determine that an oral suspension is not necessary and that the extended-release tablet is not the form ordered. The nurse may now proceed to calculate one dose from the available oral tablets pictured, either from a floor stock cabinet (Figure 10-3a) or from an ADC located in the medication room (Figure 10-3b).

FIGURE 10-3(a) Label for stock bottles of clarithromycin (Biaxin Filmtab) 250 mg and 500 mg tablets; (b) Hospital pharmacy-repackaged clarithromycin in unit dosages of 250 mg and 500 mg tablets

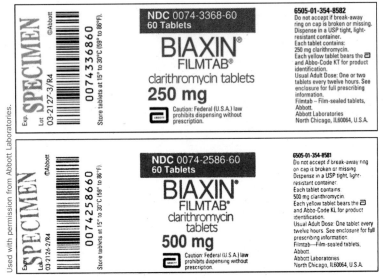
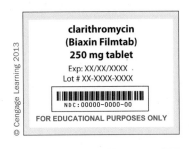
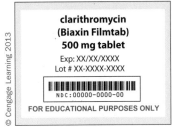

(a)   (b)

Whether the hospital uses the floor-stock distribution system or a unit-dose supply, the calculation is simple. In both instances, two dosage choices are supplied: 250 mg and 500 mg tablets. It should be obvious to the nurse that, for the ordered dosage, the best choice is to select one 500 mg tablet and administer it at the scheduled time.

Now let's consider an order that requires a little more clinical reasoning.

EXAMPLE 3 ■

The doctor's order reads: clonazepam 1.5 mg p.o. t.i.d.

Clonazepam is an anticonvulsant given to adults and children for seizures or panic disorder. There are many options for administration. It is supplied in 0.5 mg, 1 mg, and 2 mg tablets and also in 0.125 mg, 0.25 mg, 0.5 mg, 1 mg, and 2 mg orally disintegrating tablets. The usual adult dosage range is 0.5 mg 3 times a day, which may be increased gradually based on the patient's response, up to a maximum daily dosage of 20 mg if necessary. The usual dosage for children is based on weight, so the dosage varies greatly depending on the age and size of the child. As you can see, the wide range of dosage strengths is needed for this type of medication. An orally disintegrating tablet (ODT) is a solid form that is designed to be placed directly on the tongue, dissolve within 60 seconds, and then be swallowed with saliva. ODTs differ from sublingual tablets, as they are meant to be absorbed in the gastrointestinal tract and are therefore considered to be administered by the oral route. ODTs do not necessarily result in a faster therapeutic onset, but may be the preferred form for patients with difficulty in swallowing traditional solid oral-dose forms, such as pediatric and geriatric patients. It would be unusual for a specific nursing unit to stock all of the possible dose forms of this medication in the stock cabinet or the ADC. Let's consider the following potential supply in the ADC.

Figure 10-4 illustrates ADC cubbies with prepackaged unit-dose packets of the orally disintegrating tablet (ODT) form of clonazepam: (a) 0.5 mg, (b) 1 mg, (c) 2 mg, and (d) hospital pharmacy-repackaged clonidine hydrochloride 0.2 mg tablets.

ADC cubicle drawers may be customized in various configurations to meet the needs of specific nursing units. Figure 10-4 illustrates one row that would be located in a larger drawer with many different medications in individual cubbies. ADCs will often contain a combination of medications in original unit-dose packages from the manufacturer (Figure 10-4a, 10-4b, 10-4c), as well as medications the pharmacy has repackaged in unit doses (Figure 10-4d).

FIGURE 10-4 Clonazepam and clonidine unit-dose packages

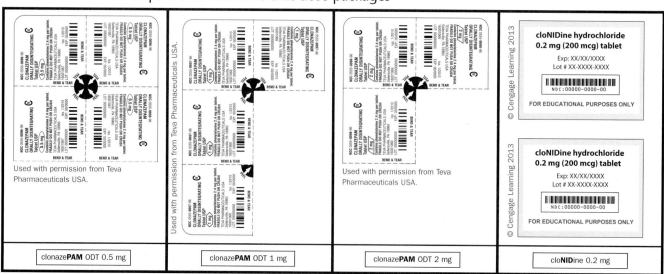

| clonazePAM ODT 0.5 mg | clonazePAM ODT 1 mg | clonazePAM ODT 2 mg | cloNIDine 0.2 mg |

(a)   (b)   (c)   (d)

The pictured drawer shows medications ordered alphabetically and by dosage strength. Did you notice something unusual in the typing of the drug names on the cubby labels? Clonazepam and clonidine, located in adjacent cubbies, are on the list of look-alike/sound-alike (LASA) drugs. To reduce the risk of mistaken drug identity, the labels have been printed with Tall Man letters. The ADC supplies only the oral disintegrating tablet (ODT) form of clonazepam. The traditional solid oral-dose form of this drug is a scored tablet and may be split into halves. Because ODTs dissolve rapidly, handling should be kept to a minimum. These tablets are not scored, which will limit the administration options.

We will be administering the medication to an adult patient. Recall that the order is for clonazepam 1.5 mg. None of the tablets is supplied in that dosage. The tablets are not scored, so the nurse can only use a combination of whole tablets to calculate the correct dose amount. The only possible option is to administer one 1 mg tablet with one 0.5 mg tablet for a total dosage of 1.5 mg.

THREE-STEP APPROACH TO DOSAGE CALCULATIONS

As the previous examples demonstrate, most of the calculations for tablets and capsules will be simple. At times, the calculations will be more complex if the dosage ordered is in a different unit than the supplied dosage or when the computations involve decimals. Additionally, medications in liquids and solutions will require more exact measurements and calculations.

The following simple Three-Step Approach has been proven to reduce anxiety about calculations and ensure that your results are accurate. Take notice that you will be asked to think or estimate before you attempt to calculate the dosage. Learn and memorize this simple Three-Step Approach, and use it for every dosage calculation every time.

REMEMBER

Three-Step Approach to Dosage Calculations

Step 1	**Convert**	Ensure that all measurements are in the same system of measurement and the same-size unit of measurement. If not, convert before proceeding.
Step 2	**Think**	Estimate what is a *reasonable amount* of the drug to administer.
Step 3	**Calculate**	Apply the formula: $\frac{D}{H} \times Q = X$

$$\frac{D \text{ (desired)}}{H \text{ (have)}} \times Q \text{ (quantity)} = X \text{ (amount)}$$

Let's carefully examine each of the three steps as essential and consecutive rules of accurate dosage calculation.

RULE

| Step 1 | **Convert** | Be sure that all measurements are in the same system and all units are in the same size, converting when necessary. |

Many medications are both ordered and supplied in the same system of measurement and in the same-size unit of measurement. This makes dosage calculation easy, because no conversion is necessary. When this is not the case, then you must convert to the same system or the same units. Let's look at two examples where conversion may be a necessary first step in dosage calculation.

EXAMPLE 1 ■

The physician's order reads: clarithromycin 0.5 g p.o. q.12h

Recall from the previous example that clarithromycin (Biaxin) is supplied in 250 mg and 500 mg tablets (Figure 10-3), but the order is written in the unit grams. This is an example of a medication order written and supplied in the same system (metric) but in different-size units (g and mg). That's not a problem. A drug order written in grams but supplied in milligrams will just have to be converted to the same-size unit. We will now perform the first step of the Three-Step Approach: Convert.

MATH TIP

In most cases, it is more practical to convert to the smaller unit (such as g to mg). This usually eliminates the decimal or fraction, keeping the calculation in whole numbers.

To continue with Example 1, you should convert 0.5 gram to milligrams. Notice that milligrams is the smaller unit and converting eliminates the decimal fraction.

Equivalent: 1 g = 1,000 mg

Remember: You are converting from a larger to a smaller unit. Therefore, you will multiply by the conversion factor of 1,000 mg/g or move the decimal point three places to the right.

Larger ↓ Smaller → Multiply (×)

0.5 g × 1,000 mg/g = 500 mg; or 0.5 g = 0.500. = 500 mg

Now you can see that the order and one of the supply choices you have on hand are in the same amount: 500 mg.

Order: clarithromycin 500 mg p.o. q.12h

Supply: clarithromycin 500 mg tablet

There is no need to proceed to steps 2 and 3. The nurse should select one 500 mg tablet of clarithromycin and administer it at the scheduled time.

EXAMPLE 2 ■

Let's now consider another situation for an order of clonazepam.

The physician's order reads: clonazepam 500 mcg p.o. t.i.d.

In a previous example, we learned that the traditional solid oral-dosage form of clonazepam is supplied in 0.5 mg, 1 mg, and 2 mg scored tablets. For this example, the pharmacy stocked the ADC with repackaged unit-dose packets in the dosages pictured in Figure 10-5.

The Three-Step Approach should be used to calculate this dose. We will again begin with the first step: Convert.

The supplied dosages of clonazepam are measured in 1 mg and 2 mg, but the order is expressed in mcg. Before proceeding with calculations, the units of measure must match. Converting the larger unit (mg) of the supplied dosage to the smaller unit (mcg) in the order will avoid the use of decimals.

Equivalent: 1 mg = 1,000 mcg

Converting from a larger to a smaller unit requires multiplying by the conversion factor of 1,000 mcg/mg or moving the decimal point three places to the right.

Larger ↓ Smaller → Multiply (×)

1 mg × 1,000 mcg/mg = 1,000 mcg; or 1 mg = 1.000. = 1,000 mcg

2 mg × 1,000 mcg/mg = 2,000 mcg; or 2 mg = 2.000. = 2,000 mcg

FIGURE 10-5 ADC with various dosages of hospital pharmacy-repackaged clonazepam and clonidine hydrochloride in individual cubbies

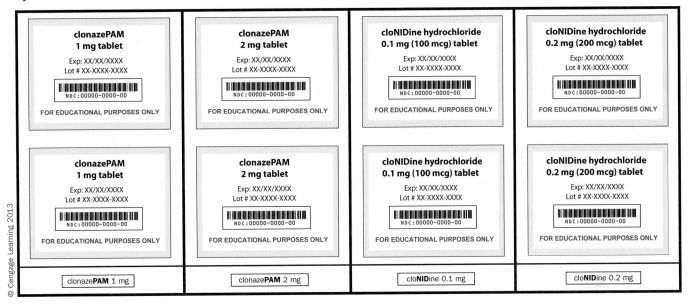

© Cengage Learning 2013

Now the order looks like this:

Order: *clonazepam 500 mcg p.o. t.i.d.*

Supply: clonazepam 1,000 mcg per tablet or clonazepam 2,000 mcg per tablet

RULE

Step 2 **Think** Carefully consider what is the reasonable amount of the drug that should be administered.

Now that the two supplied dosages are expressed in the same unit as the order, the nurse will need to decide which supplied dosage to use. Step 2 asks you to logically conclude what amount should be given. Before you go on to Step 3, you may be able to picture in your mind a reasonable amount of medication to be administered, as was demonstrated in the previous example. You know that 500 mcg is half of 1,000 mcg and is one-fourth of 2,000 mcg. The tablets are only scored in half, so it is not possible to use the 2,000 mcg tablet. You should calculate the dose using the 1,000 mcg tablet and expect that the answer will be less than one tablet or exactly one-half. *Basically, Step 2 asks you to stop and think before you go any further.*

RULE

Step 3 **Calculate** Apply the dosage calculation formula: $\frac{D}{H} \times Q = X$

Even though administration of tablets and capsules frequently will not require any calculation, when calculations are necessary, always double-check your estimated amount from Step 2 with the simple formula $\frac{D}{H} \times Q = X$.

In this formula, *D* represents the *desired* dosage or the dosage ordered. You will find this in the prescribed order. *H* represents the dosage you *have* on hand per a *quantity, Q*. Both *H* and *Q* constitute the *supply dosage* found on the label of the drug available. *X* is the unknown and represents the amount of the supply dosage form you want to give, such as *number of tablets* or *mL* of the drug available.

REMEMBER

$$\frac{D \text{ (desired)}}{H \text{ (have)}} \times Q \text{ (quantity)} = X \text{ (amount)}$$

MATH TIP

When solving dosage problems for drugs supplied in tablets or capsules, the amount on hand is always 1, because the supply dosage is per 1 tablet or capsule.

Now you are ready to complete the example with Step 3: Calculate.

Order: **clonazepam 500 mcg p.o. t.i.d.**

Supply: clonazepam 1 mg per tablet converted to 1,000 mcg

D = desired = 500 mcg

H = have = 1,000 mcg

Q = quantity = 1 tablet

X = unknown = X tablet (s)

$\frac{D}{H} \times Q = X$

$\frac{D}{H} \times Q = \frac{500 \text{ mcg}}{1,000 \text{ mcg}} \times 1 \text{ tablet} = X \text{ tablet(s)}$

$\frac{\overset{1}{\cancel{500 \text{ mcg}}}}{\underset{2}{\cancel{1,000 \text{ mcg}}}} \times 1 \text{ tablet} = \frac{1}{2} \times 1 \text{ tablet} = \frac{1}{2} \text{ tablet}$ (Notice that mcg cancels out.)

Give $\frac{1}{2}$ of the clonazepam 1 g tablet orally three times daily. The calculations verify your estimate from Step 2.

It is wise to get in the habit of always inserting the *Quantity* value in the formula, even when Q is 1. This is important for preparing you to accurately calculate dosages for oral liquid or parenteral injection drugs that may be supplied in a solution-strength quantity of more or less than 1 (such as per 5 mL).

Notice that the formula is set up with D *(desired dosage)* as the numerator and H (dosage *strength* you *have* on hand) as the denominator of a fraction. You are calculating for some portion of Q *(quantity* you have on hand). You can see that setting up a dosage calculation like this makes sense.

Let's examine three more examples of oral dosages supplied in capsules and tablets, to reinforce the three basic steps. With practice you will be ready to solve dosage calculations such as these on your own.

EXAMPLE 3 ▮

Order: **levothyroxine sodium 0.05 mg p.o. daily**

Synthroid (levothyroxine), a thyroid hormone replacement, is supplied in 25 mcg, 50 mcg, 75 mcg, 88 mcg, 100 mcg, 112 mcg, 125 mcg, 137 mcg, 150 mcg, 175 mcg, 200 mcg, and 300 mcg tablets. All Synthroid tablets are round, color coded, and scored. Levothyroxine is also given by injection. The usual dosage for adults is 50 to 125 mcg daily but may be reduced to 12.5 to 75 mcg per day for geriatric patients. It is also given to children. It would be highly unlikely that a patient unit would stock all of these supply dosages. For this example, the medication will be acquired from a stock medication cabinet. Two stock bottles of Synthroid are located side by side on the shelf in 25 mcg and 100 mcg dosage strengths (Figure 10-6). Do you know which bottle you would choose?

FIGURE 10-6 Synthroid (levothryroxine sodium) stock medication bottles containing (a) 25 mcg and (b) 100 mcg scored tablets

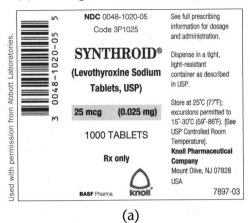 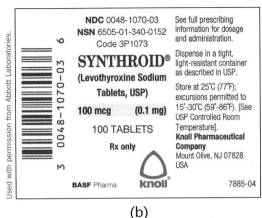

(a)   (b)

| Step 1 | **Convert** | At first look, you might think a conversion is necessary. The order is written as 0.05 mg, but the available supply dosages are 25 mcg and 100 mcg. But on these labels the dosage is provided in both mcg and mg (mg in parentheses). You have two choices. You may calculate this example using the supply dosage in mg, with no conversion needed. The computation will include decimals, and extra care must be taken to avoid a mistake. You may also convert the ordered dosage from 0.05 mg to an equivalent in mcg, which will eliminate the decimal; then you will use the supply dosage in mcg. Let's work this example by first converting. |

Convert to the same-size units. Remember the math tip: Convert larger unit (mg) to smaller unit (mcg) and you will eliminate the decimal fraction. Equivalent: 1 mg = 1,000 mcg. Conversion factor is 1,000 mcg/mg.

Larger ↓ Smaller → Multiply (×) or move decimal 3 places to the right.

0.05 m̶g̶ × 1,000 mcg/m̶g̶ = 50 mcg; or 0.05 mg = 0.050. = 50 mcg

Order: **levothyroxine sodium 0.05 mg = 50 mcg**

Supply: Synthroid (levothyroxine sodium) 25 mcg tablets

| Step 2 | **Think** | As soon as you convert the ordered dosage of Synthroid 0.05 mg to Synthroid 50 mcg, you suspect that the 25 mcg supply would be the best to use and that you want to give more than 1 tablet for each dose. In fact, you want to give twice the supply dosage, which is the same as 2 tablets. |

To avoid getting confused by the way this example is originally presented, be sure that you recognize which is the dosage ordered (D—desired) and which is the supply dosage (H—have on hand) per the quantity on hand (Q). A common error is to misread the information and mix up the calculations in Step 3. This demonstrates the importance of thinking (Step 2) before you calculate.

| Step 3 | **Calculate** | $\dfrac{\text{D}}{\text{H}} \times \text{Q} = \dfrac{50 \text{ mcg}}{25 \text{ mcg}} \times 1 \text{ tablet}$ |

$\dfrac{\overset{2}{\cancel{50 \text{ mcg}}}}{\underset{1}{\cancel{25 \text{ mcg}}}} \times 1 \text{ tablet} = 2 \times 1 \text{ tablet} = 2 \text{ tablets};$ given orally once a day

EXAMPLE 4 ■

Order: nitroglycerin 0.6 mg SL stat, repeat in 5 minutes if no relief of angina

Nitroglycerin, an antianginal, is used for the treatment of acute and long-term management of angina pectoris, characterized by episodic severe chest pain. Nitroglycerin is supplied in many different dosage forms and may be administered by a variety of routes (Figure 10-7). Sublingual tablets are available in 0.3 mg, 0.4 mg, and 0.6 mg dosages and extended-release capsules in 2.5 mg, 6.5 mg, and 9 mg dosages. Compare the dosage strengths between the sublingual tablets and oral capsules. Nitroglycerin is rapidly absorbed when given sublingually but undergoes significant metabolism when given orally, leading to decreased bioavailability, thereby requiring a higher dosage to be effective.

In this example, the nurse will provide the medication to an adult patient in an emergency department. In this hospital, the medications are located in a stock medication cabinet in a central medication room.

FIGURE 10-7 Nitroglycerin (Nitrostat) stock medication bottles containing (a) 0.3 mg sublingual tablets, (b) 6.5 mg extended-release capsules, (c) 0.4 mg sublingual tablets, and (d) 9 mg extended-release capsules

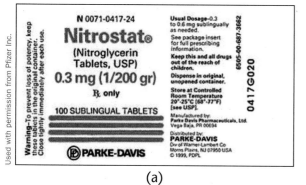

(a)

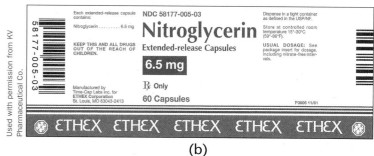

(b)

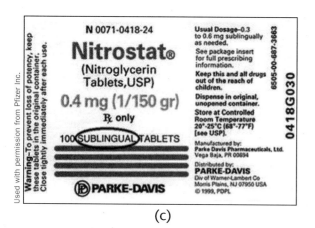

(c)

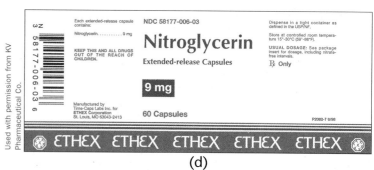

(d)

| Step 1 | Convert | Consider the dosage strength on the Nitrostat labels: 0.3 mg (1/200 gr) and 0.4 mg (1/150 gr). The order is written using the metric unit milligram. Why would the pharmaceutical company also include the dose in the apothecary unit grain (gr)? Although The Joint Commission recommends discontinuing the use of the apothecary system, this medication is an example of a drug that has traditionally been prescribed and is still labeled using apothecary notation. In this example, the order is written in milligrams and the supplied dosage strengths are all provided in the same unit of measure, so no conversion is needed. Be careful to find the metric dosage strength, and avoid being distracted by the apothecary dosage found on the labels. |

Step 2   **Think**   There are four possible supply dosages to use. You might first glance at the supply bottle with 6.5 mg capsules, but after carefully reading the label, you would realize that it is not the correct medication. It is more than ten times the dosage ordered and is in the extended-release capsule form, which cannot be given by the sublingual route. Additionally, neither of the extended-release capsules would be appropriate for a stat medication order to treat an acute condition. That leaves two possible choices. Mathematically, either 0.3 mg or 0.4 mg could be used to calculate a 0.6 mg dosage. Recall the recommendation to use whole tablets whenever possible and only divide tablets that are scored. The 0.4 mg tablet is not scored. That leaves only one choice in this situation: the 0.3 mg SL tablet. You anticipate that you will need to give more than one tablet, or exactly two.

Step 3   **Calculate**   Order: nitroglycerin 0.6 mg SL stat

Supply: nitroglycerin 0.3 mg sublingual tablets

$$\frac{D}{H} \times Q = \frac{\overset{2}{\cancel{0.6\ \text{mg}}}}{\underset{1}{\cancel{0.3\ \text{mg}}}} \times 1\ \text{tablet} = 2\ \text{tablets}$$

EXAMPLE 5 ◾

Order: Lasix 10 mg p.o. b.i.d.

Lasix (furosemide), a loop diuretic, is supplied for oral use in 20 mg, 40 mg, and 80 mg tablets or 10 mg/mL and 8 mg/mL oral solutions. It also may be given by injection. It is ordered for both adults and children with medical conditions that require a reduction in excess fluid. Depending on the indication, the usual adult oral dosage ranges from 20 to 80 mg total per day, given in one or two doses. The usual dosage for children is based on weight. In this example, the nurse will provide the medication in tablet form to an adult patient. Medications are distributed in this hospital by ADCs located in the unit medication rooms. Notice that LASA (look-alike/sound-alike) drugs are supplied in adjacent cubbies (Figure 10-8).

FIGURE 10-8   Illustrated ADC cubbies with hospital pharmacy-repackaged (a) fluoxetine (Prozac) 10 mg capsules, (b) furosemide (Lasix) 20 mg tablets, (c) furosemide (Lasix) 40 mg tablets, and (d) furosemide (Lasix) 80 mg tablets

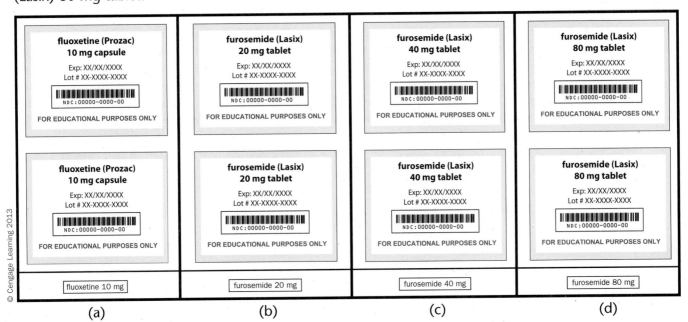

© Cengage Learning 2013

Step 1	**Convert**	No conversion is necessary. The units are in the same system (metric) and the same size (mg).
Step 2	**Think**	There are three possible supply dosages to use. You might first glance at the cubby with the fluoxetine 10 mg capsules, but after carefully reading, you would realize that it is not the correct medication, and instead you choose the furosemide 20 mg tablet. You anticipate that you will need to give less than one tablet, or exactly one-half.
Step 3	**Calculate**	Order: Lasix 10 mg p.o. b.i.d.

Supply: furosemide (Lasix) 20 mg per tablet

$$\frac{D}{H} \times Q = \frac{10 \text{ mg}}{20 \text{ mg}} \times 1 \text{ tablet} = X \text{ tablet(s)}$$

$$\frac{\overset{1}{\cancel{10 \text{ mg}}}}{\underset{2}{\cancel{20 \text{ mg}}}} \times 1 \text{ tablet} = \frac{1}{2} \times 1 \text{ tablet} = \frac{1}{2} \text{ tablet}$$

The calculations verify your estimate from Step 2. But in this case, when you go to administer the medication, you will find that the 20 mg tablet is not scored. When you look closely at the three furosemide tablets, you will find that each tablet is a different size and shape. The 20 mg tablets are white, oval, and not scored. The 40 mg tablets are white, round, and are scored in half. The 80 mg tablets are white, round, have facetted edges, and are not scored. You will not be able to split the 20 mg tablet, and the other two choices will not work for this order either. The first thing you might question is the accuracy of your calculations. However, you double-check and find that the calculations are correct. The second thing you might question is the original order. Furosemide 10 mg given twice a day will provide a total of 20 mg, which is within the usual dosage range but on the low end. Is there an alternative supply that would work for this order? You realize that furosemide is supplied in 10 mg/mL oral solution, which would provide the correct dosage. Because this form is not supplied in the ADC, it is probably not frequently administered to adult patients on this unit. You should verify the order with the prescriber, and once the order is confirmed in this dosage, ask that the hospital pharmacy deliver the oral solution for this patient.

The previous examples illustrated five different scenarios that you may encounter when calculating and preparing oral medications for administration. Now you are ready to apply all three steps of this logical approach to dosage calculations. The same three steps will be used to solve both oral and parenteral dosage calculation problems. It is most important that you develop the ability to reason for the answer or estimate before you calculate the amount to give. Health care professionals can unknowingly make errors if they rely solely on a calculation method rather than first asking themselves what the answer should be. As a nurse or allied health professional, you are expected to be able to reason sensibly, solve problems, and justify your judgments rationally. With these same skills, you gained admission to your educational program and to your profession. While you sharpen your math skills, your ability to think and estimate are your best resources for avoiding errors. Use the $\frac{D}{H} \times Q = X$ formula as a calculation tool to validate the dose amount you anticipate should be given, rather than the reverse. If your reasoning is sound, you will find that the dosages you compute make sense and are accurate. For example, you would question any calculation that directs you to administer 5 tablets of any medication.

CAUTION
The maximum number of tablets or capsules for a single dose is usually 3. Stop, think, and recheck your calculation if a single dose requires more. Question all orders that exceed that amount.

QUICK REVIEW

Simple Three-Step Approach to Dosage Calculations

Step 1	**Convert**	If necessary, convert to units of the same system and the same size.
Step 2	**Think**	Estimate a reasonable amount to give.
Step 3	**Calculate**	$\frac{D}{H} \times Q = X$

$$\frac{D \text{ (desired)}}{H \text{ (have)}} \times Q \text{ (quantity)} = X \text{ (amount)}$$

- For most dosage calculation problems, convert to smaller-size unit. Example: g → mg

- Consider the reasonableness of the calculated amount to give. Example: You would question giving more than 3 tablets or capsules per dose for oral administration.

- Carefully select the correct drug to match the order and dose amount.

- Only scored tablets may be divided in halves or quarters.

Review Set 22

Calculate the correct number of tablets or capsules to be administered per dose. Tablets are scored in half.

1. Order: Diabinese 0.1 g p.o. daily

   Supply: Diabinese 100 mg tablets

   Give: _____ tablet(s)

2. Order: Urecholine 15 mg p.o. t.i.d.

   Supply: Urecholine 10 mg tablets

   Give: _____ tablet(s)

3. Order: hydrochlorothiazide 12.5 mg p.o. t.i.d.

   Supply: hydrochlorothiazide 25 mg tablets

   Give: _____ tablet(s)

4. Order: digoxin 0.125 mg p.o. daily

   Supply: digoxin 0.25 mg tablets

   Give: _____ tablet(s)

5. Order: Motrin 600 mg p.o. b.i.d.

   Supply: Motrin 200 mg tablets

   Give: _____ tablet(s)

6. Order: Levaquin 0.5 g p.o. daily

   Supply: Levaquin 500 mg tablets

   Give: _____ tablet(s)

7. Order: Synthroid 0.1 mg p.o. daily

   Supply: Synthroid 50 mcg tablets

   Give: _____ tablet(s)

8. Order: Tranxene 7.5 mg p.o. q.i.d.

   Supply: Tranxene 3.75 mg capsules

   Give: _____ capsule(s)

Calculate 1 dose for each of the medication orders 9 through 16. The labels lettered A through I are the drugs you have available, supplied in stock medication bottles in a locked cabinet in a central medication room. Indicate the letter corresponding to the label you select.

9. Order: carbamazepine 0.2 g p.o. t.i.d.

   Select: _____

   Give: _____

10. Order: potassium chloride 20 mEq p.o. daily

    Select: _____

    Give: _____

11. Order: digoxin 375 mcg p.o. daily

    Select: _____

    Give: _____

12. Order: sulfasalazine 1 g p.o. b.i.d.

    Select: _____

    Give: _____

13. Order: levothyroxine sodium 0.2 mg p.o. daily

    Select: _____

    Give: _____

14. Order: digoxin 0.5 mg p.o. daily

    Select: _____

    Give: _____

15. Order: Neurontin 0.1 g p.o. t.i.d.

    Select: _____

    Give: _____

16. Order: Lopid 0.6 g p.o. daily

    Select: _____

    Give: _____

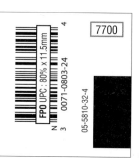

A

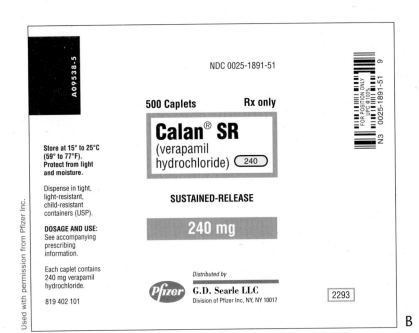

A09538-5

NDC 0025-1891-51

500 Caplets   Rx only

Calan® SR
(verapamil
hydrochloride) 240

SUSTAINED-RELEASE

240 mg

Distributed by
Pfizer **G.D. Searle LLC**
Division of Pfizer Inc, NY, NY 10017

2293

Store at 15° to 25°C
(59° to 77°F).
Protect from light
and moisture.

Dispense in tight,
light-resistant,
child-resistant
containers (USP).

DOSAGE AND USE:
See accompanying
prescribing
information.

Each caplet contains
240 mg verapamil
hydrochloride.

819 402 101

Used with permission from Pfizer Inc.

B

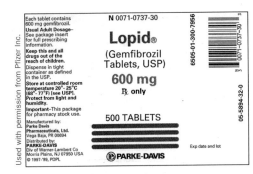

Each tablet contains
600 mg gemfibrozil.
Usual Adult Dosage–
See package insert
for full prescribing
information.
Keep this and all
drugs out of the
reach of children.
Dispense in tight
container as defined
in the USP.
Store at controlled room
temperature 20°- 25°C
[68°- 77°F] [see USP].
Protect from light and
humidity.
Important–This package
for pharmacy stock use.
Manufactured by:
Parke Davis
Pharmaceuticals, Ltd.
Vega Baja, PR 00694
Distributed by:
PARKE-DAVIS
Div of Warner-Lambert Co
Morris Plains, NJ 07950 USA
© 1997-99, PDPL

N 0071-0737-30

Lopid®
(Gemfibrozil
Tablets, USP)

600 mg
Rx only

500 TABLETS

Exp date and lot

PARKE-DAVIS

6505-01-300-7956

05-5894-32-0

Used with permission from Pfizer Inc.

C

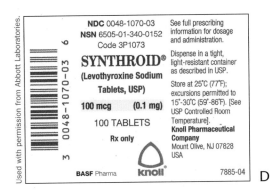

NDC 0048-1070-03
NSN 6505-01-340-0152
Code 3P1073

SYNTHROID®

(Levothyroxine Sodium
Tablets, USP)

100 mcg   (0.1 mg)

100 TABLETS

Rx only

See full prescribing
information for dosage
and administration.

Dispense in a tight,
light-resistant container
as described in USP.

Store at 25°C (77°F);
excursions permitted to
15°-30°C (59°-86°F). [See
USP Controlled Room
Temperature].
Knoll Pharmaceutical
Company
Mount Olive, NJ 07828
USA

BASF Pharma   **knoll®**   7885-04

Used with permission from Abbott Laboratories.

D

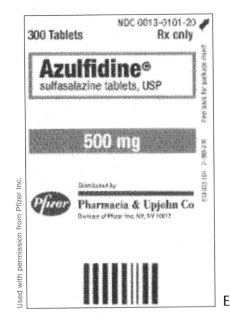

300 Tablets   Rx only

NDC 0013-0101-20

Azulfidine®
sulfasalazine tablets, USP

500 mg

Pfizer Distributed by
Pharmacia & Upjohn Co
Division of Pfizer Inc, NY, NY 10017

Used with permission from Pfizer Inc.

E

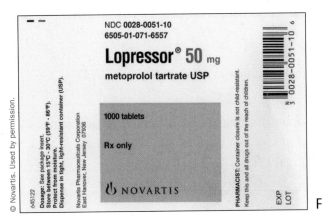

NDC 0028-0051-10
6505-01-071-6557

Lopressor® 50 mg

metoprolol tartrate USP

1000 tablets

Rx only

NOVARTIS

© Novartis. Used by permission.

A65122
Dosage: See package insert.
Store between 15°C- 30°C (59°F - 86°F).
Protect from moisture.
Dispense in tight, light-resistant container (USP).

Novartis Pharmaceuticals Corporation
East Hanover, New Jersey 07936

PHARMACIST: Container closure is not child-resistant.
Keep this and all drugs out of the reach of children.

EXP
LOT

F

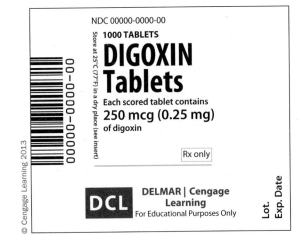

NDC 00000-0000-00

1000 TABLETS

DIGOXIN
Tablets

Each scored tablet contains
250 mcg (0.25 mg)
of digoxin

Rx only

Store at 25°C (77°F) in a dry place (see insert)

DCL **DELMAR | Cengage**
Learning
For Educational Purposes Only

© Cengage Learning 2013

Lot.
Exp. Date

G

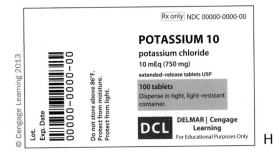

Rx only NDC 00000-0000-00

POTASSIUM 10

potassium chloride
10 mEq (750 mg)
extended-release tablets USP

100 tablets
Dispense in tight, light-resistant
container.

DCL **DELMAR | Cengage**
Learning
For Educational Purposes Only

© Cengage Learning 2013

Lot.
Exp. Date

Do not store above 86°F.
Protect from moisture.
Protect from light.

H

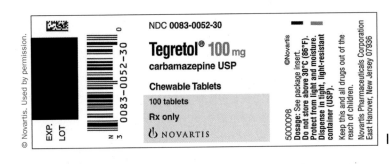

NDC 0083-0052-30

Tegretol® 100 mg

carbamazepine USP

Chewable Tablets

100 tablets

Rx only

NOVARTIS

© Novartis. Used by permission.

EXP.
LOT

©Novartis

5000098
Dosage: See package insert.
Do not store above 30°C (86°F).
Protect from light and moisture.
Dispense in tight, light-resistant
container (USP).

Keep this and all drugs out of the
reach of children.

Novartis Pharmaceuticals Corporation
East Hanover, New Jersey 07936

I

Questions 17 through 30 depict medication administration simulation exercises. The medications are stocked for each individual patient in unit-dose carts by the pharmacy once every 24 hours. Prepare the medications for each patient, using the Three-Step Approach. Refer to a nursing drug guide, such as the annual *Delmar Nurse's Drug Handbook*, to answer specific questions about the medication prior to administering.

Patient #1 (questions 17 through 19) is scheduled to receive the following medications at 0800. The patient's stocked unit-dose drawer with pharmacy-repackaged medications is pictured below. The full supply of medications needed for 24 hours should be in the ADC; therefore, multiple packets of the same medication are included in random order as stocked.

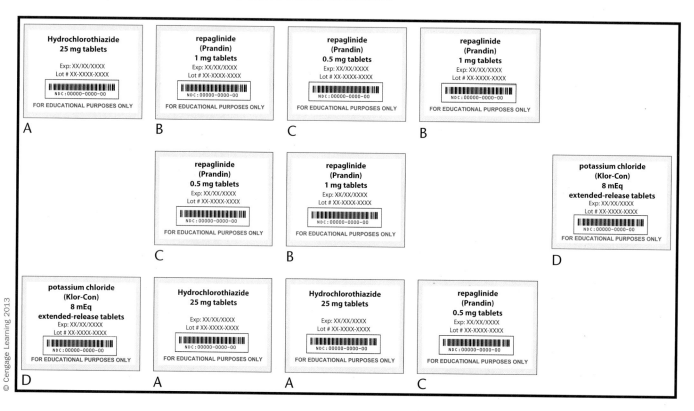

© Cengage Learning 2013

17. Order: repaglinide 1.5 mg t.i.d. with meals

    a. Look up repaglinide in your drug guide. For what condition(s) is repaglinide indicated? _____

    _____

    b. What supply dosages (dosage strengths) and forms may be available from the pharmaceutical manufacturer? _____

    c. What is the usual recommended adult dosage range? _____

    d. Identify the letter of the supplied dosage strength you will use to calculate 1 dose. _____

    e. Give: _____ tablet(s)

18. Order: hydrochlorothiazide 12.5 mg p.o. t.i.d

    a. For what condition(s) is hydrochlorothiazide indicated? _____

    b. What supply dosages (dosage strengths) and forms may be available from the pharmaceutical manufacturer? _____

    c. What is the usual recommended adult dosage range? _____

    d. Identify the letter of the supplied dosage strength you will use to calculate 1 dose. _____

    e. Give: _____ tablet(s)

19. Order: Klor-Con 16 mEq p.o. daily

   a. For what condition(s) is Klor-Con indicated? _____

   b. What supply dosages (dosage strengths) and forms may be available from the pharmaceutical manufacturer? _____

   c. What is the usual recommended adult dosage range? _____

   d. Identify the letter of the supplied dosage strength you will use to calculate 1 dose. _____

   e. Give: _____ tablet(s)

Patient #2 (questions 20 through 22) is scheduled to receive the following routine medications at 2100. The patient's unit-dose drawer is stocked with pharmacy-repackaged medications as pictured below.

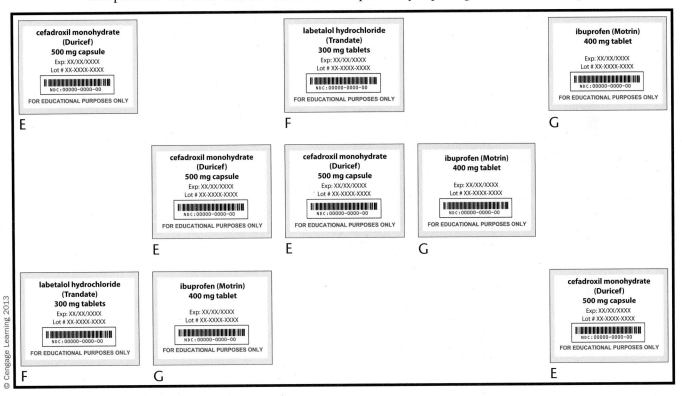

20. Order: Trandate 150 mg p.o. b.i.d.

   a. For what condition(s) is Trandate indicated? _____

   b. What supply dosages (dosage strengths) and forms may be available from the pharmaceutical manufacturer? _____

   c. What is the usual recommended adult dosage range? _____

   d. Identify the letter of the supplied dosage strength you will use to calculate 1 dose. _____

   e. Give: _____ tablet(s)

21. Order: ibuprofen 800 mg p.o. t.i.d

   a. For what condition(s) is ibuprofen indicated? _____

   b. What supply dosages (dosage strengths) and forms may be available from the pharmaceutical manufacturer? _____

   c. What is the usual recommended adult dosage range? _____

   d. Identify the letter of the supplied dosage strength you will use to calculate 1 dose. _____

   e. Give: _____ tablet(s)

22. Order: cefadroxil monohydrate 1 g p.o. b.i.d.

    a. For what condition(s) is cefadroxil indicated? _____

    b. What supply dosages (dosage strengths) and forms may be available from the pharmaceutical manufacturer? _____

    c. What is the usual recommended adult dosage range? _____

    d. Identify the letter of the supplied dosage strength you will use to calculate 1 dose. _____

    e. Give: _____ capsule(s)

Patient #3 (questions 23 through 30) complains of pain rated 8 on a 1-to-10 scale at 1800. Controlled substances are located in a double-locked medication supply cabinet with stock bottles of medications located on shelves as pictured below.

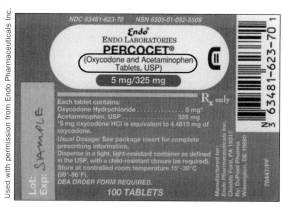

H   I

23. Order: oxycodone 5 mg/acetaminophen 325 mg 1 to 2 tablets p.o. q.6h p.r.n., moderate to moderately severe pain

    a. For what condition(s) is oxycodone indicated? _____

    b. For what condition(s) is acetaminophen indicated? _____

    c. How may dosage variations of oxycodone with acetaminophen be supplied in tablet or capsule form? _____

24. What is the usual recommended adult dosage range? _____

25. Identify the drugs that are different in the two supplied combination medications. Refer to Figure 9-8: *FDA and ISMP Lists of Look-Alike Drug Names with Recommended Tall Man Letters* (on page 189). Write the drug names, using Tall Man letters. _____

    _____

26. Identify the letter of the supplied dosage strength you will use to calculate 1 dose. _____

27. To administer the p.r.n., medication at the right time, what is the latest time the patient should have received the previous dose? _____

28. Give: _____ tablet(s)

29. What is the maximum recommended daily dosage of acetaminophen? _____

30. If this patient receives the maximum ordered dosage in 24 hours, will the maximum recommended daily dosage be exceeded? _____

After completing these problems, see pages 605–606 to check your answers.

ORAL LIQUIDS

Oral liquids are supplied in solution form and contain a specific amount of drug in a given amount of solution or suspension, as stated on the label. In solving dosage problems when the drug is supplied in solid form, you calculated the number of tablets or capsules that contained the prescribed dosage. The supply container label indicates the amount of medication per 1 tablet or 1 capsule. For medications supplied in liquid form, you must calculate the volume of the liquid that contains the prescribed dosage of the drug. The supply dosage noted on the label may indicate the amount of drug per 1 milliliter (Figure 10-9) or per multiple milliliters of solution, such as 125 mg per 5 mL (Figure 10-10a) or 20 mEq per 15 mL (Figure 10-11c).

The Three-Step Approach can be used to solve liquid oral dosage calculations in the same way that solid-form oral dosages are calculated. Let's apply the three steps to dosage calculations in a few examples.

EXAMPLE 1 ▪

Order: oxycodone 15 mg p.o. q.3h p.r.n., moderate to severe pain

Oxycodone is an opioid analgesic Schedule II controlled substance used to treat moderate to severe pain. It may be used in adults and children. The usual adult oral dosage is 5 to 10 mg q.3 to 4h as needed, but a larger dosage may be required for chronic pain relief. The patient in this example is an adult with terminal cancer, being cared for in his home by hospice. The patient has difficulty swallowing pills, and the hospice nurse has decided that an oral solution would be indicated at this time. Oral solution is available in 5 mg per 5 mL in a 500 mL bottle and in a concentrated oral solution in 20 mg/mL in a 30 mL bottle with a dropper. A stock bottle of oxycodone hydrochloride oral concentrate solution has been dispensed (Figure 10-9).

FIGURE 10-9   Stock bottle of oxycodone hydrochloride oral concentrate solution 20 mg per mL

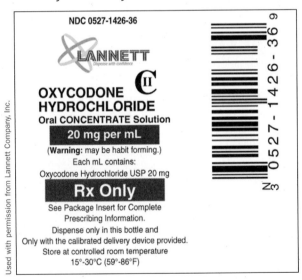

Step 1	**Convert**	The order is in the metric unit milligrams. The supply is 20 mg/mL. The ordered unit is the same as the supplied unit. No conversion needed.
Step 2	**Think**	The ordered dosage is 15 mg every 3 hours, but the usual dosage is 5 to 10 mg every 3 to 4 hours. This ordered dosage is higher than the usual dosage, but this patient has a chronic condition. Larger dosages may be required for chronic conditions. The ordered dosage of 15 mg is $1\frac{1}{2}$ times more than the high end of the usual dosage. This seems reasonable for a patient with terminal cancer pain. The supply is 20 mg/mL, so you expect the 15 mg dosage to be slightly less than 1 mL.

Step 3   **Calculate** $\dfrac{D}{H} \times Q = \dfrac{\overset{3}{\cancel{15}} \text{ mg}}{\underset{4}{\cancel{20}} \text{ mg}} \times 1 \text{ mL} = \dfrac{3}{4} \text{ mL} = 0.75 \text{ mL}$

The patient should be given 0.75 mL of the oxycodone hydrochloride oral concentrate solution, using the dropper provided with the bottle. This confirms your estimate.

EXAMPLE 2 ■

Order: *cefaclor 100 mg p.o. q.8h times 7 days*

Cefaclor is a second-generation cephalosporin, a broad-spectrum anti-infective used to treat a variety of infections. It is used in adults and children and administered only by the oral routes. It is supplied in 250 mg and 500 mg capsules; 125 mg, 187 mg, 250 mg, and 375 mg chewable tablets; 375 mg and 500 mg extended-release tablets; and 125 mg per 5 mL, 187 mg per 5 mL, 250 mg per 5 mL, and 375 mg per 5 mL strawberry flavored oral suspension. Your patient for this example is an 18-month-old child weighing 10 kg who is evaluated in an urgent care clinic and being treated for a respiratory infection. The usual child dosage is 6.7 to 13.4 mg/kg every 8 hours. In Chapter 14, you will learn how to calculate and verify dosages based on weight, but for this example, you may assume that the ordered dosage is appropriate. Medications are dispensed as a courtesy in this urgent care clinic. Four dosage strengths of cefaclor are available in stock (Figure 10-10).

FIGURE 10-10 Cefaclor oral suspension (a) 125 mg per 5 mL, (b) 187 mg per 5 mL, (c) 250 mg per 5 mL, and (d) 375 mg per 5 mL

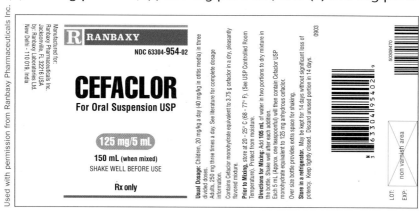

(a)

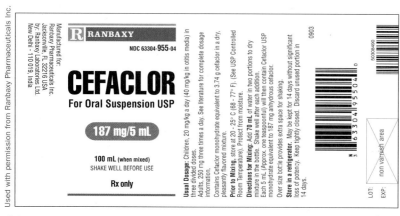

(b)

Continued

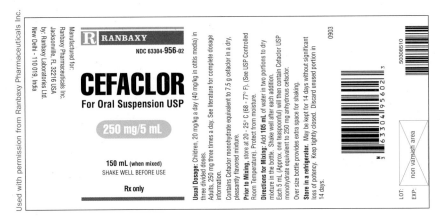

(c)

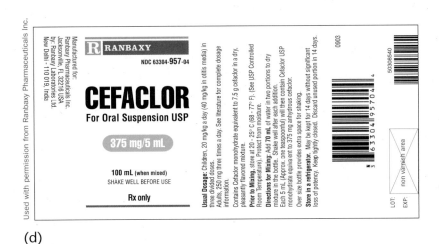

(d)

Step 1   Convert   The order is in the metric unit milligrams. All supplied dosages are also in millgrams. No conversion is needed.

Step 2   Think   Which supplied dosage will you select? All four choices could be used. The supplied dosages of 125 mg per 5 mL and 250 mg per 5 mL seem to be the easiest to calculate; but will both provide a total volume for the full 7 days of therapy? Let's check.

100 mg given 3 times per day = 300 mg

300 mg per day given for 7 days = 2,100 mg total

Both bottles contain 150 mL when mixed.

$$125 \text{ mg/5 mL} \times 150 \text{ mL} = \frac{125 \text{ mg}}{\cancel{5} \text{ mL}} \times \overset{30}{\cancel{150 \text{ mL}}} = 3{,}750 \text{ mg}$$

$$250 \text{ mg/5 mL} \times 150 \text{ mL} = \frac{250 \text{ mg}}{\cancel{5} \text{ mL}} \times \overset{30}{\cancel{150 \text{ mL}}} = 7{,}500 \text{ mg}$$

Both bottles will supply enough medication for the 7-day total dosage of 2,100 mg. Let's consider both dosage strengths in our calculations.

If the dosage strength with a concentration of 125 mg per 5 mL is used, then it would be expected that slightly less than 5 mL would be required to provide 100 mg. If the 250 mg per 5 mL concentration is selected, then less than $\frac{1}{2}$ of the 5 mL would be needed, or slightly less than 2.5 mL.

Step 3   **Calculate**   Order: *cefaclor 100 mg p.o. q.8h*

Supply: cefaclor 125 mg per 5 mL

$$\frac{D}{H} \times Q = \frac{\overset{4}{\cancel{100}\ \cancel{mg}}}{\underset{5}{\cancel{125}\ \cancel{mg}}} \times 5\ mL = \frac{20}{5}\ mL = 4\ mL$$

Order: *cefaclor 100 mg p.o. q.8h*

Supply: cefaclor 250 mg per 5 mL

$$\frac{D}{H} \times Q = \frac{\overset{2}{\cancel{100}\ \cancel{mg}}}{\underset{5}{\cancel{250}\ \cancel{mg}}} \times 5\ mL = \frac{10}{5}\ mL = 2\ mL$$

Both calculations confirm your estimates. You may choose to administer either one, depending on the equipment you select to use.

Notice that in both supplied dosage strengths in Example 2, the supply quantity is the same (5 mL), but the dosage strength (weight) of the medication is different (125 mg per 5 mL versus 250 mg per 5 mL). This results in the calculated dose volume (amount to give) being different (4 mL versus 2 mL). This difference is the result of each liquid's concentration. *Cefaclor 125 mg per 5 mL is half as concentrated as cefaclor 250 mg per 5 mL.* In other words, there is half as much drug in 5 mL of the *125 mg per 5 mL* supply as there is in 5 mL of the *250 mg per 5 mL* supply. Likewise, *cefaclor 250 mg per 5 mL* is twice as concentrated as *cefaclor 125 mg per 5 mL.* The more concentrated solution allows you to give the patient less volume per dose for the same dosage. This is significant when administering medication to infants and small children when a smaller quantity is needed. Think about this carefully until it is clear.

CAUTION

Think before you calculate. It is important to estimate before you apply any formula. In this way, if you make an error in math or if you set up the problem incorrectly, your thinking will alert you to try again.

EXAMPLE 3 ■

Order: **potassium chloride 30 mEq p.o. b.i.d for 2 doses**

Potassium is an electrolyte essential for many physiologic responses such as transmission of nerve impulses and contraction of cardiac, skeletal, and smooth muscle. Potassium supplements are administered either by the oral or intravenous route to treat or prevent potassium depletion, which may be a side effect of some medications. For the prevention of hypokalemia during diuretic therapy, the recommended adult dosage is 20 to 40 mEq in 1 to 2 divided doses, but a single dose should not exceed 20 mEq. For the treatment of hypokalemia, the recommended dosage is 40 to 100 mEq/day in divided doses. The oral form of potassium chloride is supplied in 8 mEq, 10 mEq, and 20 mEq extended-release tablets; 8 mEq, 10 mEq, and 20 mEq extended-release capsules; 20 mEq per 15 mL and 40 mEq per 15 mL oral solution; 20 mEq and 25 mEq powder packet for oral solution; and 20 mEq packets for oral suspension. As you can see, there are a number of options for the ordered dosage.

The patient for this example is an adult patient admitted to the hospital for scheduled surgery the next day. The patient has been taking diuretics and potassium supplements for a number of years. Compare the recommended dosage to the ordered dosage. What might you be able to conclude about the indication for this order? The ordered dosage falls within the dosage range for the treatment of hypokalemia, not the prevention of hypokalemia. This is likely a higher dosage than the patient usually takes at home, and the preop lab work may have revealed a low serum potassium level. The nurse should check the most recent lab results before proceeding with this order and be prepared to explain the increased dosage to the patient. Medications are distributed in this hospital by ADCs located in the unit medication rooms (Figure 10-11).

FIGURE 10-11   Illustrated ADC cubbies with hospital pharmacy-repackaged potassium chloride extended-release tablets: (a) 8 mEq, (b) 20 mEq, and (c) prepackaged unit-dose cups of 20 mEq oral solution

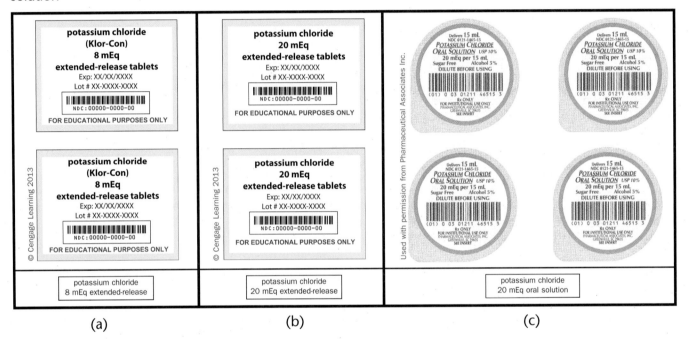

(a)	(b)	(c)

Step 1	**Convert**	The order is in a miscellaneous unit of measure, mEq (milliequivalents). Recall from Chapter 3 that there is no standard equivalent between mEq and other systems of measurement. Conversion should never be necessary, and the supplied medication used must also be measured in mEq. All three supplied dosages are measured in mEq. No conversion is needed.
Step 2	**Think**	The order is for 30 mEq of potassium chloride, but none of the supplied dosages will provide the exact amount. Using the 8 mEq or 20 mEq tablets would require whole and partial tablets to equal the ordered amount. Remember: In order to split tablets, they must be scored. Do you think the extended-release tablets are scored? Probably not. Extended-release tablets should be administered whole without crushing or chewing, so using either of these tablets is not recommended. The only option for this problem is the 20 mEq per 15 mL oral solution. You will need more than one 15 mL unit-dose cup, but less than the 30 mL contained in 2 cups. Remove two unit-dose cups from the ADC.

Step 3   **Calculate** $\dfrac{D}{H} \times Q = \dfrac{\overset{3}{\cancel{30}\ \cancel{mEq}}}{\underset{2}{\cancel{20}\ \cancel{mEq}}} \times 15\ mL = \dfrac{45}{2}\ mL = 22.5\ mL$

The patient should be given 22.5 mL of the potassium chloride oral solution. This confirms your estimate. But now how will you administer it? Can you measure 22.5 mL in a calibrated medication cup? Check the image below (Figure 10-12).

FIGURE 10-12   Calibrated medication cup showing measurements in mL and cc (recall that cc is an obsolete, prohibited unit for dosage measurement)

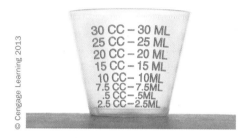

As you can see, 22.5 mL is not a calibration on a standard medication cup. You will have to think of a more accurate way to measure this dose.

You could deliver one of the unit-dose cups, then measure the extra you would need. If you use one full 15 mL unit-dose cup, how much more will you need from the second unit-dose cup?

22.5 mL − 15 mL = 7.5 mL

Can you measure this amount in a calibrated medication cup? Yes; 7.5 mL is a calibration on the medication cup. Give the patient one full unit-dose cup and measure an additional 7.5 mL from the second unit-dose cup in the calibrated medication cup. It is recommended that potassium in powdered or liquid form be further diluted in 3 to 8 fl oz of water or juice. You should consult your patient before diluting, to clarify personal preference of water or juice and the amount of fluid the patient can tolerate. If the patient is unable to finish the entire mixture, the patient will not receive the correct dosage and you will not be able to accurately document the dosage that was administered.

EXAMPLE 4 ■

Order: *potassium chloride 40 mEq p.o. daily*

The doctor orders potassium chloride for another patient on diuretic therapy in need of potassium supplement. You have potassium chloride available as shown in the ADC, Figure 10-11(c). How many fluid ounces of potassium chloride will you administer?

Step 1   **Convert**   The order is in a miscellaneous unit of measure, mEq (milliequivalents). Recall from Chapter 3 that there is no standard equivalent between mEq and other systems of measurement. Conversion should never be necessary, and the supplied medication used must also be measured in mEq. The supplied dosage is measured in mEq. No conversion is needed.

Step 2   **Think**   The order is for 40 mEq of potassium chloride, and two doses of the 20 mEq oral solution will provide exactly that amount; therefore, you would assume that you are going to be using twice the given dosage.

Step 3   **Calculate** $\dfrac{D}{H} \times Q = \dfrac{\overset{2}{\cancel{40 \text{ mEq}}}}{\underset{1}{\cancel{20 \text{ mEq}}}} \times 15 \text{ mL} = \dfrac{2}{1} \times 15 \text{ mL} = 30 \text{ mL}$

The order calls for 30 mL of potassium chloride to be administered to the patient. However, the question was to calculate how many fluid *ounces* of potassium chloride was ordered to be administered. Therefore, we must convert the 30 mL (metric measure) of potassium chloride into fluid ounces (household measure). You learned in Chapter 3 that the approximate equivalent is 30 mL = 1 fl oz. Because 30 mL is approximately 1 fl oz, you would administer 1 fl oz of potassium chloride to the patient.

For more practice, let's go back to Example 3 and calculate how many fluid ounces that dose would be equivalent to. The dose is 22.5 mL.

Convert   Approximate equivalent: 1 fl oz = 30 mL; conversion factor: 30 mL/fl oz

Smaller ↑ Larger → Divide (÷)

22.5 mL = 22.5 mL ÷ 30 mL/fl oz = 22.5 $\cancel{\text{mL}}$ × 1 fl oz/30 $\cancel{\text{mL}}$ =

$\dfrac{22.5}{30}$ fl oz = 0.75 fl oz = $\dfrac{3}{4}$ fl oz

QUICK REVIEW

Look again at Steps 1 through 3 as a valuable dosage calculation checklist.

Step 1   **Convert**   Be sure that all measurements are in the same system and all units are the same size.

Step 2   **Think**   Carefully estimate the reasonable amount of the drug that you should administer.

Step 3   **Calculate** $\dfrac{D}{H} \times Q = X$ $\dfrac{D \text{ (desired)}}{H \text{ (have)}} \times Q \text{ (quantity)} = X \text{ (amount)}$

Review Set 23

Calculate 1 dose of the drugs ordered.

1. Order: **Roxanol Oral Solution 30 mg p.o. q.4h p.r.n., pain**

   Supply: Roxanol Oral Solution 20 mg per 5 mL

   Give: _____ mL

2. Order: **penicillin V potassium 1 g p.o. 1 h pre-op dental surgery**

   Supply: penicillin V potassium oral suspension 250 mg (400,000 units) per 5 mL

   Give: _____ mL

3. Order: **amoxicillin 100 mg p.o. q.i.d.**

   Supply: 80 mL bottle of Amoxil (amoxicillin) oral pediatric suspension 200 mg per 5 mL

   Give: _____ mL

4. Order: Tylenol 0.325 g p.o. q.4h p.r.n., pain

   Supply: Tylenol 325 mg per 5 mL

   Give: _____ t

5. Order: promethazine HCl 25 mg p.o. at bedtime pre-op

   Supply: promethazine HCl 6.25 mg/t

   Give: _____ mL

6. Order: dicloxacillin 125 mg p.o. q.6h

   Supply: dicloxacillin suspension 62.5 mg per 5 mL

   Give: _____ t

7. Order: Pediazole 300 mg p.o. q.6h

   Supply: Pediazole 200 mg per 5 mL

   Give: _____ mL

8. Order: cefaclor suspension 225 mg p.o. b.i.d.

   Supply: cefaclor suspension 375 mg per 5 mL

   Give: _____ mL

9. Order: Septra suspension 400 mg p.o. b.i.d.

   Supply: Septra suspension 200 mg per 5 mL

   Give: _____ mL

10. Order: Elixophyllin liquid 0.24 g p.o. stat

    Supply: Elixophyllin liquid 80 mg per 5 mL

    Give: _____ mL

11. Order: Trilisate liquid 750 mg p.o. t.i.d.

    Supply: Trilisate liquid 500 mg per 5 mL

    Give: _____ mL

12. Order: digoxin elixir 0.25 mg p.o. daily

    Supply: digoxin elixir 50 mcg/mL

    Give: _____ mL

13. Order: Zyvox 0.6 g p.o. q.12h

    Supply: Zyvox 100 mg per 5 mL

    Give: _____ fl oz

14. Order: cephalexin 375 mg p.o. t.i.d.

    Supply: cephalexin 250 mg per 5 mL

    Give: _____ t

15. Order: oxacillin sodium 0.25 g p.o. q.8h

    Supply: oxacillin sodium 125 mg per 2.5 mL

    Give: _____ t

For questions 16 through 21, the medications are usually stocked for each individual patient in unit-dose carts by the pharmacy once every 24 hours. But these medications require refrigeration; therefore, pharmacy has supplied stock bottles labeled on the back of the bottle with individual patient names and hospital identification, and stored in the medication refrigerator as pictured below. Prepare the medications for each patient, using the Three-Step Approach. Refer to a nursing drug guide, such as the annual *Delmar Nurse's Drug Handbook,* to answer specific questions about the medication prior to administering.

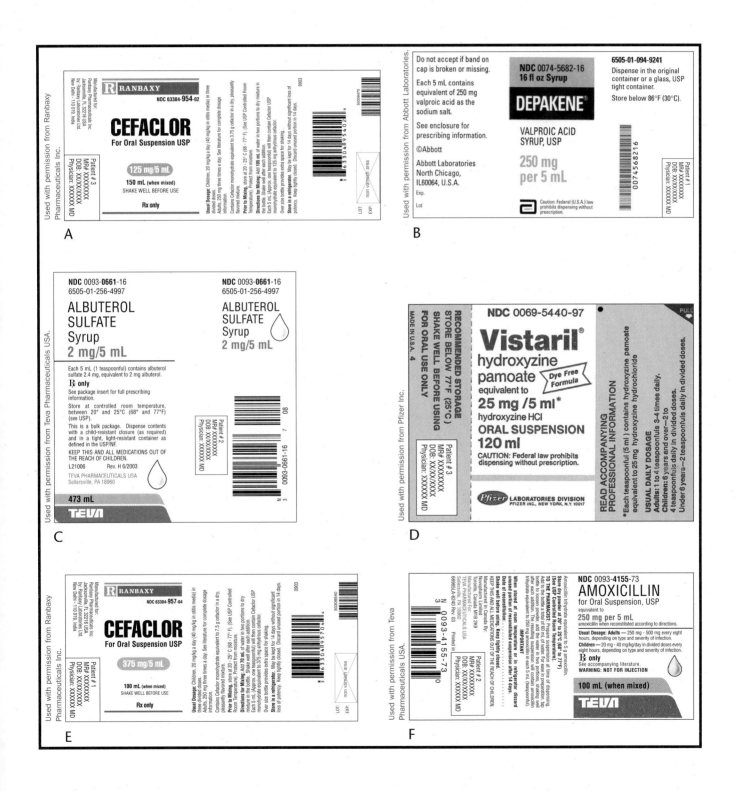

Patient #1 (questions 16 and 17) is scheduled to receive the following medications at 0800.

16. Order: *cefaclor 300 mg p.o. q.8h*

   a. For what condition(s) is cefaclor indicated? _____

   b. What oral dosage strengths of cefaclor are manufactured?

      _____

   c. Is using a tablet or capsule a possible option for this ordered dosage? _____

   d. What is the usual recommended adult dosage range? _____

   e. Identify the letter of the supplied dosage(s) you will retrieve from the stocked medication refrigerator to calculate 1 dose. _____

   f. Give: _____ mL

   Mark correct amount on the oral syringe:

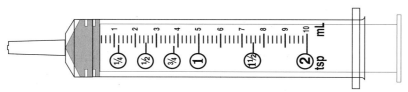

17. Order: *valproic acid 150 mg p.o. b.i.d*

   a. For what conditions(s) is valproic acid indicated? _____

   b. What oral dosage strengths of valproic acid are manufactured?

      _____

   c. Is using a tablet or capsule a possible option for this ordered dosage? _____

   d. What is the usual recommended adult dosage range? _____

   e. Identify the letter of the supplied dosage(s) you will retrieve from the stocked medication refrigerator to calculate 1 dose. _____

   f. Give: _____ mL

   Mark correct amount on the oral syringe:

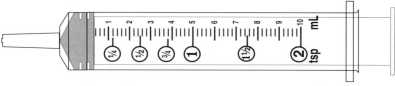

Patient #2 (questions 18 and 19) is scheduled to receive the following medications at 2100.

18. Order: *amoxicillin 500 mg p.o. q.12h*

   a. For what conditions(s) is amoxicillin indicated? _____

   b. What oral dosage strengths of amoxicillin are manufactured?

      _____

   c. Is using a tablet or capsule a possible option for this ordered dosage? _____

   d. What is the usual recommended adult dosage range? _____

   e. Identify the letter of the supplied dosage strength(s) you will retrieve from the stocked medication refrigerator to calculate 1 dose. _____

f. Give: _____ mL

Mark correct amount on the oral syringe:

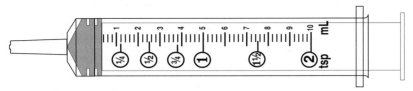

© Cengage Learning 2013

19. Order: **albuterol sulfate 5 mg p.o. t.i.d.**

   a. For what conditions(s) is albuterol sulfate indicated? _____

   b. What oral dosage strengths of albuterol are manufactured?

     _____

   c. Is using a tablet or capsule a possible option for this ordered dosage? _____

   d. What is the usual recommended adult dosage range? _____

   e. Identify the letter of the supplied dosage strength(s) you will retrieve from the stocked medication refrigerator to calculate 1 dose. _____

   f. Give: _____ mL

Mark correct amount on the oral syringe:

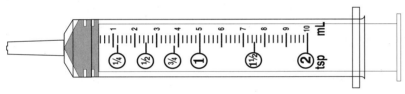

© Cengage Learning 2013

Patient #3 (questions 20 and 21) is scheduled to receive the following medications at 1400.

20. Order: **Vistaril 15 mg p.o. on call radiology**

   a. For what conditions(s) is Vistaril indicated? _____

   b. What oral dosage strengths of Vistaril are manufactured?

     _____

   c. Is using a tablet or capsule a possible option for this ordered dosage? _____

   d. What is the usual recommended adult dosage range? _____

   e. Do you think this patient is more likely an adult or a child? _____

     Why? _____

   f. Identify the letter of the supplied dosage strength(s) you will retrieve from the stocked medication refrigerator to calculate 1 dose. _____

   g. Give: _____ mL

Mark correct amount on the oral syringe:

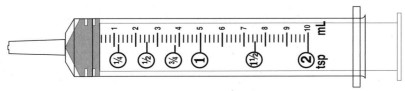

© Cengage Learning 2013

21. Order: *cefaclor 100 mg p.o. q.8h*

    a. For what condition is cefaclor indicated? *Recall from question #16.* _____

    b. What oral dosage strengths of cefaclor are manufactured? *Recall from question #16.* _____

    c. Is using a tablet or capsule a possible option for this ordered dosage? _____

    d. What is the usual recommended adult dosage range? *Recall from question #16.* _____

    e. Do you think this patient is more likely an adult or a child? _____

    f. Identify the letter of the supplied dosage(s) you will retrieve from the stocked medication refrigerator to calculate 1 dose. _____

    g. Give: _____ mL

Mark correct amount on the oral syringe:

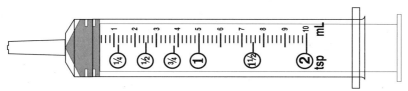

© Cengage Learning 2013

Questions 22 through 30 will give you additional practice using the Three-Step Approach to prepare dosages for oral solutions. Medications are prepared and labeled by the pharmacy in individually filled unit-dose syringes and supplied to each patient's labeled drawer in the unit-dosage cart. Use your drug guide to look up the medication orders and supplied dosages as you did in questions 16 through 21. Then calculate and confirm the measurement of each dosage.

22. Order: **metoclopramide 10 mg p.o. 30 min a.c. and at bedtime**

    Pharmacy-supplied dose:

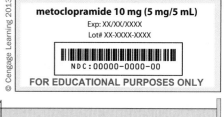

metoclopramide 10 mg (5 mg/5 mL)
Exp: XX/XX/XXXX
Lot# XX-XXXX-XXXX
NDC: 00000-0000-00
FOR EDUCATIONAL PURPOSES ONLY

© Cengage Learning 2013

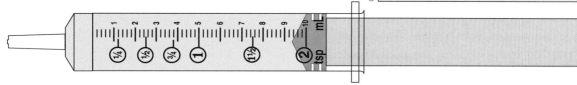

© Cengage Learning 2013

    a. Calculate correct dose:

_____

    b. Is the dispensed dosage correct? _____

23. Order: **phenytoin 200 mg p.o. t.i.d.**

    Pharmacy-supplied dose:

phenytoin 200 mg (125 mg/5 mL)
Exp: XX/XX/XXXX
Lot# XX-XXXX-XXXX
NDC: 00000-0000-00
FOR EDUCATIONAL PURPOSES ONLY

© Cengage Learning 2013

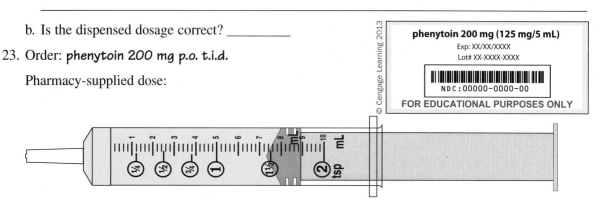

© Cengage Learning 2013

a. Calculate correct dose:

_____

b. Is the dispensed dose correct? _____

24. Order: **furosemide 40 mg p.o. b.i.d.**

Pharmacy-supplied dose:

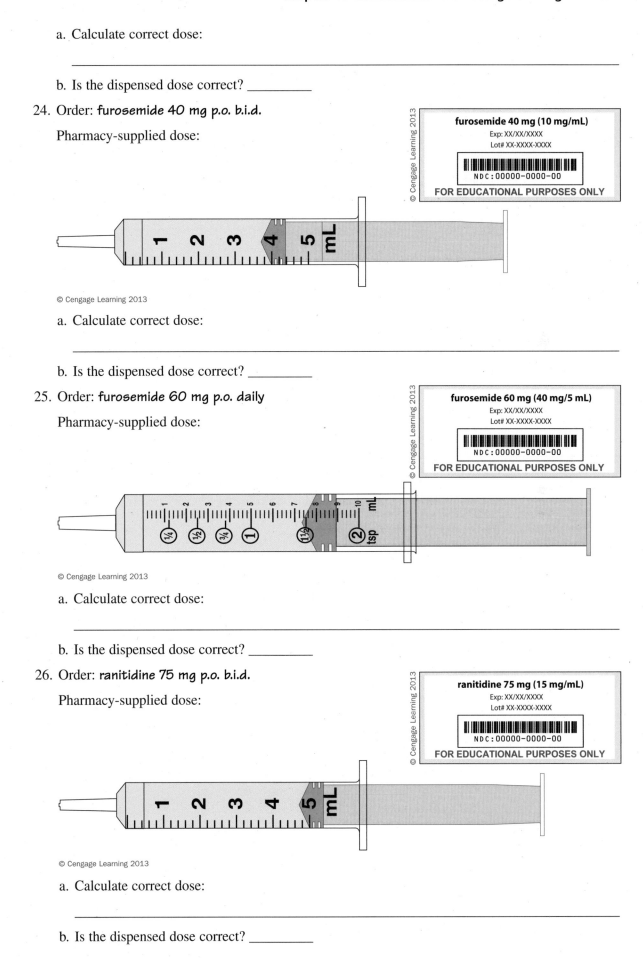

furosemide 40 mg (10 mg/mL)
Exp: XX/XX/XXXX
Lot# XX-XXXX-XXXX

N D C : 00000-0000-00
FOR EDUCATIONAL PURPOSES ONLY

© Cengage Learning 2013

© Cengage Learning 2013

a. Calculate correct dose:

_____

b. Is the dispensed dose correct? _____

25. Order: **furosemide 60 mg p.o. daily**

Pharmacy-supplied dose:

furosemide 60 mg (40 mg/5 mL)
Exp: XX/XX/XXXX
Lot# XX-XXXX-XXXX

N D C : 00000-0000-00
FOR EDUCATIONAL PURPOSES ONLY

© Cengage Learning 2013

© Cengage Learning 2013

a. Calculate correct dose:

_____

b. Is the dispensed dose correct? _____

26. Order: **ranitidine 75 mg p.o. b.i.d.**

Pharmacy-supplied dose:

ranitidine 75 mg (15 mg/mL)
Exp: XX/XX/XXXX
Lot# XX-XXXX-XXXX

N D C : 00000-0000-00
FOR EDUCATIONAL PURPOSES ONLY

© Cengage Learning 2013

© Cengage Learning 2013

a. Calculate correct dose:

_____

b. Is the dispensed dose correct? _____

27. Order: promethazine 12.5 mg p.o. a.c. and at bedtime

    Pharmacy-supplied dose:

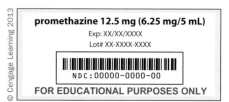

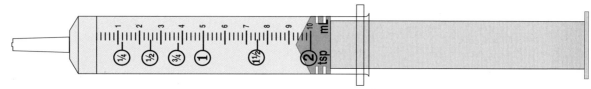

© Cengage Learning 2013

a. Calculate correct dose:

    _____

b. Is the dispensed dose correct? _____

28. Order: digoxin 250 mcg p.o. daily

    Pharmacy-supplied dose:

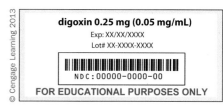

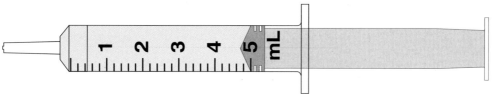

© Cengage Learning 2013

a. Calculate correct dose:

    _____

b. Is the dispensed dose correct? _____

29. Order: acetaminophen 150 mg p.o. q.4h fever greater than 102°F

    Pharmacy-supplied dose:

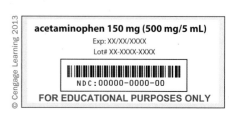

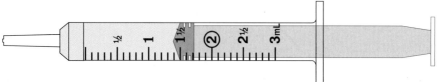

© Cengage Learning 2013

a. Calculate correct dose:

    _____

b. Is the dispensed dose correct? _____

Review Set 45

Calculate the following. Assume IV pumps measure whole milliliters.

1. If a child is receiving **chloramphenicol 400 mg IV q.6h** and the maximum concentration is 100 mg/mL, what is the minimum volume of fluid in which the medication can be safely diluted? _____ mL

2. If a child is receiving **gentamicin 25 mg IV q.8h** and the minimal concentration is 1 mg/mL, what is the maximum volume of fluid in which the medication can be safely diluted? _____ mL

3. Calculate the total volume and hourly IV flow rate for a 25 kg child receiving maintenance IV fluids. Infuse _____ mL at _____ mL/h.

4. Calculate the total volume and hourly IV flow rate for a 13 kg child receiving maintenance IV fluids. Infuse _____ mL at _____ mL/h.

5. Calculate the total volume and hourly IV flow rate for a 77 lb child receiving maintenance IV fluids. Infuse _____ mL at _____ mL/h.

6. Calculate the total volume and hourly IV flow rate for a 3,500 g infant receiving maintenance IV fluids. Infuse _____ mL at _____ mL/h.

7. A child is receiving 350 mg of a certain medication IV, and the minimal and maximal dilution range is 30 to 100 mg/mL. What is the minimum volume (maximal concentration) and the maximum volume (minimal concentration) for safe dilution? _____ mL (minimum volume); _____ mL (maximum volume). (Hint: The equipment measures whole mL; round up to the next whole mL.)

8. A child is receiving 52 mg of a certain medication IV, and the minimal and maximal dilution range is 0.8 to 20 mg/mL. What is the minimum volume and the maximum volume of fluid for safe dilution? _____ mL (minimum volume); _____ mL (maximum volume)

9. A child is receiving 175 mg of a certain medication IV, and the minimal and maximal dilution range is 5 to 75 mg/mL. What is the minimum volume and the maximum volume of fluid for safe dilution? _____ mL (minimum volume); _____ mL (maximum volume)

10. You are making rounds on your pediatric patients and you notice that a 2-year-old child who weighs 14 kg has 1,000 mL of normal saline infusing at the rate of 50 mL/h. You decide to question this order. What is your rationale? _____

_____

After completing these problems, see page 657 to check your answers.

CLINICAL REASONING SKILLS

Let's look at an example in which the nurse *prevents* a medication error by calculating the safe dosage of a medication before administering the drug to an infant.

ERROR

Dosage that is too high for an infant.

Possible Scenario

Suppose a physician ordered KCl (*potassium chloride*) 25 mEq IV per 500 mL of $D_5\frac{1}{2}NS$ to infuse at the rate of 20 mL/h.

The infant weighs $10\frac{1}{2}$ lb and is 24 in long. KCl (*potassium chloride*) for IV injection is supplied as 2 mEq/mL. The nurse looked up potassium chloride in a drug reference and noted that the safe dosage of potassium chloride is up to 3 mEq/kg or 40 mEq/m²/day. The nurse calculated the infant's dosage as 14.4 mEq/day based on body weight and 11.2 mEq/day based on BSA.

First the nurse converted lb to kg.

$10\frac{1}{2}$ lb = 10.5 lb

10.5 lb ÷ 2.2 lb/kg = 10.5 ~~lb~~ × 1 kg/2.2 ~~lb~~ = 4.77 kg = 4.8 kg

3 mEq/~~kg~~/day × 4.8 ~~kg~~ = 14.4 mEq/day

$$\text{BSA (m}^2\text{)} = \sqrt{\frac{\text{ht (in)} \times \text{wt (lb)}}{3,131}} = \sqrt{\frac{24 \times 10.5}{3,131}} = \sqrt{\frac{252}{3,131}} = \sqrt{0.080\ldots} = 0.283 \text{ m}^2 = 0.28 \text{ m}^2$$

40 mEq/~~m²~~/day × 0.28 ~~m²~~ = 11.2 mEq/day

The nurse further calculated that, at the rate ordered, the infant would receive 480 mL of IV fluid per day, which is a reasonable daily rate of pediatric maintenance IV fluids.

20 mL/~~h~~ × 24 ~~h~~/day = 480 mL/day

Maintenance pediatric IV fluids:

100 mL/kg/day for first 10 kg: 100 mL/~~kg~~/day × 4.8 ~~kg~~ = 480 mL/day

But then the nurse calculated that the infant would receive 1 mEq KCl (potassium chloride) per hour.

$$\frac{25 \text{ mEq}}{500 \text{ mL}} \diagup\!\!\!\!\diagdown \frac{X \text{ mEq}}{20 \text{ mL}}$$

500X = 500

X = 1 mEq

Finally, the nurse calculated that, at this rate, the infant would receive 24 mEq/day, which is approximately twice the safe dosage. Therefore, the order is unsafe.

1 mEq/~~h~~ × 24 ~~h~~/day = 24 mEq/day

The nurse notified the physician and questioned the order. The physician responded, "Thank you. You are correct. I intended to order one-half that amount of potassium chloride, or 25 mEq per L, which should have been 12.5 mEq per 500 mL. This was my error, and I am glad that you caught it."

Potential Outcome

If the nurse had not questioned the order, the infant would have received twice the safe dosage. The infant likely would have developed signs of hyperkalemia that could lead to ventricular fibrillation, muscle weakness progressing to flaccid quadriplegia, respiratory failure, and possibly death.

Prevention

In this instance, the nurse prevented a medication error by checking the safe dosage and notifying the physician before administering the infusion. Let this be you!

PRACTICE PROBLEMS—CHAPTER 16

Calculate the volume for one safe dosage. Refer to the BSA formulas or the West Nomogram below (Figure 16-7) as needed to answer questions 1 through 20.

FIGURE 16-7   West Nomogram for estimation of body surface area

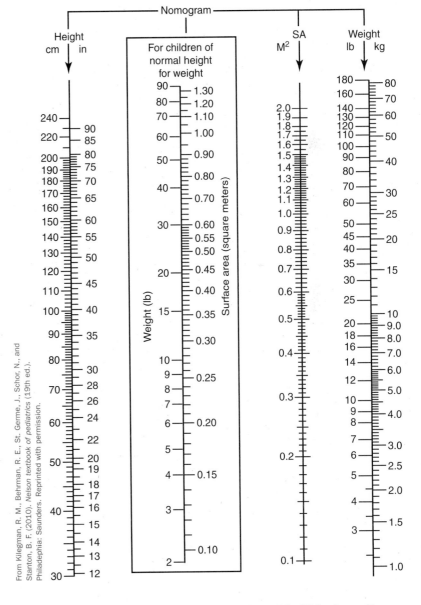

Metric:

$$BSA\ (m^2) = \sqrt{\frac{ht\ (cm) \times wt\ (kg)}{3,600}}$$

Household:

$$BSA\ (m^2) = \sqrt{\frac{ht\ (in) \times wt\ (lb)}{3,131}}$$

1. Order: **vincristine 2 mg direct IV stat** for a child who weighs 85 pounds and is 50 inches tall

   Recommended dosage of vincristine for children: 1.5 to 2 mg/m² 1 time/week; inject slowly over a period of 1 minute.

   Supply: vincristine 1 mg/mL

   BSA (per formula) of this child: _____ m²

   Recommended dosage range for this child: _____ mg to _____ mg

Is the ordered dosage safe? _____

If safe, give _____ mL/min or _____ mL per 15 sec.

If not, what should you do? _____

2. Use the BSA nomogram to calculate the safe oral dosage and amount to give of mercaptopurine for a child of normal proportions who weighs 25 pounds.

   Recommended dosage: 80 mg/m^2/day once daily p.o.

   Supply: mercaptopurine 50 mg/mL

   BSA: _____ m^2

   Safe dosage: _____ mg

   Give: _____ mL

3. Use the BSA nomogram to calculate the safe IV dosage of sargramostim for a 1-year-old child who is 25 inches tall and weighs 20 pounds.

   Recommended dosage: 250 mcg/m^2/day once daily IV

   BSA: _____ m^2

   Safe dosage: _____ mcg

4. Sargramostim is available in a solution strength of 500 mcg per 10 mL. Calculate 1 dose for the child in question 3.

   Give: _____ mL

5. Use the BSA nomogram to determine the BSA for a child who is 35 inches tall and weighs 40 pounds.

   BSA: _____ m^2

6. The child in question 5 will receive levodopa. The recommended oral dosage of levodopa is 0.5 g/m^2. What is the safe dosage for this child?

   Safe dosage: _____ mg

7. Levodopa is supplied in 100 mg and 250 mg capsules. Calculate 1 dose for the child in question 6.

   Give: _____ of the _____ mg capsule(s)

8. Use the BSA nomogram to determine the safe IM dosage of Oncaspar for a child who is 42 inches tall and weighs 45 pounds. The recommended IM dosage is 2,500 units/m^2/dose.

   BSA: _____ m^2

   Safe dosage: _____ units

9. Oncaspar is reconstituted to 750 units/mL. Calculate 1 dose for the child in question 8.

   Give: _____ mL

10. Should the Oncaspar in question 9 be given in one injection? _____

11. A child is 140 cm tall and weighs 43.5 kg. The recommended IV dosage of Adriamycin is 20 mg/m^2. Use the BSA formula to calculate the safe IV dosage of Adriamycin for this child.

    BSA: _____ m^2

    Safe dosage: _____ mg

12. Calculate the dose amount of Adriamycin for the child in question 11.

    Supply: Adriamycin 2 mg/mL

    Give: _____ mL

For questions 13 through 20, use the BSA formulas to calculate the BSA value.

13. Height: 5 ft 6 in   Weight: 136 lb   BSA: _____ m^2

14. Height: 4 ft   Weight: 80 lb   BSA: _____ m^2

15. Height: 60 cm   Weight: 6 kg   BSA: _____ m^2

16. Height: 68 in   Weight: 170 lb   BSA: _____ m^2

17. Height: 164 cm   Weight: 58 kg   BSA: _____ m^2

18. Height: 100 cm   Weight: 17 kg   BSA: _____ m^2

19. Height: 64 in   Weight: 63 kg   BSA: _____ m^2

20. Height: 85 cm   Weight: 11.5 kg   BSA: _____ m^2

21. What is the safe dosage of 1 dose of interferon alpha-2b required for a child with a BSA of 0.28 m^2 if the recommended dosage is 2 million units/m^2? _____ units

22. What is the safe dosage of calcium EDTA required for an adult with a BSA of 2.17 m^2 if the recommended dosage is 500 mg/m^2? _____ mg or _____ g

23. What is the total daily dosage range of mitomycin required for a child with a BSA of 0.19 m^2 if the recommended dosage range is 10 to 20 mg/m^2/day? _____ mg/day to _____ mg/day

24. What is the total safe daily dosage of thiotepa required for an adult with a BSA of 1.34 m^2 if the recommended dosage is 6 mg/m^2/day? _____ mg/day

25. After 5 full days of therapy receiving the recommended dosage, the patient in question 24 will have received a total of _____ mg of thiotepa.

For questions 26 through 38, the IV pump measures whole milliliters.

26. Order: **Ancef 0.42 g IV q.12 h in 30 mL D₅NS over 30 min by volume control set on an electronic infusion pump. Flush with 15 mL.**

   Supply: Ancef 500 mg per 5 mL

   Total IV fluid volume: _____ mL

   Flow rate: _____ mL/h

   Add _____ mL Ancef and _____ mL D₅NS to the chamber.

27. After 7 days of IV therapy, the patient referred to in question 26 will have received a total of _____ mL of Ancef.

28. Order: **clindamycin 285 mg IV q.8h in 45 mL D₅NS over 60 min by volume control set on an electronic infusion pump. Flush with 15 mL.**

   Supply: clindamycin 75 mg per 0.5 mL

   Total IV fluid volume: _____ mL

   Flow rate: _____ mL/h

   Add _____ mL clindamycin and _____ mL D₅NS to the chamber.

29. When the patient in item 28 has received 4 days of therapy with clindamycin, she will have received a total IV medication volume of _____ mL.

30. Order: **D₅ 0.225% NaCl IV at 65 mL/h c̄ erythromycin 500 mg IV q.6h to be infused over 40 min**

   You will use a volume control set and flush with 15 mL.

   Supply: erythromycin 50 mg/mL

   Add _____ mL of erythromycin and _____ mL D₅ 0.225% NaCl to the chamber.

31. When the patient in question 30 has received 5 days of therapy with erythromycin, he will have received a total IV medication volume of _____ mL.

32. Order: D₅ 0.45% NaCl IV at 66 mL/h with Fortaz 620 mg IV q.8h to be infused over 40 min

    You will use a volume control set and flush with 15 mL.

    Supply: Fortaz 0.5 g per 5 mL

    Add _____ mL Fortaz and _____ mL D₅ 0.45% NaCl to the chamber.

33. When the patient in question 32 has received 7 days of therapy with Fortaz, she will have received a total IV medication volume of _____ mL.

For questions 34 through 38, calculate the daily volume of pediatric maintenance IV fluids using:

    100 mL/kg/day for first 10 kg of body weight

    50 mL/kg/day for next 10 kg of body weight

    20 mL/kg/day for each kg of body weight above 20 kg

34. Calculate the total volume and hourly IV flow rate for a child who weighs 10 kg and who is receiving maintenance fluids.

    Infuse _____ mL at _____ mL/h.

35. Calculate the total volume and hourly IV flow rate for a 21 kg child receiving maintenance fluids.

    Infuse _____ mL at _____ mL/h.

36. Calculate the total volume and hourly IV flow rate for a 78 lb child receiving maintenance fluids.

    Infuse _____ mL at _____ mL/h.

37. Calculate the total volume and hourly IV flow rate for a 33 lb child receiving maintenance fluids.

    Infuse _____ mL at _____ mL/h.

38. Calculate the total volume and hourly IV flow rate for a 2,400 g infant receiving maintenance fluids.

    Infuse _____ mL at _____ mL/h.

For questions 39 through 49, verify the safety of the following pediatric dosages ordered. If the dosage is safe, calculate one dose and the IV volume to infuse one dose.

Order for a child weighing 15 kg:

D₅ 0.45% NaCl IV at 53 mL/h c̄ ampicillin 275 mg IV q.4h infused over 40 min by volume control set

Recommended dosage: ampicillin 100 to 125 mg/kg/day in 6 divided doses

Supply: ampicillin 1 g per 10 mL

39. Safe daily dosage range for this child: _____ mg/day to _____ mg/day

    Safe single dosage range for this child: _____ mg/dose to _____ mg/dose

    Is the ordered dosage safe? _____ If safe, give _____ mL/dose.

    If not safe, describe your action. _____

40. IV fluid volume to be infused in 40 min: _____ mL

    Add _____ mL ampicillin and _____ mL D₅ 0.45% NaCl to the chamber.

For questions 41 and 42, order for a child who weighs 27 lb:

D₅NS IV at 46 mL/h c̄ oxacillin 308 mg IV q.6h to be infused over 30 min by volume control set

Recommended dosage: oxacillin 100 mg/kg/day in 4 divided doses

Supply: oxacillin 500 mg per 10 mL

41. Child's weight: _____ kg

    Safe daily dosage for this child: _____ mg/day

    Safe single dosage for this child: _____ mg/dose

    Is the ordered dosage safe? _____ If safe, give _____ mL/dose.

    If not safe, describe your action. _____

42. IV fluid volume to be infused in 30 min: _____ mL

    Add _____ mL oxacillin and _____ mL D$_5$ NS to the chamber.

For questions 43 and 44, order for a child who weighs 22 kg:

D$_5$ 0.225% NaCl IV at 50 mL/h c̄ Amikin 165 mg IV q.8h to be infused over 30 min by volume control set

Recommended dosage: Amikin 15 to 22.5 mg/kg/day in 3 divided doses q.8h

Supply: Amikin 100 mg per 2 mL

43. Safe daily dosage range for this child: _____ mg/day to _____ mg/day

    Safe single dosage range for this child: _____ mg/dose to _____ mg/dose

    Is the ordered dosage safe? _____ If safe, give _____ mL/dose.

    If not safe, describe your action. _____

44. IV fluid volume to be infused in 30 min: _____ mL

    Add _____ mL Amikin and _____ mL D$_5$ 0.225% NaCl to the chamber.

For questions 45 and 46, order for a child who weighs 9 kg:

D$_5$NS IV at 38 mL/h c̄ Timentin 800 mg IV q.4h to be infused over 40 min by volume control set

Recommended dosage: Timentin 200 to 300 mg/kg/day in 6 divided doses every 4 hours

Supply: Timentin 200 mg/mL

45. Safe daily dosage range for this child: _____ mg/day to _____ mg/day

    Safe single dosage range for this child: _____ mg/dose to _____ mg/dose

    Is the ordered dosage safe? _____ If safe, give _____ mL/dose.

    If not safe, describe your action. _____

46. IV fluid volume to be infused in 40 min: _____ mL

    Add _____ mL Timentin and _____ mL D$_5$ NS to the chamber.

For questions 47 through 49, order for a child who weighs 55 lbs:

D$_5$NS IV at 60 mL/h c̄ penicillin G potassium 525,000 units q.4h to be infused over 20 min by volume control set

Recommended dosage: penicillin G potassium 100,000 to 250,000 units/kg/day in 6 divided doses q.4h

Supply: penicillin G potassium 200,000 units/mL

47. Child's weight: _____ kg

    Safe daily dosage range for this child: _____ units/day to _____ units/day

    Safe single dosage range for this child: _____ units/dose to _____ units/dose

48. Is the ordered dosage safe? _____ If safe, give _____ mL/dose.

    If not safe, describe your action. _____

49. IV fluid volume to be infused in 20 min: _____ mL

    Add _____ mL penicillin G potassium and _____ mL D$_5$ NS to the chamber.

50. Describe the clinical reasoning you would use to prevent the following medication error.

Possible Scenario

Suppose the physician came to the pediatric oncology unit to administer chemotherapy to a critically ill child whose cancer symptoms had recurred suddenly. The nurse assigned to care for the child was floated from the adult oncology unit and was experienced in administering chemotherapy to adults. The physician, recognizing the nurse, said, "Oh good, you know how to calculate and prepare chemo. Go draw up 2 mg/m^2 of vincristine for this child so I can get his chemotherapy started quickly." The nurse consulted the child's chart and saw the following weights written on his assessment sheet: 20/.45. No height was recorded.

On the adult unit, that designation means __X__ kg or __Y__ lb. The nurse took the West Nomogram and estimated the child's BSA based on his weight of 45 lb to be 0.82 m^2. The nurse calculated 2 mg/m^2 × 0.82 m^2 = 1.64 mg. Vincristine is supplied as 1 mg/1 mL, so the nurse further calculated that 1.6 mL was the dose and drew it up in a 3 mL syringe. As the nurse handed the syringe to the physician, the amount looked wrong. The physician asked the nurse how that amount was obtained. When the nurse told the physician that the estimated BSA from the child's weight (45 pounds) was 0.82 m^2 and that the dosage was 2 mg/m^2 × 0.82 m^2 = 1.64 mg, or 1.6 mL, the physician said, "No! This child's *BSA is 0.45 m^2*. I wrote it myself next to his weight—20 pounds." The physician, despite the need to give the medication as soon as possible, took the necessary extra step and examined the amount of medication in the syringe. Though the physician knew and trusted the nurse, the amount of medication in the syringe did not seem right. Perhaps the physician had figured a ballpark amount of about 1 mL and the volume the nurse brought in made the physician question what was calculated. The correct dosage calculations are:

$$2 \text{ mg/m}^2 \times 0.45 \text{ m}^2 = 0.9 \text{ mg}$$

$$\frac{D}{H} \times Q = \frac{0.9 \text{ mg}}{1 \text{ mg}} \times 1 \text{ mL} = 0.9 \text{ mL}$$

Potential Outcome

The child, already critically ill, could have received almost double the amount of medication had the physician rushed to give the dose calculated and prepared by someone else. This excessive amount of medication probably could have caused a fatal overdose. What should have been done to prevent this error?

Prevention

_____

_____

After completing these problems, see pages 658–660 to check your answers.

For additional practice, visit the online practice software at www.CengageBrain.com, using the Premium Website access code found in the front of your text.

Reference

Kliegman, R. M., Behrman, R. E., St. Germe, J., Schor, N., & Stanton, B. F. (2010). *Nelson textbook of pediatrics* (19th ed.). Philadelphia: Saunders.

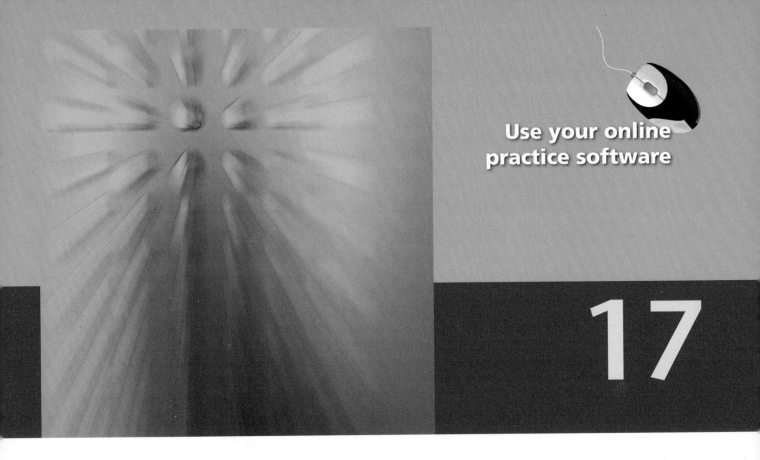

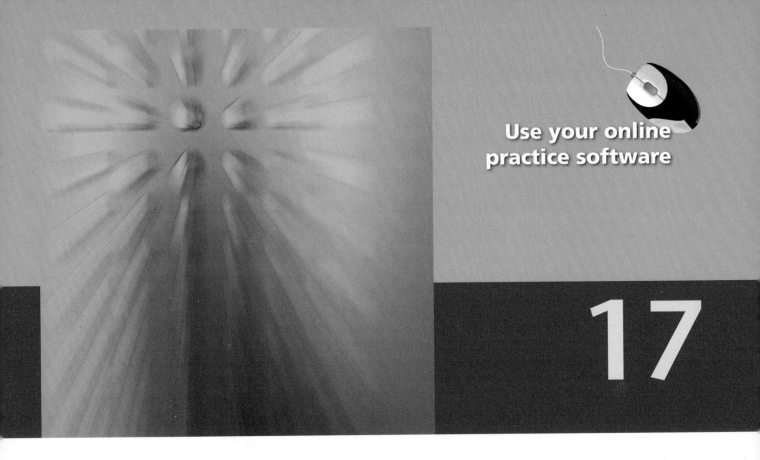

Use your online practice software

17

Advanced Adult Intravenous Calculations

OBJECTIVES

Upon mastery of Chapter 17, you will be able to perform advanced adult intravenous (IV) calculations and apply these skills to patients across the life span. To accomplish this, you will also be able to:

- Initiate and manage continuous infusions of critical medications (such as heparin and insulin) using protocol to:
  - Calculate a bolus dosage and volume.
  - Calculate a continuous infusion dosage (units/h) and rate (mL/h).
  - Monitor and make necessary adjustments to continuous intravenous therapy.
  - Observe patients for serious adverse reactions and administer antidote as needed.
- Calculate the flow rate and assess safe dosages for critical care IV medications administered over a specified time period.
- Calculate the flow rate for primary IV and IV piggyback (IV PB) solutions for patients with restricted fluid intake requirements.

Nurses are becoming increasingly more responsible for the administration of high-alert IV medications in the critical care areas as well as on general nursing units. Patients in life-threatening situations require thorough and timely interventions that frequently involve specialized, potent drugs. This chapter focuses on advanced adult IV calculations with special requirements that can be applied to patients across the life span.

CALCULATING IV DOSAGES AND FLOW RATES USING CLINICAL PROTOCOLS

Clinical protocols are preapproved orders for routine therapies, monitoring guidelines, and diagnostic procedures for patients with identified clinical problems. These orders are common in practice settings where patients' needs require immediate attention. Clinical protocols give the nurse legal protection to intervene appropriately and administer medication without contacting the prescriber each time the patient's condition changes. Heparin and insulin, two high-alert medications for which you learned to calculate dosages in Chapter 11, are examples of medications given intravenously that are ordered using standard protocols. Specific protocols will vary slightly between practitioners and agencies; however, two typical protocols (Figure 17-1 and Figure 17-5) are provided in this chapter as samples for study purposes.

Because patients vary significantly in weight, the intravenous heparin dosage is individualized based on the patient's weight. The heparin protocol orders depicted in Figure 17-1 are based on patient weight rounded to the nearest 10 kg (line 1). Some facilities use the patient's exact weight in kilograms. It is important to know the protocol for your clinical setting. When the patient's response to heparin therapy changes, as measured by the aPTT blood clotting value (activated partial thromboplastin time measured in seconds), the heparin dosage is adjusted as indicated in lines 11 to 15 of Figure 17-1.

Insulin dosage must be closely matched with insulin needs. For hospitalized patients, the dosage must be monitored and adjusted to meet special conditions such as infection, surgery, pregnancy, and drug-to-drug interactions. Nurses follow standard protocols to ensure that insulin dosage is coordinated with insulin requirements through rigorous blood glucose monitoring and insulin replacement therapy. The insulin protocol orders in Figure 17-5 provide instructions to use specific dosage grids for three levels of therapy based on potential resistance to insulin. If the patient is nondiabetic, the insulin infusion is started on the lowest level—i.e., Level 1. Diabetic patients begin insulin replacement on Level 2 and may need to move to the Level 3 insulin dosage grid if the therapy has proven ineffective.

For both the heparin and insulin protocols, as well as other protocols for critical medications, the administration process is the same and includes three sequential actions: 1) Bolus, 2) Continuous Infusion, and 3) Rebolus and/or Adjust Infusion Rate.

RULE

To administer critical intravenous medications according to protocol, follow three sequential actions:

Action 1   **Bolus:** Determine the need for a bolus dose (a large dose to rapidly achieve a therapeutic effect) according to patient condition specified in the protocol. Select the right supplied drug, calculate, and administer the right amount by IV push or direct IV infusion.

Action 2   **Continuous Infusion:** Acquire the right concentration of the continuous solution from the pharmacy (or mix the IV PB bag by selecting the right supplied drug), calculate to determine the amount required to provide the ordered dosage, and calculate and set the flow rate as determined by protocol.

Action 3   **Rebolus and/or Adjust Infusion Rate:** Based on patient monitoring, determine if additional bolus is needed or if the continuous infusion rate needs to be increased, decreased, or discontinued.

CAUTION

Remember that high-alert drugs require independent double verification (of the order, test results, calculations, and drug preparation) by two clinicians who are alone and apart from each other, and who later compare results.

Let's apply all three actions beginning with the heparin protocol, and then we will work through the same process with the insulin protocol.

IV Heparin Protocol

Heparin protocols will vary slightly between facilities. For problems in this text, we will use a sample Standard Weight-Based Heparin Protocol (Figure 17-1), but you will use the protocol that has been adopted by the specific agency where you practice.

FIGURE 17-1   Sample heparin therapy protocol

SAMPLE STANDARD WEIGHT-BASED HEPARIN PROTOCOL		
For all patients on heparin drips:		
1. Weight in KILOGRAMS. Required for order to be processed: _____ kg (round to nearest 10 kg).		
2. Heparin 25,000 units in 250 mL of $\frac{1}{2}$NS; boluses to be given as 1,000 units/mL.		
3. aPTT q.6h or 6 hours after rate change; daily after two consecutive therapeutic aPTTs.		
4. CBC initially and repeat every _____ day(s).		
5. Obtain aPTT and PT/INR on day 1 prior to initiation of therapy.		
6. Guaiac stool initially, then every _____ day(s) until heparin discontinued. Notify if positive.		
7. Neuro checks every _____ hours while on heparin. Notify physician of any changes.		
8. Discontinue aPTT and CBC once heparin drip is discontinued unless otherwise ordered.		
9. Notify physician of any bleeding problems.		
10. Bolus with 80 units/kg. Start drip at 18 units/kg/h.		
11. If aPTT is less than 35 secs:	Rebolus with 80 units/kg and increase rate by 4 units/kg/h.	
12. If aPTT is 36 to 44 secs:	Rebolus with 40 units/kg and increase rate by 2 units/kg/h.	
13. If aPTT is 45 to 75 secs:	Continue current rate.	
14. If aPTT is 76 to 90 secs:	Decrease rate by 2 units/kg/h.	
15. If aPTT is greater than 90 secs:	Hold heparin for 1 hour and decrease rate by 3 units/kg/h.	
ONLY USE 1,000 unit/mL HEPARIN FOR BOLUSES		
WEIGHT	**INITIAL BOLUS** (VOL.)	**INITIAL INFUSION** (RATE)
40 kg	3,200 units (3.2 mL)	700 units/h (7 mL/h)
50 kg	4,000 units (4 mL)	900 units/h (9 mL/h)
60 kg	4,800 units (4.8 mL)	1,100 units/h (11 mL/h)
70 kg	5,600 units (5.6 mL)	1,300 units/h (13 mL/h)
80 kg	6,400 units (6.4 mL)	1,400 units/h (14 mL/h)
90 kg	7,200 units (7.2 mL)	1,600 units/h (16 mL/h)
100 kg	8,000 units (8 mL)	1,800 units/h (18 mL/h)
110 kg	8,800 units (8.8 mL)	2,000 units/h (20 mL/h)
120 kg	9,600 units (9.6 mL)	2,200 units/h (22 mL/h)
130 kg	10,400 units (10.4 mL)	2,300 units/h (23 mL/h)
140 kg	11,200 units (11.2 mL)	2,500 units/h (25 mL/h)
150 kg	12,000 units (12 mL)	2,700 units/h (27 mL/h)

Action 1: Bolus

A bolus dosage is a large dose of a medication given to rapidly achieve the needed therapeutic concentration in the bloodstream. Notice that the heparin protocol defines the bolus dosage that should be given based on the patient's weight and the results of the patient's blood tests. Let's first consider the initial bolus dosage ordered.

EXAMPLE 1 ▪

Your patient, who weighs 110 lb, has orders to start on Standard Weight-Based Heparin Protocol. The result of the baseline aPTT is 29 secs. Refer to Figure 17-1, lines 1, 2, and 10 as we work through this example.

Protocol Order: Bolus with 80 units/kg (line 10, Figure 17-1)

Supply: Automated dispensing cabinet (ADC) cubbies with vials of heparin in various concentrations (Figure 17-2)

FIGURE 17-2   (a) Heparin 1,000 units/mL; (b) 10,000 units/mL

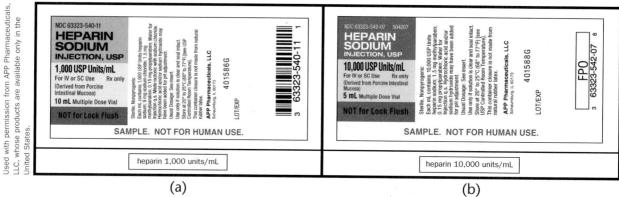

RULE

To calculate the heparin bolus:

1. Calculate the dosage (units) of the heparin bolus based on patient's weight (kg):
   units/kg × kg = units

2. Calculate the volume (mL) of the bolus to prepare using the dosage calculation formula:

   $$\frac{D}{H} \times Q = X$$

Note: This rule also applies to other bolusd rugs ordered in units/kg, milliunits/kg, mg/kg, mcg/kg, g/kg, or mEq/kg.

Let's prepare the initial IV bolus, using the Three-Step Approach to dosage calculations that you have used throughout the book.

Step 1	**Convert**	No conversion is necessary for the medications, but the patient's weight needs to be converted to kilograms to calculate the correct bolus dosage by weight.

Equivalent:1 kg = 2.2 lb; conversion factor is 2.2 lb/kg

110 lb ÷ 2.2 lb/kg = 110 l̶b̶ × 1 kg/2.2 l̶b̶ = 50 kg

Step 2	**Think**	The patient is ordered to receive an initial bolus of 80 units/kg. According to the grid provided, the initial bolus dosage for a patient weighing 50 kg is 4,000 units or 4 mL. But because heparin is supplied in various concentrations, you must know which concentration to use. You must not draw up 4 mL of just any vial of heparin. The protocol specifically requires the use of the 1,000 units/mL concentration of heparin (line 2). The grid only provides the initial bolus, so the nurse will have to calculate any additional boluses needed throughout the therapy. We will calculate the bolus now to verify the grid and then use this same calculation process for additional boluses. Carefully compare the two supplied

concentrations. Select one vial from the ADC cubby labeled 1,000 units/mL, and check the label again to be certain it is of the desired concentration.

Step 3   **Calculate**   the dosage (units) of the heparin bolus based on the patient's weight (kg)

units/kg × kg = 80 units/kg × 50 kg = 4,000 units

The patient should receive 4,000 units heparin as a bolus (verifies grid).

Calculate   the volume (mL) of the bolus to prepare.

$$\frac{D}{H} \times Q = \frac{\overset{4}{\cancel{4,000}} \text{ units}}{\underset{1}{\cancel{1,000}} \text{ units}} \times 1 \text{ mL} = 4 \text{ mL} \text{ (verifies grid)}$$

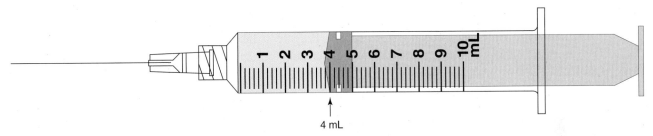

4 mL

© Cengage Learning 2013

Measure 4 mL of heparin from the 1,000 units/mL supply in a 10 mL syringe. Because 6 mL remain in the vial, label the vial with date and time opened and store safely for next use. Provide order, vial, and syringe to another nurse for independent verification and documentation.

Action 2: Continuous Infusion

A continuous infusion is a controlled method of drug administration in which the rate and quality of drug administration can be precisely adjusted over time. Often, IV solutions with heparin, insulin, or other added high-alert drugs come premixed from the hospital pharmacy. There will be times when nurses will need to mix the IV solution for the continuous infusion. Let's continue with our patient in the previous example by following the protocol to prepare the IV heparin solution and calculate the initial infusion rate.

EXAMPLE 2 ■

In addition to receiving the bolus dose, your patient from Example 1 will need to have the continuous infusion started according to protocol.

Protocol Order for Heparin Solution: Heparin 25,000 units in 250 mL $\frac{1}{2}$NS (line 2, Figure 17-1)

Supply: ADC cubbies with vials of heparin in various concentrations (Figure 17-2)

Let's prepare the IV solution using the Three-Step Approach to dosage calculations.

Step 1   **Convert**   Remember: You already know that 110 lb = 50 kg. The order and the supplied dosages are in the same unit of measurement: units. No conversion is necessary.

Step 2   **Think**   The 10,000 units/mL supply dosage is the vial that will provide 25,000 units. If there are 10,000 units in 1 mL, there are a total of 50,000 units in the 5 mL vial. This order for 25,000 units is half of the total volume in the vial, or 2.5 mL. Select one vial from the ADC cubby labeled 10,000 units/mL, and check the label again to be certain it is of the desired concentration.

Step 3   **Calculate** $\dfrac{D}{H} \times Q = \dfrac{\overset{25}{\cancel{25,000}} \text{ units}}{\underset{10}{\cancel{10,000}} \text{ units}} \times 1 \text{ mL} = \dfrac{25}{10} \text{ mL} = 2.5 \text{ mL}$ (verifies estimate)

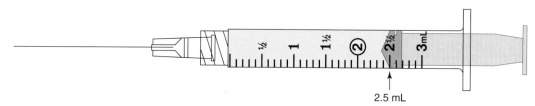

Measure 2.5 mL of heparin from the 10,000 units/mL supply in a 3 mL syringe. Provide order, vial, and syringe to another nurse for independent verification and documentation. Add to the 250 mL IV PB bag of 0.45% Sodium Chloride ($\frac{1}{2}$NS) through the injection port. There will be 2.5 mL of this highly concentrated, high-alert drug remaining in the vial. Either discard the vial immediately or label with date and time opened, and store safely. Prepare a label with the patient's name, drug name and concentration, dosage and amount added, date and time prepared, and your signature, and place the label on the IV PB bag.

Protocol Order for Initial Infusion Rate: Start drip at 18 units/kg/h (line 10, Figure 17-1)

Supply: Heparin 25,000 units in 250 mL

RULE

To calculate the continuous flow rate of the IV heparin solution in mL/h:

1. Calculate the dosage (units/h) of the initial continuous infusion based on patient's weight (kg).

units/kg/h × kg = units/h

2. Calculate the continuous infusion rate (mL/h) using a version of dosage calculation formula:

$$\frac{D \text{ (units/h desired)}}{H \text{ (units you have available)}} \times Q \text{ (mL you have available)} = R \text{ (mL/h rate)}$$

Note: This rule applies to drugs ordered in units/kg/h, milliunits/kg/h, mg/kg/h, mcg/kg/h, g/kg/h, or mEq/kg/h.

Now let's calculate the initial infusion rate using the Three-Step Approach to dosage calculations.

Step 1	**Convert**	The order and the supplied dosages are in the same unit of measurement: units. No conversion is necessary. Remember: You already know that the patient's weight of 110 lb = 50 kg.
Step 2	**Think**	According to the grid provided, the initial continuous infusion rate for a patient weighing 50 kg is 900 units/h (9 mL/h). Remember that the grid only provides the initial infusion rate, so the nurse will have to calculate any necessary infusion rate increases or decreases throughout the therapy. We will calculate the infusion rate now to verify the grid and then use this same calculation process for any needed adjustments in the rate. The solution prepared is 25,000 units per 250 mL. You need 900 units for the dose; 900 units is less than $\frac{1}{2}$ but more than $\frac{1}{3}$ of 25,000 units. So you will need less than 125 mL but more than 80 mL. You can think about this in a different way by using ratio and proportion to determine how many units are in 1 mL. If there are 25,000 units per 250 mL, how many units are there in 1 mL? Set up the ratio-proportion like this:

$$\frac{25,000 \text{ units}}{250 \text{ mL}} \diagdown \frac{X \text{ units}}{1 \text{ mL}} \quad \text{(cross-multiply)}$$

$$250X = 25,000$$

$$\frac{250X}{250} = \frac{25,000}{250} \quad \text{(solve for X)}$$

$$X = 100 \quad \text{There are 100 units of heparin per 1 mL.}$$

Now you know that with the concentration of heparin solution used for this protocol, each mL infused will contain 100 units of heparin. So if you want to administer 900 units of heparin, you want 9 times 1 mL, or 9 mL.

Step 3   **Calculate**   the dosage (units/h) of the continuous infusion increase based on the patient's weight (kg).

units/kg/h × kg = 18 units/kg/h × 50 kg = 900 units/h (verifies grid)

Calculate   the new hourly infusion rate (mL/h) using a version of the dosage calculation formula:

$$\frac{D \text{ (units/h)}}{H \text{ (units)}} \times Q \text{ (mL)} = R \text{ (mL/h)} = \frac{900 \text{ units/h}}{\underset{100}{25,000 \text{ units}}} \times \overset{1}{250} \text{ mL} = \frac{900}{100} \text{ mL/h} = 9 \text{ mL/h}$$

or

$$\frac{D \text{ (units/h)}}{H \text{ (units)}} \times Q \text{ (mL)} = R \text{ (mL/h)} = \frac{\overset{9}{900 \text{ units/h}}}{\underset{1}{100 \text{ units}}} \times 1 \text{ mL} = 9 \text{ mL/h (verifies}$$

grid and estimate)

As you can see, knowing the units per mL simplifies the calculation. In fact, for many protocols, the concentrations for the solutions are specifically chosen to help make the calculations easier, thereby reducing the risk of error. The rate on the chart included with the protocol is verified by our calculations. Remember that, while the chart is convenient to refer to when setting up the initial infusion, it is not to be used for any needed adjustment to the infusion rate throughout the therapy. This high-alert medication will be infused using an electronic IV infusion pump. For this example, we will assume that the infusion pump available is designed to infuse at the mL/h rate using whole numbers only. It is important to verify the calibration of the IV pump in your clinical setting. Some IV pumps are programmable in tenths of a milliliter. Set the rate on the pump for the initial infusion at 9 mL/h. Ask another nurse for independent verification of the initial infusion rate.

Action 3: Rebolus and/or Adjust Infusion Rate

The anticoagulant heparin is used to prevent formation of thrombi (intravenous blood clots) by suppressing clotting factors, such as thrombin. The most significant complication of treatment is life-threatening hemorrhage. The goal of heparin therapy is to reduce the body's ability to clot to a level that is low enough to prevent thrombosis but not so low that it causes spontaneous bleeding. Response to heparin therapy is highly variable from one individual patient to another. The activated partial thromboplastin time (aPTT) is a blood test that measures the time it takes blood to clot. The aPTT is used during anticoagulation therapy to determine the right dosage of the drug. It is the nurse's responsibility to monitor the patient for bleeding and adjust the dosage of heparin based on periodic measurements of aPTT and the heparin protocol. In order to have consistent monitoring from shift to shift, the nurse must document the time and dose of the bolus and any infusion rate changes. Figure 17-3 is an example of a handwritten heparin protocol worksheet that could be used for our patient.

FIGURE 17-3   Sample heparin protocol worksheet

STANDARD WEIGHT-BASED HEPARIN PROTOCOL WORKSHEET

Round patient's total body weight to nearest 10 kg: _____ kg.

DO NOT change the weight based on daily measurements.

FOUND ON THE ORDER FORM

Initial Bolus (80 units/kg): _____ units _____ mL

Initial Infusion Rate (18 units/kg/h): _____ units/h _____ mL/h

---

Make adjustments to the heparin drip rate as directed by the order form.

ALL DOSES ARE ROUNDED TO THE NEAREST 100 UNITS.

Date	Time	aPTT	Bolus	Rate Change units/h	Rate Change mL/h	New Rate	RN 1	RN 2

If aPTT is	Then
Less than 35 secs:	Rebolus with 80 units/kg and increase rate by 4 units/kg/h.
36 to 44 secs:	Rebolus with 40 units/kg and increase rate by 2 units/kg/h.
45 to 75 secs:	Continue current rate.
76 to 90 secs:	Decrease rate by 2 units/kg/h.
Greater than 90 secs:	Hold heparin for 1 hour and decrease rate by 3 units/kg/h.

Signatures   Initials

_____   _____

_____   _____

_____   _____

_____   _____

EXAMPLE 3 ▪

After 6 hours of heparin infusion, your patient on the heparin protocol has an aPTT test done (line 3, Figure 17-1). One hour later the result is reported to be 43 seconds. The clotting time measured has lengthened from 26 seconds to 43 seconds but has not reached the target time. According to the protocol, you will rebolus with 40 units/kg and increase the amount of IV heparin by 2 units/kg/h (line 12, Figure 17-1) and then recheck the aPTT in 6 hours. You will use the same calculation skills you learned in the previous examples for the initial bolus and to set the initial infusion rate.

RULE

To calculate the heparin rebolus and adjust the continuous infusion rate:

1. Calculate the dose (units) of the heparin bolus based on aPTT results and patient's weight (kg):
   units/kg × kg = units

2. Calculate the volume (mL) of the bolus to prepare using the dosage calculation formula:
   $$\frac{D}{H} \times Q = X$$

3. Calculate the dosage (units/h) of the continuous infusion adjustment based on aPTT results and patient's weight (kg).
   units/kg/h × kg = units/h

4. Calculate the adjustment to the hourly infusion rate (mL/h) using a version of the dosage calculation formula:
   $$\frac{D \text{ (units/h desired)}}{H \text{ (units you have available)}} \times Q \text{ (mL you have available)} = R \text{ (mL/h rate)}$$

5. Calculate the new hourly infusion rate (mL/h)
   current rate (mL/h) ± adjustment (mL/h) = new rate (mL/h)

Note: This rule also applies to other rebolus or continuous infusion drugs ordered in units/kg/h, milliunits/kg/h, mg/kg/h, mcg/kg/h, g/h, or mEq/kg/h.

Protocol Order: Rebolus with 40 units/kg and increase rate by 2 units/kg/h (line 12, Figure 17-1)

Supply: Vial of heparin 1,000 units/mL with 6 mL remaining; IV PB of heparin 25,000 units in 250 mL

Calculate the adjusted infusion rate using the Three-Step Approach to dosage calculations.

Step 1   **Convert**   Remember that you already know that the patient's weight of 110 lb = 50 kg and that no unit conversion is necessary.

Step 2   **Think**   The patient now needs to receive a bolus of 40 units/kg. You cannot use the grid provided, because it lists the dosage for the initial bolus of 80 units/kg. You will need to calculate the dose, so think: if the patient now needs half of the initial bolus order, the dose should be half of the bolus dose, which was 4 mL. The bolus should now be 2 mL. Additionally, the continuous infusion is set at a rate of 18 units/kg/h, or 9 mL per hour. The rate will need to be increased by 2 units/kg/h, which should provide an hourly rate of slightly more than 9 mL.

Step 3   **Calculate**   the dosage (units) of the heparin rebolus based on patient's weight (kg).

units/kg × kg = 40 units/kg × 50 kg = 2,000 units

The patient should receive 2,000 units heparin as a rebolus.

Calculate the volume (mL) of the rebolus to prepare. Remember that you will use the 1,000 units/mL supply to measure the amount of heparin for the rebolus.

$$\frac{D}{H} \times Q = \frac{\overset{2}{\cancel{2,000} \text{ units}}}{\underset{1}{\cancel{1,000} \text{ units}}} \times 1 \text{ mL} = 2 \text{ mL (verifies estimate)}$$

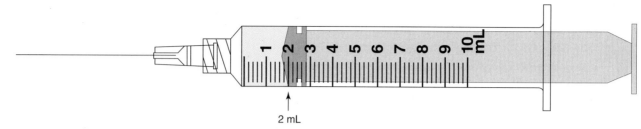

2 mL

© Cengage Learning 2013

Measure 2 mL of heparin from the 1,000 units/mL supply in a 10 mL syringe. You may use the vial with 6 mL remaining from the initial bolus if it was safely labeled and stored. There will now be 4 mL remaining, which you may store safely for the next use. Provide order, vial, and syringe to another nurse for independent verification and documentation.

Calculate the dosage (units/h) of the continuous infusion increase based on patient's weight (kg).

units/kg/h × kg = 2 units/kg/h × 50 kg = 100 units/h

The infusion rate should be increased by 100 units per hour.

Calculate the adjustment to the hourly infusion rate (mL/h).

$$\frac{D\ (units/h)}{H\ (units)} \times Q\ (mL) = R\ (mL/h) = \frac{100\ units/h}{100\ units} \times 1\ mL = 1\ mL/h$$

Calculate the new hourly infusion rate (mL/h).

9 mL/h + 1 mL/h = 10 mL/h (verifies estimate)

Increase the rate on the pump to 10 mL/h. Ask another nurse for independent verification of the infusion rate adjustment.

You have now worked through the three sequential actions needed to safely initiate, monitor, and maintain continuous intravenous infusions of high-alert medications. The principles learned with the heparin examples may be applied to calculations of boluses and continuous infusions for other critical medications.

Heparin Overdose

Intravenous infusions of high-alert medications require vigilance to ensure that the patient receives the correct dosage and that serious side effects are recognized and treated promptly. In addition to safely preparing the medication according to protocol, the nurse must be prepared to administer an antidote in the case of life-threatening adverse reactions. Adverse reactions may be the result of expected risks due to individual patient variation, but may also occur due to calculation error or intravenous pump malfunction. Protamine sulfate is the antidote to severe heparin overdose. Let's consider a potential situation when protamine sulfate might be indicated.

EXAMPLE 4 ■

Your patient on the heparin protocol has been receiving intravenous heparin according to protocol for 21 hours. After periodic adjustments, the infusion rate is currently set for 12 mL/h, which is equal to 12,000 units/h. The most recent aPTT result was 94 seconds, which according to protocol required the infusion to be stopped for 1 hour and then decreased by 3 units/kg/h (line 15, Figure 17-1). While waiting to resume the heparin infusion, the patient care technician reports to the nurse that the patient's blood pressure has dropped, pulse has increased, and that urine is very dark. Recognizing that these are all signs of possible hemorrhage, the nurse contacts the physician, who orders **protamine sulfate 12 mg slow IV push.** The recommended infusion rate is no faster than 20 mg per minute. Calculate this emergency dose using the Three-Step Approach to dosage calculations.

Order: **protamine sulfate 12 mg slow IV push**

Supply: See Figure 17-4

FIGURE 17-4 Protamine sulfate 50 mg (10 mg/mL)

Step 1 **Convert** The order and the supplied dosages are in the same unit of measurement: units. No conversion is necessary.

Step 2 **Think** There are 50 mg in the entire 5 mL vial, but the concentration is also stated as 10 mg/mL. Because 12 mg is slightly larger than 10 mg, you will need slightly more than 1 mL. The rate should be no faster than 20 mg per minute. As 12 mg is slightly larger than $\frac{1}{2}$ of 20 mg, the dose should be injected in slightly more than $\frac{1}{2}$ minute.

Step 3 **Calculate** $\dfrac{D}{H} \times Q = \dfrac{\overset{6}{\cancel{12}} \text{ mg}}{\underset{5}{\cancel{10}} \text{ mg}} \times 1 \text{ mL} = \dfrac{6}{5} \text{ mL} = 1.2 \text{ mL}$ (verifies estimate)

Draw up 1.2 mL in a 3 mL syringe and inject as an IV push.

Recall from Chapter 15 that $\dfrac{D}{H} \times T$ can be used to calculate the time required to administer IV push medications.

Rate: 20 mg/min or 20 mg per 60 sec

$\dfrac{D}{H} \times T = \dfrac{12 \text{ mg}}{\underset{1}{\cancel{20}} \text{ mg}} \times \overset{3}{\cancel{60}} \text{ sec} = \dfrac{36}{1} \text{ sec} = 36 \text{ sec}$ (verifies estimate)

Infuse 1.2 mL of protamine sulfate over at least 36 seconds.

Use ratio and proportion to calculate how much to push each 15 seconds, to slowly titrate the infusion.

$$\dfrac{1.2 \text{ mL}}{36 \text{ sec}} \diagdown\!\!\!\!\!\diagup \dfrac{X \text{ mL}}{15 \text{ sec}}$$

$$36X = 18 \text{ sec}$$

$$\dfrac{36X}{36} = \dfrac{18}{36}$$

$$X = 0.5 \text{ mL (every 15 sec)}$$

IV Insulin Protocol

It has been shown that critically ill diabetic patients who have tight management of blood glucose levels have reduced morbidity and mortality. There is increased use of intravenous insulin protocols in the intensive care units and on some medical surgical units to maintain tight control over hyperglycemia. While there is no universal protocol for intravenous insulin infusions, most are similar in approach. In this text, we will use the sample critical care intravenous insulin protocol (Figure 17-5) to calculate insulin dosage, but in your clinical practice, you will use the protocol that has been adopted by your health care agency. According to the sample protocol, the target level for blood glucose control is 70 to 110 mg/dL.

FIGURE 17-5   Sample intravenous insulin therapy protocol

	Sample Critical Care Intravenous Insulin Protocol Orders
TARGET	**BLOOD GLUCOSE LEVEL 70 to 110 mg/dL**
Insulin Solution	1. 100 units **regular insulin** in 100 mL of 0.9% NaCl, to be titrated based on grid for Levels 1, 2 ,or 3.
Initial Infusion	2. Start nondiabetic patients at Level 1. Advance to Level 2 if TARGET range not reached after 2 hours on Level 1. 3. Start diabetic patients at Level 2. Advance to Level 3 if TARGET range not reached after 2 hours on Level 2. 4. Do not initiate insulin infusion unless blood glucose greater than 110 mg/dL.
Monitoring	5. Check blood glucose prior to start of insulin infusion. 6. Check blood glucose every hour thereafter. 7. When glucose is 80 to 110 mg/dL for 3 hours, check glucose every 2 hours. 8. Resume monitoring every hour if blood glucose greater than 120 mg/dL for 2 hours.

Blood Glucose Less than 80 mg/dL	9. If patient has blood glucose less than 80 mg/dL:
	   a. Refer to regular insulin infusion rate column in grid tables for management instructions.
	   b. If necessary to reinitiate insulin infusion, start one level below previous level.
	   c. Call physician for symptomatic hypoglycemia or blood glucose less than 50 mg/dL, even if treated.

Sample Grid for Titration of Intravenous Insulin—Level 2

LEVEL 2: DO NOT INITIATE insulin drip unless blood glucose is greater than 110 mg/dL.

Blood Glucose (mg/dL)	Regular Insulin Bolus	Regular Insulin Infusion Rate
Less than 70	Give $\frac{1}{2}$ amp of 50% dextrose	HOLD Insulin Infusion × 60 minutes and check blood glucose every 15 minutes until equal to or greater than 80.
70 to 79	0	HOLD insulin infusion × 60 minutes and check blood glucose every 15 minutes until equal to or greater than 80.
80 to 110	0	2 units/h
111 to 125	0	3 units/h
126 to 149	0	4 units/h
150 to 165	0	5 units/h
166 to 179	0	6 units/h
180 to 209	0	8 units/h
210 to 239	10 units IV push	12 units/h
240 to 269	10 units IV push	16 units/h
270 to 299	10 units IV push	20 units/h
300 to 350	10 units IV push	25 units/h
greater than 350	Notify physician	

As with the heparin protocol, we will use the same three sequential actions: 1) Bolus, 2) Continuous Infusion, and 3) Rebolus and/or Adjust Infusion Rate.

EXAMPLE 1 ■

Individual patients' insulin needs vary and are regulated based on the measurement of blood glucose. The sample insulin protocol provides three levels of insulin dosage, depending on expected individual response to insulin therapy. Rapid- or short-acting insulin may be used for intravenous infusions. The sample protocol uses regular insulin but does not specify whether U-100 or U-500 insulin is needed. You learned in Chapter 11 that U-500 insulin is only used for very high doses that cannot be measured in a standard U-100 insulin syringe. Based on the dosage used to mix the solution (100 units—line 1, Figure 17-5) and the bolus dosage listed in the grid (10 units), U-500 insulin would not be needed. Choose U-100 regular insulin as pictured in Figure 17-6.

FIGURE 17-6   Humulin R regular U-100 insulin

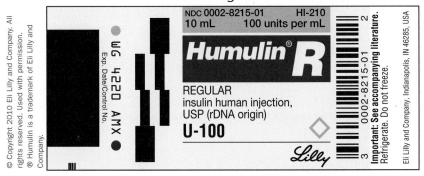

For this example, we will provide insulin coverage for an insulin-dependent diabetic who is recovering in the intensive care unit from extensive surgery. According to protocol (line 3, Figure 17-5), the sample Level 2 grid for titration of insulin will be used for this patient. (For simplicity, the Level 1 and Level 3 grids have been omitted.) The point-of-care blood glucose measurement of this patient is 226 mg/dL, as tested upon admission to the intensive care unit.

Action 1   **Bolus:** Unlike the heparin protocol, the initial insulin bolus dose is not based on patient weight, but glucose level alone. A bolus dose is not always required. In this instance, the patient's blood glucose level of 226 mg/dL falls between 210 and 239 mg/dL, which requires a bolus of 10 units U-100 regular insulin. Draw up 10 units in a 30-unit Lo-Dose insulin syringe.

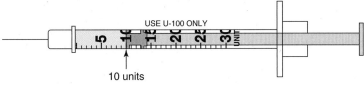

© Cengage Learning 2013

Provide the order, point-of-care glucose measurement, insulin vial, and syringe to another nurse for independent verification and documentation.

Action 2   **Continuous Infusion:** Often, insulin or other high-alert drugs come premixed from the hospital pharmacy. But there will be times when nurses will need to mix the IV solution for the continuous infusion. Let's continue with our patient example by following the protocol to prepare the IV insulin solution (line 1, Figure 17-5) and then by calculating the initial infusion rate for the blood glucose level of this patient (226 mg/dL, which is in the range on the Level 2 grid of 210 to 239 mg/dL).

Protocol Order Insulin Solution: 100 units regular insulin in 100 mL of 0.9% NaCl

Draw up 100 units of regular U-100 insulin in a standard U-100 insulin syringe.

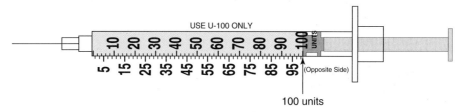

USE U-100 ONLY

(Opposite Side)

100 units

© Cengage Learning 2013

Provide the order, point-of-care glucose measurement, insulin vial, and syringe to another nurse for independent verification and documentation. Inject the 100 units into the 100 mL IV PB bag of 0.9% NaCl (NS or normal saline). Prepare a label with the patient's name, drug name and concentration, dosage and amount added, date and time prepared, and your signature. Secure the label on the IV PB bag.

Protocol Order Insulin Infusion Rate: Now we will calculate the hourly infusion rate with the same formula we used to calculate the heparin infusion.

RULE

To calculate the continuous flow rate of IV solutions in mL/h using a version of the dosage calculation formula:

$$\frac{\text{D (units/h desired)}}{\text{H (units you have available)}} \times \text{Q (mL you have available)} = \text{R (mL/h rate)}$$

Note: This rule also applies to other continuous infusion drugs ordered in units/h, milliunits/h, mg/h, mcg/h, g/h, or mEq/h.

The patient's blood glucose level of 226 mg/dL falls between 210 and 239 mg/dL, which requires an infusion rate of 12 units/h.

$$\frac{\text{D (units/h)}}{\text{H (units)}} \times \text{Q (mL)} = \text{R (mL/h)}$$

$$\frac{12 \text{ units/h}}{100 \text{ units}} \times 100 \text{ mL} = 12 \text{ mL/h}$$

Remember that you can think of this a different way by using ratio and proportion to determine how many units are in 1 mL. If there are 100 units per 100 mL, how many units are there in 1 mL? Use ratio and proportion to calculate the amount.

$$\frac{100 \text{ units}}{100 \text{ mL}} \diagdown\diagup \frac{\text{X units}}{1 \text{ mL}}$$

$$100\text{X} = 100 \text{ (cross-multiply)}$$

$$\frac{100}{100} = \frac{100\text{X}}{100} \text{ (solve for X)}$$

$$\text{X} = 1 \quad \text{There is 1 unit of insulin in 1 mL}$$

After setting up the equation, it is obvious that the prepared solution provides 1 unit of insulin in each 1 mL of solution. It is safe practice to develop intravenous infusion protocols that require the simplest possible math calculations. Use the dosage calculation formula to see how using this calculation is so much simpler.

$$\frac{\text{D (units/h)}}{\text{H (units)}} \times \text{Q (mL)} = \text{R (mL/h)}$$

$$\frac{12 \text{ units/h}}{1 \text{ unit}} \times 1 \text{ mL} = 12 \text{ mL/h}$$

For this problem, we will assume that the infusion pump available is designed to infuse at a mL/h rate using whole numbers only. Set the rate on the pump for the initial infusion at 12 mL/h. Ask another nurse for independent verification of the initial infusion rate.

Action 3   **Rebolus and/or Adjust Infusion Rate:** The insulin protocol requires hourly blood glucose monitoring until the glucose level is 80 to 110 mg/dL for 3 hours (lines 6 and 7, Figure 17-5). For the patient in this example, one hour after the infusion is started, the point-of-care blood glucose measurement is 206 mg/dL. What will you do?

Rebolus: Is a bolus necessary now? 206 mg/dL falls between 180 and 209 mg/dL. According to the grid, no bolus is needed at this time.

Adjust Infusion Rate: According to the grid, for a glucose measurement of 206 mg/dL, the rate should be set for 8 units per hour. Now that we know there is 1 unit/mL, we will give 8 times as much, or 8 mL/h. While this seems obvious, let's use the dosage calculation formula one more time to verify our estimate.

$$\frac{D\ (units/h)}{H\ (units)} \times Q\ (mL) = R\ (mL/h) \qquad \frac{8\ \cancel{units}/h}{1\ \cancel{units}} \times 1\ mL = 8\ mL/h$$

Reduce the rate on the infusion pump from 12 mL/h to 8 mL/h. Ask another nurse for independent verification of the change in infusion rate. Remember: In order to have consistent monitoring from shift to shift, the nurse must document the time and dose of the bolus and infusion rate changes on a standard worksheet.

Insulin Overdose

Hypoglycemia (blood glucose below 50 mg/dL) occurs when insulin levels exceed insulin needs. This may result from an overdose of insulin during intravenous infusion due to expected risks because of individual patient variation, but may also occur because of calculation error or intravenous pump malfunction. Rapid treatment of hypoglycemia is required to prevent irreversible brain damage or even death. For this reason, protocols for insulin and other high-alert drugs frequently include standard orders for severe adverse reactions. The sample protocol for intravenous insulin infusion provides an order for 50% dextrose in the case of hypoglycemia. It is supplied for emergency use in a prefilled ampule of 25 g per 50 mL.

EXAMPLE 2 ■

After periodic adjustments in the insulin infusion rate, the patient care technician reports that your patient in the previous example was acting confused during the point-of-care glucose monitoring, which was 65 mg/dL. According to the protocol, the nurse should give $\frac{1}{2}$ amp (ampule) of 50% dextrose, hold the insulin infusion for 60 minutes, and check blood glucose every 15 minutes until it is greater than or equal to 80 mg/dL.

Protocol Order: Give $\frac{1}{2}$ amp of 50% dextrose

Supply: 50 mL ampule of 50% dextrose

Calculate: $\frac{1}{2} \times 50\ mL = \dfrac{\overset{25}{\cancel{50}}}{\underset{1}{\cancel{2}}}\ mL = 25\ mL$

To administer $\frac{1}{2}$ amp of 50% dextrose, you will need to give 25 mL by IV push. You should discard 25 mL, leaving 25 mL in the ampule, and then push the entire amount remaining through an infusion port near the IV insertion site. It is not safe to insert the ampule with the entire amount into the port and then try to push only 25 mL. It is very difficult to push a 50% dextrose solution, and you could push forcefully and inject more than the ordered amount.

According to protocol, increase glucose monitoring to every 15 minutes until greater than 80 mg/dL. The physician must be notified for symptomatic hypoglycemia or blood glucose that is less than 50 mg/dL, even if treated (line 9c, Figure 17-5). Your patient showed the hypoglycemic symptom of confusion. Notify the physician.

QUICK REVIEW

- Many hospitals use standard protocols to initiate and maintain continuous infusion therapy for critical medications such as heparin and insulin.
- Protocols may be based on weight in kilograms, and dose adjustments are made based on blood tests or other patient data such as physical assessment findings.
- To calculate mL/h when you know units/h and units/mL, use $\frac{D}{H} \times Q = R$.
- Document boluses and changes to infusion rate on flowsheet for consistent monitoring and maintenance of infusions.
- Be prepared to administer an antidote if severe adverse reactions occur.

Review Set 46

Calculate the flow rate. The infusion pumps are calibrated to deliver whole mL.

1. Order: 0.45% NS 1,000 mL IV c̄ heparin 25,000 units to infuse at 1,000 units/h

   Flow rate: _____ mL/h

2. Order: D₅W 500 mL IV c̄ heparin 40,000 units to infuse at 1,100 units/h

   Flow rate: _____ mL/h

3. Order: 0.45% NS 500 mL IV c̄ heparin 25,000 units to infuse at 500 units/h

   Flow rate: _____ mL/h

4. Order: D₅W 500 mL IV c̄ heparin 40,000 units to infuse at 1,500 units/h

   Flow rate: _____ mL/h

5. Order: D₅W 1 L IV c̄ heparin 25,000 units to infuse at 1,200 units/h. On rounds, you assess the patient and observe that the infusion pump is set at 120 mL/h.

   At what rate should the pump be set? _____ mL/h

   What should your action be? _____

6. Order: D₅W 500 mL IV with heparin 25,000 units to infuse at 800 units/h

   Flow rate: _____ mL/h

Questions 7 through 10 refer to a patient who weighs 165 lb and has IV heparin ordered per the following Weight-Based Heparin Protocol. With this variation of the heparin protocol, you will not round the patient's weight, and instead you will use the patient's actual weight. The infusion pumps are calibrated to deliver whole mL.

Weight-Based Heparin Protocol:

Heparin IV infusion: Heparin 25,000 units in 250 mL of $\frac{1}{2}$NS

IV boluses: Use heparin 1,000 units/mL.

Calculate the patient's weight in kg. Weight: _____ kg

Bolus with heparin 80 units/kg. Then initiate heparin drip at 18 units/kg/h. Obtain aPTT every 6 hours, and adjust dosage and rate as follows:

If aPTT is less than 35 seconds: Rebolus with 80 units/kg and increase rate by 4 units/kg/h.

If aPTT is 36 to 44 seconds: Rebolus with 40 units/kg and increase rate by 2 units/kg/h.

If aPTT is 45 to 75 seconds: Continue current rate.

If aPTT is 76 to 90 seconds: Decrease rate by 2 units/kg/h.

If aPTT is greater than 90 seconds: Hold heparin for 1 hour and then decrease rate by 3 units/kg/h.

7. Convert the patient's weight to kg: _____ kg

   Calculate the initial heparin bolus dosage: _____ units

   Calculate the bolus dose: _____ mL

   Calculate the initial heparin infusion rate: _____ units/h, or _____ mL/h

8. At 0900, the patient's aPTT is 33 seconds. According to the protocol, what will your action be?

   Rebolus with _____ units, or _____ mL.

   Increase infusion rate by _____ units/h, or _____ mL/h, for a new rate of _____ mL/h.

9. At 1500, the patient's aPTT is 40 seconds. According to the protocol, what will your action be?

   Rebolus with _____ units or _____ mL.

   Increase infusion rate by _____ units/h, or _____ mL/h, for a new rate of _____ mL/h.

10. At 2100, the patient's aPTT is 60 seconds. What will your action be according to the protocol?

    _____

Questions 11 through 15 refer to a seriously ill patient in the critical care unit who has insulin dependent diabetes. Use the following grid for titration of intravenous insulin. An IV pump is used, and it is calibrated to deliver whole milliliters.

Sample Grid for Titration of Intravenous Insulin—Level 2		
LEVEL 2: DO NOT INITIATE insulin drip unless blood glucose is greater than 110 mg/dL.		
Blood Glucose mg/dL)	**Regular Insulin Bolus**	**Regular Insulin Infusion Rate**
Less than 70	Give $\frac{1}{2}$ amp of 50% dextrose	HOLD Insulin Infusion × 60 minutes and check blood glucose every 15 minutes until equal to or greater than 80.
70 to 79	0	HOLD insulin infusion × 60 minutes and check blood glucose every 15 minutes until equal to or greater than 80.
80 to 110	0	2 units/h
111 to 125	0	3 units/h
126 to 149	0	4 units/h
150 to 165	0	5 units/h
166 to 179	0	6 units/h
180 to 209	0	8 units/h
210 to 239	10 units IV push	12 units/h
240 to 269	10 units IV push	16 units/h
270 to 299	10 units IV push	20 units/h
300 to 350	10 units IV push	25 units/h
greater than 350	Notify physician	

11. The blood glucose level at the start of the infusion is 320 mg/dL. Is a bolus dose of insulin required? _____ If so, what is the required bolus dosage? _____ units

12. The insulin solution prepared for the continuous infusion is 100 units U-100 regular insulin in 100 mL of 0.9% NaCl. What should be the rate at the start of the infusion? _____ mL/h

13. One hour later, the blood glucose level is 198 mg/dL. Is a bolus dose of insulin required? _____ If so, what is the required dosage? _____ units

14. What should be the new rate for the continuous infusion? _____ mL/h

15. After monitoring and adjustment to insulin doses over 4 hours, the blood glucose level is 72 mg/dL. What should your action be at this time? _____

After completing these problems, see page 660 to check your answers.

CRITICAL CARE IV CALCULATIONS: CALCULATING FLOW RATE OF AN IV MEDICATION TO BE GIVEN OVER A SPECIFIED TIME PERIOD

With increasing frequency, medications are ordered for patients in critical care situations as a prescribed amount to be administered in a specified time period, such as *X mg per minute*. Such medications are usually administered by electronic infusion devices programmed in mL/h. Unless stated otherwise, for calculations you can assume that the IV pump is calibrated to deliver whole milliliters. Careful monitoring of patients receiving life-threatening therapies is a critical nursing skill.

IV Medication Ordered per Minute

RULE

To determine the flow rate (mL/h) for IV medications ordered per minute (such as mg/min):

Step 1   Calculate the dosage in mL/min:

$$\frac{D}{H} \times Q = R \text{ (mL/min)}$$

Step 2   Calculate the flow rate in mL/h of the volume to administer per minute

mL/min × 60 min/h = mL/h

Note: The order may specify mg/min, mcg/min, g/min, units/min, milliunits/min, or mEq/min.

In the formula $\frac{D}{H} \times Q = R$ (mL/min):

D = Dosage *desired:* mg/min

H = Dosage you *have* available: mg

Q = *Quantity* of solution you have available: mL

R = Flow *rate:* mL/min

EXAMPLE 1 ■

Order: **lidocaine 2 g IV in 500 mL D₅W at 2 mg/min via infusion pump.** You must prepare and hang 500 mL of D₅W IV solution that has 2 g of lidocaine added to it. Then, you must regulate the flow rate so the patient receives 2 mg of the lidocaine every minute. Determine the flow rate for the IV pump calibrated to deliver tenths of a mL/h.

Step 1   Calculate mL/min (change mg/min to mL/min)

Apply the formula $\frac{D}{H} \times Q = R$ (mL/min).

D = dosage desired = 2 mg/min

H = dosage you have available = 2 g = 2.000. = 2,000 mg

Q = quantity of available solution = 500 mL

$$\frac{D}{H} \times Q = \frac{2 \text{ mg/min}}{2,000 \text{ mg}} \times 500 \text{ mL} = R \text{ (mL/min)}$$

MATH TIP

$\dfrac{\text{mg/min}}{\text{mg}} \times \text{mL} = \text{mL/min}$, because mg cancel out

$$\frac{2 \text{ mg/min}}{2,000 \text{ mg}} \times \frac{\overset{1}{\cancel{500}} \text{ mL}}{1} = \frac{\overset{1}{\cancel{2}}}{\underset{2}{\cancel{4}}} \text{ mL/min} = \frac{1}{2} \text{ mL/min} = 0.5 \text{ mL/min}$$

Step 2   Determine the flow rate in mL/h. You know there are 60 minutes per hour, so you can multiply by 60 min/h.

mL/min × 60 min/h = mL/h

0.5 mL/min × 60 min/h = X mL/h

MATH TIP

$\dfrac{\text{mL}}{\text{min}} \times \dfrac{\text{min}}{\text{h}} = \text{mL/h}$, because min cancel out

$$\frac{0.5 \text{ mL}}{\cancel{\text{min}}} \times \frac{60 \cancel{\text{min}}}{\text{h}} = 30 \text{ mL/h, or } 0.5 \text{ mL/}\cancel{\text{min}} \times 60 \cancel{\text{min}}/\text{h} = 30 \text{ mL/h}$$

Rate is 30 mL/h.

Regulate the flow rate to 30 mL/h to deliver 2 mg/min of lidocaine that is prepared at the concentration of 2 g per 500 mL of D₅W IV solution.

EXAMPLE 2 ■

Order: **nitroglycerin 125 mg IV in 500 mL D₅W to infuse at 42 mcg/min**

Calculate the flow rate in mL/h to program the infusion pump calibrated to deliver tenths of a mL/h.

Step 1   Calculate mL/min (change mcg/min to mL/min)

First, convert mg to mcg: 1 mg = 1,000 mcg; 125 mg = 125.000. = 125,000 mcg

Then, calculate mL/min:

$$\frac{D}{H} \times Q = \frac{42 \text{ mcg/min}}{\underset{250}{\cancel{125,000}} \text{ mcg}} \times \overset{1}{\cancel{500}} \text{mL} = \frac{42}{250} \text{ mL/min} = 0.168 \text{ mL/min} = 0.17 \text{ mL/min}$$

Step 2   Determine the flow rate in mL/h (change mL/min to mL/h). You know that 1 h = 60 min.

mL/min × 60 min/h = mL/h

0.17 mL/$\cancel{\text{min}}$ × 60 $\cancel{\text{min}}$/h = 10.2 mL/h

Rate is 10.2 mL/h, not 10 mL/h, because the IV pump is calibrated in tenths.

Regulate the flow rate to 10 mL/h to deliver 42 mcg/min of nitroglycerin, which is prepared at the concentration of 125 mg per 500 mL of D₅W IV solution.

IV Medication Ordered per Kilogram per Minute

The physician may also order the amount of medication in an IV solution that a patient should receive in a specified time period per kilogram of body weight. An electronic infusion device is usually used to administer these orders.

RULE

To determine the flow rate (mL/h) for IV medications ordered per minute (such as mg/kg/min):

Step 1   Convert to like units, such as mg to mcg or lb to kg.

Step 2   Calculate desired dosage per minute: mg/kg/min × kg = mg/min.

Step 3   Calculate the dosage flow rate in mL/min: $\frac{D}{H} \times Q = R$ (mL/min)

Step 4   Calculate the flow rate in mL/h of the volume to administer per minute:
mL/min × 60 min/h = mL/h

Note: The order may specify mg/min, mcg/min, g/min, units/min, milliunits/min, or mEq/min; or it may specify mg/h, mcg/h, g/h, units/h, milliunits/h, or mEq/h.

EXAMPLE ■

Order: **250 mL of IV solution with 225 mg of a medication to infuse at 3 mcg/kg/min via infusion pump** for a person who weighs 110 lb.

Determine the flow rate for the IV pump calibrated in whole mL/h.

Step 1   Convert mg to mcg: 1 mg = 1,000 mcg; 225 mg = 225.000. = 225,000 mcg

Convert lb to kg: 1 kg = 2.2 lb; 110 lb ÷ 2.2 lb/kg = 110 lb × 1 kg/2.2 lb = 50 kg

Step 2   Calculate desired mcg/min.

3 mcg/kg/min × 50 kg = 150 mcg/min

Step 3   Calculate mL/min.

$$\frac{D}{H} \times Q = \frac{150 \text{ mcg/min}}{\underset{900}{225,000 \text{ mcg}}} \times \overset{1}{250} \text{ mL} = \frac{150}{900} \text{ mL/min} = 0.166 \text{ mL/min} = 0.17 \text{ mL/min}$$

Step 4   Calculate mL/h. You know that 1 h = 60 min.

mL/min × 60 min/h = 0.17 mL/min × 60 min/h = 10.2 mL/h = 10 mL/h

Rate is 10 mL/h. Remember: The IV pump is calibrated in whole mL/h.

For a person who weighs 110 lb, or 50 kg, regulate the IV flow rate to 10 mL/h to deliver 150 mcg/min (3 mcg/kg/min) of the drug, which is prepared at the concentration of 225 mg per 250 mL of IV solution.

Titrating IV Drugs

Sometimes IV medications may be prescribed to be administered at an initial dosage over a specified time period and then continued at a different dosage and time period. These situations are common in obstetrics and critical care. Medications such as magnesium sulfate, dopamine, Isuprel, and Pitocin are ordered to be *titrated*, or *regulated*, to obtain measurable physiologic responses. Dosages will be adjusted until the desired effect is achieved. In some cases, a loading or bolus dose is infused and monitored closely. Most IV medications that require titration usually start at the lowest dosage and are increased or decreased as needed. An upper titration limit is usually set and is not exceeded unless the desired response is not obtained. A new drug order is then required.

Let's look at some of these situations.

RULE

To calculate flow rate (mL/h) for IV medications ordered over a specific time period (such as mg/min):

Step 1 Calculate mg/mL.

Step 2 Calculate mL/h.

Note: The order may specify mg/min, mcg/min, g/min, units/min, milliunits/min, or mEq/min; or it may specify mg/h, mcg/h, g/h, units/h, milliunits/h, or mEq/h.

EXAMPLE 1 ▪

Order: RL 1,000 mL IV c̄ magnesium sulfate 20 g. Start with bolus of 4 g for 30 min, then maintain a continuous infusion at 2 g/h

1. What is the flow rate in whole mL/h for the bolus order?

Step 1 Calculate the bolus dosage in g/mL.

There are 20 g in 1,000 mL. How many mL are necessary to infuse 4 g?

Desired (D) = 4 g   Have (H) = 20 g per 1,000 mL Quantity (Q)

$$\frac{D}{H} \times Q = \frac{4\ \cancel{g}}{\underset{1}{\cancel{20}\ \cancel{g}}} \times \overset{50}{\cancel{1,000}}\ mL = 200\ mL$$

Therefore, 200 mL contain 4 g, to be administered over 30 min.

Step 2 Calculate the bolus rate in mL/h.

What is the flow rate in mL/h to infuse 200 mL (which contain 4 g of magnesium sulfate)? Remember: 1 h = 60 min.

$$\frac{Total\ mL}{Total\ min} \times 60\ min/h = \frac{200\ mL}{\underset{1}{\cancel{30}\ \cancel{min}}} \times \frac{\overset{2}{\cancel{60}\ \cancel{min}}}{1\ h} = 400\ mL/h$$

Rate is 400 mL/h.

Set the infusion pump at 400 mL/h to deliver the bolus of 4 g per 30 min as ordered.

Now calculate the continuous IV rate in mL/h.

2. What is the flow rate in mL/h for the continuous infusion of magnesium sulfate of 2 g/h? You know from the bolus dosage calculation that 200 mL contain 4 g.

Desired (D) = 2 g/h   Have (H) = 4 g per 200 mL Quantity (Q)

$$\frac{D}{H} \times Q = \frac{2\ \cancel{g}/h}{\underset{1}{\cancel{4}\ \cancel{g}}} \times \overset{50}{\cancel{200}}\ mL = 100\ mL/h$$

After the bolus has infused in the first 30 min, reset the infusion pump to 100 mL/h to deliver the continuous infusion of 2 g/h.

Let's look at an example using Pitocin (a drug used to induce or augment labor) measured in units and milliunits.

EXAMPLE 2 ▪

A drug order is written to induce labor: LR 1,000 mL IV c̄ Pitocin 20 units. Begin a continuous infusion IV at 1 milliunit/min, increase by 1 milliunit/min q.15 min to a maximum of 20 milliunits/min

1. What is the flow rate in whole mL/h to deliver 1 milliunit/min?

   In this example, the medication is measured in units (instead of g or mg).

   Step 1   Calculate milliunits/mL.

   Convert: 1 unit = 1,000 milliunits; 20 units = 20.000. = 20,000 milliunits

   Desired (D) = 1 milliunit   Have (H) = 20,000 milliunits per 1,000 mL Quantity (Q)

   $$\frac{D}{H} \times Q = \frac{1 \text{ milliunit}}{\underset{20}{20,000 \text{ milliunits}}} \times \overset{1}{1,000} \text{ mL} = \frac{1}{20} \text{ mL} = 0.05 \text{ mL}$$

   Therefore, 0.05 mL contains 1 milliunit of Pitocin, or there is 1 milliunit per 0.05 mL.

   Step 2   Calculate mL/h.

   What is the flow rate in mL/h to infuse 0.05 mL/min (which is 1 milliunit Pitocin/min)?

   $$\frac{\text{Total mL}}{\text{Total min}} \times 60 \text{ min/h} = \frac{0.05 \text{ mL}}{1 \text{ min}} \times \frac{60 \text{ min}}{1 \text{ h}} = 3 \text{ mL/h}$$

   Set the infusion pump at 3 mL/h to infuse Pitocin 1 milliunit/min as ordered.

2. What is the maximum flow rate in mL/h at which the Pitocin infusion can be set for the titration as ordered? Notice that the order allows a maximum of 20 milliunits/min. You know from the bolus dosage calculation that there is 1 milliunit per 0.05 mL.

   Desired (D) = 20 milliunits/min   Have (H) = 1 milliunit per 0.05 mL Quantity (Q)

   $$\frac{D}{H} \times Q = \frac{20 \text{ milliunits/min}}{1 \text{ milliunit}} \times 0.05 \text{ mL} = 1 \text{ mL/min}$$

   Now convert mL/min to mL/h so you can program the electronic infusion device.

   mL/min × 60 min/h = 1 mL/min × 60 min/h = 60 mL/h

   Rate of 60 mL/h will deliver 20 milliunits/min.

Verifying Safe IV Medication Dosage Recommended per Minute

It is also a critical nursing skill to be sure that patients are receiving safe dosages of medications. Therefore, you must also be able to convert critical care IVs with additive medications to **mg/h** or **mg/min** to check safe or normal dosage ranges.

RULE

To check safe dosage of IV medications ordered in mL/h:

Step 1   Calculate mg/h.

Step 2   Calculate mg/min.

Step 3   Compare recommended dosage and ordered dosage to decide if the dosage is safe.

Note: The ordered and recommended dosages may specify mg/min, mcg/min, g/min, units/min, milliunits/min, or mEq/min.

EXAMPLE ▪

The drug reference states that the recommended dosage of lidocaine is 1 to 4 mg/min. The patient has an order for D₅W 500 mL IV c̄ lidocaine 1 g to infuse at 30 mL/h. Is the lidocaine dosage within the safe range?

Step 1   Calculate mg/h

Convert: 1 g = 1,000 mg

The unknown in the formula is D (mg/h).

Desired (D) = D mg/h   Have (H) = 1,000 mg per 500 mL Quantity (Q)
Rate (R) = 30 mL/h

$$\frac{D}{H} \times Q = \frac{D \text{ mg/h}}{\underset{2}{\cancel{1,000} \text{ mg}}} \times \overset{1}{\cancel{500}} \text{ mL} = 30 \text{ mL/h}$$

$$\frac{D}{2} = 30$$

$$\frac{D}{2} \underset{1}{\overset{30}{\times}}$$

X = 60 mg/h (You know the answer is in mg/h because D is measured in mg/h.)

Step 2   Calculate mg/min. THINK: It is obvious that 60 mg/h is the same as 60 mg per 60 min or 1 mg/min.

1 h = 60 min

$$\frac{\text{mg/h}}{60 \text{ min/h}} = \text{mg/min}$$

$$\frac{\overset{1}{\cancel{60} \text{ mg/}\cancel{h}}}{\underset{1}{\cancel{60} \text{ min/}\cancel{h}}} = 1 \text{ mg/min}$$

Rate is 1 mg/min.

Step 3   Compare ordered and recommended dosages.

1 mg/min is within the safe range of 1 to 4 mg/min. The dosage is safe.

Likewise, IV medications ordered as mL/h and recommended in mg/kg/min require verification of their safety or normal dosage range.

RULE

To check safe dosage of IV medications recommended in mg/kg/min and ordered in mL/h:

Step 1   Convert to like units, such as mg to mcg or lb to kg.

Step 2   Calculate recommended mg/min.

Step 3   Calculate ordered mg/h.

Step 4   Calculate ordered mg/min.

Step 5   Compare ordered and recommended dosages. Decide if the dosage is safe.

Note: The ordered and recommended dosages may specify mg/kg/min, mcg/kg/min, g/kg/min, units/kg/min, milliunits/kg/min, or mEq/kg/min.

EXAMPLE ▪

The recommended dosage range of Nitropress for adults is 0.3 to 10 mcg/kg/min. The patient has an order for D₅W 100 mL IV with Nitropress 420 mg to infuse at 1 mL/h. The patient weighs 154 lb. Is the Nitropress dosage within the normal range?

Step 1   Convert lb to kg: 154 lb ÷ 2.2 lb/kg = 154 l̶b̶ × 1 kg/2.2 l̶b̶ = 70 kg

         Convert mg to mcg: 420 mg = 420.000. = 420,000 mcg

Step 2   Calculate recommended mcg/min range.

         Minimum: 0.3 mcg/k̶g̶/min × 70 k̶g̶ = 21 mcg/min

         Maximum: 10 mcg/k̶g̶/min × 70 k̶g̶ = 700 mcg/min

Step 3   Calculate ordered mcg/h.

         Desired (D) = D mcg/h   Have (H) = 420,000 mcg per 100 mL Quantity (Q)
Rate (R) = 1 mL/h

$$\frac{D}{H} \times Q = R$$

$$\frac{D \ \text{mcg/h}}{\underset{4,200}{420,000 \ \text{mcg}}} \times \overset{1}{100} \ \text{mL} = 1 \ \text{mL/h}$$

$$\frac{D}{4,200} = 1$$

$$\frac{D}{4,200} \times\!\!\!\!\times \frac{1}{1}$$

           D = 4,200 mcg/h (You know the answer is in mcg/h because D is measured in mcg/h.)

Step 4   Calculate ordered mcg/min: 4,200 mcg/h = 4,200 mcg per 60 min

$$\frac{4,200 \ \text{mcg}}{60 \ \text{min}} = 70 \ \text{mcg/min}$$

Step 5   Compare ordered and recommended dosages. Decide if the dosage is safe. Because 70 mcg/min is within the allowable range of 21 to 700 mcg/min, the ordered dosage is safe.

QUICK REVIEW

■ For IV medications ordered in mg/min:
Step 1 Calculate mL/min.
Step 2 Calculate mL/h.

■ To check safe dosages of IV medications recommended in mg/min and ordered in mL/h:
Step 1 Calculate mg/h.
Step 2 Calculate mg/min.
Step 3 Compare recommended and ordered dosages. Decide if the dosage is safe.

■ To check safe dosage of IV medications recommended in mg/kg/min and ordered in mL/h:
Step 1 Convert to like units, such as mg to mcg or lb to kg.
Step 2 Calculate recommended mg/min.
Step 3 Calculate ordered mg/h.
Step 4 Calculate ordered mg/min.
Step 5 Compare ordered and recommended dosages. Decide if the dosage is safe.

Review Set 47

For questions 1 to 5, compute the flow rate for the medications to be administered by IV pump calibrated in tenths of a mL/h.

1. Order: lidocaine 2 g IV per 1,000 mL D₅W at 4 mg/min

    Rate: _____ mL/min and _____ mL/h

2. Order: Pronestyl 0.5 g IV per 250 mL D₅W at 2 mg/min

   Rate: _____ mL/min and _____ mL/h

3. Order: Isuprel 2 mg IV per 500 mL D₅W at 6 mcg/min

   Rate: _____ mL/min and _____ mL/h

4. Order: Medication X 450 mg IV per 500 mL NS at 4 mcg/kg/min

   Weight: 198 lb

   Weight: _____ kg   Give: _____ mcg/min

   Rate: _____ mL/min and _____ mL/h

5. Order: dopamine 800 mg in 500 mL NS IV at 15 mcg/kg/min

   Weight: 70 kg

   Give: _____ mcg/min

   Rate: _____ mL/min and _____ mL/h

Refer to this order for questions 6 through 8.

Order: D₅W 500 mL IV c̄ dobutamine hydrochloride 500 mg to infuse at 15 mL/h. The patient weighs 125 lb. Recommended range: 2.5 to 10 mcg/kg/min

6. What mcg/min range of dobutamine should this patient receive? _____ to _____ mcg/min

7. What mg/min range of dobutamine should this patient receive? _____ to _____ mg/min

8. Is the dobutamine as ordered within the safe range? _____

Refer to this order for questions 9 and 10.

Order: D₅W 500 mL IV c̄ Pronestyl 2 g to infuse at 60 mL/h. Normal range: 2 to 6 mg/min

9. How many mg/min of Pronestyl is the patient receiving? _____ mg/min

10. Is the dosage of Pronestyl within the normal range? _____

11. Order: magnesium sulfate 20 g IV in LR 500 mL. Start with a bolus of 2 g to infuse over 30 min. Then maintain a continuous infusion at 1 g/h. IV pump delivers whole mL/h.

    Rate: _____ mL/h for bolus

    _____ mL/h for continuous infusion

12. The following order is to induce labor. The IV pump delivers whole mL/h.

    Pitocin 15 units IV in 250 mL LR. Begin a continuous infusion at the rate of 1 milliunit/min.

    Rate: _____ mL/h

Refer to this order for questions 13 through 15.

Order: D₅W 1,000 mL IV with terbutaline sulfate 10 mg to infuse at 150 mL/h

Normal dosage range: 10 to 80 mcg/min

13. How many mg/min of terbutaline is the patient receiving? _____ mg/min

14. How many mcg/min of terbutaline is the patient receiving? _____ mcg/min

15. Is the dosage of terbutaline within the normal range? _____

After completing these problems, see pages 661–662 to check your answers.

LIMITING INFUSION VOLUMES

Calculating IV rates to include the IV piggyback (IV PB) volume may be necessary to limit the total volume of IV fluid a patient receives. To do this, you must calculate the flow rate for both the regular IV and the piggyback IV. In such instances of restricted fluids, the piggyback IVs are to be included as part of the total prescribed IV volume and time.

RULE

Follow these six steps to calculate the flow rate of an IV, which includes IV PB.

Step 1   IV PB flow rate: $\dfrac{V}{T} \times C = R$

         or use $\dfrac{mL/h}{\text{Drop factor constant}} = R$

Step 2   Total IV PB time: Time for 1 dose $\times$ # of doses in 24 h

Step 3   Total IV PB volume: Volume of 1 dose $\times$ # of doses in 24 h

Step 4   Total regular IV volume: Total volume − IV PB volume = Regular IV volume

Step 5   Total regular IV time: Total time − IV PB time = Regular IV time

Step 6   Regular IV flow rate: $\dfrac{V}{T} \times C = R$

         or use $\dfrac{mL/h}{\text{Drop factor constant}} = R$

EXAMPLE 1 ■

Order: D_5LR 3,000 mL IV for 24 h with cefazolin 1 g IV PB per 100 mL D_5W q.6h to run 1 hour. Limit total fluids to 3,000 mL daily.

The drop factor is 10 gtt/mL.

Note: The order intends that the patient receive a maximum of 3,000 mL in 24 hours. Remember: When fluids are restricted, the piggybacks are to be *included* in the total 24-hour intake, not added to it.

Step 1   Calculate the flow rate of the IV PB.

$$\frac{V}{T} \times C = \frac{100 \text{ mL}}{\underset{6}{60} \text{ min}} \times \overset{1}{10} \text{ gtt/mL} = \frac{100 \text{ gtt}}{6 \text{ min}} = 16.6 \text{ gtt/min} = 17 \text{ gtt/min}$$

or $\dfrac{mL/h}{\text{Drop factor constant}}$ = gtt/min (drop factor constant is 6)

$$\frac{100 \text{ mL/h}}{6} = 16.6 \text{ gtt/min} = 17 \text{ gtt/min}$$

Set the flow rate for the IV PB at 17 gtt/min to infuse 1 g cefazolin in 100 mL over 1 hour, or 60 min.

Step 2   Calculate the total time the IV PB will be administered.

q.6h = 4 times per 24 h; 4 $\times$ 1 h = 4 h

Step 3   Calculate the total volume of the IV PB.

100 mL $\times$ 4 = 400 mL IV PB per 24 hours

Step 4   Calculate the volume of the regular IV fluids to be administered between IV PB doses. Total volume of regular IV minus total volume of IV PB: 3,000 mL − 400 mL = 2,600 mL

Step 5   Calculate the total regular IV fluid time or the time between IV PB doses. Total IV time minus total IV PB time: 24 h − 4 h = 20 h

Step 6   Calculate the flow rate of the regular IV.

$$mL/h = \frac{2,600 \text{ mL}}{20 \text{ h}} = 130 \text{ mL/h}$$

$$\frac{V}{T} \times C = \frac{130 \text{ mL}}{\underset{6}{60 \text{ min}}} \times \overset{1}{10} \text{ gtt/mL} = \frac{130 \text{ gtt}}{6 \text{ min}} = 21.6 \text{ gtt/min} = 22 \text{ gtt/min}$$

or $\dfrac{mL/h}{\text{Drop factor constant}} = $ gtt/min (drop factor constant is 6)

$$\frac{130 \text{ mL/h}}{6} = 21.6 \text{ gtt/min} = 22 \text{ gtt/min}$$

Set the regular IV of D_5LR at the flow rate of 22 gtt/min. Then after 5 hours, switch to the cefazolin IV PB at the flow rate of 17 gtt/min for 1 hour. Repeat this process 4 times in 24 hours.

EXAMPLE 2 ■

Order: **NS 2,000 mL IV for 24 h with 80 mg gentamycin in 80 mL IV PB q.8h to run for 30 min. Limit fluid intake to 2,000 mL daily.**

Drop factor: 15 gtt/mL

Calculate the flow rate for the regular IV and for the IV PB. IV pump is calibrated in whole mL/h.

Step 1   IV PB flow rate:

$$\frac{V}{T} \times C = \frac{80 \text{ mL}}{\underset{2}{30 \text{ min}}} \times \overset{1}{15} \text{ gtt/mL} = \; = \frac{80 \text{ gtt}}{2 \text{ min}} = 40 \text{ gtt/min}$$

Step 2   Total IV PB time: q.8h = 3 times per 24 h; $3 \times 30 \text{ min} = 90 \text{ min}$

$$90 \text{ min} \div 60 \text{ min/h} = 90 \text{ min} \times 1 \text{ h/60 min} = 1\frac{1}{2} \text{ h}$$

Step 3   Total IV PB volume: $80 \text{ mL} \times 3 = 240 \text{ mL}$

Step 4   Total regular IV volume: $2,000 \text{ mL} - 240 \text{ mL} = 1,760 \text{ mL}$

Step 5   Total regular IV time: $24 \text{ h} - 1\frac{1}{2} \text{ h} = 22\frac{1}{2} \text{ h} = 22.5 \text{ h}$

Step 6   Regular IV flow rate:

$$mL/h = \frac{1,760 \text{ mL}}{22.5 \text{ h}} = 78.2 \text{ mL/h} = 78 \text{ mL/h}$$

$$\frac{V}{T} \times C = \frac{78 \text{ mL}}{\underset{4}{60 \text{ min}}} \times \overset{1}{15} \text{ gtt/mL} = \; = \frac{78 \text{ gtt}}{4 \text{ min}} = 19.5 \text{ gtt/min} = 20 \text{ gtt/min}$$

or $\dfrac{mL/h}{\text{Drop factor constant}} = R$ (drop factor constant is 4)

$$\frac{78 \text{ mL/h}}{4} = 19.5 \text{ gtt/min} = 20 \text{ gtt/min}$$

Set the regular IV of NS at the flow rate of 20 gtt/min. After $7\frac{1}{2}$ hours, switch to the gentamycin IV PB at the flow rate of 40 gtt/min for 30 minutes. Repeat this process 3 times in 24 hours.

Patients receiving a primary IV at a specific rate via an electronic infusion pump may require that the infusion rate be altered when a secondary (piggyback) medication is being administered. To do this, calculate the flow rate of the secondary medication in mL/h as you would the primary IV, and reset the infusion device.

Some infusion pumps allow you to set the flow rate for the secondary IV independent of the primary IV. Upon completion of the secondary infusion, the infusion device automatically returns to the original flow rate. If this is not the case, be sure to manually readjust the primary flow rate after the completion of the secondary set.

QUICK REVIEW

- To calculate the flow rate of a regular IV with an IV PB and restricted fluids, calculate:

Step 1	IV PB flow rate
Step 2	Total IV PB time
Step 3	Total IV PB volume
Step 4	Total regular IV volume
Step 5	Total regular IV time
Step 6	Regular IV flow rate

Review Set 48

Calculate the flow rates for the IV and IV PB orders. These patients are on limited fluid volume (restricted fluids). IV pumps are calibrated in whole mL.

1. Orders: NS 3,000 mL IV for 24 h

   Limit total IV fluids to 3,000 mL daily

   penicillin G potassium 1,000,000 units IV PB q.4h in 100 mL NS to run for 30 min

   Drop factor: 10 gtt/mL

   IV PB flow rate: _____ gtt/min

   IV flow rate: _____ gtt/min

2. Orders: D_5W 1,000 mL IV for 24 h

   Limit total IV fluids to 1,000 mL daily

   gentamicin 40 mg q.i.d. in 40 mL IV PB to run 1 h

   Drop factor: 60 gtt/mL

   IV PB flow rate: _____ gtt/min

   IV flow rate: _____ gtt/min

3. Orders: D_5LR 3,000 mL IV for 24 h

   Limit total IV fluids to 3,000 mL daily

   ampicillin 0.5 g q.6h IV PB in 50 mL D_5W to run 30 min

   Drop factor: 15 gtt/mL

   IV PB flow rate: _____ gtt/min

   IV flow rate: _____ gtt/min

4. Orders: $\frac{1}{2}$NS 2,000 mL IV for 24 h

   Limit total IV fluids to 2,000 mL daily

   Chloromycetin 500 mg per 50 mL NS IV PB q.6h to run 1 h

   Drop factor: 60 gtt/mL

   IV PB flow rate: _____ gtt/min

   IV flow rate: _____ gtt/min

5. Orders: LR 1,000 mL IV for 24 h

   Limit total IV fluids to 1,000 mL daily

   cefazolin 250 mg IV PB per 50 mL D₅W q.8h to run 1 h

   Drop factor: 60 gtt/mL

   IV PB flow rate: _____ gtt/min

   IV flow rate: _____ gtt/min

6. Orders: D₅LR 2,400 mL IV for 24 h

   Limit total IV fluids to 2,400 mL daily

   Ancef 1 g IV PB q.6h in 50 mL D₅W to run 30 min

   Drop factor: On electronic infusion pump

   IV PB flow rate: _____ mL/h

   IV flow rate: _____ mL/h

7. Orders: NS 2,000 mL IV for 24 h

   Limit total IV fluids to 2,000 mL daily

   gentamicin 100 mg IV PB q.8h in 100 mL D₅W to run in over 30 min

   Drop factor: On electronic infusion pump

   IV PB flow rate: _____ mL/h

   IV flow rate: _____ mL/h

8. Orders: D₅ 0.45% NS3,000 mL IV to run 24 h

   Limit total IV fluids to 3,000 mL daily

   Zantac 50 mg q.6h in 50 mL D₅W to infuse 15 min

   Drop factor: On electronic infusion pump

   IV PB flow rate: _____ mL/h

   IV flow rate: _____ mL/h

9. Orders: D₅NS 1,500 mL IV to run 24 h

   Limit total IV fluids to 1,500 mL daily

   cefazolin 500 mg IV PB per 50 mL D₅W q.8h to run 1 h

   Drop factor: 20 gtt/mL

   IV PB flow rate: _____ gtt/min

   IV flow rate: _____ gtt/min

10. Orders: NS 2,700 mL IV for 24 h

   Limit total IV fluids to 2,700 mL per day

   gentamicin 60 mg in 60 mL D₅W IV PB q.8h to run for 30 min

   Drop factor: On electronic infusion pump

   IV PB flow rate: _____ mL/h

   IV flow rate: _____ mL/h

After completing these problems, see pages 662–664 to check your answers.

CLINICAL REASONING SKILLS

Knowing the therapeutic dosage of a given medication is a critical nursing skill. Let's look at an example in which the order was unclear and the nurse did not verify the order with the appropriate person.

ERROR

Failing to clarify an order.

Possible Scenario

Suppose the physician ordered a heparin infusion for a patient with thrombophlebitis who weighs 100 kg. The facility uses the Standard Weight-Based Heparin Protocol as seen in Figure 17-1. The order was written this way:

heparin 25,000 units in 250 mL $\frac{1}{2}$NS IV at 18000/h

The order was difficult to read, and the nurse asked a coworker to help her decipher it. They both agreed that it read 18,000 units per hour. The nurse calculated mL/h to be:

$$\frac{18,000 \text{ units/h}}{25,000 \text{ units}} \times 250 \text{ mL} = 180 \text{ mL/h} \quad \textbf{INCORRECT}$$

The nurse proceeded to start the heparin drip at 180 mL/h. The patient's aPTT prior to initiation of the infusion was 37 seconds. Six hours into the infusion, an aPTT was drawn according to protocol. The nurse was shocked when the results returned and were 95 seconds, which is abnormally high. The nurse called the physician, who asked, "What is the rate of the heparin drip?" The nurse replied, "I have the infusion set at 180 mL/h so that the patient receives the prescribed amount of 18,000 units per hour." The physician was astonished and replied, "I ordered the drip at 1,800 units per hour, not 18,000 units per hour."

Potential Outcome

The physician would likely have discontinued the heparin; ordered protamine sulfate, the antidote for heparin overdosage; and obtained another aPTT. The patient may have started to show signs of abnormal bleeding, such as blood in the urine, bloody nose, and increased tendency to bruise.

Prevention

When the physician wrote the order for 1800 U/h, the *U* for "units" looked like an 0, and the nurse misinterpreted the order as 18,000 units. The nurse missed three opportunities to prevent this error. The order as written is unclear, unsafe, and incomplete. Contacting the physician and requesting a clarification of the order is an appropriate action for several reasons. First, the writing is unclear and does not follow The Joint Commission guidelines, which are automatic cautions to contact the prescribing practitioner for clarification. The prescriber should have used commas to write amounts of 1,000 and greater, and the prescriber should have spelled out *units* rather than use the *U* abbreviation. Guessing about the exact meaning of an order is dangerous, as this scenario demonstrates.

Second, the Standard Weight-Based Heparin Protocol recommends a safe heparin infusion rate of 1,800 units/h, or 18 mL/h (with a supply dosage of 25,000 units per 250 mL or 100 units/mL), for an individual weighing 100 kg. It is the responsibility of the individual administering a medication to be sure the Six Rights of medication administration are observed. The first three rights state that the *"right patient must receive the right drug in the right amount."* The order of 18,000 units as understood by the nurse was unsafe. The patient was overdosed by 10 times the recommended amount of heparin.

Third, if the nurse clearly interpreted the order as 18,000, then no unit of measure was specified, which is a medication error that requires contact with the physician for correction. An incomplete order must not be filled.

PRACTICE PROBLEMS—CHAPTER 17

Unless stated otherwise, IV pumps are calibrated in whole mL/h.

Refer to the following patient information for questions 1 through 5. You are working on the day shift, 0700–1500 hours. You observe that one of the patients assigned to you has an IV infusion with a volume control set (as shown in Figure 16-3). His orders include:

D₅W IV at 50 mL/h for continuous infusion

piperacillin 1 g IV q.6h

The pharmacy supplies the piperacillin in a prefilled syringe labeled *1 g per 5 mL,* with instructions to *add piperacillin to volume control set, and infuse over 30 minutes.* Answer questions 1 through 5.

1. What is the drop factor of the volume control set? _____ gtt/mL

2. What amount of piperacillin will you add to the chamber? _____ mL

3. How much D₅W IV fluid will you add to the chamber with the piperacillin? _____ mL

4. To maintain the flow rate at 50 mL/h, you will time the IV piperacillin to infuse at _____ gtt/min.

5. The medication administration record indicates that the patient received his last dose of IV piperacillin at 0600. How many doses of piperacillin will you administer during your shift? _____

6. Order: **heparin 25,000 units in 250 mL 0.45% NS to infuse at 1,200 units/h**

   Drop factor: On electronic infusion pump

   Flow rate: _____ mL/h

7. Order: **thiamine 100 mg per L D₅W IV to infuse at 5 mg/h**

   Drop factor: On electronic infusion pump

   Flow rate: _____ mL/h

8. Order: **magnesium sulfate 4 g in 500 mL D₅W at 500 mg/h**

   Drop factor: On electronic infusion pump

   Flow rate: _____ mL/h

9. A patient is to receive **D₅W 500 mL c̄ heparin 20,000 units at 1,400 units/h.**

   Set the infusion pump at _____ mL/h.

10. At the rate of 4 mL/min, how long will it take to administer 1.5 L of IV fluid?
    _____ h and _____ min

11. Order: **lidocaine 2 g in 500 mL D₅W IV to run at 4 mg/min**

    Drop factor: On electronic infusion pump calibrated in tenths of a mL/h

    Flow rate: _____ mL/h

12. Order: **Xylocaine 1 g IV in 250 mL D₅W at 3 mg/min**

    Drop factor: On electronic infusion pump calibrated in tenths of a mL/h

    Flow rate: _____ mL/h

13. Order: **procainamide 1 g IV in 500 mL D₅W to infuse at 2 mg/min**

    Drop factor: On electronic infusion pump calibrated in tenths of a mL/h

    Flow rate: _____ mL/h

14. Order: **dobutamine 250 mg IV in 250 mL D$_5$W to infuse at 5 mcg/kg/min**

    Weight: 80 kg

    Drop factor: On electronic infusion pump calibrated in tenths of a mL/h

    Flow rate: _____ mL/h

15. Your patient has an order for D$_5$W 1 L IV with **2 g lidocaine added infusing at 75 mL/h**. The recommended continuous IV dosage of lidocaine is 1 to 4 mg/min. Is this dosage safe? _____

16. Orders: **Restricted fluids: 3,000 mL D$_5$NS IV for 24 h**

    Chloromycetin 1 g IV PB in 100 mL NS q.6h to run 1 h

    Drop factor: 10 gtt/mL

    Flow rate: _____ gtt/min IV PB and _____ gtt/min primary IV

17. Order: **Restricted fluids: 3,000 mL D$_5$W IV for 24 h**

    ampicillin 500 mg in 50 mL D$_5$W IV PB q.i.d. for 30 min

    Drop factor: On electronic infusion pump

    Flow rate: _____ mL/h IV PB and _____ mL/h primary IV

18. Order: **50 mg Nitropress IV in 500 mL D$_5$W to infuse at 3 mcg/kg/min**

    Weight: 125 lb

    Drop factor: On electronic infusion pump calibrated in tenths of a mL/h

    Flow rate: _____ mL/h

19. Order: **KCl 40 mEq to each liter IV fluid**

    Situation: IV discontinued with 800 mL remaining

    How much KCl infused? _____

20. A patient's infusion rate is 125 mL/h. The rate is equivalent to _____ mL/min.

21. Order: $\frac{1}{2}$NS **1,500 mL IV to run at 100 mL/h.** Calculate the infusion time. _____ h

22. Order: **KCl 40 mEq/L D$_5$W IV to infuse at 2 mEq/h**

    Rate: _____ mL/h

23. Order: **heparin 50,000 units/L D$_5$W IV to infuse at 1,250 units/h**

    Rate: _____ mL/h

24. If the minimal dilution for tobramycin is 5 mg/mL and you are giving 37 mg, what is the least amount of fluid in which you could safely dilute the dosage? _____ mL

25. Order: **oxytocin 10 units IV in 500 mL NS. Infuse 4 milliunits/min for 20 min, followed by 6 milliunits/min for 20 min. Use electronic infusion pump.**

    Rate: _____ mL/h for first 20 min

    Rate: _____ mL/h for next 20 min

26. Order: magnesium sulfate 20 g IV in 500 mL of LR solution. Start with a bolus of 3 g to infuse over 30 min. Then maintain a continuous infusion at 2 g/h.

    You will use an electronic infusion pump.

    Rate: _____ mL/h for bolus

    Rate: _____ mL/h for continuous infusion

27. Order: Pitocin 15 units IV in 500 mL of LR solution. Infuse at 1 milliunit/min.

    You will use an electronic infusion pump.

    Rate: _____ mL/h

28. Order: heparin drip 40,000 units/L D₅W IV to infuse at 1,400 units/h

    Drop factor: On infusion pump

    Flow rate: _____ mL/h

Refer to this order for questions 29 and 30.

Order: magnesium sulfate 4 g IV in 500 mL D₅W at 500 mg/h on an infusion pump

29. What is the solution concentration? _____ mg/mL

30. What is the hourly flow rate? _____ mL/h

Calculate the drug concentration of the following IV solutions as requested.

31. A solution containing 80 units of oxytocin in 1,000 mL of D₅W: _____ milliunits/mL

32. A solution containing 200 mg of nitroglycerin in 500 mL of D₅W: _____ mg/mL

33. A solution containing 4 mg of Isuprel in 1,000 mL of D₅W: _____ mcg/mL

34. A solution containing 2 g of lidocaine in 500 mL of D₅W: _____ mg/mL

Refer to this order for questions 35 through 37.

Order: venuronium bromide IV 1 mg/kg/min to control respirations for a patient who is ventilated

35. The patient weighs 220 pounds, which is equal to _____ kg.

36. The available venuronium bromide 20 mg is dissolved in 100 mL NS. This available solution concentration is _____ mg/mL, which is equivalent to _____ mcg/mL.

37. The IV is infusing at the rate of 1 mcg/kg/min on an infusion pump calibrated in tenths of a mL/h. The hourly rate is _____ mL/h.

Refer to these orders for questions 38 through 43.

Orders: Restricted fluids: 3,000 mL per 24 h. Primary IV of D₅LR running via infusion pump
          ampicillin 3 g IV PB q.6h in 100 mL of D₅W over 30 min
          gentamicin 170 mg IV PB q.8h in 50 mL of D₅W to infuse in 1 h

38. Calculate the IV PB flow rates. ampicillin: _____ mL/h; gentamicin: _____ mL/h

39. Calculate the total IV PB time. _____ h

40. Calculate the total IV PB volume. _____ mL

41. Calculate the total regular IV volume. _____ mL

42. Calculate the total regular IV time. _____ h

43. Calculate the regular IV flow rate. _____ mL/h

44. A patient who weighs 190 lb receives **dopamine 800 mg in 500 mL of D₅W IV at 4 mcg/kg/min.** As the patient's blood pressure drops, the nurse titrates the drip to **12 mcg/kg/min** as ordered.

    What is the initial flow rate for the IV pump calibrated in tenths of a mL/h? _____ mL/h

    After titration, what is the flow rate? _____ mL/h

Questions 45 through 49 refer to your patient who has left-leg deep vein thrombosis. He has orders for IV heparin therapy. He weighs 225 lb. On admission, his aPTT is 25 seconds. You initiate therapy at 1130 on 5/10/xx. Follow the Standard Weight-Based Heparin Protocol (Figure 17-7), and record your answers on the Standard Weight-Based Heparin Protocol Worksheet (Figure 17-8).

FIGURE 17-7

Standard Weight-Based Heparin Protocol
For all patients on heparin drips:
1. Weight in kilograms (round to nearest 10 kg). Required for order to be processed: _____ kg
2. Heparin 25,000 units in 250 mL of ½NS. Boluses to be given as 1,000 units/mL.
3. aPTT q.6h or 6 hours after rate change; daily after two consecutive therapeutic aPTTs.
4. CBC initially and repeat every _____ days(s).
5. Obtain aPTT and PT/INR on day 1 prior to initiation of therapy.
6. Guaiac stool initially, then every _____ day(s) until heparin discontinued. Notify if positive.
7. Neuro checks every _____ hours while on heparin. Notify physician of any changes.
8. Discontinue aPTT and CBC once heparin drip is discontinued, unless otherwise ordered.
9. Notify physician of any bleeding problems.
10. Bolus with 80 units/kg. Start drip at 18 units/kg/h.
11. If aPTT is less than 35 secs: Rebolus with 80 units/kg and increase rate by 4 units/kg/h.
12. If aPTT is 36 to 44 secs: Rebolus with 40 units/kg and increase rate by 2 units/kg/h.
13. If aPTT is 45 to 75 secs: Continue current rate.
14. If aPTT is 76 to 90 secs: Decrease rate by 2 units/kg/h.
15. If aPTT is greater than 90 secs: Hold heparin for 1 hour and decrease rate by 3 units/kg/h.

© Cengage Learning 2013.

45. What is the patient's weight in kilograms? Calculate the weight as instructed in the protocol and record weight on the worksheet. _____ kg.

    What does the protocol indicate for the standard bolus dosage of heparin? _____ units/kg

46. Calculate the dosage of heparin that should be administered for the bolus for this patient, and record your answer on the worksheet. _____ units

    What does the protocol indicate as the required solution concentration (supply dosage) of heparin to use for the bolus? _____ units/mL

    Calculate the dose volume of heparin that should be administered for the bolus for this patient, and record your answer on the worksheet. _____ mL

FIGURE 17-8

STANDARD WEIGHT-BASED HEPARIN PROTOCOL WORKSHEET

Round patient's total body weight to nearest 10 kg: _____ kg.

DO NOT change the weight based on daily measurements.

FOUND ON THE ORDER FORM

Initial Bolus (80 units/kg): _____ units _____ mL

Initial Infusion Rate (18 units/kg/h): _____ units/h _____ mL/h

Make adjustments to the heparin drip rate as directed by the order form.

ALL DOSES ARE ROUNDED TO THE NEAREST 100 UNITS.

Date	Time	aPTT	Bolus	Rate Change units/h	Rate Change mL/h	New Rate	RN 1	RN 2

If aPTT is	Then
Less than 35 secs:	Rebolus with 80 units/kg and increase rate by 4 units/kg/h.
36 to 44 secs:	Rebolus with 40 units/kg and increase rate by 2 units/kg/h.
45 to 75 secs:	Continue current rate.
76 to 90 secs:	Decrease rate by 2 units/kg/h.
Greater than 90 secs:	Hold heparin for 1 hour and decrease rate by 3 units/kg/h.

Signatures _____ Initials _____

_____

_____

_____

_____

47. What does the protocol indicate for the initial infusion rate? _____ units/kg/h

    Calculate the dosage of heparin this patient should receive each hour, and record your answer on the worksheet. _____ units/h

    What does the protocol indicate as the required solution concentration (supply dosage) of heparin to use for the initial infusion? _____ units/mL

    Calculate the heparin solution volume this patient should receive each hour to provide the correct infusion for his weight, and record your answer on the worksheet. _____ mL/h

48. According to the protocol, how often should the patient's APTT be checked? q. _____ h

    At 1730, the patient's APTT is 37 seconds. Calculate the new heparin bolus and record your answer on the worksheet. Give _____ units/kg or _____ units measured as _____ mL

    Calculate the change in heparin infusion rate (increase or decrease) and record on worksheet. How much should you change the infusion rate? _____ by _____ units/kg/h or _____ units/h for a rate of _____ mL/h

    Calculate the new infusion rate and record on worksheet. _____ mL/h

49. At 2330, the patient's APPT is 77 seconds. What should you do now?

    _____

    Calculate the new infusion rate and record your answer on the worksheet. _____ mL/h

50. Describe the strategy you would implement to prevent this medication error.

Possible Scenario

Suppose the physician writes an order to induce labor, as follows: **Pitocin 20 U IV added to 1 liter of LR beginning at 1 mU/min, then increase by 1 mU/min q 15 min to a maximum of 20 mU/min until adequate labor is reached.** The labor and delivery unit stocks Pitocin ampules 10 units per mL in boxes of 50 ampules. The nurse preparing the IV solution misread the order as "20 mL of Pitocin added to 1 liter of lactated Ringer's . . ." and pulled 20 ampules of Pitocin from the supply shelf. Another nurse, seeing this nurse drawing up medication from several ampules, asked what the nurse was preparing. When the nurse described the IV solution being prepared, he suddenly realized he had misinterpreted the order.

Potential Outcome

The amount of Pitocin that was being drawn up (20 mL) to be added to the IV solution would have been 10 units/mL × 20 mL = 200 units of Pitocin, 10 times the ordered amount of 20 units. Starting this Pitocin solution, even at the usual slow rate, would have delivered an excessively high amount of Pitocin that could have led to fatal consequences for both the fetus and laboring mother. What should the nurse have done to avoid this type of error?

Prevention

_____

_____

After completing these problems, see pages 664–667 to check your answers.

🔍 For additional practice, visit the online practice software at www.CengageBrain.com, using the Premium Website access code found in the front of your text.

SECTION 4 SELF-EVALUATION

Chapter 15—Intravenous Solutions, Equipment, and Calculations

1. Which of the following IV solutions is normal saline?

_____ 0.45% NaCl   _____ 0.9% NaCl   _____ D_5W

2. What is the solute and concentration of 0.9% NaCl? _____

3. What is the solute and concentration of 0.45% NaCl? _____

Use the following information to answer questions 4 and 5.

Order: D_5 0.45% NaCl 1,000 mL IV q.8h

4. The IV solution contains _____ g dextrose.

5. The IV solution contains _____ g sodium chloride.

6. Order: 0.45% NaCl 500 mL IV q.6h. The IV solution contains _____ g sodium chloride.

Refer to this order for questions 7 and 8.

Order: D_{10} 0.9% NaCl 750 mL IV q.8h

7. The IV solution contains _____ g dextrose.

8. The IV solution contains _____ g sodium chloride.

9. Are most electronic infusion devices calibrated in gtt/min, mL/h, mL/min, or gtt/mL? _____

Use the following information to answer questions 10 and 11.

Mrs. Wilson has an order to receive 2,000 mL of D_5NS IV fluids over 24 h. The IV tubing is calibrated for a drop factor of 15 gtt/mL.

10. Calculate the watch-count flow rate for Mrs. Wilson's IV. _____ gtt/min

11. An electronic infusion pump calibrated to deliver whole mL/h becomes available, and you decide to use it to regulate Mrs. Wilson's IV. Set the pump at _____ mL/h.

12. Mrs. Hawkins returns from the delivery room at 1530 with 400 mL D_5LR infusing at 24 gtt/min, with your hospital's standard macrodrop infusion control set calibrated at 15 gtt/mL. You anticipate that Mrs. Hawkins's IV will be complete at _____ hours.

13. You start your shift at 3:00 PM. On your nursing assessment rounds, you find that Mr. Johnson has an IV of $D_5 \frac{1}{2}NS$ infusing at 32 gtt/min. The tubing is calibrated for 10 gtt/mL. Mr. Johnson will receive _____ mL during your 8-hour shift.

Use the following information to answer questions 14 through 16.

As you continue on your rounds, you find Mr. Boyd with an infiltrated IV and decide to restart it and regulate it on an electronic infusion pump calibrated in whole mL/h. The orders specify:

NS 1,000 mL IV c̄ 20 mEq KCl q.8h

cefazolin 250 mg IV PB per 100 mL NS q.8h over 30 min

Limit IV total fluids to 3,000 mL daily

14. Interpret Mr. Boyd's IV and medication orders. _____

_____

15. Regulate the electronic infusion pump for Mr. Boyd's standard IV at _____ mL/h.

16. Regulate the electronic infusion pump for Mr. Boyd's IV PB at _____ mL/h.

17. Order: **D₅LR 1,200 mL IV at 100 mL/h.** You start this IV at 1530 and, during your nursing assessment at 2200, you find 650 mL remaining. The flow rate is 100 gtt/min using a microdrip infusion set. Describe your action now. _____

_____

Chapter 16—Body Surface Area and Advanced Pediatric Calculations

Calculate the hourly maintenance IV rate for the children described in questions 18 through 21. Use the following recommendations:

First 10 kg of body weight: 100 mL/kg/day

Next 10 kg of body weight: 50 mL/kg/day

Each additional kg over 20 kg of body weight: 20 mL/kg/day

18. A child who weighs 40 lb requires _____ mL/day for maintenance IV fluids.

19. The infusion rate for the same child who weighs 40 lb is _____ mL/h.

20. An infant who weighs 1,185 g requires _____ mL/day for maintenance IV fluids.

21. The infusion rate for the same infant who weighs 1,185 g is _____ mL/h.

Use the BSA formula method on the following page to answer questions 22 through 24.

22. Height: 30 in   Weight: 24 lb   BSA: _____ m²

23. Height: 155 cm   Weight: 39 kg   BSA: _____ m²

24. Height: 52 in   Weight: 65 lb   BSA: _____ m²

Questions 25 through 31 refer to the following situation.

A child who is 28 in tall and weighs 25 lb will receive 1 dosage of cisplatin IV. The recommended dosage is 37 to 75 mg/m² once every 2 to 3 weeks. The order reads **cisplatin 18.5 mg IV at 1 mg/min today at 1500 hours.** You have available a 50 mg vial of cisplatin. Reconstitution directions state to *add 50 mL of sterile water to yield 1 mg/mL*. Minimal dilution instructions require 2 mL of IV solution for every 1 mg of cisplatin.

25. According to the nomogram on the following page, the child's BSA is _____ m².

26. The safe dosage range for this child is _____ mg to _____ mg.

27. Is this dosage safe? _____.

28. If safe, you will prepare _____ mL. If not, describe your action. _____

_____

29. How many mL of IV fluid are required for safe dilution of the cisplatin? _____ mL

30. Given the ordered rate of 1 mg/min, set the infusion pump at _____ mL/h.

31. How long will this infusion take? _____ min

WEST NOMOGRAM

Metric:

$$\text{BSA (m}^2) = \sqrt{\frac{\text{ht (cm)} \times \text{wt (kg)}}{3{,}600}}$$

Household:

$$\text{BSA (m}^2) = \sqrt{\frac{\text{ht (in)} \times \text{wt (lb)}}{3{,}131}}$$

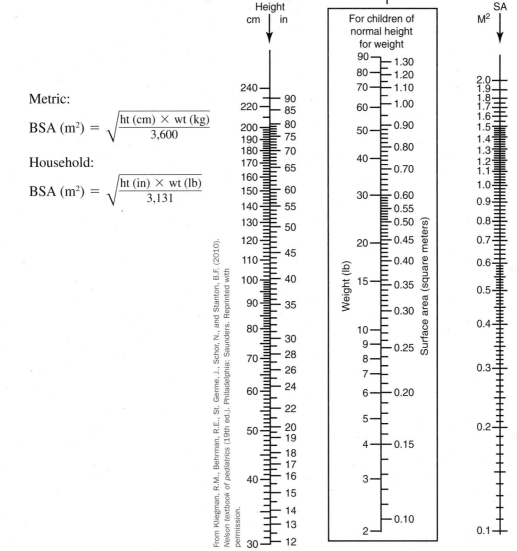

From Kliegman, R.M., Behrman, R.E., St. Germe, J., Schor, N., and Stanton, B.F. (2010). *Nelson textbook of pediatrics* (19th ed.). Philadelphia: Saunders. Reprinted with permission.

Questions 32 through 35 refer to the following situation.

Order: **Vincasar 1.6 mg IV stat.** The child is 50 inches tall and weighs 40 lb. The following label represents the Vincasar solution you have available. The recommended dosage of Vincasar is 2 mg/m² daily.

32. According to the nomogram on the previous page, the child's BSA is _____ m².

33. The recommended safe dosage for this child is _____ mg.

34. Is the dosage ordered safe? _____

35. If safe, you will prepare _____ mL Vincasar to add to the IV. If not safe, describe your action.

_____

36. Order: **NS IV for continuous infusion at 40 mL/h c̄ Ancef 250 mg IV q.8h over 30 min by volume control set**

    Available: Ancef 125 mg/mL

    Add _____ mL NS and _____ mL Ancef to the chamber to infuse at 40 mL/h.

37. Order: **Timentin 750 mg IV q.6h.** Recommended minimal dilution (maximal concentration) is 100 mg/mL. Calculate the number of mL to be used for minimal dilution of the Timentin as ordered. _____ mL

Chapter 17—Advanced Adult Intravenous Calculations

Unless stated otherwise, IV pumps are calibrated to deliver whole mL/h.

Use the following information to answer questions 38 through 41.

Mr. Smith is on restricted fluids. His IV order is: **NS 1,500 mL IV q.24h c̄ 300,000 units penicillin G potassium IV PB in 100 mL NS q.4h over 30 min.** The infusion set is calibrated at 60 gtt/mL.

38. Set Mr. Smith's regular IV at _____ gtt/min.

39. Set Mr. Smith's IV PB at _____ gtt/min.

Later during your shift, an electronic infusion pump becomes available. You decide to use it to regulate Mr. Smith's IVs.

40. Regulate Mr. Smith's regular IV at _____ mL/h.

41. Regulate Mr. Smith's IV PB at _____ mL/h.

42. Order: **KCl 40 mEq/L D₅W IV at 2 mEq/h**

    Regulate the infusion pump at _____ mL/h.

43. Order: **nitroglycerin 25 mg/L D₅W IV at 5 mcg/min**

    Regulate the infusion pump calibrated in tenths of a mL/h at _____ mL/h.

Refer to this order for questions 44 through 47.

Order: **Induce labor c̄ Pitocin 15 units/L LR IV continuous infusion at 2 milliunits/min; increase by 1 milliunit/min q.30 min to a maximum of 20 milliunits/min**

44. The initial concentration of Pitocin is _____ milliunits/mL.

45. The initial Pitocin order will infuse at the rate of _____ mL/min.

46. Regulate the electronic infusion pump at _____ mL/h to initiate the order.

NDC 0703-4402-11

VINCASAR PFS®
(vincristine sulfate injection, USP)
PRESERVATIVE FREE SOLUTION
1 mg/mL
FATAL IF GIVEN INTRATHECALLY
FOR INTRAVENOUS USE ONLY
Single Dose Vial
REFRIGERATE
Protect From Light
sicor™
SICOR Pharmaceuticals, Inc.,
Irvine, CA 92618

(01)00307034402115

440202

Used with permission from Teva Pharmaceuticals USA.

47. The infusion pump will be regulated at a maximum of _____ mL/h to infuse the maximum of 20 milliunits/min.

Use the following information to answer questions 48 and 49.

Order for Ms. Hill, who weighs 150 lb, to stabilize her blood pressure: **dopamine 400 mg per 0.5 L D₅W at 4 mcg/kg/min titrated to 12 mcg/kg/min**

48. Regulate the electronic infusion pump calibrated in tenths of a mL/h for Ms. Hill's IV at _____ mL/h to initiate the order.

49. Anticipate that the maximum flow rate for Ms. Hill's IV to achieve the maximum safe titration would be _____ mL/h.

50. Mr. Black has a new order for **heparin 10,000 units in 500 mL NS IV at 750 units/h**. Regulate the infusion pump at _____ mL/h.

Section 4 Board Examination Practice

To obtain licensure, you will be required to pass a board examination. The following problems represent the various types of items on the NCLEX-RN (National Council Licensure Examination for Registered Nurses) and NCLEX-PN (National Council Licensure Examination for Practical Nurses) exams. Whether you will be taking one of these board examinations or one from another licensure board, alternate test items such as these are good practice. For additional practice, go to the online practice software that accompanies this text, to respond to more interactive test items, including those using the calculator tool.

51. NCLEX *Fill-in-the-Blank* Item

The antidote drug for heparin overdosage is _____.

Answer: _____

52. NCLEX *Multiple-Response* Item

Before administering high-alert medications, the nurse should perform independent double verification. What does this process require? (Place a check mark beside all that apply.)

Answer:

a. Two clinicians checking volume in syringe separately from each other.   _____

b. One nurse isolated, away from distractions, reviewing calculations twice.   _____

c. Independent review of order, lab tests, calculations, and amount prepared.   _____

d. Comparison of previous dose and current dose.   _____

53. NCLEX *Exhibit* Item

Patient scenario: Diabetic patient with blood glucose level of 310 mg/dL. According to the following IV insulin protocol on the following page, the nurse should administer a bolus of:

a. $\frac{1}{2}$ amp of 50% dextrose

b. 10 units IV push

c. 100 units regular insulin in 100 mL of 0.9% NaCl

d. 25 units/hour

Critical Care Intravenous Insulin Protocol Orders	
TARGET	**BLOOD GLUCOSE LEVEL 70 to 110 mg/dL**
Insulin Solution	1. 100 units regular insulin in 100 mL of 0.9% NaCl, to be titrated based on grid for Levels 1, 2, or 3.
Initial Infusion	2. Start nondiabetic patients at Level 1. Advance to Level 2 if TARGET range not reached after 2 hours on Level 1.
	3. Start diabetic patients at Level 2. Advance to Level 3 if TARGET range not reached after 2 hours on Level 2.
	4. Do not initiate insulin infusion unless blood glucose greater than 110 mg/dL.
Monitoring	5. Check blood glucose prior to start of insulin infusion.
	6. Check blood glucose every hour thereafter.
	7. When glucose is 80 to 110 mg/dL for 3 hours, check glucose every 2 hours.
	8. Resume monitoring every hour if blood glucose greater than 120 mg/dL for 2 hours.
Blood Glucose less than 80 mg/dL	9. If patient has blood glucose less than 80 mg/dL:
	a. Refer to regular insulin infusion rate column in grid tables for management instructions.
	b. If necessary to reinitiate insulin infusion, start one level below previous level.
	c. Call physician for symptomatic hypoglycemia or blood glucose less than 50 mg/dL, even if treated.

Grid for Titration of Intravenous Insulin—Level 2

LEVEL 2: DO NOT INITIATE insulin drip unless blood glucose is greater than 110 mg/dL.

Blood Glucose (mg/dL)	Regular Insulin Bolus	Regular Insulin Infusion Rate
Less than 70	Give $\frac{1}{2}$ amp of 50% dextrose	HOLD insulin infusion × 60 minutes and check blood glucose every 15 minutes until equal to or greater than 80.
70 to 79	0	HOLD insulin infusion × 60 minutes and check blood glucose every 15 minutes until equal to or greater than 80.
80 to 110	0	2 units/h
111 to 125	0	3 units/h
126 to 149	0	4 units/h
150 to 165	0	5 units/h
166 to 179	0	6 units/h
180 to 209	0	8 units/h
210 to 239	10 units IV push	12 units/h
240 to 269	10 units IV push	16 units/h
270 to 299	10 units IV push	20 units/h
300 to 350	10 units IV push	25 units/h
Greater than 350	Notify physician	

54. NCLEX *Drag-and-Drop / Ordered-Response* **Item**

Copy the tasks from the box onto the list in the proper sequence to *administer high-alert intravenous heparin by a standard weight-based protocol.*

Answer:

Check aPTT test results.
Start continuous infusion, if required.
Record weight in kilograms.
Administer bolus, if required.
Adjust infusion rate, if required.
Check aPTT test results.
Administer rebolus, if required.

_____

_____

_____

_____

_____

_____

_____

55. NCLEX *Hot Box* **Item**

Place an X on the label(s) that the nurse could reasonably select from the ADC cubby to prepare the following order.

Order: D₅W 500 mL with heparin 25,000 units IV at 1,000 units/h

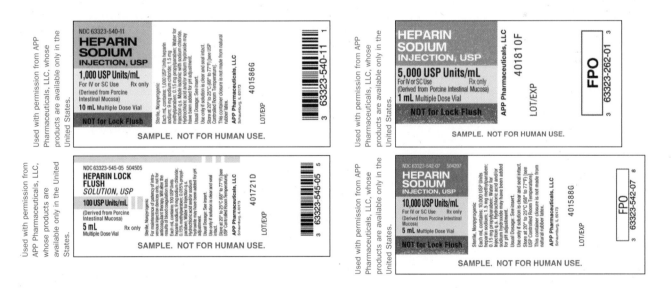

After completing these problems, refer to pages 667–669 to check your answers. Give yourself 1.8 points for each correct answer.

Perfect score = 100   My score = _____

Minimum mastery score = 86 (48 correct)

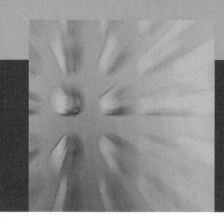

Essential Skills Evaluation: Posttest

G o back to the **Essential Skills Evaluation: Pretest** on page 3 and rework the questions as a Posttest to evaluate your mastery of the essential skills of dosage calculations. Record your answers here and compare with the results of your pretest.

ESSENTIAL SKILLS EVALUATION: POSTTEST ANSWER SHEET

1. Give: _____ tablet(s)   Frequency: _____

2. Give: _____ tablet(s)   Frequency: _____

3. Choose: _____ mg capsules   Give: _____ capsule(s)   Frequency: _____

4. Give: _____ tablet(s)   Frequency: _____

5. Give: _____ tablet(s)   Frequency: _____

6. Give: _____ mL   Frequency: _____

© Cengage Learning 2013

7. Give: _____ mL   Frequency: _____

© Cengage Learning 2013

8. Give: _____ mL   Frequency: _____

9. Give: _____ mL   Frequency: _____

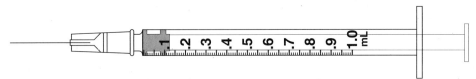

© Cengage Learning 2013

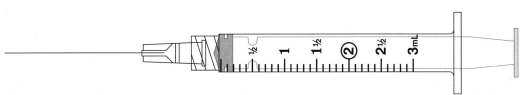

© Cengage Learning 2013

10. Give: _____ mL   Frequency: _____

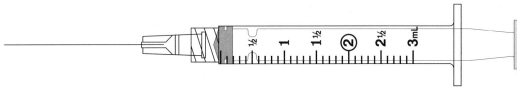

© Cengage Learning 2013

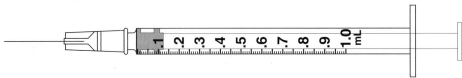

© Cengage Learning 2013

11. Give: _____ mL   Frequency: _____

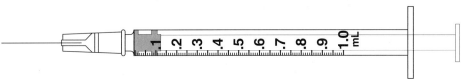

© Cengage Learning 2013

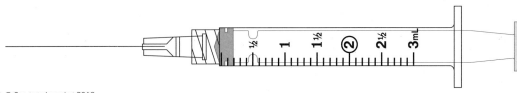

© Cengage Learning 2013

12. Give: _____ mL   Frequency: _____

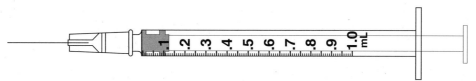

13. Give: _____ mL   Frequency: _____

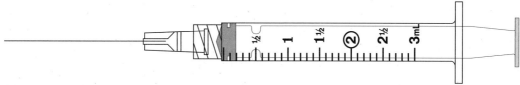

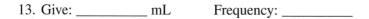

14. Give: _____ mL   Frequency: _____

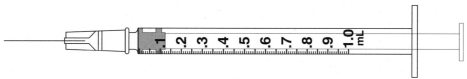

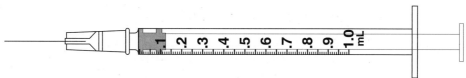

15. Give: _____ mL   Frequency: _____

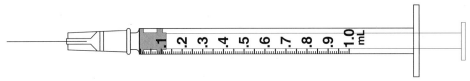

© Cengage Learning 2013

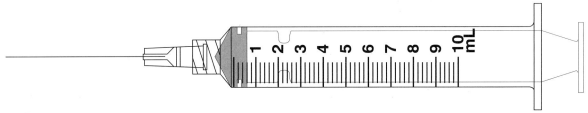

© Cengage Learning 2013

16. Give: _____ mL   Frequency: _____

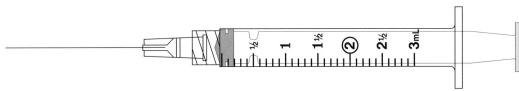

© Cengage Learning 2013

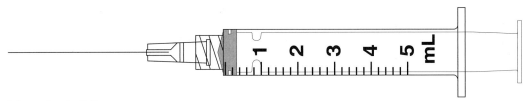

© Cengage Learning 2013

17. Give: _____ mL at _____ mL/min, which equals _____ mL per 15 sec
    Frequency: _____

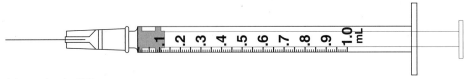

© Cengage Learning 2013

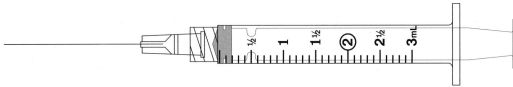

© Cengage Learning 2013

18. Add: _____ mL to the IV PB bag, and set the drip rate on the tubing to _____ gtt/min

Frequency: _____

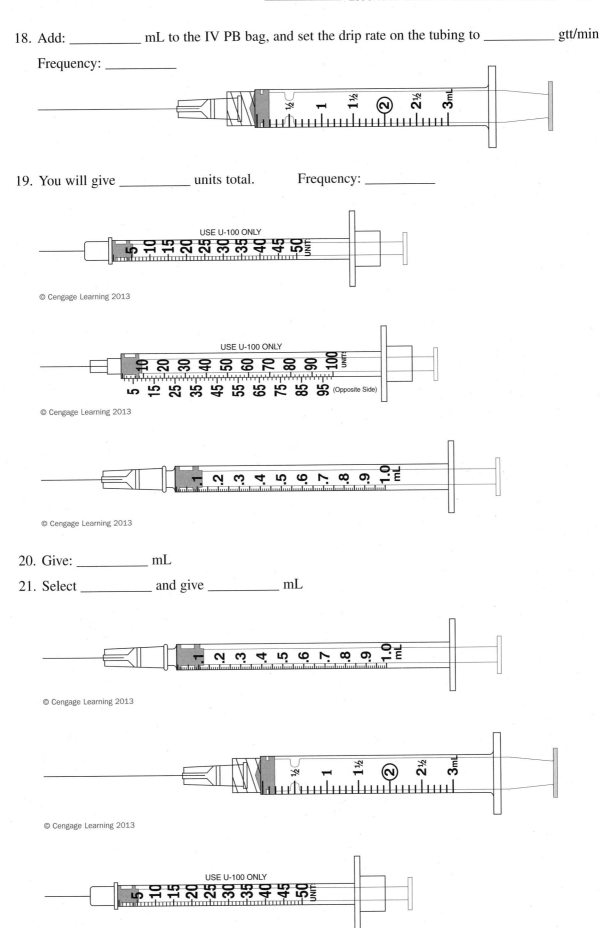

© Cengage Learning 2013

19. You will give _____ units total.   Frequency: _____

© Cengage Learning 2013

© Cengage Learning 2013

© Cengage Learning 2013

20. Give: _____ mL

21. Select _____ and give _____ mL

© Cengage Learning 2013

© Cengage Learning 2013

© Cengage Learning 2013

22. Medication: _____ Give _____ mL

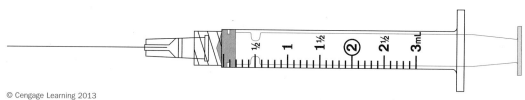

© Cengage Learning 2013

23. Yes or No: _____ Explain: _____

_____

24. _____ tablet(s)

25. _____ mL; _____ gtt/min

26. _____ mL/h

27. _____ mL diluent; give _____ mL

28. _____ tablet(s); _____, _____, and _____ hours

29. _____ units; _____ route

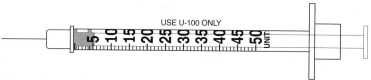

© Cengage Learning 2013

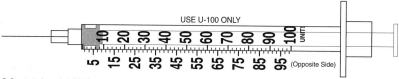

© Cengage Learning 2013

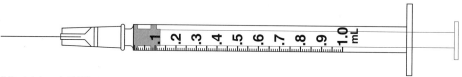

© Cengage Learning 2013

30. _____ mL

31. Yes or No: _____ Explain: _____

_____

32. _____ mL

33. Yes or No: _____ Explain: _____

_____

34. _____ mL Next Action: _____

35. _____ °F

36. _____ mg/dose to _____ mg/dose

37. _____ mL

38. _____ mg/dose to _____ mg/dose; Yes or No: _____

39. _____ mL; _____ gtt/min

40. _____ mL

41. _____ gtt/min

42. _____ mL

43. _____ mg; _____ mL

44. _____ dose(s)

45. _____ hours; _____ (AM/PM)

46. _____ mL

47. _____ mg per _____ mL

48. _____ mL

49.

50. **Prevention:** _____

_____

After completing these problems, see the same Answers from the Pretest on pages 581–587 to check your answers. Give yourself 2 points for each correct answer.

Perfect score = 100   My score = _____

Minimum mastery score = 90 (45 correct)

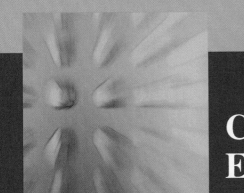

Comprehensive Skills Evaluation

This evaluation is a comprehensive assessment of your mastery of the concepts presented in all 17 chapters of *Dosage Calculations.*

Donna Smith, a 46-year-old patient of Dr. J. Physician, has been admitted to the Progressive Care Unit (PCU) with complaints of an irregular heartbeat, shortness of breath, and chest pain (relieved by nitroglycerin). Questions 1 through 14 refer to the admitting orders on page 567 for Mrs. Smith. The following labels represent the available medications and infusion set.

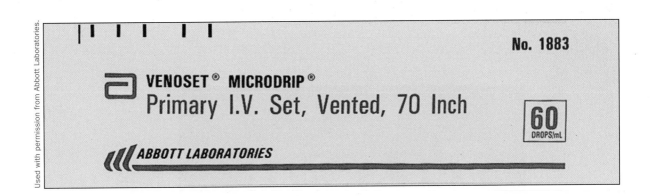

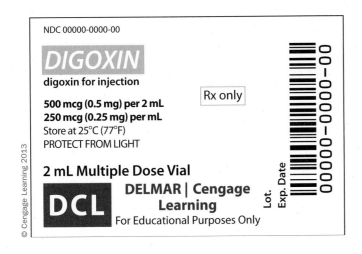

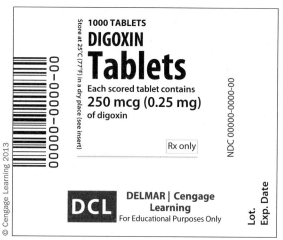

1000 TABLETS
DIGOXIN
Tablets
Each scored tablet contains
250 mcg (0.25 mg)
of digoxin

Rx only

Store at 25°C (77°F) in a dry place (see insert)

NDC 00000-0000-00

© Cengage Learning 2013

DCL DELMAR | Cengage **Learning**
For Educational Purposes Only

Lot.
Exp. Date

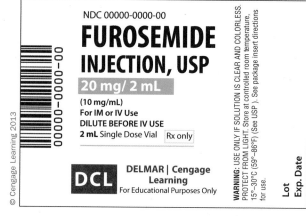

NDC 00000-0000-00

FUROSEMIDE
INJECTION, USP
20 mg/ 2 mL
(10 mg/mL)
For IM or IV Use
DILUTE BEFORE IV USE
2 mL Single Dose Vial   Rx only

WARNING: USE ONLY IF SOLUTION IS CLEAR AND COLORLESS. PROTECT FROM LIGHT. Store at controlled room temperature, 15°–30°C (59°–86°F) (See USP.). See package insert directions for use.

© Cengage Learning 2013

DCL DELMAR | Cengage **Learning**
For Educational Purposes Only

Lot
Exp. Date

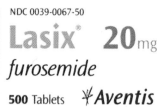

Used with permission from Aventis Pharmaceuticals.

NDC 0039-0067-50

Lasix® 20mg

furosemide

500 Tablets   ✲*Aventis*

3 0039-0067-50 9

℞ ONLY
Each LASIX® Tablet contains 20mg furosemide. **Dosage and Administration:** See package insert for dosage information. **WARNING:** Keep out of reach of children. Do not use if bottle closure seal is broken. **Pharmacist:** Dispense in well-closed, light-resistant container with child-resistant closure. **Store at room temperature.**
Hoechst-Roussel Pharmaceuticals
Division of **Aventis** Pharmaceuticals Inc.
Kansas City, MO 64137 USA   ©2000
www.aventispharma-us.com

50058803 50058803 **50058803**

Used with permission from McNeil Consumer and Specialty Pharmaceuticals.

Used with permission from KV Pharmaceutical Co.

N 3 58177-005-04 6

Each extended-release capsule contains:

Nitroglycerin . . . . 6.5 mg

KEEP THIS AND ALL DRUGS OUT OF THE REACH OF CHILDREN.

Manufactured by
Time-Cap Labs Inc. for
ETHEX Corporation
St. Louis, MO 63043-2413

NDC 58177-005-04

Nitroglycerin
Extended-release Capsules

6.5 mg

℞ Only
100 Capsules

Dispense in a tight container as defined in the USP/NF.

Store at controlled room temperature 15°–30°C (59°–86°F).

USUAL DOSAGE: See package insert for dosage, including nitrate-free intervals.

P3808 12/01

 ETHEX ETHEX *ETHEX* ETHEX ETHEX

			ENTERED	FILLED	CHECKED	VERIFIED
						—

NOTE: A NON-PROPRIETARY DRUG OF EQUAL QUALITY MAY BE DISPENSED - IF THIS COLUMN IS NOT CHECKED!

DATE	TIME WRITTEN	PLEASE USE BALL POINT - PRESS FIRMLY	✓	TIME NOTED	NURSES SIGNATURE
9/3/xx	1600	Admit to PCU, monitored bed			
		Bedrest c̄ bathroom privileges			
		nitroglycerin ER 13 mg p.o. q.8h			
		furosemide 20 mg IV Push stat, then 20 mg p.o. b.i.d.			
		digoxin 0.25 mg IV Push stat, repeat in 4 hours,	✓	1610 GP	
		then 0.125 mg p.o. daily			
		KCl 10 mEq per L D$_5$ $\frac{1}{2}$NS IV at 80 mL/h			
		Tylenol 1 g p.o. q.4h p.r.n, headache	✓		
		Labwork: Electrolytes and CBC in am			
		Soft diet, advance as tolerated			
		J. Physician, MD			

AUTO STOP ORDERS: UNLESS REORDERED, FOLLOWING WILL BE D/C'D AT 0800 ON:

DATE	ORDER		
		☐ CONT	PHYSICIAN SIGNATURE
		☐ D/C	
		☐ CONT	PHYSICIAN SIGNATURE
		☐ D/C	
		☐ CONT	PHYSICIAN SIGNATURE
		☐ D/C	

CHECK WHEN ANTIBIOTICS ORDERED   ☐ Prophylactic   ☐ Empiric   ☐ Therapeutic

Allergies: None Known

Chest Pain

PATIENT DIAGNOSIS

Smith, Donna

ID #257-226-3

HEIGHT   5' 6"   WEIGHT   110 lb

PHYSICIAN'S ORDER   Reynolds + Reynolds   LITHO IN U.S.A. K41814 (7-90) D339080

FORM 959-708 (8xx)

①

© Cengage Learning 2013

1. The progressive care unit (PCU) is short on IV pumps because of unscheduled repairs. The nurse implements a backup plan and starts a straight gravity flow IV on Mrs. Smith at 1630 hours. Calculate the watch-count flow rate for the IV fluid ordered. _____ gtt/min

2. Estimate the time and date when the nurse should plan to hang the next liter of $D_5\frac{1}{2}NS$. _____ hours on _____ (date)

3. At the present infusion rate, how much $D_5\frac{1}{2}NS$ will Mrs. Smith receive in a 24-hour period? _____ mL/day

4. How many mEq of KCl will Mrs. Smith receive per hour and per day? _____ mEq/h; _____ mEq/day

5. Both digoxin and furosemide are ordered "stat."

   a. What does this mean? _____

   b. How frequently should the nurse administer these two stat orders? _____

6. Prior to administering the IV digoxin, the nurse consults the drug guide, which states that the recommended rate for direct IV administration of digoxin is 0.25 mg in 4 mL NS administered at the rate of 0.25 mg per 5 min.

   a. How much digoxin should the nurse administer for the stat IV order? At what rate?

   Prepare: _____ mL digoxin and add _____ mL NS for a total of _____ mL. Administer at the rate of _____ mL/min or _____ mL per 15 sec.

   b. Draw an arrow on the appropriate syringe to indicate how much digoxin to prepare.

© Cengage Learning 2013

© Cengage Learning 2013

7. In addition to manual IV push administration, what other method(s) could the nurse choose for administering the direct IV digoxin order, if available?

   a. IV PB on an IV infusion pump

   b. Syringe pump

   c. Volume control device, such as Buretrol

   d. All of the above

   e. b and c

8. The nurse consults the drug guide for more information about the furosemide ordered. The recommended rate for direct IV administration is 40 mg per 2 min.

   a. How much furosemide should the nurse administer for Mrs. Smith's stat dose? At what rate?

   Give: _____ mL at the rate of _____ mL/min or _____ mL per 15 sec

   b. Draw an arrow on the appropriate syringe to indicate how much furosemide to prepare.

© Cengage Learning 2013

© Cengage Learning 2013

9. How many digoxin tablets will Mrs. Smith need for a 24-hour period for the p.o. digoxin order? _____ tablet(s)

10. After the initial dose of furosemide, how many tablets should the nurse give Mrs. Smith for each subsequent dose? _____ tablet(s)

11. How much nitroglycerin should the nurse give Mrs. Smith for one dose? _____ capsule(s)

12. Mrs. Smith has a headache.

    a. How much Tylenol should the nurse give her for one dose? _____ tablet(s)

    b. When should the nurse give her the next dose? _____

13. Compare the drug labels for Mrs. Smith, and identify the drug(s) that is (are) supplied as generic(s).

    _____

14. An IV infusion pump that is programmable in whole milliliters becomes available for Mrs. Smith. At what rate should the nurse now set the IV pump for the continuous infusion? _____ mL/h

    Despite excellent care, Mrs. Smith's condition worsens and she is transferred into the coronary care unit (CCU) with the medical orders on page 570. CCU IV infusion pumps are programmable in tenths of a milliliter. Questions 15 through 20 refer to these orders.

		ENTERED	FILLED	CHECKED	VERIFIED

NOTE: A NON-PROPRIETARY DRUG OF EQUAL QUALITY MAY BE DISPENSED - IF THIS COLUMN IS NOT CHECKED!

DATE	TIME WRITTEN	PLEASE USE BALL POINT - PRESS FIRMLY	✓	TIME NOTED	NURSES SIGNATURE
9/4/xx	2230	Transfer to CCU			
		NPO			
		Discontinue nitroglycerin			
		lidocaine bolus 50 mg IV stat, then begin			
		lidocaine drip 2 g IV in 500 mL D_5W			
		at 2 mg/min by infusion pump			
		Increase lidocaine to 4 mg/min IV if PVCs			
		(premature ventricular contractions)			
		persist		2235 MS	
		dopamine 400 mg IV PB in 250 mL D_5W			
		at 500 mcg/min by infusion pump			
		Increase KCl to 20 mEq per L D_5W $\frac{1}{2}$NS IV at 50 mL/h			
		Increase furosemide to 40 mg IV q.12h			
		O_2 at 30% p̄ ABGs (arterial blood gases)			
		Labwork: Electrolytes stat and in am and			
		ABGs stat and p.r.n.			
		J. Physician, MD			

AUTO STOP ORDERS: UNLESS REORDERED, FOLLOWING WILL BE D/C'D AT 0800 ON:

DATE	ORDER		
		☐ CONT	PHYSICIAN SIGNATURE
		☐ D/C	
		☐ CONT	PHYSICIAN SIGNATURE
		☐ D/C	
		☐ CONT	PHYSICIAN SIGNATURE
		☐ D/C	

CHECK WHEN ANTIBIOTICS ORDERED   ☐ Prophylactic   ☐ Empiric   ☐ Therapeutic

Allergies:
None Known

Chest Pain
PATIENT DIAGNOSIS

Smith, Donna
ID #257-226-3

HEIGHT 5' 6"   WEIGHT 110 lb

FORM 959-708 (8XX)   **PHYSICIAN'S ORDER**   Reynolds + Reynolds LITHO IN U.S.A. K41614 (7-00) D339060

①

15. Lidocaine is supplied in the 10 mg/mL dosage strength for Mrs. Smith. The nurse is familiar with lidocaine and knows the order is safe.

    a. How much lidocaine should the nurse administer to Mrs. Smith for the bolus? _____ mL

    b. Draw an arrow on the appropriate syringe to indicate the amount to prepare.

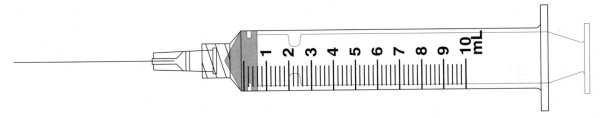

© Cengage Learning 2013

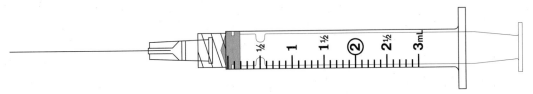

© Cengage Learning 2013

16. The CCU IV pumps are programmed in tenths of a milliliter. At what rate should the nurse initially set the IV infusion pump for the lidocaine drip? _____ mL/h

17. Dopamine is supplied for Mrs. Smith in the dosage strength of 80 mg/mL. The nurse checks the drug guide and finds that the recommended dosage of dopamine is 5 to 10 mcg/kg/min.

    a. Is the dosage ordered for Mrs. Smith safe? _____ Explain: _____

    _____

    b. If it is safe, how much dopamine should the nurse add to mix the IV PB dopamine drip?
    _____ mL

    c. If the dosage ordered is safe, draw an arrow on the appropriate syringe to indicate the amount to add to the IV PB.

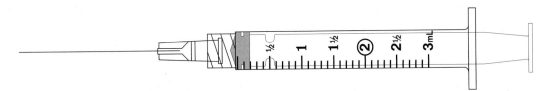

© Cengage Learning 2013

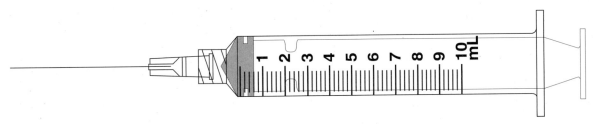

© Cengage Learning 2013

18. Calculate the rate for the IV infusion pump for the dopamine drip. _____ mL/h

19. How much dopamine will Mrs. Smith receive per hour? _____ mcg/h or _____ mg/h

20. Mrs. Smith is having increasing amounts of premature ventricular contractions (PVCs). To increase her lidocaine drip to 4 mg/min, the nurse should reprogram the IV infusion pump to _____ mL/h.

21. Julie Thomas is a 6-year-old pediatric patient who weighs 33 lb. She is in the hospital for fever of unknown origin. Julie complains of burning on urination, and her urinalysis shows *E. coli* bacterial infection. The doctor prescribes **Kantrex 75 mg IV q.8h to be administered by volume control set on an infusion pump in 25 mL D$_5$$\frac{1}{2}$NS followed by 15 mL flush over 1 hour.** The drug guide indicates that the maximum recommended dosage of Kantrex is 15 mg/kg/day IV in 3 divided doses.

NDC 0015-3512-20
EQUIVALENT TO NSN 6505-00-926-9202
75 mg KANAMYCIN per 2 mL
KANTREX®
Kanamycin Sulfate Injection, USP
Pediatric Injection
FOR I.M. OR I.V. USE
CAUTION: Federal law prohibits dispensing without prescription.

a. Is the order safe? _____

   Explain: _____

b. If safe, add _____ mL Kantrex and _____ mL D$_5$$\frac{1}{2}$NS to the chamber, and set the flow rate for _____ mL/h.

Jamie Smith is hospitalized with a staphylococcal bone infection. He weighs 66 lb. The nurse intends to use an IV pump for Jamie. The pump is programmable in tenths of a milliliter. Questions 22 through 24 refer to Jamie.

Orders: **D$_5$ $\frac{1}{2}$NS IV at 50 mL/h for continuous infusion**

vancomycin 300 mg IV q.6h

Supply in the ADC cubby: vancomycin 500 mg per 10 mL with instructions that state, "add to volume control set and infuse over 60 min."

Recommended dosage from drug guide: vancomycin 40 mg/kg/day IV in 4 divided doses.

22. Is this drug order safe? _____. Explain: _____

23. a. If safe, how much vancomycin should the nurse add to the chamber? _____ mL

    b. How much IV fluid should the nurse add to the chamber with the vancomycin? _____ mL

    c. How much IV fluid will Jamie receive in 24 hours? _____ mL

24. Use the following recommendations to calculate the hourly maintenance IV rate for Jamie.

    First 10 kg of body weight: 100 mL/kg/day

    Second 10 kg of body weight: 50 mL/kg/day

    Each additional kg over 20 kg of body weight: 20 mL/kg/day

    a. Jamie requires _____ mL/day for maintenance IV fluids.

    b. The infusion rate should be set at _____ mL/h.

    c. Does the recommended rate match the ordered rate? _____

Use the following related orders and labels to answer questions 25 through 29. Select the appropriate syringe, and mark it with the dose volume as indicated.

25. Order: Unasyn 500 mg IV q.6h in 50 mL D₅W IV PB over 30 min

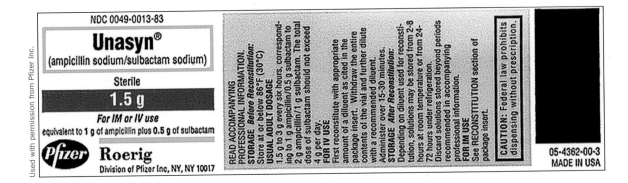

Package insert directions state:

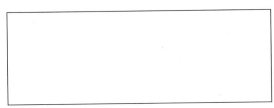

Unasyn Vial Size	Volume Diluent to Be Added	Withdrawal Volume
1.5 g	3.2 mL	4.0 mL
3.0 g	6.4 mL	8.0 mL

To reconstitute the Unasyn, the nurse should add _____ mL diluent.

26. Prepare a reconstitution label for the Unasyn.

Reconstitution label

27. To prepare the IV PB for administration, the nurse should add _____ mL Unasyn to the 50 mL D₅W IV PB. Choose and mark the appropriate syringe.

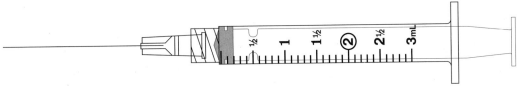

© Cengage Learning 2013

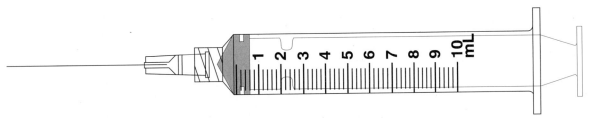

© Cengage Learning 2013

28. The IV PB Unasyn is regulated on an IV infusion pump. The nurse should set the flow rate at _____ mL/h.

29. Order: heparin 10,000 units IV in 500 mL D₅W to infuse at 1,200 units/h

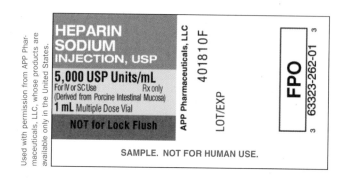

a. Add _____ mL heparin to the IV solution. Mark the dose amount on the syringe.

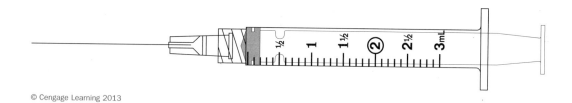

© Cengage Learning 2013

b. Set the flow rate to _____ mL/h on an IV infusion pump.

Questions 30 and 31 refer to a patient who weighs 125 lb and is receiving IV heparin therapy.

30. Use the Weight-Based Heparin Protocol to calculate bolus dosage and infusion rate. The IV pump delivers tenths of a milliliter.

Weight-Based Heparin Protocol:

Heparin IV infusion: heparin 25,000 units IV in 250 mL of ½NS

IV boluses: Use heparin 1,000 units/mL

Bolus with heparin 80 units/kg. Then initiate heparin drip at 18 units/kg/h. Obtain aPTT every 6 hours, and adjust dosage and rate as follows:

If aPTT is less than 35 seconds: Rebolus with 80 units/kg and increase rate by 4 units/kg/h.

If aPTT is 36 to 44 seconds: Rebolus with 40 units/kg and increase rate by 2 units/kg/h.

If aPTT is 45 to 75 seconds: Continue current rate.

If aPTT is 76 to 90 seconds: Decrease rate by 2 units/kg/h.

If aPTT is greater than 90 seconds: Hold heparin for 1 hour and then decrease rate by 3 units/kg/h.

---

a. Convert the patient's weight to kg (rounded to tenths): _____ kg

b. Calculate the initial heparin bolus dosage: _____ units

c. Calculate the bolus dose: _____ mL

d. Calculate the initial heparin infusion rate: _____ units/h or _____ mL/h

31. At 0930, the patient's aPTT is 77 seconds.

a. According to the protocol, what action should the nurse implement?

_____

_____

b. The nurse should decrease infusion rate by _____ units/h or _____ mL/h.

c. The nurse should reset infusion rate to _____ mL/h.

32. Order: **Novolin R regular U-100 insulin subcut ac per sliding scale**
The patient's blood sugar at 1730 hours is 238.

Blood Glucose mg/dL	Insulin Dosage
0 to 150	0 units
151 to 250	8 units
251 to 350	13 units
351 to 400	18 units
greater than 400	Call MD

Give: _____ units, which equals _____ mL (Mark dose on appropriate syringe.)

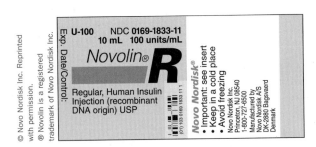

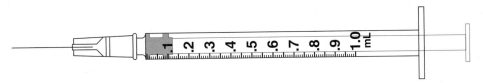

© Cengage Learning 2013

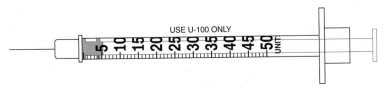

© Cengage Learning 2013

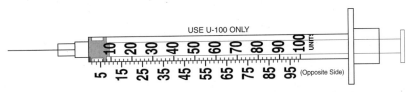

© Cengage Learning 2013

33. Order: Humulin R regular U-100 insulin 15 units c̄ Humulin N NPH U-100 insulin 45 units subcut at 0730

    a. The nurse should give a total of _____ units insulin. (Remember, nurse will get independent verification after drawing up each insulin.)

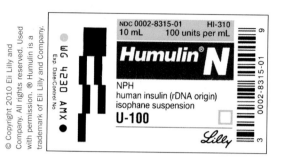

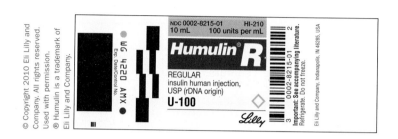

b. Mark dose on appropriate syringe, designating measurement of both regular and NPH insulins.

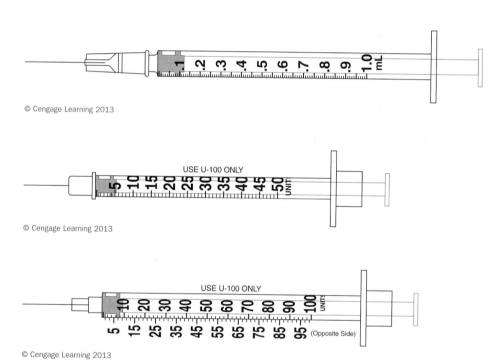

© Cengage Learning 2013

© Cengage Learning 2013

© Cengage Learning 2013

34. A patient is receiving an insulin drip of Humulin R regular U-100 insulin 300 units added to 150 mL NS IV infusing at 10 mL/h. How many units/h of insulin is this patient receiving? _____ units/h

Questions 35 and 36 refer to a child who weighs 16 lb and is admitted to the pediatric unit with vomiting and diarrhea of 3 days' duration.

Order: $\frac{1}{4}$ strength Isomil 80 mL q.3h for 4 feedings; if tolerated, increase Isomil to $\frac{1}{2}$ strength 80 mL q.3h for 4 feedings

Supply: Isomil ready-to-feed formula in 8-fluid-ounce cans

35. To reconstitute a full 8-fluid-ounce can of Isomil ready-to-feed to $\frac{1}{4}$ strength, the nurse should add _____ mL water to mix a total of _____ mL of $\frac{1}{4}$ strength reconstituted Isomil.

36. The child is not tolerating the oral feedings. Calculate this child's allowable daily and hourly IV maintenance fluids using the following recommendation.

> Daily rate of pediatric maintenance IV fluids:
>
> 100 mL/kg for first 10 kg of body weight
>
> 50 mL/kg for next 10 kg of body weight
>
> 20 mL/kg for each kg above 20 kg of body weight
>
> Allowance: _____ mL/day or _____ mL/h

Use the following information and order to answer questions 37 through 39.

Metric: $\text{BSA (m}^2) = \sqrt{\dfrac{\text{ht (cm)} \times \text{wt (kg)}}{3{,}600}}$ Household: $\text{BSA (m}^2) = \sqrt{\dfrac{\text{ht (in)} \times \text{wt (lb)}}{3{,}131}}$

Order: **mitomycin 28 mg IV push stat**

Recommended dosage is 10 to 20 mg/m²/single IV dose.

Patient is 5 ft 2 in tall and weighs 103 lb.

Mitomycin is available in a 40 mg vial with directions to reconstitute with 80 mL sterile water for injection and inject slowly over 10 minutes.

37. The patient's BSA is _____ m².

38. a. What is the recommended dosage range of mitomycin for this patient?

     _____ mg to _____ mg

    b. Is the ordered dosage safe? _____ Explain _____

    _____

39. a. What is the concentration of mitomycin after reconstitution? _____ mg/mL

    b. If the order is safe, administer _____ mL mitomycin at the rate of _____ mL/min

       or _____ mL per 15 sec.

40. A child's IV is **1 L D₅ 0.45% NaCl.** Calculate the amount of solute in this IV solution.

    _____ g dextrose and
    _____ g NaCl

Used with permission from Teva Pharmaceuticals USA.

TEVA

NDC 0703-0335-01 ℞only

Ceftriaxone for Injection, USP

1 gram

For I.M. or I.V. Use
Single Use Vial

Each vial contains: ceftriaxone sodium powder equivalent to 1 gram ceftriaxone. **For I.M. Administration :** Reconstitute with 2.1 mL 1% Lidocaine Hydrochloride Injection (USP) or Sterile Water for Injection (USP). Each 1 mL of solution contains approximately 350 mg equivalent of ceftriaxone. **For I.V. Administration :** See Package Insert

Usual Dosage: See Package Insert

Iss. 9/2007
39C1701450907

Storage Prior to Reconstitution: Store powder at 20° to 25°C (68° to 77°F) [See USP Controlled Room Temperature]. **Protect from Light. Storage After Reconstitution:** See Package Insert
Mfd for: Teva Parenteral Medicines Irvine, CA 92618

Use the following order and ceftriaxone label for the available drug to answer questions 41 and 42.

Order: **Ceftriaxone 600 mg IV q.12h for total volume of 50 mL to infuse over 1 h via volume control set**

The package insert states, "For IV administration, reconstitute with 9.6 mL of the specified IV diluent and each 1 mL of solution contains 100 mg of ceftriaxone."

41. The nurse should add _____ mL ceftriaxone and _____ mL IV fluid to the chamber.

42. The package insert states, ". . . recommended dilution concentration is 10 mg/mL to 40 mg/mL . . ." Is the ordered amount of IV fluid sufficient to safely dilute the ceftriaxone? _____

    Explain: _____

    _____

Use the following order and Pfizerpen label to answer questions 43 and 44.

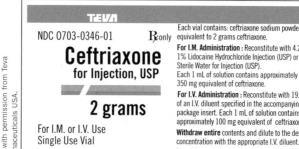

NDC 0049-0510-83

Buffered

Pfizerpen®

penicillin G potassium

For Injection

ONE MILLION UNITS

CAUTION: Federal law prohibits
dispensing without prescription.

ROERIG *Pfizer*

A division of Pfizer Inc., N.Y., N.Y. 10017

43. Order: **penicillin G potassium 400,000 units IV PB q.6h** for a child who weighs 10 kg.
    Recommended dosage for children: Give penicillin G potassium 150,000 to 250,000 units/kg/day
    in divided doses q.6h; dilute with 100 mL NS and infuse over 60 minutes.

    a. How many units per day of penicillin G potassium will this child receive with this order?
       _____ units/day

    b. Is the ordered dosage safe? _____ Explain: _____

    _____

    c. If safe, reconstitute with _____ mL diluent for a concentration of _____ units/mL
       and prepare a reconstitution label.

    Reconstitution label

    d. Prepare to give _____ mL.

    e. If the order is not safe, what should the nurse do? _____

44. The child's IV is infusing on an IV pump programmable in whole milliliters. If the dosage is safe,
    set the IV flow rate at _____ mL/h.

Use the following patient information, orders, labels, and package insert to answer questions
45 through 48.

A patient has been admitted to the hospital with fever and chills, productive cough with yellow-
green sputum, shortness of breath, malaise, and anorexia. Laboratory tests and X-rays confirm a
diagnosis of pneumonia. The patient is complaining of nausea. The physician writes the following
orders. The labels represent the drugs you have available.

NS 1,000 mL IV at 125 mL/h

ceftriaxone 1,500 mg IV PB q.8h in 100 mL NS over 30 min

promethazine 12.5 mg IV push q.4h p.r.n., nausea and vomiting

NDC 0703-2191-01

Promethazine
Hydrochloride
Injection, USP

25 mg/mL

FOR DEEP IM OR IV USE
1 mL Single Dose Vial
PROTECT FROM LIGHT
sicor™
SICOR Pharmaceuticals, Inc.,
Irvine, CA 92618

(01)03007092191017

00150B

TEVA

NDC 0703-0346-01   ℞only

Ceftriaxone
for Injection, USP

2 grams

For I.M. or I.V. Use
Single Use Vial

Each vial contains: ceftriaxone sodium powder
equivalent to 2 grams ceftriaxone.
For I.M. Administration : Reconstitute with 4.2 mL
1% Lidocaine Hydrochloride Injection (USP) or
Sterile Water for Injection (USP).
Each 1 mL of solution contains approximately
350 mg equivalent of ceftriaxone.
For I.V. Administration : Reconstitute with 19.2 mL
of an I.V. diluent specified in the accompanying
package insert. Each 1 mL of solution contains
approximately 100 mg equivalent of ceftriaxone.
Withdraw entire contents and dilute to the desired
concentration with the appropriate I.V. diluent.
Usual Dosage: See Package Insert

Storage Prior to Reconstitution:
Store powder at 20° to 25°C (68° to 77°F)
[See USP Controlled Room Temperature].
Protect from Light.
Storage After Reconstitution:
See Package Insert
Mfd for:
Teva Parenteral Medicines
Irvine, CA 92618
Iss. 9/2007
39C2302450907

Intravenous Administration

Ceftriaxone for injection, USP should be administered intravenously by infusion over a period of 30 minutes. Concentrations between 10 mg/mL and 40 mg/mL are recommended; however, lower concentrations may be used if desired. Reconstitute vials with an appropriate IV diluent (see **COMPATIBILITY AND STABILITY**).

Vial Dosage Size	Amount of Diluent to be Added
250 mg	2.4 mL
500 mg	4.8 mL
1 g	9.6 mL
2 g	19.2 mL

After reconstitution, each 1 mL of solution contains approximately 100 mg equivalent of ceftriaxone. Withdraw entire contents and dilute to the desired concentration with the appropriate IV diluent.

---

45. The nurse starts the primary IV at 1:15 PM on an IV infusion pump. When do you estimate (using international time) that the primary IV and one IV PB administration will be completely infused and the primary IV will have to be replaced? _____ hours

46. For the direct IV administration of promethazine, the drug guide states, "not to exceed 25 mg/min." The nurse should give _____ mL of promethazine per min or _____ mL per 15 sec.

47. Calculate one dose of ceftriaxone: _____ mL

48. Calculate the IV PB flow rate for each dose of ceftriaxone: _____ mL/h

49. Describe the clinical reasoning that you would use to prevent this medication error.

Possible Scenario

A student nurse was preparing for medication administration. One of the orders on the medication administration record (MAR) was written as **Lanoxin 0.125 mg od.** The student nurse crushed the Lanoxin tablet. Prior to giving the medication, the nursing instructor checked the medications that the student had prepared. The instructor asked the student to explain the rationale for crushing the Lanoxin tablet. The student explained to the instructor that the Lanoxin order was for the right eye ("O.D." is an outdated abbreviation for right eye). The student planned to add a small amount of sterile water to the crushed tablet and put it in the patient's eye.

Potential Outcome

What is wrong with the Lanoxin order? _____

_____

What could be the result? _____

Prevention

_____

_____

50. Describe the clinical reasoning you would use to prevent this medication error.

Possible Scenario

Order: **Quinapril 30 mg p.o. daily**

Supply: quinidine 300 mg tablets

A student nurse administering medications noted the difference between the order and the supply drug and questioned the staff nurse about the order and what had been administered. The staff nurse at first dismissed it as only the brand name versus the generic name of the drug. Later, the nurse realized that the student was exactly right to question the order and the drug supplied, and the nurse admitted to the student that the patient had been receiving the wrong drug all week. Not only was the wrong drug supplied, the nurse also did not notice the supply was not the correct dosage.

Potential Outcome

The student referred to a drug reference book and compared the therapeutic and side effects of both drugs. The quinapril was correctly ordered for hypertension. Quinidine is an antiarrhythmic heart medication. The physician was notified of the medication error and ordered a stat electrocardiogram. Indeed, on the electrocardiogram, the patient had a long QT interval, putting the patient at grave risk for a fatal arrythmia.

Prevention

_____

_____

After completing these problems, see pages 670–675 to check your answers. Give yourself 2 points for each correct answer.

Perfect score = 100   My score = _____

Minimum mastery score = 90 (45 correct)

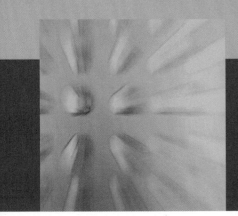

Answers

Essential Skills Evaluation: Pretest and Posttest from pages 4–20

1) $\frac{1}{2}$; 3 times a day 2) 3; 2 times a day 3) 10; 2; once a day 4) $\frac{1}{2}$; every 3 hours as needed for moderate pain

5) 2; once every morning 6) 2.5; every 8 hours

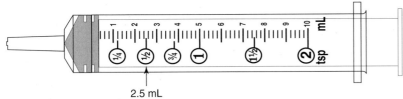

2.5 mL

© Cengage Learning 2013

7)   0.5; every 4 hours as needed for nausea

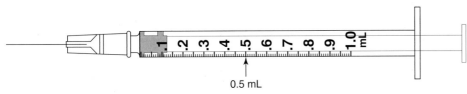

0.5 mL

© Cengage Learning 2013

8)   0.8; once, immediately

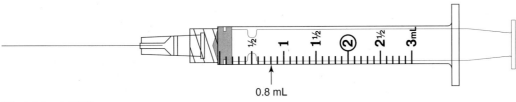

0.8 mL

© Cengage Learning 2013

9)   0.4; every 4 hours as needed for severe pain

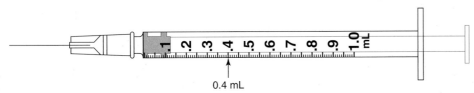

0.4 mL

© Cengage Learning 2013

10)   1.5; once, immediately

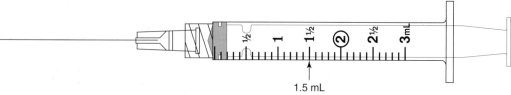

1.5 mL

11)   1.4; every 8 hours

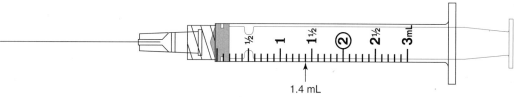

1.4 mL

12)   0.88; once, immediately

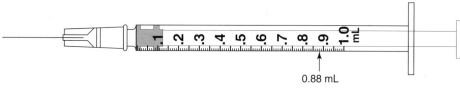

0.88 mL

13)   1; once, immediately; either syringe is appropriate

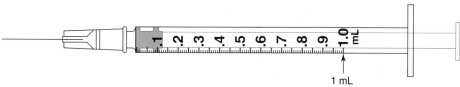

1 mL

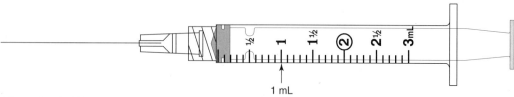

1 mL

14)   0.5; once, every morning; either syringe is appropriate

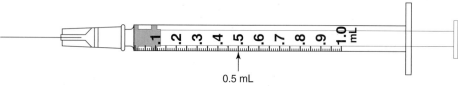

0.5 mL

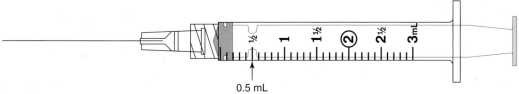

0.5 mL

© Cengage Learning 2013

15) 8; every 12 hours

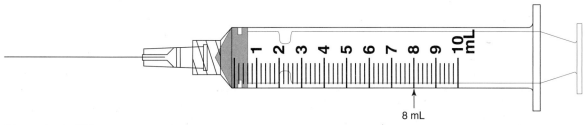

8 mL

© Cengage Learning 2013

16) 4; every 12 hours

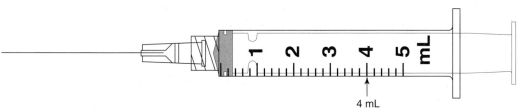

4 mL

© Cengage Learning 2013

17) 1; 1; 0.25; every 8 hours

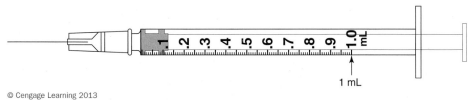

1 mL

© Cengage Learning 2013

18) 1.4; 75; every 6 hours

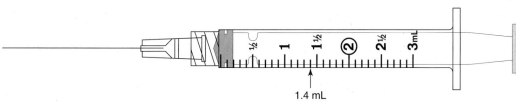

1.4 mL

© Cengage Learning 2013

19)   68; once a day before breakfast

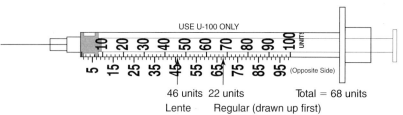

© Cengage Learning 2013

20)   1

21)   Benadryl; 0.7; either syringe is appropriate

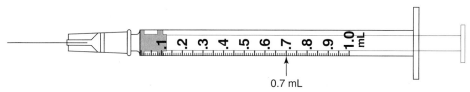

© Cengage Learning 2013

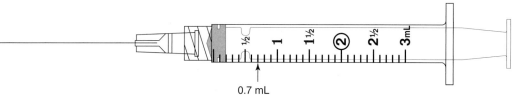

© Cengage Learning 2013

22)   Narcan; 1

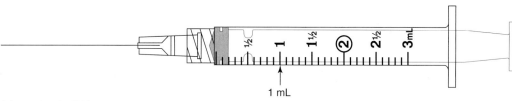

© Cengage Learning 2013

23) Yes. Her temperature is 102.2°F. Tylenol every 4 hours as needed is indicated for fever greater than 101°F. It has been 5 hours and 5 minutes since her last dose. **24)** 2 **25)** 18.8; 138 **26)** 138 **27)** 8; 2 **28)** 1; 0700; 1200; 1700

29) 18; subcutaneous

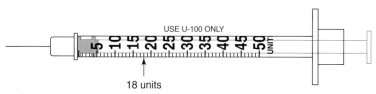

© Cengage Learning 2013

30)   113

31)   Yes; the usual dosage is 20–40 mg/kg/day divided into 3 doses q.8h, which is equivalent to 67–133 mg per dose for a 22 lb (10 kg) child.

32)   4

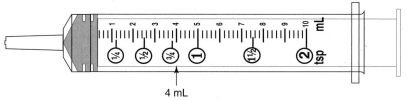

4 mL

© Cengage Learning 2013

33) Yes; the usual dosage is 40 mg/kg/day divided into 3 doses q.8h, which is equivalent to 240 mg per dose for a 40 lb (approx. 18 kg) child.

34) 3; dosage is safe **35)** 103.3 **36)** 282; 423 **37)** 9.4 **38)** 250–375; Yes **39)** 1.7; 26 **40)** 880 **41)** 25 **42)** 1 **43)** 5; 5 **44)** 50

45) 0030; 12:30 AM the next day **46)** 10 **47)** 100; 1 **48)** 5

49)

> 1/30/XX, 1500, reconstituted
>
> as 100 mg/mL. Expires
>
> 1/31/XX, 1500. G.D.P.

50) Prevention: The importance of checking a medication label at least three times to verify supply dosage cannot be overemphasized. It is also important NEVER to assume that the supply dosage is the same as a supply dosage used to calculate previously. Always read the label carefully. Writing the calculation down will also help improve accuracy.

Solutions—Essential Skills Evaluation: Pretest and Posttest

1) $\dfrac{D}{H} \times Q = \dfrac{\overset{1}{\cancel{40} \text{ mg}}}{\underset{2}{\cancel{80} \text{ mg}}} \times 1 \text{ tablet} = \dfrac{1}{2} \text{ tablet}$

2) $\dfrac{D}{H} \times Q = \dfrac{1.5 \text{ mg}}{0.5 \text{ mg}} \times 1 \text{ tablet} = 3 \text{ tablets}$

3) Use 10 mg capsules; 40 mg capsule cannot be split to provide the 20 mg dose.

$\dfrac{D}{H} \times Q = \dfrac{\overset{2}{\cancel{20} \text{ mg}}}{\underset{1}{\cancel{10} \text{ mg}}} \times 1 \text{ capsule} = 2 \text{ capsules}$

4) $\dfrac{D}{H} \times Q = \dfrac{2.5 \text{ mg}}{5 \text{ mg}} \times 1 \text{ tablet} = \dfrac{2.5}{5.0} \text{ tabs} = \dfrac{1}{2} \text{ tablet}$

5) $\dfrac{D}{H} \times Q = \dfrac{0.3 \text{ mg}}{0.15 \text{ mg}} \times 1 \text{ tablet} = \dfrac{0.30}{0.15} \text{ tabs} = 2 \text{ tablets}$

6) $\dfrac{D}{H} \times Q = \dfrac{\overset{1}{\cancel{100} \text{ mg}}}{\underset{2}{\cancel{200} \text{ mg}}} \times 5 \text{ mL} = \dfrac{5}{2} \text{ mL} = 2.5 \text{ mL}$

7) $\dfrac{D}{H} \times Q = \dfrac{12.5 \text{ mg}}{25 \text{ mg}} \times 1 \text{ mL} = \dfrac{12.5}{25.0} \text{ mL} = 0.5 \text{ mL}$

8) $\dfrac{D}{H} \times Q = \dfrac{40 \text{ mg}}{50 \text{ mg}} \times 1 \text{ mL} = 0.8 \text{ mL}$

9) $\dfrac{D}{H} \times Q = \dfrac{4 \text{ mg}}{10 \text{ mg}} \times 1 \text{ mL} = 0.4 \text{ mL}$

10) $\dfrac{D}{H} \times Q = \dfrac{3 \text{ mg}}{2 \text{ mg}} \times 1 \text{ mL} = 1.5 \text{ mL}$

11) $\dfrac{D}{H} \times Q = \dfrac{350 \text{ mg}}{500 \text{ mg}} \times 2 \text{ mL} = \dfrac{700}{500} \text{ mL} = 1.4 \text{ mL}$

12) $\dfrac{D}{H} \times Q = \dfrac{35 \text{ mg}}{80 \text{ mg}} \times 2 \text{ mL} = \dfrac{70}{80} \text{ mL} = 0.875 \text{ mL} = 0.88 \text{ mL}$

13) 1 mg = 1,000 mcg (known equivalent)

0.2 mg × 1,000 mcg/mg = 0.200. = 200 mcg

$\dfrac{D}{H} \times Q = \dfrac{200 \text{ mcg}}{200 \text{ mcg}} \times 1 \text{ mL} = 1 \text{ mL}$

14) 1 mg = 1,000 mcg (known equivalent)

0.125 mg × 1,000 mcg/mg = 0.125. = 125 mcg

$\dfrac{D}{H} \times Q = \dfrac{125 \text{ mcg}}{500 \text{ mcg}} \times 2 \text{ mL} = \dfrac{\overset{1}{\cancel{250}}}{\underset{2}{\cancel{500}}} \text{ mL} = 0.5 \text{ mL}$

15) $\dfrac{D}{H} \times Q = \dfrac{80 \text{ mg}}{\underset{10}{\cancel{100} \text{ mg}}} \times \overset{1}{\cancel{10}} \text{ mL} = \dfrac{\overset{8}{\cancel{80}}}{\underset{1}{\cancel{10}}} \text{ mL} = 8 \text{ mL}$

16) 1 g = 1,000 mg (known equivalent)

0.4 g × 1,000 mg/g = 0.400. = 400 mg

$\dfrac{D}{H} \times Q = \dfrac{\overset{4}{\cancel{400} \text{ mg}}}{\underset{1}{\cancel{100} \text{ mg}}} \times 1 \text{ mL} = 4 \text{ mL}$

17) $\dfrac{D}{H} \times Q = \dfrac{\overset{1}{\cancel{50 \text{ mg}}}}{\underset{5}{\cancel{250 \text{ mg}}}} \times 5 \text{ mL} = \dfrac{5}{5} \text{ mL} = 1 \text{ mL}$

250 mg/5 mL = 50 mg/1 mL

Do not exceed 50 mg/1 min. The 1 mL dose = 50 mg. Administer at 1 mL/1 min or 0.25 mL/15 seconds.

$\dfrac{1 \text{ mL}}{60 \text{ sec}} \diagdown\!\!\!\diagup \dfrac{X \text{ mL}}{15 \text{ sec}}$

$60X = 15$

$\dfrac{60X}{60} = \dfrac{15}{60}$

$X = \dfrac{1}{4} \text{ mL} = 0.25 \text{ mL}$

Either syringe could measure the amount, but the 1 mL syringe will provide greater control for pushing medication at the rate recommended.

18) $\dfrac{D}{H} \times Q = \dfrac{35 \text{ mg}}{25 \text{ mg}} \times 1 \text{ mL} = \dfrac{35}{25} \text{ mL} = 1.4 \text{ mL}$

$\dfrac{V \text{ (mL)}}{T \text{ (min)}} \times C \text{ (gtt/mL)} = \dfrac{100 \text{ mL}}{20 \text{ min}} \times 15 \text{ gtt/mL}$

$= \dfrac{1,500}{20} \text{ gtt/min} = 75 \text{ gtt/min}$

19)   46 units + 22 units = 68 units (total)

20) $\dfrac{D}{H} \times Q = \dfrac{\overset{1}{\cancel{30 \text{ mg}}}}{\underset{2}{\cancel{60 \text{ mg}}}} \times 2 \text{ mL} = \dfrac{2}{2} \text{ mL} = 1 \text{ mL}$

21) $\dfrac{D}{H} \times Q = \dfrac{\overset{7}{\cancel{35 \text{ mg}}}}{\underset{10}{\cancel{50 \text{ mg}}}} \times 1 \text{ mL} = \dfrac{7}{10} \text{ mL} = 0.7 \text{ mL}$

22) $\dfrac{D}{H} \times Q = \dfrac{\cancel{0.4 \text{ mg}}}{\cancel{0.4 \text{ mg}}} \times 1 \text{ mL} = 1 \text{ mL}$

23)   °F = 1.8°C + 32 = (1.8 × 39) + 32 = 70.2 + 32 = 102.2°F;

102.2°F is greater than 101°F;

2400 − 2110 = 0250 or 2 h 50 min;

0215 = 2 h 15 min after 2400;

2 h 50 min + 2 h 15 min = 5 h 5 min

24) $\dfrac{D}{H} \times Q = \dfrac{\overset{2}{\cancel{650 \text{ mg}}}}{\underset{1}{\cancel{325 \text{ mg}}}} \times 1 \text{ tablet} = 2 \text{ tablets}$

25) $\dfrac{D}{H} \times Q = \dfrac{100 \text{ mg}}{\underset{16}{\cancel{80 \text{ mg}}}} \times \overset{3}{\cancel{15}} \text{ mL} = \dfrac{300}{16} \text{ mL} = 18.75 \text{ mL}$

$= 18.8 \text{ mL}$

Measure the 18.8 mL precisely to add to the IV PB bag. But for the drip-rate calculation, such a precise measurement is not necessary. You may round the 18.8 mL to 19 mL for the computation of the drip rate only.

50 mL + 19 mL = 69 mL

$\dfrac{V \text{ (mL)}}{T \text{ (min)}} \times C \text{ (gtt/mL)} = \dfrac{69 \text{ mL}}{\underset{1}{\cancel{30 \text{ min}}}} \times \overset{2}{\cancel{60}} \text{ gtt/mL} = 138 \text{ gtt/min}$

26)   Pump measured in mL/h. 69 mL in 30 min = 138 mL in 60 min.

$\dfrac{69 \text{ mL}}{30 \text{ min}} \diagdown\!\!\!\diagup \dfrac{X \text{ mL}}{60 \text{ min}}$

$30X = 4,140$

$\dfrac{30X}{30} = \dfrac{4,140}{30}$

$X = 138 \text{ mL}$

27) $\dfrac{D}{H} \times Q = \dfrac{\overset{1}{\cancel{125 \text{ mg}}}}{\underset{4}{\cancel{500 \text{ mg}}}} \times 8 \text{ mL} = \dfrac{\overset{2}{\cancel{8}}}{\underset{1}{\cancel{4}}} \text{ mL} = 2 \text{ mL}$

28) $\dfrac{D}{H} \times Q = \dfrac{\cancel{1 \text{ g}}}{\cancel{1 \text{ g}}} \times 1 \text{ tablet} = 1 \text{ tablet}$

31)   1 kg = 2.2 lb (known equivalent)

22 lb ÷ 2.2 lb/kg = 22 $\cancel{\text{lb}}$ × 1 kg/2.2 $\cancel{\text{lb}}$ = 10 kg

Minimum dosage: 20 mg/kg/day × 10 $\cancel{\text{kg}}$ = 200 mg/day
200 mg/day ÷ 3 doses/day = 200 $\cancel{\text{mg/day}}$ × 1 $\cancel{\text{day}}$/3 doses
= 66.6 mg/dose = 67 mg/dose
Maximum dosage: 40 mg/kg/day × 10 $\cancel{\text{kg}}$ = 400 mg/day
400 mg/day ÷ 3 doses/day = 400 $\cancel{\text{mg/day}}$ × 1 $\cancel{\text{day}}$/3 doses
= 133.3 mg/dose = 133 mg/dose

32) $\dfrac{D}{H} \times Q = \dfrac{\overset{4}{\cancel{100 \text{ mg}}}}{\underset{5}{\cancel{125 \text{ mg}}}} \times 5 \text{ mL} = \dfrac{20}{5} \text{ mL} = 4 \text{ mL}$

33)   1 kg = 2.2 lb (known equivalent)

40 lb ÷ 2.2 lb/kg = 40 $\cancel{\text{lb}}$ × 1 kg/2.2 $\cancel{\text{lb}}$ = 18.18 kg = 18.2 kg

40 mg/kg/day × 18.2 $\cancel{\text{kg}}$ = 728 mg/day

728 mg/day ÷ 3 doses/day = 728 $\cancel{\text{mg/day}}$ × 1 $\cancel{\text{day}}$/3 doses
= 242.6 mg/dose = 243 mg/dose
close approximation to ordered dosage of 240 mg; dosage is safe.

34) $\dfrac{D}{H} \times Q = \dfrac{240 \text{ mg}}{\underset{80}{\cancel{400 \text{ mg}}}} \times \overset{1}{\cancel{5}} \text{ mL} = \dfrac{240}{80} \text{ mL} = 3 \text{ mL}$

35)   °F = 1.8 °C + 32 = (1.8 × 39.6) + 32 = 71.28 + 32
= 103.28°F = 103.3°F

36)   1 kg = 2.2 lb (known equivalent)

62 lb ÷ 2.2 lb/kg = 62 $\cancel{\text{lb}}$ × 1 kg/2.2 $\cancel{\text{lb}}$ = 28.18 kg = 28.2 kg
Minimum dosage: 10 mg/kg × 28.2 $\cancel{\text{kg}}$ = 282 mg
Maximum dosage: 15 mg/kg × 28.2 $\cancel{\text{kg}}$ = 423 mg

37) $\dfrac{D}{H} \times Q = \dfrac{\overset{30}{\cancel{300 \text{ mg}}}}{\underset{8}{\cancel{80 \text{ mg}}}} \times 2.5 \text{ mL} = \dfrac{75}{8} \text{ mL} = 9.37 \text{ mL} = 9.4 \text{ mL}$

38) 1 kg = 2.2 lb (known equivalent)

110 lb ÷ 2.2 lb/kg = 110 l̶b̶ × 1 kg/2.2 l̶b̶ = 50 kg

Minimum dosage: 20 mg/k̶g̶/day × 50 k̶g̶ = 1,000 mg/day

1,000 mg/day ÷ 4 doses/day = 1,000 mg/d̶a̶y̶ × 1 d̶a̶y̶/4 doses

= 250 mg/dose

Maximum dosage: 30 mg/k̶g̶/day × 50 k̶g̶ = 1,500 mg/day

1,500 mg/day ÷ 4 doses/day = 1,500 mg/d̶a̶y̶ × 1 d̶a̶y̶/4 doses

= 375 mg/dose

39) $\frac{D}{H} \times Q = \frac{\overset{5}{250\text{ m̶g̶}}}{\underset{6}{300\text{ m̶g̶}}} \times 2\text{ mL} = \frac{10}{6}\text{ mL} = 1.66\text{ mL} = 1.7\text{ mL}$

1.7 mL (medication) + 50 mL (IV fluid) = 51.7 mL = 52 mL
(to be infused)

$\frac{V\text{ (mL)}}{T\text{ (min)}} \times C\text{ (gtt/mL)} = \frac{52\text{ m̶L̶}}{\underset{2}{20\text{ min}}} \times \overset{1}{1̶0̶}\text{ gtt/m̶L̶}$

$= \frac{52}{2}\text{ gtt/min} = 26\text{ gtt/min}$

40)   IV fluid: 50 mL + 50 mL = 100 mL

Gelatin: 4 fl oz = 4 f̶l̶ ̶o̶z̶ × 30 mL/f̶l̶ ̶o̶z̶ = 120 mL

Water: 3 fl oz × 2 = 6 fl oz = 6 f̶l̶ ̶o̶z̶ × 30 mL/f̶l̶ ̶o̶z̶ = 180 mL

Apple juice: 16 fl oz = 16 f̶l̶ ̶o̶z̶ × 30 mL/f̶l̶ ̶o̶z̶ = 480 mL

Total = 880 mL

41) $\frac{V\text{ (mL)}}{T\text{ (min)}} \times C\text{ (gtt/mL)} = \frac{600\text{ m̶L̶}}{\underset{24}{240\text{ min}}} \times \overset{1}{1̶0̶}\text{ gtt/m̶L̶}$

$= \frac{600}{24}\text{ gtt/min} = 25\text{ gtt/min}$

42) $\frac{D}{H} \times Q = \frac{1\text{ m̶g̶}}{\underset{1}{50\text{ m̶g̶}}} \times \overset{1}{5̶0̶}\text{ mL} = 1\text{ mL}$

43) 1 mg/d̶o̶s̶e̶ × 5 d̶o̶s̶e̶s̶ = 5 mg

1 mL/d̶o̶s̶e̶ × 5 d̶o̶s̶e̶s̶ = 5 mL

44) 50 mg ÷ 1 mg/dose = 50 m̶g̶ × 1 dose/1 m̶g̶ = 50 doses

45) 50 doses ÷ 5 doses/h = 50 d̶o̶s̶e̶s̶ × 1 h/5 d̶o̶s̶e̶s̶ = 10 h;

1430 h + 1000 h = 2430 h = 0030 = 12:30 AM

(or 30 min after midnight, the next day)

46) 1 g = 1,000 mg (known equivalent)

1,000 mg ÷ 100 mg/mL = 1,000 m̶g̶ × 1 mL/100 m̶g̶

= 10 mL;

therefore, after adding 9.2 mL to the vial, the resulting volume
totals 10 mL.

47) 100; 1

48) 1 g = 1,000 mg (known equivalent)

0.5 g̶ × 1,000 mg/g̶ = 0.500. = 500 mg

$\frac{D}{H} \times Q = \frac{\overset{5}{500\text{ m̶g̶}}}{\underset{1}{100\text{ m̶g̶}}} \times 1\text{ mL} = 5\text{ mL}$

49) Clinical reasoning indicates that the full reconstituted solution
will be used up within 2 doses, so storage unrefrigerated for
24 hours is satisfactory.

Mathematics Diagnostic Evaluation from pages 28–30

1) 1,517.63 **2)** 20.74 **3)** 100.66 **4)** $323.72 **5)** 46.11 **6)** 754.5 **7)** 16.91 **8)** 19,494.7 **9)** $173.04 **10)** 403.26 **11)** 36

12) 2,500 **13)** $\frac{2}{3}$ **14)** 6.25 **15)** $\frac{4}{5}$ **16)** 40% **17)** 0.4% **18)** 0.05 **19)** 1:3 **20)** 0.02 **21)** $1\frac{1}{4}$ **22)** $6\frac{13}{24}$ **23)** $1\frac{11}{18}$ **24)** $\frac{3}{5}$ **25)** $14\frac{7}{8}$

26) $\frac{1}{100}$ **27)** 0.009 **28)** 320 **29)** 3 **30)** 0.05 **31)** 4 **32)** 0.09 **33)** 0.22 **34)** 25 **35)** 4 **36)** 0.75 **37)** 3 **38)** 500 **39)** 18.24

40) 2.4 **41)** $\frac{1}{5}$ **42)** 1:50 **43)** 5 tablets **44)** 2 milligrams **45)** 30 kilograms **46)** 3.3 pounds **47)** 6.67 centimeters

48) 7.5 centimeters **49)** 90% **50)** 5:1

Solutions—Mathematics Diagnostic Evaluation

3)
```
    9.50
   17.06
   32.00
   41.11
  + 0.99
  ------
  100.66
```

6)
```
  1,005.0
  - 250.5
  -------
    754.5
```

10)
```
    17.16
  × 23.5
  ------
   8580
   5148
   3432
  --------
  403.260 = 403.26
```

12)
$$0.001\overline{)2.500.} = 2,500$$
with quotient 2500.

19) $33\frac{1}{3}\% = \frac{33\frac{1}{3}}{100} = \frac{\frac{100}{3}}{100} = \frac{100}{3} \div \frac{100}{1} = \frac{\cancel{100}}{3} \times \frac{1}{\cancel{100}} = \frac{1}{3} = 1:3$

23)
$$
\begin{array}{r}
1\frac{5}{6} = 1\frac{15}{18} \\
-\frac{2}{9} = -\frac{4}{18} \\
\hline
1\frac{11}{18}
\end{array}
$$

25) $4\frac{1}{4} \times 3\frac{1}{2} = \frac{17}{4} \times \frac{7}{2} = \frac{119}{8} = 14\frac{7}{8}$

29) $\dfrac{0.02 + 0.16}{0.4 - 0.34}$

$$
\begin{array}{rr}
0.02 & 0.40 \\
+0.16 & -0.34 \\
\hline
0.18 & 0.06
\end{array}
$$

$\dfrac{0.18}{0.06} = 0.06\overline{)0.18} = 3$

32) $\frac{1}{2}\% = 0.5\% = 0.005$

$$
\begin{array}{r}
18 \\
\times 0.005 \\
\hline
0.090 = 0.09
\end{array}
$$

34) $\dfrac{1:1,000}{1:100} \times 250 =$

$\dfrac{\frac{1}{1,000}}{\frac{1}{100}} \times 250 = \frac{1}{1,000} \times \frac{\overset{1}{\cancel{100}}}{1} \times \frac{250}{1} = \frac{250}{10} = 25$

45) 66 pounds $= \frac{66}{2.2} = 30$ kilograms or

$\dfrac{2.2 \text{ pounds}}{1 \text{ kilogram}} \times\!\!\times \dfrac{66 \text{ pounds}}{\text{X kilograms}}$

$2.2\text{X} = 66$

$\dfrac{2.2\text{X}}{2.2} = \dfrac{66}{2.2}$

$\text{X} = 30$ kilograms

49)
$$
\begin{array}{r}
50 \text{ items} \\
- 5 \text{ incorrect} \\
\hline
45 \text{ correct}
\end{array}
$$
$\dfrac{45}{50} = \dfrac{9}{10} = 90\%$ (correct)

Review Set 1 from pages 37–38

1) $\frac{6}{6}, \frac{7}{5}$ **2)** $\frac{\frac{1}{100}}{\frac{1}{150}}$ **3)** $\frac{1}{4}, \frac{1}{14}$ **4)** $1\frac{2}{9}, 1\frac{1}{4}, 5\frac{7}{8}$ **5)** $\frac{3}{4} = \frac{6}{8}, \frac{1}{5} = \frac{2}{10}, \frac{3}{9} = \frac{1}{3}$ **6)** $\frac{13}{2}$ **7)** $\frac{6}{5}$ **8)** $\frac{32}{3}$ **9)** $\frac{47}{6}$ **10)** $\frac{411}{4}$ **11)** 2 **12)** 1

13) $3\frac{1}{3}$ **14)** $1\frac{1}{3}$ **15)** $2\frac{3}{4}$ **16)** $\frac{6}{8}$ **17)** $\frac{4}{16}$ **18)** $\frac{8}{12}$ **19)** $\frac{4}{10}$ **20)** $\frac{6}{9}$ **21)** $\frac{1}{100}$ **22)** $\frac{1}{10,000}$ **23)** $\frac{5}{9}$ **24)** $\frac{3}{10}$ **25)** $\frac{2}{5}$ bottle **26)** $1\frac{1}{2}$ bottles

27) $\frac{2}{5}$ of the students are men **28)** $\frac{9}{10}$ of the questions were answered correctly **29)** $\frac{1}{2}$ dose **30)** $\frac{1}{2}$ teaspoon

Solutions—Review Set 1

8) $10\frac{2}{3} = \frac{(10 \times 3) + 2}{3} = \frac{32}{3}$

14) $\frac{100}{75} = 1\frac{25}{75} = 1\frac{1}{3}$

18) $\frac{2}{3} \times \frac{4}{4} = \frac{8}{12}$

25) 10 ounces − 6 ounces = 4 ounces remaining

$\dfrac{\overset{2}{\cancel{4}}}{\underset{5}{\cancel{10}}} = \dfrac{2}{5}$ bottle remaining

27)
$$
\begin{array}{r}
24 \\
+36 \\
\hline
60 \quad \text{people in class}
\end{array}
$$

The men represent $\frac{24}{60}$ or $\frac{2}{5}$ of the students in the class.

29) $\frac{80}{160} = \frac{1}{2}$ of a dose

30) $\frac{1}{2}$ of 1 teaspoon $= \frac{1}{2}$ teaspoon

Review Set 2 from pages 40–41

1) $8\frac{7}{15}$ **2)** $1\frac{5}{12}$ **3)** $17\frac{5}{24}$ **4)** $1\frac{1}{24}$ **5)** $32\frac{5}{6}$ **6)** $5\frac{7}{12}$ **7)** $1\frac{1}{3}$ **8)** $5\frac{53}{72}$ **9)** 43 **10)** $5\frac{118}{119}$ **11)** $2\frac{8}{15}$ **12)** $\frac{53}{132}$ **13)** $\frac{1}{2}$ **14)** $4\frac{5}{6}$ **15)** $\frac{1}{24}$ **16)** $63\frac{2}{3}$

17) $299\frac{4}{5}$ **18)** $\frac{1}{6}$ **19)** $1\frac{2}{5}$ **20)** $7\frac{1}{16}$ **21)** $7\frac{2}{9}$ **22)** $1\frac{1}{4}$ **23)** $24\frac{6}{11}$ **24)** $\frac{7}{12}$ **25)** $\frac{1}{25}$ **26)** $5\frac{5}{6}$ fluid ounces **27)** $1\frac{1}{8}$ inches **28)** 8 inches

29) $21\frac{1}{2}$ pints **30)** $13\frac{1}{4}$ pounds

Solutions—Review Set 2

1)
$$
\begin{array}{r}
7\frac{4}{5} + \frac{2}{3} \qquad 7\frac{12}{15} \\
+\frac{10}{15} \\
\hline
7\frac{22}{15} = 8\frac{7}{15}
\end{array}
$$

3)
$$
\begin{array}{r}
4\frac{2}{3} + 5\frac{1}{24} + 7\frac{1}{2} \qquad 4\frac{16}{24} \\
5\frac{1}{24} \\
+7\frac{12}{24} \\
\hline
16\frac{29}{24} = 17\frac{5}{24}
\end{array}
$$

4) $\frac{3}{4} + \frac{1}{8} + \frac{1}{6} = \frac{18}{24} + \frac{3}{24} + \frac{4}{24} = \frac{18 + 3 + 4}{24} =$

$\frac{25}{24} = 1\frac{1}{24}$

14) $8\frac{1}{12} - 3\frac{1}{4} = 8\frac{1}{12} - 3\frac{3}{12}$ $\quad\begin{array}{r} 7\frac{13}{12} \\ -3\frac{3}{12} \\ \hline 4\frac{10}{12} = 4\frac{5}{6} \end{array}$

25) 50 pounds − 48 pounds = 2 pounds lost

$\frac{2}{50} = \frac{1}{25}$ of weight lost

26) $2\frac{1}{2}$ fluid ounces $+ 3\frac{1}{3}$ fluid ounces $=$

$2\frac{3}{6} + 3\frac{2}{6} = 5\frac{5}{6}$ fluid ounces

29) $56 - 34\frac{1}{2}$ $\quad\begin{array}{r} 55\frac{2}{2} \\ -34\frac{1}{2} \\ \hline 21\frac{1}{2} \text{ pints} \end{array}$

30) $20\frac{1}{2} - 7\frac{1}{4}$ $\quad\begin{array}{r} 20\frac{2}{4} \\ -7\frac{1}{4} \\ \hline 13\frac{1}{4} \text{ pounds} \end{array}$

Review Set 3 from pages 45–46

1) $\frac{1}{40}$ **2)** $\frac{36}{125}$ **3)** $\frac{35}{48}$ **4)** $\frac{3}{100}$ **5)** 3 **6)** $1\frac{2}{3}$ **7)** $\frac{4}{5}$ **8)** $6\frac{8}{15}$ **9)** $\frac{1}{2}$ **10)** $23\frac{19}{36}$ **11)** $\frac{3}{32}$ **12)** $254\frac{1}{6}$ **13)** 3 **14)** $1\frac{34}{39}$ **15)** $\frac{3}{14}$ **16)** $\frac{1}{11}$ **17)** $\frac{1}{2}$ **18)** $\frac{1}{30}$ **19)** $3\frac{1}{3}$ **20)** $\frac{3}{20}$ **21)** $\frac{1}{3}$ **22)** $\frac{7}{12}$ **23)** $1\frac{1}{9}$ **24)** 60 calories **25)** 560 seconds **26)** 40 doses **27)** $31\frac{1}{2}$ tablets **28)** 1,275 milliliters **29)** $52\frac{1}{2}$ ounces **30)** 6 full days

Solutions—Review Set 3

3) $\frac{5}{8} \times 1\frac{1}{6} = \frac{5}{8} \times \frac{7}{6} = \frac{35}{48}$

5) $\dfrac{\frac{1}{6}}{\frac{1}{4}} \times \dfrac{\frac{3}{2}}{\frac{2}{3}} = \left(\frac{1}{6} \times \frac{4}{1}\right) \times \left(\frac{3}{1} \times \frac{3}{2}\right) = \frac{\overset{2}{\cancel{4}}}{\cancel{6}} \times \frac{\overset{3}{\cancel{18}}}{\cancel{6}}_{\,3}{}_{\,1} = 3$

16) $\frac{1}{33} \div \frac{1}{3} = \frac{1}{33} \times \frac{3}{1} = \frac{\overset{1}{\cancel{3}}}{\cancel{33}}_{11} = \frac{1}{11}$

19) $2\frac{1}{2} \div \frac{3}{4} = \frac{5}{2} \div \frac{3}{4} = \frac{5}{\cancel{2}} \times \frac{\overset{2}{\cancel{4}}}{3} = \frac{10}{3} = 3\frac{1}{3}$

27) $3 \times 7 = 21$ doses

$21 \times 1\frac{1}{2} = \frac{21}{1} \times \frac{3}{2} = \frac{63}{2} = 31\frac{1}{2}$ tablets

28) Pitcher is $\frac{1}{3}$ full; $\frac{2}{3}$ was consumed.

$850 \div \frac{2}{3} = \frac{\overset{425}{\cancel{850}}}{1} \times \frac{3}{\cancel{2}}_{1} = 1,275$ milliliters

30)

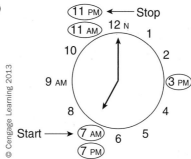

Daily doses would be taken at: 7 AM, 11 AM, 3 PM, 7 PM, and 11 PM for 5 doses/day.

5 doses/day $\times \frac{1}{2}$ fluid ounce/dose $= \frac{5}{2} =$

$2\frac{1}{2}$ fluid ounces/day

16 fluid ounces $\div 2\frac{1}{2}$ fluid ounces/day $= \frac{16}{1} \div \frac{5}{2} =$

$\frac{16}{1} \times \frac{2}{5} = \frac{32}{5} = 6\frac{2}{5}$ days or 6 full days

Review Set 4 from pages 52–53

1) 0.2, two tenths **2)** $\frac{17}{20}$, 0.85 **3)** $1\frac{1}{20}$, one and five hundredths **4)** $\frac{3}{500}$, six thousandths **5)** 10.015, ten and fifteen thousandths **6)** $1\frac{9}{10}$, one and nine tenths **7)** $5\frac{1}{10}$, 5.1 **8)** 0.8, eight tenths **9)** $250\frac{1}{2}$, two hundred fifty and five tenths **10)** 33.03, thirty-three and three hundredths **11)** $\frac{19}{20}$, ninety-five hundredths **12)** 2.75, two and seventy-five hundredths **13)** $7\frac{1}{200}$, 7.005 **14)** 0.084, eighty-four thousandths **15)** $12\frac{1}{8}$, twelve and one hundred twenty-five thousandths **16)** $20\frac{9}{100}$, twenty and nine hundredths **17)** $22\frac{11}{500}$, 22.022 **18)** $\frac{3}{20}$, fifteen hundredths **19)** 1,000.005, one thousand and five thousandths **20)** $4,085\frac{3}{40}$, 4,085.075 **21)** 0.0170 **22)** 0.25 **23)** 0.75 **24)** $\frac{9}{200}$ **25)** 0.12 **26)** 0.063 **27)** False **28)** False **29)** True **30)** 0.8 gram and 1.25 grams

Solutions—Review Set 4

4) $0.006 = \frac{6}{1,000} = \frac{3}{500}$

8) $\frac{4}{5} = 5\overline{)4.0}^{\,0.8}$

14) $\frac{21}{250} = 250\overline{)21.000}^{\,0.084}$
$$\begin{array}{r} 2\,000 \\ \overline{1\,000} \\ \underline{1\,000} \end{array}$$

15) $12.125 = 12\frac{125}{1,000} = 12\frac{1}{8}$

18) $0.15 = \frac{15}{100} = \frac{3}{20}$

30) Safe dosages include amounts greater than or equal to 0.5 gram but less than or equal to 2 grams. Safe dosages: 0.8 gram and 1.25 grams

Review Set 5 from pages 55–56

1) 22.585 **2)** 44.177 **3)** 12.309 **4)** 11.3 **5)** 175.199 **6)** 25.007 **7)** 0.518 **8)** $9.48 **9)** $18.91 **10)** $22.71 **11)** 6.403
12) 0.27 **13)** 4.15 **14)** 1.51 **15)** 10.25 **16)** 2.517 **17)** 374.35 **18)** 604.42 **19)** 27.449 **20)** 23.619 **21)** 0.697 gram
22) 66.25 milliliters **23)** $2,058.06 **24)** 10.3 grams **25)** 8.1 hours

Solutions—Review Set 5

2)
$$\begin{array}{r} 7.517 \\ 3.200 \\ 0.160 \\ + 33.300 \\ \hline 44.177 \end{array}$$

9)
$$\begin{array}{r} {}^{8\ 9\ 10}\\ \$19.0\,\cancel{0}\,\cancel{0} \\ -0.09 \\ \hline \$18.91 \end{array}$$

25)
$$\begin{array}{r} 3\text{ h }20\text{ min} \\ 40\text{ min} \\ 3\text{ h }30\text{ min} \\ 24\text{ min} \\ + \ 12\text{ min} \\ \hline \end{array}$$
6 h 126 min = 6 h + 2 h 6 min = 8 h 6 min (60 min/h)
$$= 8\frac{6}{60}\text{ h} = 8\frac{1}{10}\text{ h} = 8.1\text{ h (hours)}$$

Review Set 6 from page 60

1) 5.83 **2)** 2.2 **3)** 42.75 **4)** 0.15 **5)** 403.14 **6)** 75,100.75 **7)** 32.86 **8)** 2.78 **9)** 348.58 **10)** 0.02 **11)** 400 **12)** 3.74 **13)** 5
14) 2.98 **15)** 4,120 **16)** 5.45 **17)** 272.67 **18)** 1.5 **19)** 50,020 **20)** 300 **21)** 562.50. = 56,250 **22)** 16.0. = 160
23) .025. = 0.025 **24)** .032.005 = 0.032005 **25)** .00.125 = 0.00125 **26)** 23.2.5 = 232.5 **27)** 71.7.717 = 71.7717
28) 83.1.6 = 831.6 **29)** 0.33. = 33 **30)** 14.106. = 14,106

Solutions—Review Set 6

2) $0.314 \times 7 = 2.198 = 2.20 = 2.2$ **10)** $1.14 \times 0.014 = 0.01596 = 0.02$ **14)** $45.5 \div 15.25 = 2.983 = 2.98$

Practice Problems—Chapter 1 from pages 60–62

1) $\frac{7}{20}$ **2)** 0.375 **3)** LCD = 21 **4)** LCD = 55 **5)** LCD = 18 **6)** LCD = 15 **7)** $3\frac{7}{15}$ **8)** $7\frac{29}{60}$ **9)** $\frac{1}{2}$ **10)** $2\frac{7}{24}$ **11)** $\frac{7}{27}$
12) $10\frac{1}{8}$ **13)** $4\frac{4}{17}$ **14)** $\frac{39}{80}$ **15)** $5\frac{1}{55}$ **16)** $5\frac{5}{18}$ **17)** $2\frac{86}{87}$ **18)** $\frac{3}{20}$ **19)** $\frac{1}{3,125}$ **20)** $\frac{1}{4}$ **21)** $1\frac{5}{7}$ **22)** $16\frac{1}{32}$ **23)** 60.27 **24)** 66.74
25) 42.98 **26)** 4,833.92 **27)** 190.8 **28)** 19.17 **29)** 9.48 **30)** 7.7 **31)** 42.75 **32)** 300 **33)** 12,930.43 **34)** 3,200.63 **35)** 2
36) 150.96 **37)** 9.716. = 9,716 **38)** .50.25 = 0.5025 **39)** 0.25. = 25 **40)** 5.750. = 5,750 **41)** .0.25 = 0.025
42) 11.5.25 = 115.25 **43)** 147 fluid ounces **44)** 138 nurses; 46 maintenance/cleaners; 92 technicians; 92 others **45)** False
46) $1,082.79 **47)** $1.46 **48)** 0.31 gram **49)** 800 milliliters **50)** 2.95 kilograms

Solutions—Practice Problems—Chapter 1

43) $3\frac{1}{2}$ fluid ounces/feeding $\times$ 6 feedings/day =

21 fluid ounces/day, and 21 fluid ounces/day $\times$

7 days/week = 147 fluid ounces in one week

44) $\frac{3}{8} \times \frac{368}{1} = \frac{1,104}{8} = 138$ nurses

$\frac{1}{8} \times \frac{368}{1} = \frac{368}{8} = 46$ maintenance/cleaners

$\frac{1}{4} \times \frac{368}{1} = \frac{368}{4} = 92$ technicians and 92 others

45) $1\frac{2}{32} = 1.0625$; False, it's greater than normal.

46) 40 hours $\times$ \$20.43/hour = $817.20

6.5 hours overtime $\times$ \$40.86 =   +265.59

(Overtime rate = \$20.43 $\times$ 2 = \$40.86)   \$1,082.79

47) A case of 12 boxes with 12 catheters/box =

144 catheters

By case: \$975 ÷ 144 = \$6.77/catheter

By box: \$98.76 ÷ 12 = \$8.23/catheter

  \$8.23
  −6.77
 \$1.46 savings/catheter

48) 0.065 gram/ounce $\times$ 4.75 ounces = 0.31 gram

49) 1,200 milliliters $\times \frac{2}{3} = \frac{\overset{400}{\cancel{1,200}}}{1} \times \frac{2}{\underset{1}{\cancel{3}}} = 800$ milliliters

50)   6.65 kilograms
  −3.70 kilograms
  2.95 kilograms gained

Review Set 7 from pages 67–68

1) $\frac{1}{50}$ **2)** $\frac{3}{5}$ **3)** $\frac{1}{3}$ **4)** $\frac{4}{7}$ **5)** $\frac{3}{4}$ **6)** 0.5 **7)** 0.15 **8)** 0.14 **9)** 0.07 **10)** 0.24 **11)** 25% **12)** 40% **13)** 12.5% **14)** 70% **15)** 50%

16) $\frac{9}{20}$ **17)** $\frac{3}{5}$ **18)** $\frac{1}{200}$ **19)** $\frac{1}{100}$ **20)** $\frac{2}{3}$ **21)** 0.03 **22)** 0.05 **23)** 0.06 **24)** 0.33 **25)** 0.01 **26)** 4:25 **27)** 1:4 **28)** 1:2 **29)** 9:20

30) 3:50 **31)** 0.9 **32)** $\frac{1}{5}$ **33)** 0.25% **34)** 0.5 **35)** $\frac{1}{100}$

Solutions—Review Set 7

1) $3:150 = \frac{3}{150} = \frac{\overset{1}{\cancel{3}}}{\underset{50}{\cancel{150}}} = \frac{1}{50}$

3) $0.05:0.15 = \frac{\overset{1}{\cancel{0.05}}}{\underset{3}{\cancel{0.15}}} = \frac{1}{3}$

7) $\frac{1}{1,000} : \frac{1}{150} = \frac{\frac{1}{1,000}}{\frac{1}{150}} = \frac{1}{\underset{100}{\cancel{1,000}}} \times \frac{\overset{15}{\cancel{150}}}{1} = \frac{15}{100} = 0.15. = 0.15$

12) $2:5 = \frac{2}{5} = 0.4; 0.4 = 0.40. = 40\%$

13) $0.08:0.64 = \frac{0.08}{0.64} = \frac{1}{8} = 0.125;$
$0.125 = 0.12.5 = 12.5\%$

17) $60\% = \frac{60}{100} = \frac{3}{5}$

18) $0.5\% = \frac{0.5}{100} = 0.5 \div 100 = 0.00.5 = 0.005 = \frac{5}{1,000} = \frac{1}{200}$

21) $2.94\% = \frac{2.94}{100} = 2.94 \div 100 = 0.02.94 = 0.0294 = 0.03$

30) $6\% = \frac{6}{100} = \frac{3}{50} = 3:50$

31) Convert to decimals and compare:
$0.9\% = 0.009$
$0.9\ \ = 0.900$ (largest)
$1:9\ \ = 0.111$
$1:90 = 0.011$

Review Set 8 from pages 71–72

1) 3 **2)** 3.3 **3)** 1.25 **4)** 5.33 **5)** 0.56 **6)** 1.8 **7)** 0.64 **8)** 12.6 **9)** 40 **10)** 0.48 **11)** 1 **12)** 0.96 **13)** 4.5 **14)** 0.94 **15)** 10

16) 0.4 **17)** 1.5 **18)** 10 **19)** 20 **20)** 1.8

Solutions—Review Set 8

2)

$$\frac{\frac{3}{4}}{\frac{1}{2}} \times 2.2 = X$$

$$\frac{3}{4} \div \frac{1}{2} \times \frac{2.2}{1} = X$$

$$\frac{3}{\underset{2}{4}} \times \frac{\overset{1}{2}}{1} \times \frac{2.2}{1} = X$$

$$\frac{6.6}{2} = X$$

$$X = 3.3$$

4)

$$\frac{40\%}{60\%} \times 8 = X$$

$$\frac{\overset{2}{0.4}}{\underset{3}{0.6}} \times 8 = X$$

$$\frac{2}{3} \times \frac{8}{1} = X$$

$$\frac{16}{3} = X$$

$$X = 5.33\overline{3}$$

$$X = 5.33$$

6)

$$\frac{0.15}{0.1} \times 1.2 = X$$

$$\frac{\overset{3}{0.15}}{\underset{2}{0.10}} \times \frac{1.2}{1} = X$$

$$\frac{3}{2} \times \frac{1.2}{1} = X$$

$$\frac{3.6}{2} = X$$

$$X = 1.8$$

8)

$$\frac{\overset{3}{1,200,000}}{\underset{1}{400,000}} \times 4.2 = X$$

$$\frac{3}{1} \times \frac{4.2}{1} = X$$

$$\frac{12.6}{1} = X$$

$$X = 12.6$$

10)

$$\frac{\overset{3}{30}}{\underset{5}{50}} \times 0.8 = X$$

$$\frac{3}{5} \times \frac{0.8}{1} = X$$

$$\frac{2.4}{5} = X$$

$$X = 0.48$$

14)

$$\frac{\overset{1}{250,000}}{\underset{8}{2,000,000}} \times 7.5 = X$$

$$\frac{1}{8} \times \frac{7.5}{1} = X$$

$$\frac{7.5}{8} = X$$

$$X = 0.937$$

$$X = 0.94$$

20)

$$\frac{\frac{1}{100}}{\frac{1}{150}} \times 1.2 = X$$

$$\frac{1}{100} \div \frac{1}{150} \times \frac{1.2}{1} = X$$

$$\frac{1}{\underset{2}{100}} \times \frac{\overset{3}{150}}{1} \times \frac{1.2}{1} = X$$

$$\frac{1}{2} \times \frac{3}{1} \times \frac{1.2}{1} = X$$

$$\frac{3.6}{2} = X$$

$$X = 1.8$$

Review Set 9 from pages 75–76

1) 0.25 **2)** 1 **3)** 0.56 **4)** 1,000 **5)** 0.7 **6)** 8 **7)** 21.43 **8)** 500 **9)** 200 **10)** 10.5 **11)** 3 **12)** 0.63 **13)** 10 **14)** 0.67 **15)** 1.25 **16)** 31.25 **17)** 16.67 **18)** 240 **19)** 0.75 **20)** 2.27 **21)** 1 **22)** 6 **23)** 108 nurses **24)** 72 calories **25)** 81.82 milligrams/hour

Solutions—Review Set 9

4)

$$\frac{0.5}{2} \diagdown \diagup \frac{250}{X}$$

$$0.5X = 500$$

$$\frac{0.5X}{0.5} = \frac{500}{0.5}$$

$$X = 1,000$$

6)

$$\frac{40}{X} \times 12 = 60$$

$$\frac{40}{X} \times \frac{12}{1} = 60$$

$$\frac{480}{X} \diagdown \diagup \frac{60}{1}$$

$$60X = 480$$

$$\frac{60X}{60} = \frac{480}{60}$$

$$X = 8$$

9)

$$\frac{15}{500} \times X = 6$$

$$\frac{15X}{500} \diagdown \diagup \frac{6}{1}$$

$$15X = 3,000$$

$$\frac{15X}{15} = \frac{3,000}{15}$$

$$X = 200$$

10)

$$\frac{5}{X} \diagdown \diagup \frac{10}{21}$$

$$10X = 105$$

$$\frac{10X}{10} = \frac{105}{10}$$

$$X = 10.5$$

11)

$$\frac{250}{1} \diagdown \diagup \frac{750}{X}$$

$$250X = 750$$

$$\frac{250X}{250} = \frac{750}{250}$$

$$X = 3$$

14)

$$\frac{\frac{1}{100}}{1} \diagdown \diagup \frac{\frac{1}{150}}{X}$$

$$\frac{1}{100}X = \frac{1}{150}$$

$$\frac{\frac{1}{100}X}{\frac{1}{100}} = \frac{\frac{1}{150}}{\frac{1}{100}}$$

$$X = \frac{1}{150} \div \frac{1}{100}$$

$$X = \frac{1}{\underset{3}{150}} \times \frac{\overset{2}{100}}{1}$$

$$X = \frac{2}{3} = 0.666 = 0.67$$

22)

$$\frac{25\%}{30\%} = \frac{5}{X}$$

$$\frac{0.25}{0.3} \diagdown \diagup \frac{5}{X}$$

$$0.25X = 1.5$$

$$\frac{0.25X}{0.25} = \frac{1.5}{0.25}$$

$$X = 6$$

23)

$$\frac{45}{100} \diagdown \diagup \frac{X}{240}$$

$$100X = 10,800$$

$$\frac{100X}{100} = \frac{10,800}{100}$$

$$X = 108$$

Review Set 10 from page 77

1) 1.3 **2)** 4.75 **3)** 56 **4)** 0.43 **5)** 26.67 **6)** 15 **7)** 0.8 **8)** 2.38 **9)** 37.5 **10)** 112.5 **11)** 8 pills **12)** 720 milliliters
13) $3,530.21 **14)** 7.2 ounces **15)** 700 calories

Solutions—Review Set 10

1) $0.25\% = 0.00.25 = 0.0025;\ 0.0025 \times 520 = 1.3$

8) $7\% = 0.07. = 0.07;\ 0.07 \times 34 = 2.38$

11) $40\% = 0.40. = 0.4;\ 0.4 \times 20 \text{ pills} = 8 \text{ pills}$

13) $80\% \text{ of } \$17,651.07 = 0.8 \times \$17,651.07 = \$14,120.86$

   $\begin{aligned}
   \$17,651.07 &\quad \text{total bill}\\
   -14,120.86 &\quad \text{paid by insurance co.}\\
   \hline
   \$3,530.21 &\quad \text{paid by patient}
   \end{aligned}$

14) $40\% = 0.40. = 0.4;$
   $0.4 \times 18 \text{ ounces} = 7.2 \text{ ounces}$

15) $20\% = 0.20. = 0.2;$
   $0.2 \times 3,500 \text{ calories} = 700 \text{ calories}$

Practice Problems—Chapter 2 from pages 78–79

1) 0.4, 40%, 2:5 **2)** $\frac{1}{20}$, 5%, 1:20 **3)** 0.17, $\frac{17}{100}$, 17:100 **4)** 0.25, $\frac{1}{4}$, 25% **5)** 0.06, $\frac{3}{50}$, 3:50 **6)** 0.17, 17%, 1:6 **7)** 0.5, $\frac{1}{2}$, 1:2

8) 0.01, $\frac{1}{100}$, 1% **9)** $\frac{9}{100}$, 9%, 9:100 **10)** 0.38, 38%, 3:8 **11)** 0.67, $\frac{2}{3}$, 67% **12)** 0.33, 33%, 1:3 **13)** $\frac{13}{25}$, 52%, 13:25

14) 0.45, $\frac{9}{20}$, 45% **15)** 0.86, 86%, 6:7 **16)** 0.3, $\frac{3}{10}$, 30% **17)** 0.02, 2%, 1:50 **18)** $\frac{3}{5}$, 60%, 3:5 **19)** $\frac{1}{25}$, 4%, 1:25

20) 0.1, $\frac{1}{10}$, 1:10 **21)** 0.04 **22)** 1:40 **23)** 7.5% **24)** $\frac{1}{2}$ **25)** 3:4 **26)** 262.5 **27)** 3.64 **28)** 1.97 **29)** 1:4 **30)** 1:10 **31)** 84

32) 90,000 **33)** 1 **34)** 1.1 **35)** 100 **36)** 39 **37)** 0.75 **38)** 21 **39)** 120 **40)** 90 **41)** 25 grams protein; 6.25 grams fat

42) 231 points **43)** 60 minutes **44)** 50 milliliters **45)** 27 milligrams **46)** 5.4 grams **47)** 283.5 milligrams **48)** 6.5 pounds

49) $10.42 **50)** 6 total doses

Solutions—Practice Problems—Chapter 2

36) $\dfrac{3}{9} \diagdown\!\!\!\diagup \dfrac{X}{117}$

   $9X = 351$

   $\dfrac{9X}{9} = \dfrac{351}{9}$

   $X = 39$

41) $20\% = 0.20. = 0.2$

   $0.2 \times 125 \text{ grams} = 25 \text{ grams (of protein)}$

   $5\% = 0.05. = 0.05$

   $0.05 \times 125 \text{ grams} = 6.25 \text{ grams (of fat)}$

   $\begin{array}{r}
   125 \\
   \times\ 0.2 \\
   \hline
   25.0 = 25
   \end{array}$

   $\begin{array}{r}
   125 \\
   \times\ 0.05 \\
   \hline
   6.25
   \end{array}$

43) $\dfrac{90}{27} \diagdown\!\!\!\diagup \dfrac{200}{X}$

   $90X = 5,400$

   $\dfrac{90X}{90} = \dfrac{5,400}{90}$

   $X = 60$

45) $45\% = 0.45. = 0.45$

   $0.45 \times 60 \text{ milligrams} = 27 \text{ milligrams}$

   $\begin{array}{r}
   60 \\
   \times\ 0.45 \\
   \hline
   300 \\
   240 \\
   \hline
   27.00 = 27
   \end{array}$

46) $\dfrac{3}{4} = 0.75$

   $1\frac{1}{2} = 1.5$

   $\dfrac{2.7}{0.75} \diagdown\!\!\!\diagup \dfrac{X}{1.5}$

   $0.75X = 4.05$

   $\dfrac{0.75X}{0.75} = \dfrac{4.05}{0.75}$

   $X = 5.4$

47) $\dfrac{6.75}{1} \diagdown\!\!\!\diagup \dfrac{X}{42}$

   $X = 283.5$

48) $5\% = 0.05. = 0.05$

   $0.05 \times 130 \text{ pounds} = 6.5 \text{ pounds}$

   $\begin{array}{r}
   130 \\
   \times\ 0.05 \\
   \hline
   6.50 = 6.5
   \end{array}$

49) $17\% = 0.17. = 0.17;\ 0.17 \times \$12.56 = \$2.14$

   $\begin{array}{r}
   \$12.56 \\
   -\ 2.14 \\
   \hline
   \$10.42
   \end{array}$

50) $10\% = 0.10. = 0.10;\ 0.10 \times 150 = 15$

   $\begin{aligned}
   150 \text{ milligrams} &\quad \text{first dose}\\
   -\ 15 \text{ milligrams} &\\
   \hline
   135 \text{ milligrams} &\quad \text{second dose}\\
   -\ 15 \text{ milligrams} &\\
   \hline
   120 \text{ milligrams} &\quad \text{third dose}\\
   -\ 15 \text{ milligrams} &\\
   \hline
   105 \text{ milligrams} &\quad \text{fourth dose}\\
   -\ 15 \text{ milligrams} &\\
   \hline
   90 \text{ milligrams} &\quad \text{fifth dose}\\
   -\ 15 \text{ milligrams} &\\
   \hline
   75 \text{ milligrams} &\quad \text{sixth dose}
   \end{aligned}$

   6 total doses

Section 1—Self-Evaluation from pages 80–82

1) 3.05 **2)** 4,002.5 **3)** 0.63 **4)** 723.27 **5)** LCD = 12 **6)** LCD = 110 **7)** $\frac{11}{12}$ **8)** $\frac{47}{63}$ **9)** 1 **10)** $\frac{1}{2}$ **11)** 45.78 **12)** 0.02 **13)** 59.24 **14)** 0.09 **15)** 12 **16)** $\frac{2}{3}$ **17)** $\frac{1}{10}, \frac{1}{6}, \frac{1}{5}, \frac{1}{3}, \frac{1}{2}$ **18)** $\frac{2}{3}, \frac{3}{4}, \frac{5}{6}, \frac{7}{8}, \frac{9}{10}$ **19)** 0.009, 0.125, 0.1909, 0.25, 0.3 **20)** $\frac{1}{2}$ %, 0.9%, 50%, 100%, 500% **21)** 1:3 **22)** 1:600 **23)** 0.01 **24)** 0.9% **25)** $\frac{1}{3}$ **26)** 5:9 **27)** $\frac{1}{20}$ **28)** 1:200 **29)** $\frac{2}{3}$ **30)** 75% **31)** 40% **32)** 0.17 **33)** 1.21 **34)** 1.3 **35)** 2.5 **36)** 100 **37)** 4 **38)** 8.33 **39)** 24 participants **40)** 2 holidays **41)** $2.42 **42)** 12 cans of water **43)** 8 centimeters **44)** 950 milliliters **45)** 23.1 fluid ounces **46)** 17.7 **47)** Milk **48)** 0.049, 0.05, 0.175, 2.25, 2.5, 5, 5.075 **49)** 2.104, 2.06, 2.4 **50)** 0.913

.913	X 0.913
0.9130	9.130

Solutions—Section 1—Self-Evaluation

16) $\frac{1}{150} \div \frac{1}{100} = \frac{1}{150} \times \frac{100}{1} = \frac{\overset{2}{100}}{\underset{3}{150}} = \frac{2}{3}$

30) $3:4 = \frac{3}{4} = 4\overline{)3.0}\,^{0.75} = 75\%$

34) $\dfrac{0.3}{2.6} \diagdown \diagup \dfrac{0.15}{X}$
$0.3X = 2.6 \times 0.15$
$0.3X = 0.39$
$\dfrac{0.3X}{0.3} = \dfrac{0.39}{0.3}$
$X = 1.3$

39) $4\% = 0.04. = 0.04;$
0.04×600 participants $= 24$ participants
$$\begin{array}{r} 600 \\ \times\ 0.04 \\ \hline 24.00 = 24 \end{array}$$

Review Set 11 from pages 88–89

1) metric **2)** volume **3)** weight **4)** length **5)** $\frac{1}{1,000}$ or 0.001 **6)** 1,000 **7)** microgram **8)** kilogram **9)** milligram **10)** 1,000 **11)** 1 **12)** 1,000 **13)** 10 **14)** 0.3 g **15)** 1.33 mL **16)** 5 kg **17)** 1.5 mm **18)** 10 mg **19)** microgram **20)** milliliter **21)** milligram **22)** gram **23)** millimeter **24)** kilogram **25)** centimeter

Review Set 12 from page 93

1) 3 quarts **2)** 10 pounds **3)** 10 milliequivalents **4)** $2\frac{1}{2}$ pounds **5)** 10 tablespoons **6)** 75 lb **7)** 30 mEq **8)** 5 T **9)** $1\frac{1}{2}$ t **10)** 14 units **11)** False **12)** False **13)** True **14)** units **15)** 3 **16)** 2 **17)** 1 **18)** 1 **19)** 1 **20)** milliequivalent; mEq

Practice Problems—Chapter 3 from pages 94–96

1) milli **2)** micro **3)** centi **4)** kilo **5)** 1 milligram **6)** 1 kilogram **7)** 1 microgram **8)** 1 centimeter **9)** meter **10)** gram **11)** liter **12)** fluid ounce **13)** ounce **14)** milligram **15)** microgram **16)** pound **17)** milliequivalent **18)** teaspoon **19)** quart **20)** milliliter **21)** pint **22)** tablespoon **23)** millimeter **24)** gram **25)** centimeter **26)** liter **27)** meter **28)** kilogram **29)** pound **30)** 325 mcg **31)** $\frac{1}{2}$ t **32)** 2 t **33)** $\frac{1}{3}$ fl oz **34)** 5,000,000 units **35)** 0.5 L **36)** 0.05 mg **37)** 600 mL **38)** 2.5 cm **39)** 0.08 mL **40)** 5.5 kg **41)** eight and one-quarter ounces **42)** three hundred and seventy-five grams **43)** one-half kilogram **44)** two and six tenths milliliters **45)** twenty milliequivalents **46)** four tenths liter **47)** three and five hundredths micrograms **48)** seventeen hundredths milligram **49)** fourteen and one-half pounds

50) Prevention: This type of error can be prevented by avoiding the use of a decimal point or trailing zero when not necessary. In this instance, the decimal point and zero serve no purpose and can easily be misinterpreted, especially if the decimal point is difficult to see. Question any order that is unclear or unreasonable.

51) Prevention: This type of error can be prevented by asking the prescribing physician for clarification. If you see grains prescribed or if you are unclear as to what the prescriber is ordering, *do not guess—always ask for clarification*. Ideally, grains and other apothecary units will be on the "Do Not Use" list for this health care facility.

Review Set 13 from page 104

1) 0.5 **2)** 15 **3)** 0.008 **4)** 0.01 **5)** 0.06 **6)** 0.3 **7)** 200 **8)** 1,200 **9)** 2.5 **10)** 65 **11)** 5 **12)** 1,500 **13)** 0.1 **14)** 0.25
15) 2,000 **16)** 750 **17)** 5 **18)** 1,000 **19)** 1,000 **20)** 3 **21)** 0.023 **22)** 0.00105 **23)** 0.018 **24)** 400 **25)** 2.625 **26)** 0.5
27) 10,000 **28)** 0.45 **29)** 0.005 **30)** 30,000

Solutions—Review Set 13

2) 0.015. g = 15 mg; g is larger than mg. To convert from larger smaller unit, multiply. It takes more of mg (smaller) unit to make equivalent amount of g (larger) unit. Equivalent: 1 g = 1,000 mg. Therefore, multiply by 1,000 or move decimal point 3 places to right.

3) .008. mg = 0.008 g; mg is smaller unit than g. To convert from smaller to larger unit, divide. It takes fewer of g (larger) unit to make equivalent amount of mg (smaller) unit. Therefore, divide by 1,000 or move decimal point 3 places to left.

9) 0.002.5 kg = 2.5 g

16) 0.750. L = 750 mL

20) 3.000. mL = 3 L

23) .018. mcg = 0.018 mg

Review Set 14 from pages 107–108

1) 0.003; 1 kg = 1,000 g **2)** 65; 1 t = 5 mL **3)** $\frac{1}{2}$; 1 fl oz = 30 mL **4)** 75; 1 fl oz = 30 mL **5)** $\frac{3}{4}$; 1 qt = 1,000 mL
6) 4; 1 t = 5 mL **7)** 60; 1 T = 15 mL **8)** 19.8; 1 kg = 2.2 lb **9)** 113.64; 1 kg = 2.2 lb **10)** 3; 1 L = 1 qt
11) 121; 1 kg = 2.2 lb **12)** 30; 1 in = 2.5 cm **13)** 2; 1 qt = 1 L **14)** 15; 1 t = 5 mL **15)** 45; 1 kg = 2.2 lb
16) 500; 1 pt = 500 mL **17)** 360; 1 cup = 240 mL **18)** 5; 1 m = 100 cm; 1 in = 2.5 cm; 1 ft = 12 in
19) 12; 1 in = 2.5 cm **20)** 2; 1 fl oz = 30 mL **21)** 80; 1 in = 2.5 cm **22)** 14; 1 in = 2.5 cm **23)** 3; 1 in = 2.5 cm
24) 50; 1 in = 2.5 cm; 1 cm = 10 mm **25)** 88; 1 kg = 2.2 lb **26)** 15.75 or $15\frac{3}{4}$; 1 kg = 2.2 lb **27)** 50; 1 kg = 2.2 lb
28) 7.7; 1 kg = 2.2 lb **29)** 28.64; 1 kg = 2.2 lb **30)** 53.75 **31)** 4; $\frac{1}{2}$ **32)** Yes **33)** 2,430 **34)** 1.25 **35)** 10 **36)** Dissolve
2 teaspoons of Betadine concentrate in 1 pint, or 2 cups, of warm water. **37)** 2 **38)** 3 **39)** 16 **40)** 93.64

Solutions—Review Set 14

4) fl oz → mL; Larger ↓ Smaller → (×)
$2\frac{1}{2}$ fl oz × 30 mL/fl oz = 75 mL

6) mL → t; Smaller ↑ Larger → (÷)
20 mL ÷ 5 mL/t = 20 mL × 1 t/5 mL = 4 t

11) kg → lb; Larger ↓ Smaller → (×)
55 kg × 2.2 lb/kg = 121 lb

15) lb → kg; Smaller ↑ Larger → (÷)
99 lb ÷ 2.2 lb/kg = 99 lb × 1 kg/2.2 lb = 45 kg

18) 1.5 m = 1.50. = 150 cm

1 in = 2.5 cm

150 cm ÷ 2.5 cm/in = 150 cm × 1 in/2.5 cm

   = 60 in

1 ft = 12 in

60 in ÷ 12 in/ft = 60 in × 1 ft/12 in = 5 ft

20) mL → fl oz; Smaller ↑ Larger → (÷)

60 mL ÷ 30 mL/fl oz = 60 mL × 1 fl oz/30 mL

   = 2 fl oz

24) in → cm; Larger ↓ Smaller → (×)

2 in × 2.5 cm/in = 5 cm

cm → mm; Larger ↓ Smaller → (×)

5 cm × 10 mm/cm = 50 mm

31) mL → fl oz; Smaller ↑ Larger → (÷)

120 mL ÷ 30 mL/fl oz = 120 mL × 1 fl oz/30 mL

   = 4 fl oz

fl oz → cups; Smaller ↑ Larger → (÷)

4 fl oz ÷ 8 fl oz/cup = 4 fl oz × 1 cup/8 fl oz

   = $\frac{1}{2}$ cup

32) lb → kg; Smaller ↑ Larger → (÷)

250 lb − 10 lb = 240 lb

240 lb ÷ 2.2 lb/kg = 240 lb × 1 kg/2.2 lb = 109 kg;

240 lb = 109 kg

Patient now weighs 108 kg. Yes, goal met.

33) Add up the fluid ounces: 81 fl oz

fl oz → mL; Larger ↓ Smaller → (×)

81 fl oz × 30 mL/fl oz = 2,430 mL

34) lb → kg; Smaller ↑ Larger → (÷)

55 lb ÷ 2.2 lb/kg = 55 lb × 1 kg/2.2 lb = 25 kg

0.05 mg/kg × 25 kg = 1.25 mg

35) Find the total number of mL per day and the total number of mL per bottle.

Per day: 12 mL/dose × 4 doses/day = 48 mL/day

Per bottle: 16 fl oz × 30 mL/fl oz = 480 mL

480 mL ÷ 48 mL/day = 480 mL × 1 day/48 mL

   = 10 days

36) mL → t; mL → fl oz; Smaller ↑ Larger → (÷)

10 mL ÷ 5 mL/t = 10 mL × 1 t/5 mL = 2 t

480 mL ÷ 30 mL/fl oz = 480 mL × 1 fl oz/30 mL

   ÷ 16 fl oz

Add 2 t Betadine concentrate to 16 fl oz, or 2 cups, of water.

38) 1 qt = 32 fl oz (per container)

4 fl oz/feeding × 8 feedings/day = 32 fl oz per day

She needs 3 containers for 3 days.

Practice Problems—Chapter 4 from pages 110–112

1) 500 **2)** 10 **3)** 0.0075 **4)** 3 **5)** 4,000 **6)** 0.5 **7)** $\frac{1}{2}$ **8)** 0.3 **9)** 70 **10)** 149.6 **11)** 4.46 **12)** 105 **13)** 2.39 **14)** 6.4 **15)** 2 **16)** 1.63 **17)** 32.05 **18)** 7.99 **19)** 0.008 **20)** 0.45 **21)** 95 **22)** 500 **23)** 600 **24)** 4.05 **25)** 68.18 **26)** $7\frac{1}{2}$ **27)** 10 **28)** 480 **29)** 2 **30)** 3 **31)** 0.375 **32)** 30 **33)** 1 **34)** 1 **35)** 1 **36)** 1,500 **37)** 45 **38)** $1\frac{1}{2}$ **39)** 4.4 **40)** 0.025 **41)** 4,300 **42)** 0.06 **43)** 15 **44)** 3 **45)** 250 **46)** 9 **47)** 8 **48)** 840 **49)** 11.55 or $11\frac{1}{2}$

50) Prevention: The nurse didn't use the conversion rules correctly. The nurse divided instead of multiplying. This type of medication error is avoided by double-checking your dosage calculations and asking yourself, "Is this dosage reasonable?" Certainly you know that if there are 1,000 mg in 1 g and you want to give 2 g, then you need *more* than 1,000 milligrams, not less. The correct calculations are:

   Convert: g → mg; Larger ↓ Smaller → (×)

      2 g × 1,000 mg/g = 2,000 mg

To give 2,000 mg, you would need twice the amount of the available strength. Therefore, you would need 20 mL of the 1,000 mg per 10 mL strength.

Solutions—Practice Problems—Chapter 4

13) 5 lb 4 oz

4 oz ÷ 16 oz/lb = 4 oz × 1 lb/16 oz = $\frac{1}{4}$ lb = 0.25 lb

5 lb 4 oz = 5.25 lb

1 kg = 2.2 lb

5.25 lb ÷ 2.2 lb/kg = 5.25 lb × 1 kg/2.2 lb = 2.39 kg

46) Per bottle: 4 fl oz × 30 mL/fl oz = 120 mL

(1 fl oz = 30 mL)

Each dose: $2\frac{1}{2}$ t × 5 mL/t = 12.5 mL (1 t = 5 mL)

Bottle holds 120 mL; each dose is 12.5 mL

120 mL ÷ 12.5 mL/dose = 120 mL × 1 dose/12.5 mL

   = 9.6 doses or *9 full* doses

47) 120 mL ÷ 15 mL/dose = 120 mL × 1 dose/15 mL

   = 8 doses (1 T = 15 mL)

48) 4 + 8 + 6 + 10 = 28 fl oz; 28 fl oz × 30 mL/fl oz

   = 840 mL (1 fl oz = 30 mL)

49) 5,250 g ÷ 1,000 g/kg = 5,250 g × 1 kg/1,000 g

   = 5.25 kg

5.25 kg × 2.2 lb/kg = 11.55 (or $11\frac{1}{2}$) lb

Review Set 15 from page 116

1) 12:32 AM **2)** 7:30 AM **3)** 4:40 PM **4)** 9:21 PM **5)** 11:59 PM **6)** 12:15 PM **7)** 2:20 AM **8)** 10:10 AM **9)** 1:15 PM **10)** 6:25 PM **11)** 1330
12) 0004 **13)** 2145 **14)** 1200 **15)** 2315 **16)** 0345 **17)** 2400 **18)** 1530 **19)** 0620 **20)** 1745 **21)** *zero six twenty-three* **22)** *zero-zero forty-one*
23) *nineteen zero three* **24)** *twenty-three eleven* **25)** *zero three hundred*

Review Set 16 from pages 118–119

1) 38 **2)** 101.1 **3)** 97.2 **4)** 89.6 **5)** 37 **6)** 37.2 **7)** 39.8 **8)** 104 **9)** 102 **10)** 97.5 **11)** 37.8 **12)** 102.2 **13)** 99.3 **14)** 34.6 **15)** 39.3 **16)** 35.3
17) 44.6 **18)** 31.1 **19)** 98.6 **20)** 39.7

Solutions—Review Set 16

1)
$$°C = \frac{°F - 32}{1.8}$$
$$°C = \frac{100.4 - 32}{1.8}$$
$$°C = \frac{68.4}{1.8}$$
$$°C = 38°$$

2)
$$°F = 1.8°C + 32$$
$$°F = (1.8 \times 38.4) + 32$$
$$°F = 69.12 + 32$$
$$°F = 101.12 = 101.1°$$

Practice Problems—Chapter 5 from pages 120–121

1) 2:57 AM **2)** 0310 **3)** 1622 **4)** 8:01 PM **5)** 11:02 AM **6)** 0033 **7)** 0216 **8)** 4:42 PM **9)** 11:56 PM **10)** 0420 **11)** 1931 **12)** 2400 or 0000
13) 0645 **14)** 9:15 AM **15)** 9:07 PM **16)** 6:23 PM **17)** 5:40 AM **18)** 1155 **19)** 2212 **20)** 2106 **21)** 4 h **22)** 7 h **23)** 8 h 30 min **24)** 12 h 15 min
25) 14 h 50 min **26)** 4 h 12 min **27)** 4 h 48 min **28)** 3 h 41 min **29)** 6 h 30 min **30)** 16 h 38 min **31)** False **32)** a. AM; b. PM; c. AM; d. PM
33) 37.6 **34)** 97.7 **35)** 102.6 **36)** 37.9 **37)** 36.7 **38)** 99.3 **39)** 100.8 **40)** 40 **41)** 36.6 **42)** 95.7 **43)** 39.7 **44)** 102.2 **45)** 98.4 **46)** 38.6
47) 36.2 **48)** 37.2, 99 (98.96° rounds to 99.0°F) **49)** True

50) Prevention: Such situations can easily be prevented by accurately applying the complete formula for temperature conversion. Guessing is not acceptable in medical and health care calculations. Temperature conversion charts are readily available in most health care settings, but when they are not, the conversion formulas should be used. It may be wise to try to memorize the common fever temperature conversions between 98.6°F (37°C) and 104°F (40°C).

Solutions—Practice Problems—Chapter 5

24)
$$\begin{array}{r} 2150 \\ -0935 \\ \hline 1215 = 12\text{ h }15\text{ min} \end{array}$$

26) 2316 = 11:16 PM, 0328 = 3:28 AM
11:16 PM → 3:16 AM = 4 h
$$\begin{array}{r} 3\text{:}16\text{ AM} \rightarrow 3\text{:}28\text{ AM} = 12\text{ min} \\ \hline 4\text{ h }12\text{ min} \end{array}$$

28) 4:35 PM → 7:35 PM = 3 h
$$\begin{array}{r} 7\text{:}35\text{ PM} \rightarrow 8\text{:}16\text{ PM} = 41\text{ min} \\ \hline 3\text{ h }41\text{ min} \end{array}$$

48)
$$\frac{37.6 + 35.5 + 38.1 + 37.6}{4} = \frac{148.8}{4} = 37.2°C \text{ (average)}$$
$$°F = (1.8 \times 37.2) + 32 = 98.96 = 99.0 = 99°$$
(rounded; zero dropped)

Review Set 17 from pages 131–134

1) 1 mL **2)** Round 1.25 to 1.3 and measure on the mL scale as 1.3 mL **3)** No **4)** 0.5 mL **5** a) False; **5** b) The size of the drop varies according to the diameter of the tip of the dropper. **6)** No **7)** Measure the oral liquid in a 3 mL syringe, which is not intended for injections. **8)** 5 **9)** Discard the excess prior to injecting the patient. In some cases (such as for controlled substances), the nurse may need a witness to observe the discarding of the excess. **10)** To prevent needlestick injury

11)

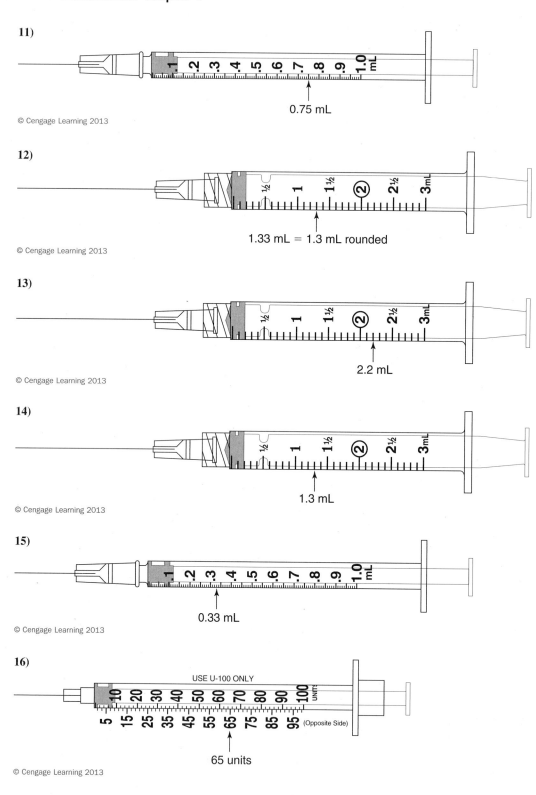

0.75 mL

© Cengage Learning 2013

12)

1.33 mL = 1.3 mL rounded

© Cengage Learning 2013

13)

2.2 mL

© Cengage Learning 2013

14)

1.3 mL

© Cengage Learning 2013

15)

0.33 mL

© Cengage Learning 2013

16)

USE U-100 ONLY

(Opposite Side)

65 units

© Cengage Learning 2013

17)

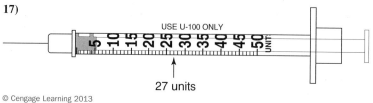

USE U-100 ONLY

27 units

© Cengage Learning 2013

18)

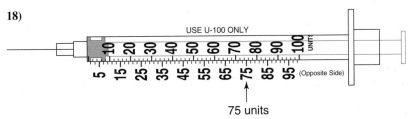

USE U-100 ONLY

75 units

© Cengage Learning 2013

19)

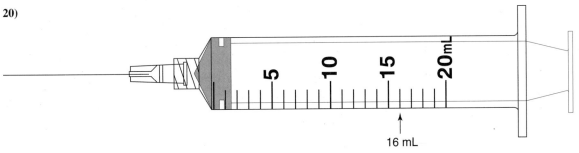

4.4 mL

© Cengage Learning 2013

20)

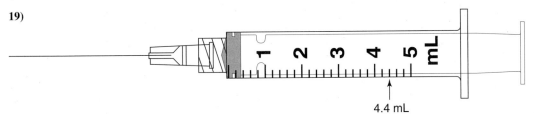

16 mL

© Cengage Learning 2013

21) 0.2 mL **22)** 1 mL **23)** 0.2 mL

Practice Problems—Chapter 6 from pages 136–139

1) 1 **2)** hundredths or 0.01 **3)** No. The tuberculin syringe has a maximum capacity of 1 mL. **4)** Round to 1.3 mL and measure at 1.3 mL. **5)** 30; 1 **6)** 1 mL **7)** 0.75 **8)** False **9)** False **10)** True **11)** To prevent accidental needlesticks during intravenous administration **12)** top ring **13)** 10 **14)** False **15)** 3 mL, 1 mL, and insulin

16)

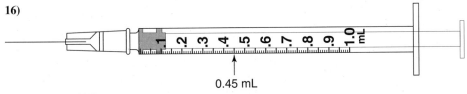

0.45 mL

© Cengage Learning 2013

17)

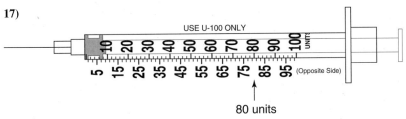

USE U-100 ONLY

80 units

© Cengage Learning 2013

18)

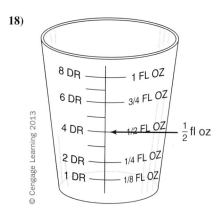

19)

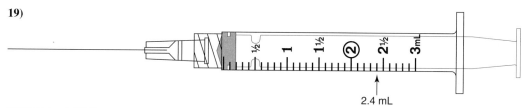

2.4 mL

© Cengage Learning 2013

20)

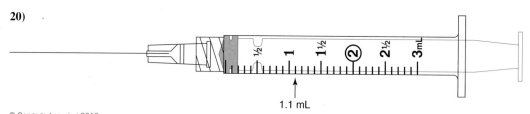

1.1 mL

© Cengage Learning 2013

21)

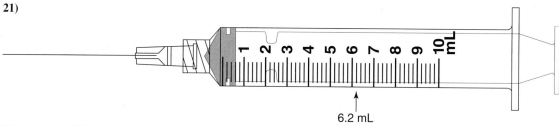

6.2 mL

© Cengage Learning 2013

22)

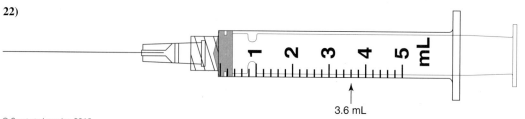

3.6 mL

© Cengage Learning 2013

23)

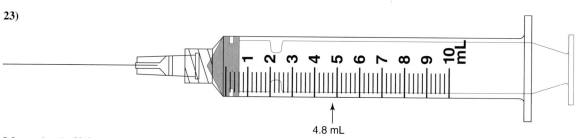

4.8 mL

© Cengage Learning 2013

24)

12 mL

© Cengage Learning 2013

25) Prevention: This error could have been avoided by following a simple principle: Don't put oral drugs in syringes intended for injection. Instead, place the medication in an oral syringe to which a needle cannot be attached. In addition, the medication should have been labeled for oral use only. The medication was ordered orally, not by injection. An alert nurse should have noticed the discrepancy. Finally, but just as important, a medication should be administered only by the nurse who prepared it.

26) Prevention: The nurse should ask for assistance to learn how to use unfamiliar equipment. Do not put the patient at risk. The nurse must remove the cap on the oral syringe prior to administering the medication, so that the child cannot choke on the cap.

Review Set 18 from pages 144–145

1) Give 250 milligrams of naproxen orally 2 times a day. **2)** Give 30 units of Humulin N NPH insulin subcutaneously every day 30 minutes before breakfast. **3)** Give 500 milligrams of cefaclor orally immediately, and then give 250 milligrams every 8 hours. **4)** Give 25 micrograms of Synthroid orally once a day. **5)** Give 10 milligrams of Ativan intramuscularly every 4 hours as necessary for agitation. **6)** Give 20 milligrams of furosemide intravenously slowly immediately. **7)** Give 10 milliliters of Mylanta orally after meals and at bedtime. **8)** Instill 2 drops of 1% atropine sulfate ophthalmic in the right eye every 15 minutes for 4 applications. **9)** Give 15 milligrams of morphine sulfate intramuscularly every 3 hours as needed for pain. **10)** Give 0.25 milligram of digoxin orally once a day. **11)** Give 250 milligrams of tetracycline orally 4 times a day. **12)** Give 150 micrograms of nitroglycerin sublingually immediately. **13)** Instill 2 drops of Cortisporin otic suspension in both ears 3 times a day and at bedtime. **14)** The abbreviation t.i.d. means 3 times a day with no specific interval between times. An attempt is made to give the 3 doses during waking hours. The abbreviation q.8h means every 8 hours. These doses would be given around the clock at 8-hour intervals. For example, administration times for t.i.d. might be 0800, 1200, 1700; administration times for q.8h could be 0600, 1400, 2200. **15)** Contact the physician for clarification. **16)** No, q.i.d. orders are given 4 times in 24 hours with no specific interval between times indicated in order, typically during waking hours; whereas q.4h orders are given 6 times in 24 hours at 4-hour intervals. **17)** They are determined by hospital or institutional policy. **18)** Patient, drug, dosage, route, frequency, date and time written, signature of physician/prescriber. **19)** Parts 1–5: patient's name, drug, dosage, route, frequency **20)** The right patient must receive the right drug in the right amount by the right route at the right time, followed by the right documentation.

Review Set 19 from pages 150–151

1) 9 AM, 9 PM **2)** 9 AM **3)** 7:30 AM, 11:30 AM, 4:30 PM, 9 PM **4)** 9 AM, 9 PM **5)** every 6 hours, as needed for severe pain **6)** 9/7/xx at 0900, or 9 AM **7)** sublingual, under the tongue **8)** once a day **9)** 125 mcg **10)** nitroglycerin, Darvocet-N 100, ketorolac **11)** subcutaneous injection **12)** once **13)** cephalexin **14)** before breakfast (at 7:30 AM) **15)** milliequivalent **16)** cephalexin and K-Dur **17)** Tylenol **18)** twice **19)** 0900 and 2100 **20)** 2400, 0600, 1200, and 1800 **21)** In the "One-Time Medication Dosage" section, lower left corner.

Practice Problems—Chapter 7 from pages 152–156

1) twice a day **2)** per rectum **3)** before meals **4)** after **5)** 3 times a day **6)** every 4 hours **7)** when necessary **8)** by mouth, orally **9)** intravenous **10)** 4 times a day **11)** immediately **12)** freely, as desired **13)** after meals **14)** intramuscular **15)** without **16)** noct **17)** gtt **18)** mL **19)** SL **20)** g **21)** q.i.d. **22)** c̄ **23)** subcut **24)** t **25)** b.i.d. **26)** q.3h **27)** p.c. **28)** ā **29)** kg **30)** Give 60 milligrams of Toradol intravenously immediately and every 6 hours when necessary for pain. **31)** Give 300,000 units of procaine penicillin G intravenously 4 times a day. **32)** Give 5 milliliters of Mylanta orally 1 hour before and 1 hour after meals, at bedtime, and every 2 hours as needed at night for gastric upset. **33)** Give 25 milligrams of Librium orally every 6 hours when necessary for agitation. **34)** Give 5,000 units of heparin subcutaneously immediately. **35)** Give 5 milligrams of morphine sulfate intravenously every 4 hours when necessary for moderate to severe pain. **36)** Give 0.25 milligram of digoxin orally every day. **37)** Instill 2 drops of 10% Neo-Synephrine ophthalmic solution in the left eye every 30 minutes for 2 applications. **38)** Give 40 milligrams of Lasix intramuscularly immediately. **39)** Give 4 milligrams of Decadron intravenously twice a day. **40)** 12:00 midnight, 8:00 AM, 4:00 PM **41)** 20 units **42)** subcut: subcutaneous **43)** Give 500 milligrams of Cipro orally every 12 hours. **44)** 8:00 AM, 12:00 noon, 6:00 PM **45)** digoxin (Lanoxin) 0.125 mg p.o. daily at 1700 **46)** with, c̄ **47)** Give 150 milligrams of ranitidine tablets orally twice daily with breakfast and supper. **48)** Vancomycin **49)** 12 hours

50) Prevention: This error could have been avoided by paying careful attention to the ordered frequency as well as the scheduled times each time a medication was administered.

Review Set 20 from pages 167–169

1) B **2)** D **3)** C **4)** A **5)** E **6)** F **7)** G **8)** 5 mL **9)** oral **10)** A, B, C, D, E, F, G **11)** Filmtab means *film-sealed tablet.* **12)** 1 mg/mL **13)** 2 tablets **14)** D **15)** It is a Schedule IV drug. It has limited potential for abuse and is clinically useful. **16)** penicillin G potassium **17)** Pfizerpen **18)** 5,000,000 units per vial; reconstituted to 250,000 units/mL, 500,000 units/mL, or 1,000,000 units/mL **19)** IM or IV **20)** 0049-0520-83 **21)** Pfizer-Roerig **22)** 1 **23)** 1 **24)** 10

Practice Problems—Chapter 8 from pages 171–174

1) 50 mEq per 50 mL (or 1 mEq/mL) **2)** 50 mL **3)** 4,200 mg per 50 mL (or 84 mg/mL) **4)** cefpodoxime proxetil **5)** "Shake bottle to loosen granules. Add approximately half the total amount of distilled water required for constitution (total water = 29 mL). Shake vigorously to wet the granules. Add remaining water and shake vigorously." **6)** Pharmacia **7)** 10 mL **8)** 250 mg per 10 mL (25 mg/mL) **9)** 1 mL **10)** Depo-Provera **11)** medroxyprogesterone acetate **12)** 0009-0626-01 **13)** injection solution **14)** 10 mL **15)** intramuscular **16)** Akrimax Pharmaceuticals, LLC **17)** capsule **18)** 20° to 25°C (68°–77°F) **19)** 1 mg per 4 mL (or 0.25 mg/mL) **20)** 1 mg (per 4 mL vial) **21)** I **22)** H **23)** H **24)** oral **25)** H **26)** III **27)** 2% **28)** 2; 20

29) Prevention: This error could have been prevented by carefully comparing the drug label and dosage to the MAR drug and dosage three times while preparing the medication. In this instance, both the incorrect drug and the incorrect dosage strength sent by the pharmacy should have been noted by the nurse. Further, the nurse should have asked for clarification of the order.

30 a) Prevention: The nurse should have recognized that the patient was still complaining of signs and symptoms that the medication was ordered to treat. **30 b)** If the order was difficult to read, the physician should have been called to clarify the order. Was the dosage of 100 mg a usual dosage for Celexa? The nurse should have consulted a drug guide to ensure that the dosage was appropriate. Also, if the patient wasn't complaining of or diagnosed with depression, the nurse should have questioned why Celexa was ordered.

Review Set 21 from page 193–194

1) Right patient, right drug, right amount (dosage or dose), right route, right time, right documentation **2)** *NPH insulin 20 units SC daily. NPH insulin 20 units subcut daily* (preferred). The abbreviation SC is included on the ISMP list of error-prone abbreviations and, while not restricted by The Joint Commission, many hospitals have included this on their Do Not Use list. The ISMP recommends "subcut" or "subcutaneously." Know the local policy. **3)** After preparing the drug, just prior to administration **4)** Patient name and date of birth, or patient name and ID number **5)** True **6)** a **7)** Removing medication for more than one patient at a time from the ADC **8)** On the patient identification band and on the medication **9)** Insulin, opiates and narcotics, injectable potassium chloride, and intravenous anticoagulants; high-alert medications **10)** Write the order down on the patient's chart or enter it into the computer record, then read the order back, and finally get confirmation from the prescriber that it is correct. Before administering the medication, verify the safety of the order by consulting a reputable drug reference if you are unfamiliar with the order.

Practice Problems—Chapter 9 from pages 195–197

1) d **2)** False **3)** True **4)** True **5)** True **6)** Patient, drug (or medication), amount (or dosage or dose), route, time, documentation **7)** Prescription, transcription, administration **8)** Upon first contact with the drug, while measuring the dosage, and just prior to administration **9)** 0.75 mg **10)** Write out the order, read it back, and get confirmation from the prescriber. **11)** Any four of these: patient injury; loss of life; increased health care costs; additional technology expenses to prevent error; liability defense; increased length of stay; harm to the nurse involved in regard to his or her personal and professional status, confidence, and practice

12) Prevention: The health care professional originating the order should not have used "q.d." to indicate the frequency of administration. The employee transcribing the order and the nurse signing off on the order both erroneously interpreted the "q.d." notation as "q.i.d." They should have been alert to the risk of errors associated with the use of this notation and should have been especially cautious in transcribing the order correctly.

Section 2—Self-Evaluation from pages 199–204

1) 0.6 g **2)** 4 t **3)** 250,000 units **4)** 0.5 mL **5)** $\frac{1}{2}$ fl oz **6)** four drops **7)** twenty-five hundredths of a milligram **8)** one hundred twenty-five micrograms **9)** two tablespoons **10)** twenty-five hundredths of a liter **11)** 0.35; 0.00035 **12)** 1,200; 1,200,000 **13)** 12; 60 **14)** 150; 0.15 **15)** 3.5 or $3\frac{1}{2}$; 1.59 **16)** 5.62; 2.25 or $2\frac{1}{4}$ **17)** 90; 90,000 **18)** 11,590; 25.5 or $25\frac{1}{2}$ **19)** 2.5 **20)** 10 **21)** No **22)** 480 **23)** 2335 **24)** 6:44 PM **25)** 0803 **26)** 100.4 **27)** 38.6 **28)** 99

29)

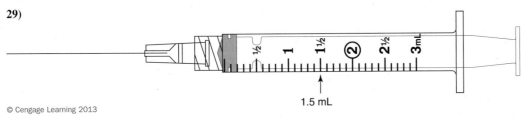

1.5 mL

© Cengage Learning 2013

30)

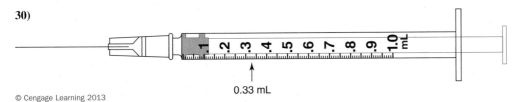

0.33 mL

© Cengage Learning 2013

31)

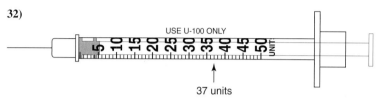

44 units

© Cengage Learning 2013

32)

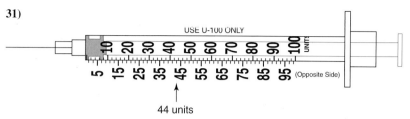

37 units

© Cengage Learning 2013

33)

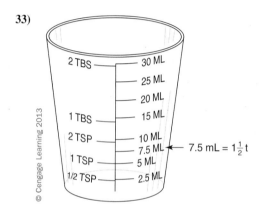

7.5 mL = $1\frac{1}{2}$ t

© Cengage Learning 2013

34) nitroglycerin **35)** under the tongue **36)** Give 400 micrograms of nitroglycerin by the sublingual route immediately.

37) 5,000 units per mL **38)** 63323-262-01 **39)** Give 3,750 units of heparin subcutaneously every 8 hours. **40)** neomycin sulfate

41) 125 mg per 5 mL **42)** *heparin 5,000 units subcut daily* **43)** The right patient must receive the right drug, in the right

amount, by the right route, at the right time, with the right documentation. **44)** 250 mcg **45)** c. DOBUTamine – DOPamine

46) 2100 **47)** c. 1.2 mL **48)** acetaminophen (Tylenol); 650 mg; p.o.; q.4h; p.r.n; fever greater than 101° F **49)** b. 0730, 1330,

1830, 2230; e. 7:00 AM, 12:00 PM, 5:00 PM, 10:00 PM

50)

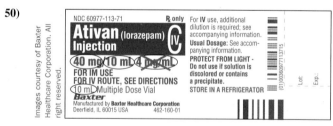

Solutions—Section 2—Self-Evaluation

12)   1,000 mg/g; g → mg; Larger ↓ Smaller → (×)

1.2 g × 1,000 mg/g = 1.200.g = 1,200 mg

1,000 mcg/mg; mg → mcg; Larger ↓ Smaller → (×)

1,200 mg × 1,000 mcg/mg = 1,200.000.mcg = 1,200,000 mcg

15)   16 oz/lb; oz → lb; Smaller ↑ Larger → (÷)

56 oz ÷ 16 oz/lb = 56 oz × 1 lb/16 oz = 3.5 lb or $3\frac{1}{2}$ lb

2.2 lb/kg; lb → kg; Smaller ↑ Larger → (÷)

3.5 lb ÷ 2.2 lb/kg = 3.5 lb × 1 kg/2.2 lb = 1.59 kg

21)   16 oz/lb; oz → lb; Smaller ↑ Larger → (÷)

4 oz ÷ 16 oz/lb = 4 o̶z̶ × 1 lb/16 o̶z̶ = 0.25 lb; 6 lb 4 oz = 6.25 lb

2.2 lb/kg; lb → kg; Smaller ↑ Larger → (÷)

6.25 lb ÷ 2.2 lb/kg = 6.25 l̶b̶ × 1 kg/2.2 l̶b̶ = 2.84 kg

1,000 g/kg; kg → g; Larger ↓ Smaller → (×)

2.84 k̶g̶ × 1,000 g/k̶g̶ = 2.840. kg = 2,840 g

This full-term newborn weighs 2,840 g, which is more than 2,500 g, the weight considered small for gestational age.

45)   Rationale for correct answer c: The dissimilarities in the LASA drugs are printed in uppercase letters. Rationale for incorrect answers a, b, d: Similarities are printed in uppercase letters; red type is a recommendation, but all letters are in uppercase; underlining is a recommendation, but all letters are in uppercase.

Review Set 22 from pages 221–226

1) 1   **2)** $1\frac{1}{2}$ **3)** $\frac{1}{2}$ **4)** $\frac{1}{2}$ **5)** 3   **6)** 1   **7)** 2   **8)** 2   **9)** I, 2 tablets   **10)** H, 2 tablets   **11)** G, $1\frac{1}{2}$ tablets   **12)** E, 2 tablets
13) D, 2 tablets   **14)** G, 2 tablets   **15)** A, 1 capsule   **16)** C, 1 tablet

Note: For questions 17 through 30 the *201 Delmar Nurse's Drug Handbook* was used as reference. Answers may vary slightly if another resource was used.

17)   a) type 2 diabetes mellitus; b) 0.5 mg, 1 mg, 2 mg tablets; c) 0.5 to 4 mg taken with meals, 16 mg maximum daily dose; d) B and C; e) one 1 mg tablet and one 0.5 mg tablet

18)   a) hypertension, edema; b) 12.5 mg capsules, 12.5 mg, 25 mg, 50 mg, 100 mg tablets; c) 12.5 mg to 100 mg per day in one or two daily doses depending on condition; d) A, need to check to see if scored; e) one-half scored tablet

19)   a) treat or prevent hypokalemia; b) 8 mEq and 10 mEq extended-release capsules; c) 16 to 24 mEq/day prophylaxis, treatment highly individualized; d) D; e) two 8 mEq capsules

20)   a) hypertension; b) 100 mg, 200 mg, 300 mg tablets; c) 100 mg to 400 mg twice a day up to 1,200 to 2,400 mg/day for severe cases; d) F, need to check to see if scored; e) one-half 300 mg scored tablets

21)   a) mild to moderate pain, rheumatoid arthritis, and osteoarthritis; b) OTC 100 mg and 200 mg tablets, 200 mg capsules, RX 400 mg, 600 mg, 800 mg tablets; c) 200 mg to 800 mg every 3 to 6 hours depending on condition; d) G; e. two 400 mg tablets

22)   a) infections of the skin, urinary tract, and respiratory tract; b) 500 mg capsules, 1 g tablets; c) 1 to 2 g/day in single or 2 divided doses depending on condition; d) E; e) two 500 mg capsules

23)   a) moderate to moderately severe pain; b) temporary relief of fever and minor aches and pains;

c) 2.5 mg/325 mg, 2.5 g/300 mg, 2.5 g/400 mg, 5 mg/325 mg, 5 mg/300 mg, 5 mg/400 mg, 5 mg/500 mg, 7.5 mg/300 mg, 7.5 mg/325 mg, 7.5 mg/400 mg, 7.5 mg/500 mg, 10 mg/300 mg, 10 mg/325 mg, 10 mg/400 mg, 10 mg/650 mg

24)   1 caplet, capsule, or tablets q.6h as needed for pain; 6 to 12 may be taken per day depending on dosage

25)   HYDROcodone—OXYcodone   **26)** H   **27)** 1200   **28)** 2   **29)** 4,000 mg   **30)** No

Solutions—Review Set 22

17)   Order: repaglinide 1.5 mg t.i.d. with meals

Convert: Order and supply in same unit. No conversion needed.

Think: Look at all the supplied dosages in the drawer. Both 0.5 mg and 1 mg unscored tablets are supplied. Using only 1 mg tablets would require splitting an unscored tablet, which is wrong. Using a combination of dosages will allow administering whole tablets. Use combination of supplied dosages.

Calculate:

1 mg + 0.5 mg = 1.5 mg (verifies estimate)

18) Order: hydrochlorothiazide 12.5 mg p.o. t.i.d

Convert: Order and supply in same unit. No conversion needed.

Think: 25 mg scored tablets are supplied. Will need a partial dose of 1 tablet.

Calculate:

$$\frac{D}{H} \times Q = \frac{\overset{1}{\cancel{12.5 \text{ mg}}}}{\underset{2}{\cancel{25 \text{ mg}}}} \times 1 \text{ tablet} = \frac{1}{2} \text{ tablet (verifies estimate)}$$

Discard the leftover $\frac{1}{2}$ tablet in designated container.

19) Order: Klor-Con 16 mEq p.o. daily

Convert: Order and supply in same unit, and mEq should not be converted. No conversion needed.

Think: 8 mEq tablets are supplied. Will need more than 1 tablet, or exactly 2 tablets.

Calculate:

$$\frac{D}{H} \times Q = \frac{\overset{2}{\cancel{16 \text{ mEq}}}}{\underset{1}{\cancel{8 \text{ mEq}}}} \times 1 \text{ tablet} = 2 \text{ tablets (verifies estimate)}$$

20) Order: Trandate 150 mg p.o. b.i.d.

Convert: Order and supply in same unit. No conversion needed.

Think: 300 mg scored tablets are supplied. Will need a partial dose of 1 tablet.

Calculate:

$$\frac{D}{H} \times Q = \frac{\overset{1}{\cancel{150 \text{ mg}}}}{\underset{2}{\cancel{300 \text{ mg}}}} \times 1 \text{ tablet} = \frac{1}{2} \text{ tablet (verifies estimate)}$$

21) Order: ibuprofen 800 mg p.o. t.i.d

Convert: Order and supply in same unit. No conversion needed.

Think: 400 mg tablets are supplied. Will need more than 1 tablet, or exactly 2 tablets.

Calculate:

$$\frac{D}{H} \times Q = \frac{\overset{2}{\cancel{800 \text{ mg}}}}{\underset{1}{\cancel{400 \text{ mg}}}} \times 1 \text{ tablet} = 2 \text{ tablets (verifies estimate)}$$

22) Order: cefadroxil monohydrate 1 g p.o. b.i.d.

Convert: Order expressed in grams and supply is in mg. Conversion needed.

1 g = 1,000 mg (known equivalent)

Think: 500 mg capsules are supplied. Will need more than 1 capsule, or exactly 2 capsules.

Calculate:

$$\frac{D}{H} \times Q = \frac{\overset{2}{\cancel{1,000 \text{ mg}}}}{\underset{1}{\cancel{500 \text{ mg}}}} \times 1 \text{ capsule} = 2 \text{ capsules (verifies estimate)}$$

23) Order: oxycodone 5 mg/acetaminophen 325 mg 1 to 2 tablets p.o. q.6h p.r.n., moderate to moderately severe pain

Once the correct supplied dose is identified, no calculation is required. Patient rates pain as moderately severe on scale. Offer patient 2 tablets.

Maximum daily dose of acetaminophen = 4,000 mg

Dose of acetaminophen per tablet = 325 mg

325 mg/$\cancel{\text{tab}}$ × 2 $\cancel{\text{tab}}$/dose = 650 mg/dose

650 mg/$\cancel{\text{dose}}$ × 4 $\cancel{\text{doses}}$/day = 2,600 mg/day

2,600 mg does not exceed maximum daily dose of 4,000 mg

Review Set 23 from pages 233–241

1) 7.5 **2)** 20 **3)** 2.5 **4)** 1 **5)** 20 **6)** 2 **7)** 7.5 **8)** 3 **9)** 10 **10)** 15 **11)** 7.5 **12)** 5 **13)** 1 **14)** $1\frac{1}{2}$ **15)** 1

Note: For questions 16 through 30 the *2011 Delmar Nurse's Drug Handbook* was used as reference. Answers may vary slightly if another resource was used.

16) a) broad-spectrum anti-infective, treats variety of infections; b) 250 mg and 500 mg capsules; 125 mg, 187 mg, 250 mg, and 375 mg chewable tablets; 250 mg, 375 mg, and 500 mg extended-release tablets; and 125 mg/5 mL, 187 mg/5 mL, 250 mg/5 mL, and 375 mg/5 mL strawberry-flavored oral suspension; c) No. Capsules are only in 250 mg and 500 mg doses; d) 250 mg q.8h, may double for severe infections; e) E; f) 4

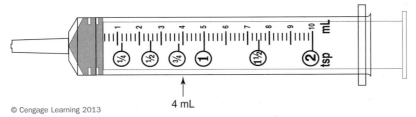

4 mL

© Cengage Learning 2013

17) a) seizures; b) 250 mg capsules, 250 mg/5 mL syrup, 100 mg concentrate; c) No; d) 10 to 15 mg/kg/day up to maximum of 60 mg/kg/day; e) B; f) 3

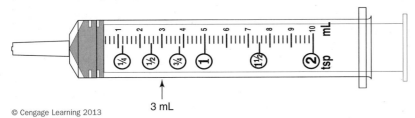

3 mL

© Cengage Learning 2013

18) a) broad-spectrum anti-infective, treats variety of infections; 250 mg and 500 mg capsules; 500 mg and 875 mg tablets; 125 mg, 200 mg, 250 mg, and 400 mg chewable tablets; 775 mg extended-release tablets; 200 mg, 400 mg, and 600 mg tablets for oral suspension; 50 mg/mL, 125 mg/5 mL, 200 mg/5 mL, and 250 mg/5 mL powder for oral suspension; c) Yes; d) 250 mg to 875 mg q.8h to q.12h; e) F; f) 10

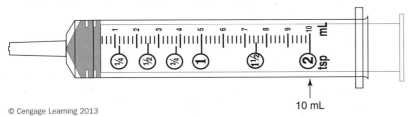

10 mL

© Cengage Learning 2013

19) a) prevention and treatment of bronchospasm; b) 2 mg and 4 mg tablets, 4 mg and 8 mg extended-release tablets, 2 mg/5 mL syrup; c) No; d) 2 mg to 4 mg 3 to 4 times a day, maximum 8 mg 4 times a day; e) C; f) 12.5

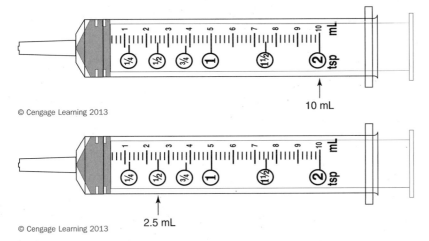

10 mL

© Cengage Learning 2013

2.5 mL

© Cengage Learning 2013

20)   a) sedation, anxiety, pruritus; b) 10 mg, 25 mg, and 50 mg tablets, 25 mg, 50 mg, and 100 mg capsules, 10 mg/5 mL and 25 mg/5 mL syrup; c) No; d) 50 mg to 100 mg as premedication; e) child; This order for 15 mg is below the recommended adult dosage listed in d. f) D; g) 3

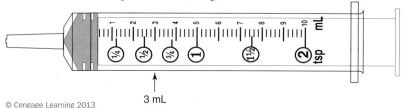

3 mL

© Cengage Learning 2013

21)   a) see question 16; b) see question 16; c) No; d) See question 16; e) child; f) A; g) 4

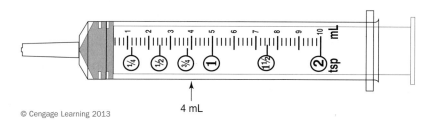

4 mL

© Cengage Learning 2013

22) a) 10 mL; b) Yes **23)** a) 8 mL; b) Yes **24)** a) 4 mL; b) Yes **25)** a) 7.5 mL; b) No **26)** a) 5 mL; b) Yes

27) a) 10 mL; b) Yes **28)** a) 5 mL; b) Yes **29)** a) 1.5 mL; b) Yes **30)** a) 0.8 mL; b) No

Solutions—Review Set 23

16)   Order: cefaclor 300 mg p.o. q.8h

Convert: Order and supply in same unit. No conversion needed.

Think: Look at all the supplied bottles in refrigerator. There are 2 bottles of cefaclor. The bottle with 375 mg/5 mL is labeled for Patient #1. 300 mg is a little less than 375 mg, so the amount needed should be a little less than 5 mL. Calculate:

$$\frac{D}{H} \times Q = \frac{\overset{4}{\cancel{300 \text{ mg}}}}{\underset{5}{\cancel{375 \text{ mg}}}} \times 5 \text{ mL} = \frac{20}{5} \text{ mL} = 4 \text{ mL (verifies estimate)}$$

17)   Order: valproic acid 150 mg p.o. b.i.d.

Convert: Order and supply in same unit. No conversion needed.

Think: Valproic acid is supplied as 250 mL per 5 mL. 150 mg is a little more than one-half 250 mg, so the amount needed should be a little more than 2.5 mL (a little more than $\frac{1}{2} \times 5$ mL).

$$\frac{D}{H} \times Q = \frac{150 \text{ mg}}{\underset{50}{\cancel{250 \text{ mg}}}} \times \overset{1}{\cancel{5}} \text{ mL} = \frac{150}{50} \text{ mL} = 3 \text{ mL (verifies estimate)}$$

18)   Order: amoxicillin 500 mg p.o. q.12h

Convert: Order and supply in same unit. No conversion needed.

Think: Amoxicillin is supplied in 250 mg/5 mL. 500 mg is twice as much as 250 mg, so the amount needed will be 10 mL (2×5 mL).

Calculate:

$$\frac{D}{H} \times Q = \frac{\overset{2}{\cancel{500 \text{ mg}}}}{\underset{1}{\cancel{250 \text{ mg}}}} \times 5 \text{ mL} = 10 \text{ mL (verifies estimate)}$$

19)   Order: albuterol sulfate 5 mg p.o. t.i.d.

Convert: Order and supply in same unit. No conversion needed.

Think: Albuterol is supplied as 2 mg/5 mL. 5 mg is a little more than twice as large as 2 mg. Will need a little more than 10 mL (a little more than 2×5 mL).

Calculate:

$$\frac{D}{H} \times Q = \frac{5 \text{ mg}}{2 \text{ mg}} \times 5 \text{ mL} = \frac{25}{2} \text{ mL} = 12.5 \text{ mL (verifies estimate)}$$

20)   Order: Vistaril 15 mg p.o. on call radiology

Convert: Order and supply in same unit. No conversion needed.

Think: Vistaril is supplied in 25 mg/5 mL. 15 mg is a little more than one-half 25 mg, so the amount needed should be a little more than 2.5 mL (a little more than $\frac{1}{2} \times 5$ mL).

Calculate:

$$\frac{D}{H} \times Q = \frac{15 \text{ mg}}{\underset{5}{25 \text{ mg}}} \times \overset{1}{5} \text{ mL} = \frac{15}{5} \text{ mL} = 3 \text{ mL (verifies estimate)}$$

21)   Order: cefaclor 100 mg p.o. q.8h

Convert: Order and supply in same unit. No conversion needed.

Think: Look at all the supplied bottles in refrigerator. There are 2 bottles of cefaclor. The bottle with 125 mg/5 mL is labeled for Patient #3. 100 mg is a little less than 125 mg, so the amount needed should be a little less than 5 mL.

Calculate:

$$\frac{D}{H} \times Q = \frac{100 \text{ mg}}{\underset{25}{125 \text{ mg}}} \times \overset{1}{5} \text{ mL} = \frac{100}{25} \text{ mL} = 4 \text{ mL (verifies estimate)}$$

22)   Order: metoclopramide 10 mg p.o. 30 min a.c. and at bedtime

Pharmacy-supplied dose: 5 mg/5 mL; syringe filled to 10 mL

Convert: Order and supply in same unit. No conversion needed.

Think: 10 mg is twice as large as 5 mg, so the 10 mL amount supplied (2×5 mL) appears to be correct.

Calculate:

$$\frac{D}{H} \times Q = \frac{\overset{2}{10 \text{ mg}}}{\underset{1}{5 \text{ mg}}} \times 5 \text{ mL} = 10 \text{ mL (verifies pharmacy-supplied dose)}$$

23)   Order: phenytoin 200 mg p.o. t.i.d.

Pharmacy-supplied dose: 125 mg/5 mL; syringe filled to 8 mL

Convert: Order and supply in same unit. No conversion needed.

Think: 200 mg is almost twice as much as 125 mg, so the amount needed should be almost twice as much as 5 mL.

Calculate:

$$\frac{D}{H} \times Q = \frac{200 \text{ mg}}{\underset{25}{125 \text{ mg}}} \times \overset{1}{5} \text{ mL} = \frac{200}{25} \text{ mL} = 8 \text{ mL (verifies pharmacy-supplied dose)}$$

24)   Order: furosemide 40 mg p.o. b.i.d.

Pharmacy-supplied dose: 10 mg/mL; syringe filled to 4 mL

Convert: Order and supply in same unit. No conversion needed.

Think: 40 mg is 4 times as much as 10 mg, so the amount needed is 4 mL (4×1 mL).

Calculate:

$$\frac{D}{H} \times Q = \frac{\overset{4}{40 \text{ mg}}}{\underset{1}{10 \text{ mg}}} \times 1 \text{ mL} = 4 \text{ mL (verifies pharmacy-supplied dose)}$$

25) Order: furosemide 60 mg p.o. daily

Pharmacy-supplied dose: 40 mg/5 mL; syringe filled to 8 mL

Convert: Order and supply in same unit. No conversion needed.

Think: 60 mg is $1\frac{1}{2}$ times 40 mg, so the amount needed should be 7.5 mL (1.5 × 5 mL). Appears pharmacy supplied too large of a dose.

Calculate:

$$\frac{D}{H} \times Q = \frac{\overset{3}{\cancel{60 \text{ mg}}}}{\underset{2}{\cancel{40 \text{ mg}}}} \times 5 \text{ mL} = \frac{15}{2} \text{ mL} = 7.5 \text{ mL (verifies pharmacy-supplied dose is too large)}$$

Notify pharmacy. Complete medication variance.

26) Order: ranitidine 75 mg p.o. b.i.d.

Pharmacy-supplied dose: 15 mg/mL; syringe filled to 5 mL

Convert: Order and supply in same unit. No conversion needed.

Think: 75 mg is 5 times more than 15 mg, so the amount needed should be 5 mL (5 × 1 mL).

Calculate:

$$\frac{D}{H} \times Q = \frac{\overset{5}{\cancel{75 \text{ mg}}}}{\underset{1}{\cancel{15 \text{ mg}}}} \times 1 \text{ mL} = 5 \text{ mL (verifies pharmacy-supplied dose)}$$

27) Order: promethazine 12.5 mg p.o. a.c. and at bedtime

Pharmacy-supplied dose: 6.25 mg/5 mL; syringe filled to 10 mL

Convert: Order and supply in same unit. No conversion needed.

Think: 12.5 mg is twice as large as 6.25 mg, so the amount should be 10 mL (2 × 5 mL).

Calculate:

$$\frac{D}{H} \times Q = \frac{12.5 \text{ mg}}{6.25 \text{ mg}} \times 5 \text{ mL} = \frac{62.5}{6.25} \text{ mL} = 10 \text{ mL (verifies pharmacy-supplied dose)}$$

28) Order: digoxin 250 mcg p.o. daily

Pharmacy-supplied dose: 0.05 mg/mL; syringe filled to 5 mL

Convert: Order is expressed in mcg, but supply is in mg. Conversion needed. Best to work without zeros.

1 mg = 1,000 mcg (known equivalent)

0.05 mg × 1,000 mcg/mg = 0.050 = 50 mcg

Supply now: 50 mcg/mL

Think: 250 mcg is five times 50 mcg, so the amount needed should be 5 mL (5 × 1 mL).

Calculate:

$$\frac{D}{H} \times Q = \frac{\overset{5}{\cancel{250 \text{ mcg}}}}{\underset{1}{\cancel{50 \text{ mcg}}}} \times 1 \text{ mL} = 5 \text{ mL (verifies pharmacy-supplied dose)}$$

29) Order: acetaminophen 150 mg p.o. q.4h fever greater than 102°F

Pharmacy-supplied dose: 500 mg/5 mL; syringe filled to 1.5 mL

Convert: Order and supply in same unit. No conversion needed.

Think: 150 mg is a little less than half of 500 mg, so the amount needed should be a little less than 2.5 mL (a little less than $\frac{1}{2}$ × 5 mL).

Calculate:

$$\frac{D}{H} \times Q = \frac{150 \text{ mg}}{\underset{100}{\cancel{500 \text{ mg}}}} \times \overset{1}{\cancel{5}} \text{ mL} = \frac{150}{100} \text{ mL} = 1.5 \text{ mL (verifies pharmacy-supplied dose)}$$

30) Order: acetaminophen 80 mg p.o. q.6h times four doses today

Pharmacy-supplied dose: 100 mg/mL; syringe filled to 1 mL

Convert: Order and supply in same unit. No conversion needed.

Think: 80 mg is a little less than 100 mg, so the amount needed should be a little less than 1 mL. Appears pharmacy supplied too large of a dose.

Calculate:

$$\frac{D}{H} \times Q = \frac{80 \text{ mg}}{100 \text{ mg}} \times 1 \text{ mL} = \frac{8}{10} \text{ mL} = 0.8 \text{ mL (verifies pharmacy-supplied dose is too large)}$$

Notify pharmacy. Complete medication variance.

Practice Problems—Chapter 10 from pages 244–253

1) $\frac{1}{2}$ 2) 2 3) $\frac{1}{2}$ 4) 2.5 5) 10 6) 2 7) 8 8) $1\frac{1}{2}$ 9) 500 mg; 2 10) $\frac{1}{2}$ 11) $1\frac{1}{2}$ 12) 1 13) $1\frac{1}{2}$ 14) 2 15) 2 16) 5; $1\frac{1}{2}$ 17) 7.5

18) 2 19) 2 20) 1.5 21) 0.75; 1 22) $\frac{1}{2}$ 23) 2 24) 2 25) 2 26) 2 27) 15 mg and 30 mg; one of each 28) 2.4 29) 2.5

30) 3 31) D; 2 tablets 32) A; 1 capsule 33) C; 1 tablet 34) B; 1 capsule 35) I; 2 tablets 36) G; 2 tablets 37) F; 2 tablets

38) H; 1 tablet 39) M; 2 tablets 40) L; 2 tablets 41) E; 30 mL 42) K; 1 tablet 43) I; 2 tablets 44) N; 2 tablets

45) O; 1 tablet 46) Q; 2 tablets 47) P; 1 capsule 48) J; 1 tablet 49) R; 2 tablets

50)   Prevention: This medication error could have been prevented if the nurse had more carefully read the physician's order and the medication label. The doctor's order misled the nurse by noting the volume first and then the drug dosage. If confused by the order, the nurse should have clarified the intent with the physician. By focusing on the volume, the nurse failed to follow the steps in dosage calculation. Had the nurse noted 250 mg as the desired dosage and the supply (or on-hand) dosage as 125 mg per 5 mL, the correct amount to be administered would have been clear. Slow down and take time to compare the order with the labels. Calculate each dose carefully before preparing and administering both solid- and liquid-form medications.

Solutions—Practice Problems—Chapter 10

1)   Order: tolbutamide 250 mg p.o. t.i.d.

Supply: tolbutamide 0.5 g scored tablets

Convert: Order expressed in grams and supply is in mg. Conversion needed. Convert supply to avoid use of decimals.

1 g = 1,000 mg (known equivalent)

0.5 g × 1,000 mg/g = 0.500. = 500 mg

Think: 500 mg scored tablets are supplied. Will need less than 1 tablet, or exactly $\frac{1}{2}$ tablet.

Calculate: $\frac{D}{H} \times Q = \frac{\overset{1}{\cancel{250} \text{ mg}}}{\underset{2}{\cancel{500} \text{ mg}}} \times 1 \text{ tablet} = \frac{1}{2}$ tablet (verifies estimate)

Discard the leftover $\frac{1}{2}$ tablet in designated container.

9)   Order: acetaminophen 1 g p.o. q.6h p.r.n., pain

Supply: acetaminophen 325 mg unscored and 500 mg unscored tablets

Convert: Order expressed in grams and supply is in mg. Conversion needed. Convert supply to avoid use of decimals.

1 g = 1,000 mg (known equivalent)

Think: Must give whole tablets. 1,000 mg is a multiple of 500 mg but not of 325 mg. Will need more than one 500 mg tablet, or exactly two tablets.

Calculate: $\frac{D}{H} \times Q = \frac{\overset{2}{\cancel{1,000} \text{ mg}}}{\underset{1}{\cancel{500} \text{ mg}}} \times 1 \text{ tablet} = 2$ tablets (verifies estimate)

17) Order: penicillin V potassium 375 mg

Supply: penicillin V potassium 250 mg per 5 mL

Convert: No conversion needed.

Think: 375 mg is more than 250 mg, actually $1\frac{1}{2}$ times larger. Will need more than 5 mL but less than 10 mL.

Calculate:

$$\frac{D}{H} \times Q = \frac{375\ \cancel{mg}}{\underset{50}{\cancel{250\ mg}}} \times \overset{1}{\cancel{5}}\ mL = \frac{375}{50}\ mL = 7.5\ mL\ \text{(verifies estimate)}$$

24) Order: Erythrocin 0.5 g

Supply: Erythrocin 250 mg unscored tablets

Convert: Order expressed in grams and supply is in mg. Conversion needed.

1 g = 1,000 mg (known equivalent)

0.5 g × 1,000 mg/g = 0.500. = 500 mg

Think: Must give whole tablets. Will need more than 1 tablet, or exactly 2 tablets.

Calculate:

$$\frac{D}{H} \times Q = \frac{\overset{2}{\cancel{500\ mg}}}{\underset{1}{\cancel{250\ mg}}} \times 1\ \text{tablet} = 2\ \text{tablets (verifies estimate)}$$

27) Order: phenobarbital 45 mg

Supply: 15 mg scored, 30 mg scored, 60 mg scored tablets

Convert: No conversion needed.

Think: Need more than 30 mg but less than 60 mg. Even though tablets are scored, best to use whole tablets when possible. Using a combination of 15 mg and 30 mg tablets will give the desired 45 mg dose.

Calculate: 15 mg + 30 mg = 45 mg (verifies estimate)

Select: One 15 mg tablet and one 30 mg tablet for 45 mg total dosage.

29) Order: acetaminophen 80 mg

Supply: acetaminophen 160 mg/t

Convert: Equipment chosen is measured in mL and supply volume is in teaspoons. Conversion needed.

1 t = 5 mL (known equivalent)

Supply: acetaminophen 160 mg/5 mL

Think: 80 mg is half of 160 mg. Will need $\frac{1}{2}$ of 5 mL, or exactly 2.5 mL.

Calculate:

$$\frac{D}{H} \times Q = \frac{\overset{1}{\cancel{80\ mg}}}{\underset{2}{\cancel{160\ mg}}} \times 5\ mL = \frac{5}{2}\ mL = 2.5\ mL\ \text{(verifies estimate)}$$

Review Set 24 from 267–276

Note to student: *2011 Delmar Nurse's Drug Handbook* was used as reference. Answers may vary slightly if another resource was used.

1) 0.75 mL

0.75 mL

2) 1 mL

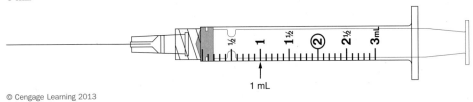

© Cengage Learning 2013

3) 1.7 mL

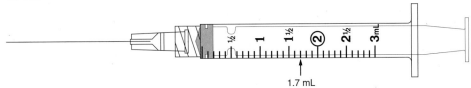

© Cengage Learning 2013

4) 0.63 mL

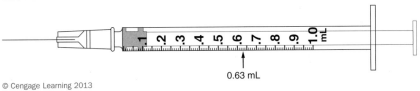

© Cengage Learning 2013

5) 0.2 mL

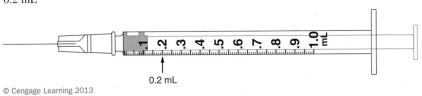

© Cengage Learning 2013

6) 1.7 mL

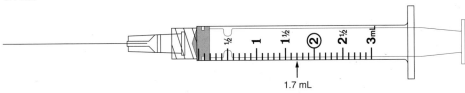

© Cengage Learning 2013

7) a) treatment of megaloblastic anemias due to folic acid deficiency; b) 5,000 mcg/mL; c) deep subcut, IM, IV;
d) 250 to 1,000 mcg/day; e) A; f) 0.2 mL;

g)

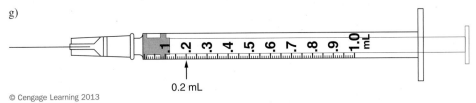

© Cengage Learning 2013

8)   a) secondary amenorrhea, abnormal endometrial bleeding, adjunctive treatment for endometrial or renal cancer, contraceptive; b) 104 mg per 0.65 mL, 150 mg/mL, 400 mg/mL; c) subcut, IM; d) 400 mg to 1,000 mg/week, 150 mg q.3 months, 104 mg q.3 months, e) C; f) 2.5 mL;

g)

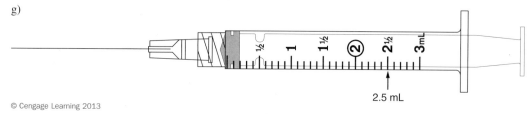

2.5 mL

© Cengage Learning 2013

9)   a) nausea and vomiting postoperatively or due to chemotherapy; b) 2 mg/mL, 32 mg per 50 mL (premixed); c) IM, IV; d) 4 mg IV undiluted over 2 to 5 min, 32 mg single dose over 15 min prior to chemotherapy; e) B; f) 1.5 mL;

g)

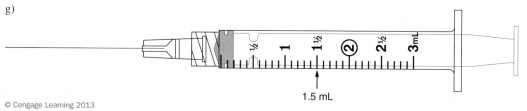

1.5 mL

© Cengage Learning 2013

10)   a) serious infections; b) 10 mg/mL, 40 mg/mL; c) IM, IV; d) 1 mg/kg q.8h up to 5 mg/kg/day for life-threatening infection; e) C; f) 1.8 mL;

g)

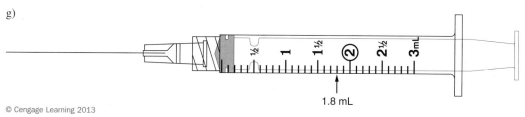

1.8 mL

© Cengage Learning 2013

11)   a) serious infections; b) 150 mg/mL; c) IM, IV; d) 600 to 1,200 mg per day in 2 to 4 divided doses; e) A; f) 4 mL;

g)

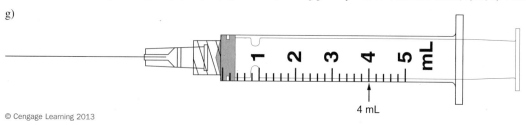

4 mL

© Cengage Learning 2013

12)   a) moderate to severe pain; b) 10 mg/mL, 20 mg/mL; c) subcut, IM, IV; d) 10 mg q.3 to 6h single dose not to exceed 20 mg; e) B; f) 0.25 mL;

g)

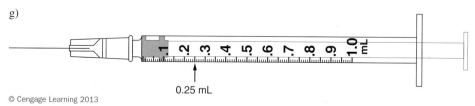

0.25 mL

© Cengage Learning 2013

13) a) prevention and treatment of bronchospasm associated with asthma, bronchitis, and emphysema, preterm labor (investigational); b) 1 mg/mL; c) subcut only; d) 0.25 mg subcut, repeat q.15 to 30 min as needed, do not exceed 0.5 mg in 4 h; e) B; f) 0.25 mL;

g)

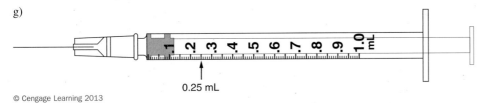

0.25 mL

© Cengage Learning 2013

14) a) treatment of edema associated with CHF, nephrotic syndrome, hepatic disease, and acute pulmonary edema; b) 0.25 mg/mL; c) IM, IV; d) 0.5 mg to 1 mg, may repeat q.3 to 4 h, do not exceed 10 mg/day; e) E; f) 2 mL;

g)

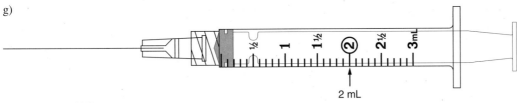

2 mL

© Cengage Learning 2013

15) a) treatment of duodenal and gastric ulcers, hypersecretory conditions, gastroesophageal reflux; b) 1 mg/mL (premixed), 25 mg/mL; c) IM, IV; d) 50 mg q.6 to 8h, dilute 50 mg to a concentration no greater than 2.5 mg/mL; e) D; f) 1.4 mL;

g)

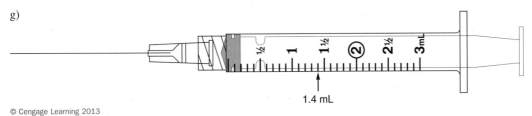

1.4 mL

© Cengage Learning 2013

16) a) treatment of seizures; b) 100 mg/mL; c) IV; d) 10 to 15 mg/kg/day, increase as needed, maximum 60 mg/kg/day; e) A; f) 4.2 mL;

g)

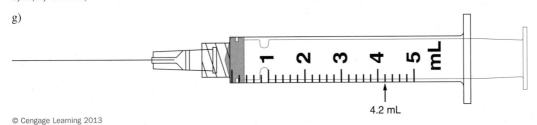

4.2 mL

© Cengage Learning 2013

17) a) oral – hypertension, angina pectoris, and migraine headaches, IV – life-threatening arrhythmias; b) 1 mg/mL; c) IV; d) 1 to 3 mg not to exceed 1 mg per minute; e) F; f) 2 mL;

g)

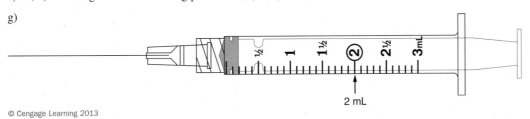

2 mL

© Cengage Learning 2013

18) a) life-threatening ventricular arrhythmias, b) 50 mg/mL, 150 mg per 3 mL, 450 mg per 9 mL, 900 mg per 18 mL;

c) IV; d) initial loading dose 150 mg over 10 minutes then 360 mg over 6 h; e) G; f) 7.2 mL;

g)

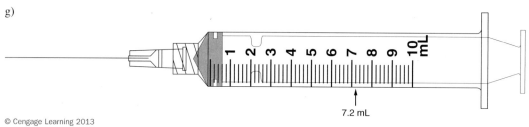

7.2 mL

© Cengage Learning 2013

19) a) short-term prevention and treatment of generalized seizures and status epilepticus; b) 50 mg/mL, 75 mg/mL;

c) IM, IV; d) maintenance 4 to 6 mg/kg/day; e) H; f) 5.6 mL;

g)

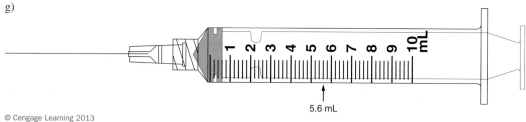

5.6 mL

© Cengage Learning 2013

20) a) oral – angina and hypertension, IV – atrial arrhythmias and supraventricular tachycardia; b) 5 mg/mL; c) IV;

d) 1st IV bolus 0.25 mg/kg over 2 min, 2nd bolus 0.35 mg/kg over 2 min; e) C; f) 3.6 mL;

g)

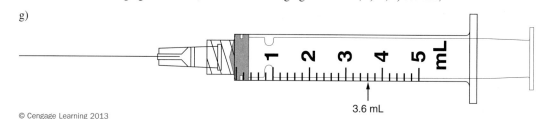

3.6 mL

© Cengage Learning 2013

Solutions Review Set 24

1) Order: Dilaudid 1.5 mg IM q.6h p.r.n., severe pain

Supply: 2 mg/mL

Convert: Order and supply in same unit. No conversion needed.

Think: 1.5 mg is less than 2 mg but not less than half.

Amount needed will be less than 1 mL but more than $\frac{1}{2}$ of a mL.

Calculate: $\frac{D}{H} \times Q = \frac{1.5 \text{ mg}}{2 \text{ mg}} \times 1 \text{ mL} = \frac{1.5}{2} \text{ mL}$

$= 0.75 \text{ mL (verifies estimate)}$

2) Order: digoxin 0.25 mg IV daily

Supply: 500 mcg/2 mL

Convert: Order expressed in mg, and supply is in mcg. Conversion needed.

1 mg = 1,000 mcg (known equivalent)

$0.25 \text{ mg} \times 1,000 \text{ mcg/mg} = 0.250. = 250 \text{ mcg}$

Order now: 250 mcg

Think: 250 mcg is less than 500 mcg, or exactly half.

Amount needed will be $\frac{1}{2}$ of 2 mL or 1 mL.

Calculate: $\frac{D}{H} \times Q = \frac{\overset{1}{250 \text{ mcg}}}{\underset{2}{500 \text{ mcg}}} \times 2 \text{ mL} = \frac{2}{2} \text{ mL}$

$= 1 \text{ mL (verifies estimate)}$

3)   Order: ketorolac 25 mg IM q.6h p.r.n., severe pain

Supply: 15 mg/mL

Convert: Order and supply in same unit. No conversion needed.

Think: 25 mg is more than 15 mg but not twice as much. Amount needed will be more than 1 mL but less than 2 mL.

Calculate: $\frac{D}{H} \times Q = \frac{\overset{5}{\cancel{25}\ \cancel{mg}}}{\underset{3}{\cancel{15}\ \cancel{mg}}} \times 1\ mL = \frac{5}{3}\ mL$

$= 1.66\ mL = 1.7\ mL$ (verifies estimate)

4)   Order: Robinul 125 mcg, IM stat

Supply: 0.2 mg/mL

Convert: Order expressed in mcg, and supply is in mg. Conversion needed.

1 mg = 1,000 mcg (known equivalent)

$0.2\ \cancel{mg} \times 1,000\ mcg/\cancel{mg} = 0.200. = 200\ mcg$

Supply now: 200 mcg/mL

Think: 125 mcg is less than 200 mcg, but not less than $\frac{1}{2}$. Amount needed will be less than 1 mL but more than $\frac{1}{2}$ of a mL.

Calculate: $\frac{D}{H} \times Q = \frac{\overset{5}{\cancel{125}\ \cancel{mcg}}}{\underset{8}{\cancel{200}\ \cancel{mcg}}} \times 1\ mL = \frac{5}{8}\ mL$

$= 0.625\ mL = 0.63\ mL$ (verifies estimate)

5)   Order: diphenhydramine 10 mg IM q.6h p.r.n., itching

Supply: 50 mg/mL

Convert: Order and supply in same unit. No conversion needed.

Think: 10 mg is quite a bit smaller than 50 mg. Amount needed will be quite a bit less than 1 mL.

Calculate: $\frac{D}{H} \times Q = \frac{\overset{1}{\cancel{10}\ \cancel{mg}}}{\underset{5}{\cancel{50}\ \cancel{mg}}} \times 1\ mL = \frac{1}{5}\ mL$

$= 0.2\ mL$ (verifies estimate)

6)   Order: Ativan 3.4 mg IM × 1 dose pre-op

Supply: 2 mg/mL

Convert: Order and supply in same unit. No conversion needed.

Think: 3.4 mg is more than 2 mg but not twice as much. Amount needed will be more than 1 mL but less than 2 mL.

Calculate: $\frac{D}{H} \times Q = \frac{3.4\ \cancel{mg}}{2\ \cancel{mg}} \times 1\ mL = \frac{3.4}{2}\ mL$

$= 1.7\ mL$ (verifies estimate)

7)   Order: folic acid 1,000 mcg IM daily for 10 days

Supply: 5 mg/mL

Convert: Order expressed in mcg, and supply is in mg. Conversion needed.

1 mg = 1,000 mcg (known equivalent)

$5\ \cancel{mg} \times 1,000\ mcg/\cancel{mg} = 5.000. = 5,000\ mcg$

Supply now: 5,000 mcg/mL

Think: 1,000 mcg is quite a bit smaller than 5,000 mg. Amount needed will be quite a bit less than 1 mL.

Calculate: $\frac{D}{H} \times Q = \frac{\overset{1}{\cancel{1,000}\ \cancel{mcg}}}{\underset{5}{\cancel{5,000}\ \cancel{mcg}}} \times 1\ mL = \frac{1}{5}\ mL$

$= 0.2\ mL$ (verifies estimate)

8)   Order: medroxyprogesterone acetate 1 g IM now

Supply: 400 mg/mL

Convert: 1 g = 1,000 mg (known equivalent)

Order now: 1,000 mg

Think: 1,000 mg is more than twice as large as 400 mg but less than 3 times. Amount needed will be more than 2 mL but less than 3 mL.

Calculate: $\frac{D}{H} \times Q = \frac{\overset{5}{\cancel{1,000}\ \cancel{mg}}}{\underset{2}{\cancel{400}\ \cancel{mg}}} \times 1\ mL = \frac{5}{2}\ mL$

$= 2.5\ mL$ (verifies estimate)

9)   Order: ondansetron 3 mg slow IV push × 1 dose stat

Supply: 2 mg/mL

Convert: Order and supply in same unit. No conversion needed.

Think: 3 mg is $1\frac{1}{2}$ times 2 mg. Amount needed will be $1\frac{1}{2}$ mL.

Calculate: $\frac{D}{H} \times Q = \frac{3\ \cancel{mg}}{2\ \cancel{mg}} \times 1\ mL = \frac{3}{2}\ mL$

$= 1.5\ mL$ (verifies estimate)

10)   Order: gentamicin 70 mg IV PB q.8h

Supply: 80 mg/2 mL

Convert: Order and supply in same unit. No conversion needed.

Think: 70 mg is slightly less than 80 mg. Amount needed will be slightly less than 2 mL.

Calculate: $\frac{D}{H} \times Q = \frac{\overset{7}{\cancel{70}\ \cancel{mg}}}{\underset{8}{\cancel{80}\ \cancel{mg}}} \times 2\ mL = \frac{14}{8}\ mL$

$= 1.75\ mL = 1.8\ mL$ (verifies estimate)

11) Order: clindamycin 0.6 g IV PB q.12h

Supply: 150 mg/mL

Convert: Order expressed in g, and supply is in mg. Conversion needed.

1 g = 1,000 mg (known equivalent)

0.6 g × 1,000 mg/g = 0.600. = 600 mg

Order now: 600 mg

Think: 600 mg is 4 times as much as 150 mg. Amount needed will be 4 times 1 mL, or exactly 4 mL.

Calculate: $\dfrac{D}{H} \times Q = \dfrac{\overset{4}{600 \text{ mg}}}{\underset{1}{150 \text{ mg}}} \times 1 \text{ mL} = 4 \text{ mL}$

(verifies estimate)

12) Order: nalbuphine HCl 5 mg subcut q.4h p.r.n., pain

Supply: 20 mg/mL

Convert: Order and supply in same unit. No conversion needed.

Think: 5 mg is $\frac{1}{4}$ of 20 mg. Amount needed will be $\frac{1}{4}$ of a mL.

Calculate: $\dfrac{D}{H} \times Q = \dfrac{\overset{1}{5 \text{ mg}}}{\underset{4}{20 \text{ mg}}} \times 1 \text{ mL} = \dfrac{1}{4} \text{ mL}$

= 0.25 mL (verifies estimate)

13) Order: terbutaline 250 mcg

Supply: terbutatline 1 mg/mL

Convert: Order expressed in mcg, and supply is in mg. Conversion needed.

1 mg = 1,000 mcg (known equivalent)

Supply now: 1,000 mcg/mL

Think: 250 mcg is $\frac{1}{4}$ of 1,000 mcg. Amount needed will be $\frac{1}{4}$ of a mL.

Calculate: $\dfrac{D}{H} \times Q = \dfrac{\overset{1}{250 \text{ mcg}}}{\underset{4}{1,000 \text{ mcg}}} \times 1 \text{ mL} = \dfrac{1}{4} \text{ mL}$

= 0.25 mL (verifies estimate)

14) Order: bumetanide 500 mcg

Supply: 0.25 mg/mL

Convert: Order expressed in mcg, and supply is in mg. Conversion needed.

1 mg = 1,000 mcg (known equivalent)

0.25 mg × 1,000 mcg//mg = 0.250. = 250 mcg

Supply now: 250 mcg/mL

Think: 500 mcg is twice as much as 250 mcg. Amount needed will be 2 times 1 mL, or exactly 2 mL.

Calculate: $\dfrac{D}{H} \times Q = \dfrac{\overset{2}{500 \text{ mcg}}}{\underset{1}{250 \text{ mcg}}} \times 1 \text{ mL} = 2 \text{ mL}$

(verifies estimate)

15) Order: ranitidine 35 mg IV q.6h

Supply: 25 mg/mL

Convert: Order and supply in same unit. No conversion needed.

Think: 35 mg is more than 25 mg but not twice as much. Amount needed will be more than 1 mL but less than 2 mL.

Calculate: $\dfrac{D}{H} \times Q = \dfrac{\overset{7}{35 \text{ mg}}}{\underset{5}{25 \text{ mg}}} \times 1 \text{ mL} = \dfrac{7}{5} \text{ mL}$

= 1.4 mL (verifies estimate)

16) Order: valproate sodium 420 mg

Supply: 500 mg/5 mL

Convert: Order and supply in same unit. No conversion needed.

Think: 420 mg is slightly less than 500 mg. Amount needed will be slightly less than 5 mL.

Calculate: $\dfrac{D}{H} \times Q = \dfrac{420 \text{ mg}}{500 \text{ mg}} \times 5 \text{ mL} = \dfrac{\overset{21}{2,100}}{\underset{5}{500}} \text{ mL}$

= $\dfrac{21}{5}$ mL = 4.2 mL (verifies estimate)

17) Order: propranolol 2 mg IV slow push stat

Supply: 1 mg/mL

Convert: Order and supply in same unit. No conversion needed.

Think: 2 mg is twice as much as 1 mg. Amount needed will be 2 times 1 mL, or exactly 2 mL.

Calculate: $\dfrac{D}{H} \times Q = \dfrac{2 \text{ mg}}{1 \text{ mg}} \times 1 \text{ mL} = 2 \text{ mL}$

(verifies estimate)

18) Order: amiodarone 360 mg IV PB (over 6 h at 1 mg/min)

Supply: 50 mg/mL

Convert: Order and supply in same unit. No conversion needed.

Think: 360 mg is more than 7 times 50 mg. Needed amount will be more than 7 times 1 mL, or more than 7 mL.

Calculate: $\dfrac{D}{H} \times Q = \dfrac{\overset{36}{360 \text{ mg}}}{\underset{5}{50 \text{ mg}}} \times 1 \text{ mL} = \dfrac{36}{5} \text{ mL}$

= 7.2 mL (verifies estimate)

19) Order: fosphenytoin 280 mg IV daily until tolerating PO fluids

Supply: 50 mg/mL

Convert: Order and supply in same unit. No conversion needed.

Think: 280 mg is more than 5 times 50 mg. Needed amount will be more than 5 times 1 mL, or more than 5 mL.

Calculate: $\frac{D}{H} \times Q = \frac{\overset{28}{\cancel{280}} \text{ mg}}{\underset{5}{\cancel{50}} \text{ mg}} \times 1 \text{ mL} = \frac{28}{5} \text{ mL}$

= 5.6 mL (verifies estimate)

20) Order: diltiazem 18 mg IV bolus stat

Supply: 5 mg/mL in 10 mL vial

Convert: Order and supply in same unit. No conversion needed.

Think: 18 mg is more than 3 times 5 mg, and closer to but less than 4 times 5 mg. Needed amount will be more than 3 times 1 mL (or more than 3 mL), but less than 4 times 1 mL (or less than 4 mL).

Calculate: $\frac{D}{H} \times Q = \frac{18 \cancel{\text{mg}}}{5 \cancel{\text{mg}}} \times 1 \text{ mL} = \frac{18}{5} \text{ mL}$

= 3.6 mL (verifies estimate)

Review Set 25 from pages 303–310

1) A **2)** C **3)** D **4)** B, D **5)** Humulin R, regular, short-acting, 100 units/mL, U-100 insulin syringe **6)** Novolin N, NPH, intermediate-acting, 100 units/mL, U-100 insulin syringe **7)** NovoLog, aspart, rapid-acting, 100 units/mL, U-100 insulin syringe **8)** Humalog, lispro, rapid-acting, 100 units/mL, U-100 insulin syringe **9)** Humulin R, regular, short-acting, 500 units/mL, 1 mL syringe **10)** Lantus, glargine, long-acting, 100 units/mL, U-100 insulin syringe **11)** standard, dual-scale 100 unit/mL U-100 syringe; Lo-Dose, 50 unit/0.5 mL U-100 syringe; Lo-Dose, 30 unit/0.3 mL U-100 syringe **12)** Lo-Dose, 50-unit U-100 syringe **13)** 0.6 **14)** 0.25 **15)** False **16)** 20 **17)** 30,000 **18)** 6,400 **19)** No; order is for 67 units and syringe amount is 68 units **20)** No; order is for Humulin R regular U-100 insulin and drug supplied is Humulin R regular U-500 insulin **21)** No; order is for 23 units of Novolog 70/30 U-100 insulin and drug supplied is 23 units of Novolog U-100 insulin **22)** Yes

23)

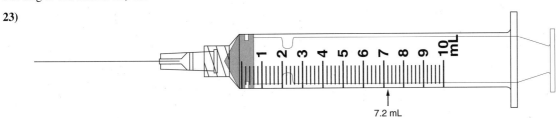

7.2 mL

© Cengage Learning 2013

24)

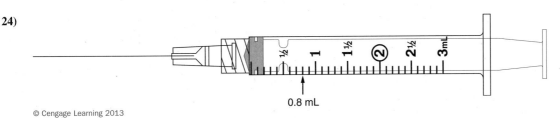

0.8 mL

© Cengage Learning 2013

25)

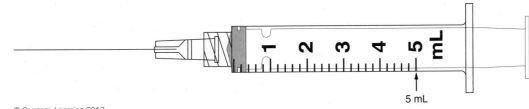

5 mL

© Cengage Learning 2013

26)

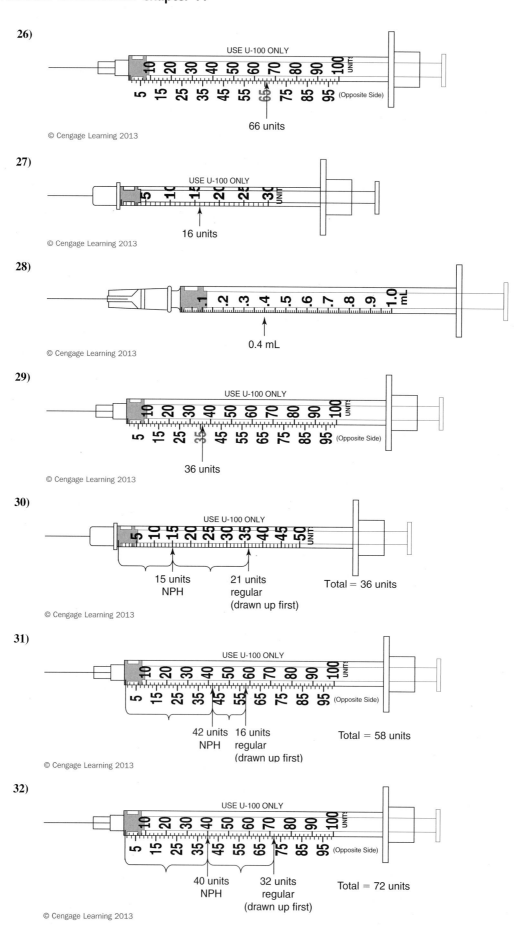

USE U-100 ONLY

(Opposite Side)

66 units

© Cengage Learning 2013

27)

USE U-100 ONLY

16 units

© Cengage Learning 2013

28)

0.4 mL

© Cengage Learning 2013

29)

USE U-100 ONLY

(Opposite Side)

36 units

© Cengage Learning 2013

30)

USE U-100 ONLY

15 units
NPH

21 units
regular
(drawn up first)

Total = 36 units

© Cengage Learning 2013

31)

USE U-100 ONLY

(Opposite Side)

42 units
NPH

16 units
regular
(drawn up first)

Total = 58 units

© Cengage Learning 2013

32)

USE U-100 ONLY

(Opposite Side)

40 units
NPH

32 units
regular
(drawn up first)

Total = 72 units

© Cengage Learning 2013

33)

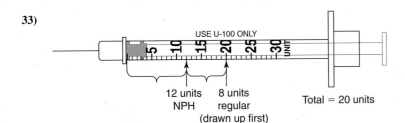

USE U-100 ONLY

12 units   8 units
NPH   regular
(drawn up first)   Total = 20 units

© Cengage Learning 2013

34) 5

35) 39

36) Before meals (before insulin administration).

37) Blood glucose levels of 160–400.

38) Administer 4 units of Humulin R regular U-100 insulin.

39) None; do not administer insulin.

40) Contact the physician immediately for further instructions.

Solutions—Review Set 25

13) Recall that U-100 = 100 units per mL

$$\frac{D}{H} \times Q = \frac{\overset{6}{\cancel{60 \text{ units}}}}{\underset{10}{\cancel{100 \text{ units}}}} \times 1 \text{ mL} = \frac{6}{10} \text{ mL} = 0.6 \text{ mL}$$

14) Recall that U-500 = 500 units/mL

$$\frac{D}{H} \times Q = \frac{\overset{1}{\cancel{125 \text{ units}}}}{\underset{4}{\cancel{500 \text{ units}}}} \times 1 \text{ mL} = \frac{1}{4} \text{ mL} = 0.25 \text{ mL}$$

Measure 0.25 mL of U-500 insulin in a 1 mL syringe to administer 125 units.

16) $\frac{D}{H} \times Q = \frac{D \text{ units}}{10 \text{ units}} \times 1 \text{ mL} = 2 \text{ mL}$

Apply ratio-proportion:

$$\frac{D}{10} \overset{2}{\underset{1}{\times}}$$

$$D = 20 \text{ units}$$

17) $\frac{D}{H} \times Q = \frac{D \text{ units}}{10,000 \text{ units}} \times 1 \text{ mL} = 3 \text{ mL}$

$$\frac{D}{10,000} \overset{3}{\underset{1}{\times}}$$

$$D = 30,000 \text{ units}$$

28) Recall that U-500 = 500 units/mL

$$\frac{D}{H} \times Q = \frac{\overset{2}{\cancel{200 \text{ units}}}}{\underset{5}{\cancel{500 \text{ units}}}} \times 1 \text{ mL} = \frac{2}{5} \text{ mL} = 0.4 \text{ mL}$$

Measure 0.4 mL of U-500 insulin in a 1 mL syringe to administer 200 units.

29) U-500 insulin is five times more concentrated than U-100 insulin. To use U-100 syringe for the more concentrated U-500 insulin, you should divide the units ordered by 5.

$\frac{180 \text{ units}}{5} = 36$ units (of U-500 insulin measured in a U-100 insulin syringe).

You can also use ratio-proportion:

$$\frac{180 \text{ units}}{500 \text{ units}} \underset{}{\times} \frac{X \text{ units}}{100 \text{ units}}$$

$$500X = 18,000$$

$$\frac{500X}{500} = \frac{18,000}{500}$$

$$X = 36 \text{ units (of U-500 insulin measured in a U-100 insulin syringe)}$$

Teach your patient to draw up 36 units of U-500 insulin in a U-100 syringe to provide 180 units of U-500 insulin.

Practice Problems—Chapter 11 from pages 312–320

1) 0.4; 1 mL **2)** 1.5; 3 mL **3)** 2.4; 3 mL **4)** 0.6; 1 mL or 3 mL **5)** 2; 3 mL **6)** 10; 10 mL **7)** 0.8; 1 mL or 3 mL

8) 1; 3 mL **9)** 1; 3 mL **10)** 5.6; 10 mL **11)** 1.5; 3 mL **12)** 0.6; 1 mL or 3 mL **13)** 0.6; 1 mL or 3 mL **14)** 1.9; 3 mL

15) 0.6; 1 mL or 3 mL **16)** 0.75; 1 mL **17)** 0.67; 1 mL **18)** 1; 3 mL **19)** 0.3; 1 mL **20)** 1.6; 3 mL **21)** 0.75; 1 mL; The route is IM; the needle may need to be changed to an appropriate gauge and length. **22)** 0.5; 1 mL or 3 mL

23) 0.7; 1 mL or 3 mL **24)** 0.8; 1 mL or 3 mL **25)** 1.3; 3 mL **26)** 1.6; 3 mL **27)** 6; 10 mL **28)** 0.8; 1 mL or 3 mL

29) 1.5; 3 mL **30)** 1.6; 3 mL **31)** 0.7; 1 mL or 3 mL **32)** 0.5; 1 mL or 3 mL **33)** 10; 10 mL **34)** 16; 30-unit Lo-Dose U-100 insulin **35)** 25; 50-unit Lo-Dose U-100 insulin **36)** 5.8; 10 mL

37) 1.5; F

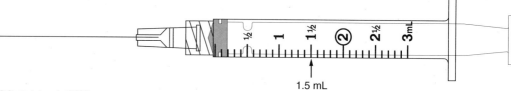

© Cengage Learning 2013

↑
1.5 mL

38) 1.3; B

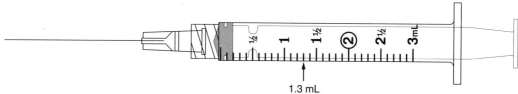

© Cengage Learning 2013

↑
1.3 mL

39) 0.4; H

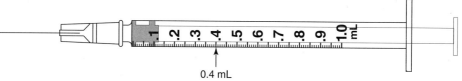

© Cengage Learning 2013

↑
0.4 mL

40) 1.5; A

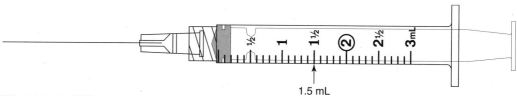

© Cengage Learning 2013

↑
1.5 mL

41) 0.5; J

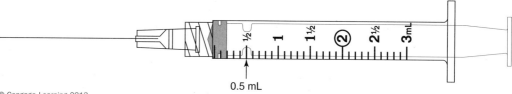

© Cengage Learning 2013

↑
0.5 mL

42) 22; I

USE U-100 ONLY

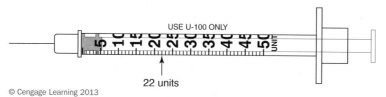

↑
22 units

© Cengage Learning 2013

43) 0.8; C

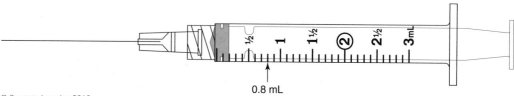

↑
0.8 mL

© Cengage Learning 2013

44) 0.6; G

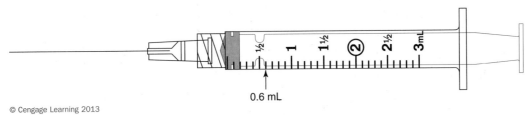

0.6 mL

© Cengage Learning 2013

45) 5; L

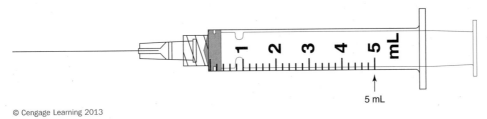

5 mL

© Cengage Learning 2013

46) 0.5; K

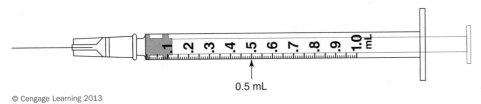

0.5 mL

© Cengage Learning 2013

47) 86; D and M

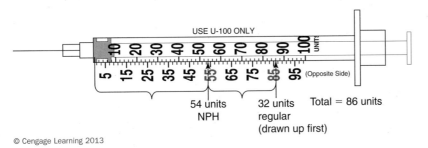

USE U-100 ONLY

54 units
NPH

32 units
regular
(drawn up first)

Total = 86 units

(Opposite Side)

© Cengage Learning 2013

48) 46; E

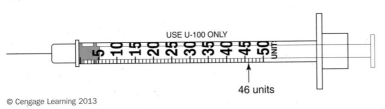

USE U-100 ONLY

46 units

© Cengage Learning 2013

49) **Prevention:** This error could have been avoided had the nurse been more careful checking the label of the insulin vial and comparing the label to the order. The nurse should have checked the label three times. In addition, the nurse should have asked another nurse to perform an independent verification after each insulin was drawn up, as required. Such hospital policies and procedures are written to protect the patient and the nurse.

50) **Prevention:** This insulin error should never occur. It is obvious that the nurse did not use Step 2 of the Three-Step Approach. The nurse did not stop to think of the reasonable dosage. If so, the nurse would have realized that the supply dosage of U-100 insulin is 100 units/mL, not 10 units/mL.

If you are unsure of what you are doing, you need to ask before you act. Insulin should only be given in an insulin syringe. The likelihood of the nurse needing to give insulin in a tuberculin syringe because an insulin syringe is unavailable is almost nonexistent today. The nurse chose the incorrect syringe. Whenever you are in doubt, you should ask for help. Further, if the nurse had asked another nurse to perform an independent verification as required, the error could have been found before the patient received the wrong dosage of insulin. After giving the insulin, it is too late to rectify the error.

Solutions—Practice Problems—Chapter 11

3) Order: 0.6 mg = 0.600. = 600 mcg

Supply: 500 mcg per 2 mL

$$\frac{D}{H} \times Q = \frac{\overset{6}{\cancel{600}} \text{ mcg}}{\underset{5}{\cancel{500}} \text{ mcg}} \times 2 \text{ mL} = \frac{12}{5} \text{ mL} = 2.4 \text{ mL}$$

6) Order: 50 mg

Supply: 5 mg/mL

$$\frac{D}{H} \times Q = \frac{\overset{10}{\cancel{50}} \text{ mg}}{\underset{1}{\cancel{5}} \text{ mg}} \times 1 \text{ mL} = 10 \text{ mL}$$

Note: route is IV, so this large dose is acceptable.

14) Order: 75 mg

Supply: 40 mg/mL

$$\frac{D}{H} \times Q = \frac{\overset{15}{\cancel{75}} \text{ mg}}{\underset{8}{\cancel{40}} \text{ mg}} \times 1 \text{ mL} = \frac{15}{8} \text{ mL}$$

$$= 1.87 \text{ mL} = 1.9 \text{ mL}$$

19) Order: 3 mg

Supply: 10 mg/mL

$$\frac{D}{H} \times Q = \frac{3 \text{ mg}}{10 \text{ mg}} \times 1 \text{ mL} = \frac{3}{10} \text{ mL} = 0.3 \text{ mL}$$

26) Order: 0.4 mg = 0.400. = 400 mcg

Supply: 500 mcg per 2 mL

$$\frac{D}{H} \times Q = \frac{\overset{4}{\cancel{400}} \text{ mcg}}{\underset{5}{\cancel{500}} \text{ mcg}} \times 2 \text{ mL} = \frac{8}{5} \text{ mL} = 1.6 \text{ mL}$$

36) Order: 5,800 units

Supply: 1,000 units/mL

$$\frac{D}{H} \times Q = \frac{\overset{58}{\cancel{5,800}} \text{ units}}{\underset{10}{\cancel{1,000}} \text{ units}} \times 1 \text{ mL} = \frac{58}{10} \text{ mL} = 5.8 \text{ mL}$$

38) Order: 50 mg

Supply: 80 mg/2 mL

$$\frac{D}{H} \times Q = \frac{50 \text{ mg}}{80 \text{ mg}} \times 2 \text{ mL} = \frac{100}{80} \text{ mL} = 1.25 \text{ mL}$$

$$= 1.3 \text{ mL}$$

39) Order: 1 mg

Supply: 2.5 mg/1 mL

$$\frac{D}{H} \times Q = \frac{1 \text{ mg}}{2.5 \text{ mg}} \times 1 \text{ mL} = \frac{1}{2.5} \text{ mL} = 0.4 \text{ mL}$$

41) Order: 0.2 mg

Supply: 0.4 mg/mL

$$\frac{D}{H} \times Q = \frac{\overset{1}{\cancel{0.2}} \text{ mg}}{\underset{2}{\cancel{0.4}} \text{ mg}} \times 1 \text{ mL} = \frac{1}{2} \text{ mL} = 0.5 \text{ mL}$$

45) Order: 25 mg

Supply: 5 mg/mL

$$\frac{D}{H} \times Q = \frac{\overset{5}{\cancel{25}} \text{ mg}}{\underset{1}{\cancel{5}} \text{ mg}} \times 1 \text{ mL} = 5 \text{ mL}$$

46) Order: digoxin 0.125 mg

Supply: digoxin 500 mcg/2 mL

1 g = 1,000 mg (known equivalent)

0.125 mg × 1,000 mcg/mg = 0.125. = 125 mcg

$$\frac{D}{H} \times Q = \frac{\overset{1}{\cancel{125}} \text{ mcg}}{\underset{4}{\cancel{500}} \text{ mcg}} \times 2 \text{ mL} = \frac{2}{4} \text{ mL} = 0.5 \text{ mL}$$

Review Set 26 from pages 339–351

1) 20; 50; 10; 2

> *2/6/xx, 0800, reconstituted as IV solution*
> *50 mg/mL. Expires 2/6/xx, 2000.*
> *Keep refrigerated. Redissolve precipitate,*
> *if present, at room temperature. G.D.P.*

© Cengage Learning 2013

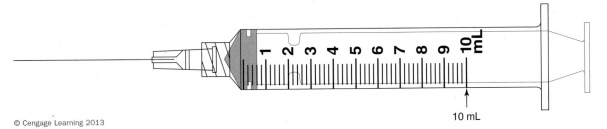

© Cengage Learning 2013

10 mL

2) 23; 200,000; 0.75

18; 250,000; 0.6

8; 500,000; 0.3

3; 1,000,000; 0.15

250,000; 0.6

The 250,000 units/mL concentration can be measured at exactly 0.6 mL in a 3 mL syringe, and 0.6 mL is a reasonable dose amount to measure in a 3 mL syringe. The 0.75 mL dose would require rounding to measure in a 3 mL syringe. The 0.75, 0.3 mL, and 0.15 mL doses are more risky to measure in a 3 mL syringe. The nurse could measure them in a 1 mL syringe, but this would not be necessary with the solution-strength choices available. 33 full doses are available. At 2 doses per day, 14 doses will be used before expiration.

> *2/6/xx, 0800, reconstituted as*
> *250,000 units/mL. Expires 2/13/xx,*
> *0800. Keep refrigerated. G.D.P.*

© Cengage Learning 2013

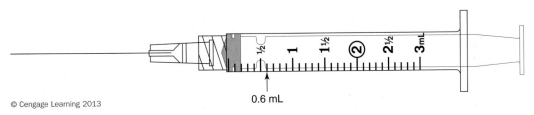

© Cengage Learning 2013

0.6 mL

3) 1.7; 250; 1.5

One full dose is available. No reconstitution label would be needed, because there is only 1 full dose available and the alert says to use solution within 1 hour; the next dose is not due for 6 more hours.

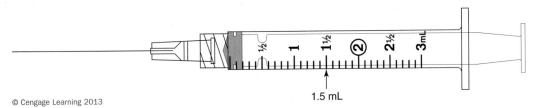

© Cengage Learning 2013

1.5 mL

4) 4.8; 100; 5; 1

No reconstitution label is required; all of the medication will be used for 1 dose.

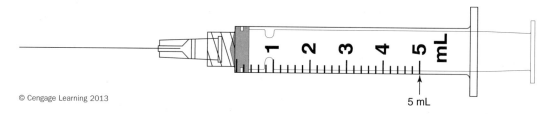

© Cengage Learning 2013

5 mL

5) 10; 10; 5; 2

© Cengage Learning 2013

*2/6/xx, 0800, reconstituted as
10 mg/mL. Expires 2/9/xx, 0800.
Refrigerate and protect from light. G.D.P.*

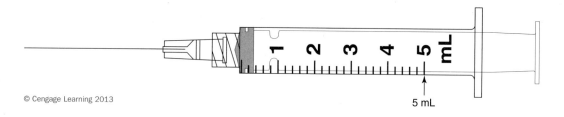

© Cengage Learning 2013

5 mL

6) 18.2; 250,000; 4

8.2; 500,000; 2

3.2; 1,000,000; 1

Select 1,000,000 units per mL and give 1 mL. Select this reconstitution concentration, because the amount to give is then obvious. No calculation is necessary.

Five full doses are available in vial.

© Cengage Learning 2013

*2/6/xx, 0800, reconstituted as
1,000,000 units/mL. Expires 2/13/xx,
0800. Keep refrigerated. G.D.P.*

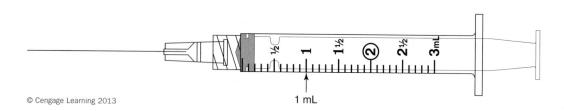

© Cengage Learning 2013

1 mL

7) 8; 500; 8; 62.5; 2.8; 2

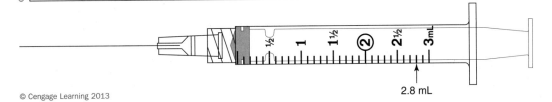

2/6/xx, 0800, reconstituted as 62.5 mg/mL. Expires 2/8/xx, 0800. Keep at room temperature and protect from light. G.D.P.

© Cengage Learning 2013

2.8 mL

© Cengage Learning 2013

8) 10; 50; 4; 2

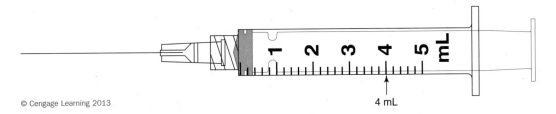

2/6/xx, 0800, reconstituted as 50 mg/mL. Expires 2/8/xx, 0800. Store at room temperature. Discard if slight haze develops. G.D.P.

© Cengage Learning 2013

4 mL

© Cengage Learning 2013

9) 20; 50,000; 10

10; 100,000; 5

4; 250,000; 2

1.8; 500,000; 1

Select 500,000 units/mL and give 1 mL. As this is an IV route, the dose would require further dilution before IV administration.

2 doses available

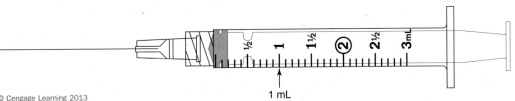

2/6/xx, 0800, reconstituted as 500,000 units/mL. Expires 2/13/xx, 0800. Keep refrigerated. G.D.P.

© Cengage Learning 2013

1 mL

© Cengage Learning 2013

10) 3.2; 1.5; 4; 375; 4; 1

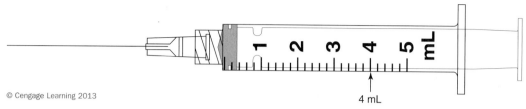

© Cengage Learning 2013

4 mL

11) 1.2; 40; 0.6; 1

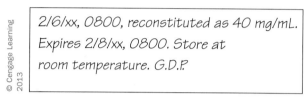

*2/6/xx, 0800, reconstituted as 40 mg/mL.
Expires 2/8/xx, 0800. Store at
room temperature. G.D.P.*

© Cengage Learning 2013

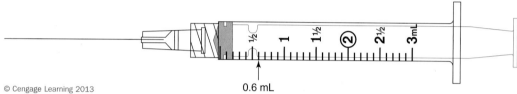

© Cengage Learning 2013

0.6 mL

12) 9.6; 1; 10; 100; 7.5; 1; yes; there is a remainder of 2.5 mL available for the next q.12h dose; solution is stable at room temperature for 24 h.

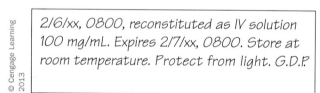

*2/6/xx, 0800, reconstituted as IV solution
100 mg/mL. Expires 2/7/xx, 0800. Store at
room temperature. Protect from light. G.D.P.*

© Cengage Learning 2013

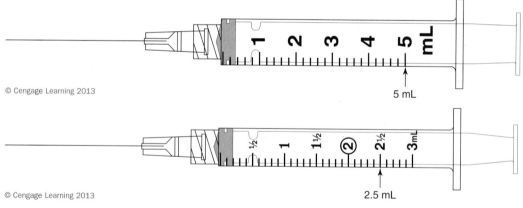

© Cengage Learning 2013

5 mL

© Cengage Learning 2013

2.5 mL

13) 10; 2; 12.5; 160; 9.4; 1

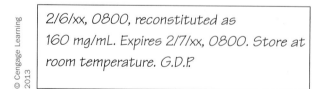

*2/6/xx, 0800, reconstituted as
160 mg/mL. Expires 2/7/xx, 0800. Store at
room temperature. G.D.P.*

© Cengage Learning 2013

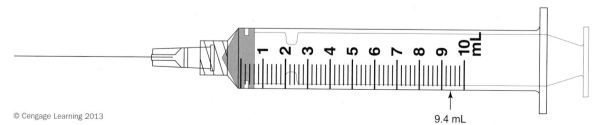

© Cengage Learning 2013

9.4 mL

14)   5; 50; 5; 1

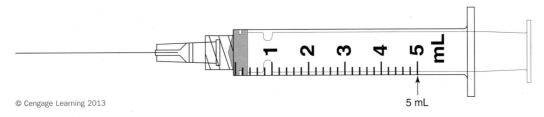

© Cengage Learning 2013

5 mL

15)   2; 225; 1.1; 2

2/6/xx, 0800, reconstituted as
225 mg/mL. Expires 2/7/xx, 0800, when
kept at room temperature. G.D.P.

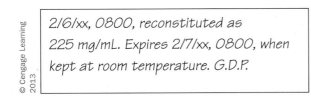

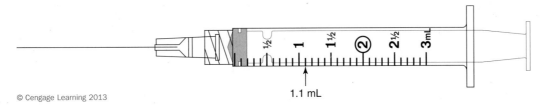

© Cengage Learning 2013

1.1 mL

Solutions—Review Set 26

1)   Order: 0.5 g

Supply: 50 mg/mL

1 g = 1,000 mg (known equivalent)

0.5 g × 1,000 mg/g = 0.500. = 500 mg

$\dfrac{D}{H} \times Q = \dfrac{\overset{10}{\cancel{500}\ \text{mg}}}{\underset{1}{\cancel{50}\ \text{mg}}} \times 1\ \text{mL} = 10\ \text{mL}$

1,000 mg/vial ÷ 500 mg/dose

= 1,000 mg/vial × 1 dose/500 mg = 2 doses/vial

2)   Order: 150,000 units

Supply: 250,000 units/mL

$\dfrac{D}{H} \times Q = \dfrac{\overset{3}{\cancel{150,000}\ \text{units}}}{\underset{5}{\cancel{250,000}\ \text{units}}} \times 1\ \text{mL} = \dfrac{3}{5}\ \text{mL} = 0.6\ \text{mL}$

5,000,000 units/vial ÷ 150,000 units/dose

= 5,000,000 units/vial × 1 dose/150,000 units

= 33.33 doses/vial or 33 full doses/vial

2 doses/day × 7 days = 14 doses will be used before expiration

3)   Order: 375 mg

Supply: 250 mg/mL

$\dfrac{D}{H} \times Q = \dfrac{375\ \text{mg}}{250\ \text{mg}} \times 1\ \text{mL} = 1.5\ \text{mL}$

500 mg/vial ÷ 375 mg/dose

= 500 mg/vial × 1 dose/375 mg

= 1.33 doses/vial or 1 full dose/vial

5)   Order: 50 mg

Supply: 10 mg/mL

$\dfrac{D}{H} \times Q = \dfrac{\overset{5}{\cancel{50}\ \text{mg}}}{\underset{1}{\cancel{10}\ \text{mg}}} \times 1\ \text{mL} = 5\ \text{mL}$

100 mg/vial ÷ 50 mg/dose

= 100 mg/vial × 1 dose/50 mg = 2 doses/vial

6)   Order: 1,000,000 units

Supply: 250,000 units/mL

$\dfrac{D}{H} \times Q = \dfrac{\overset{4}{\cancel{1,000,000}\ \text{units}}}{\underset{1}{\cancel{250,000}\ \text{units}}} \times 1\ \text{mL} = 4\ \text{mL}$

Order: 1,000,000 units

Supply: 500,000 units/mL

$\dfrac{D}{H} \times Q = \dfrac{\overset{2}{\cancel{1,000,000}\ \text{units}}}{\underset{1}{\cancel{500,000}\ \text{units}}} \times 1\ \text{mL} = 2\ \text{mL}$

Order: 1,000,000 units

Supply: 1,000,000 units/mL

$\dfrac{D}{H} \times Q = \dfrac{\overset{1}{\cancel{1,000,000}\ \text{units}}}{\underset{1}{\cancel{1,000,000}\ \text{units}}} \times 1\ \text{mL} = 1\ \text{mL}$

5,000,000 units/vial ÷ 1,000,000 units/dose

= 5,000,000 units/vial × 1 dose/1,000,000 units

= 5 doses/vial

7) Order: 175 mg

Supply: 500 mg per 8 mL

$$\frac{500 \text{ mg}}{8 \text{ mL}} = 62.5 \text{ mg/mL}$$

$$\frac{D}{H} \times Q = \frac{175 \text{ mg}}{62.5 \text{ mg}} \times 1 \text{ mL} = 2.8 \text{ mL}$$

500 mg/vial ÷ 175 mg/dose

= 500 mg/vial × 1 dose/175 mg = 2.85 doses/vial

or 2 full doses/vial

8) Order: 200 mg

Supply: 50 mg/mL

$$\frac{D}{H} \times Q = \frac{\overset{4}{200 \text{ mg}}}{\underset{1}{50 \text{ mg}}} \times 1 \text{ mL} = 4 \text{ mL}$$

2 g/vial = 2.000. = 2,000 mg/vial

2,000 mg/vial ÷ 200 mg/dose

= 2,000 mg/vial × 1 dose/200 mg = 10 doses/vial;

but only 8 doses can be used before expiration date

12) Order: 750 mg

Supply: 100 mg/mL

$$\frac{D}{H} \times Q = \frac{750 \text{ mg}}{100 \text{ mg}} \times 1 \text{ mL} = \frac{75}{10} \text{ mL} = 7.5 \text{ mL}$$

1,000 mg/vial ÷ 750 mg/dose

= 1,000 mg/vial × 1 dose/750 mg

= 1.33 doses/vial or 1 full dose/vial

13) Order: 1,500 mg

Supply: 160 mg/mL

$$\frac{D}{H} \times Q = \frac{1,500 \text{ mg}}{160 \text{ mg}} \times 1 \text{ mL} = \frac{150}{16} \text{ mL} = 9.37 \text{ mL}$$

= 9.4 mL

2,000 mg/vial ÷ 1,500 mg/dose

= 2,000 mg/vial × 1 dose/1,500 mg

= 1.33 doses/vial or 1 full dose/vial

14) Order: 25 mg

Supply: 250 mg per 5 mL

$$\frac{D}{H} \times Q = \frac{250 \text{ mg}}{250 \text{ mg}} \times 5 \text{ mL} = 5 \text{ mL}$$

You need to give the entire vial. The reconstituted amount may actually yield a little more than the 5 mL. There is only 1 full dose, so withdraw the entire amount in the vial.

Review Set 27 from page 356

1) 160 mL hydrogen peroxide (solute) + 320 mL saline (solvent) = 480 mL $\frac{1}{3}$ strength solution.

2) 1 fl oz hydrogen peroxide + 3 fl oz saline = 4 fl oz $\frac{1}{4}$ strength solution.

3) 180 mL hydrogen peroxide + 60 mL saline = 240 mL $\frac{3}{4}$ strength solution.

4) 8 fl oz hydrogen peroxide + 8 fl oz saline = 16 fl oz $\frac{1}{2}$ strength solution.

5) 300 mL Ensure + 600 mL water = 900 mL $\frac{1}{3}$ strength Ensure; one 12 fl oz can. Discard 2 fl oz (60 mL).

6) 6 fl oz (180 mL) Isomil + 18 fl oz (540 mL) water = 24 fl oz (720 mL) $\frac{1}{4}$ strength Isomil; one 6 fl oz can. None discarded.

7) 1,200 mL needed for daily supply. 800 mL Sustacal + 400 mL water = 1,200 mL $\frac{2}{3}$ strength Sustacal; three 10 fl oz cans. Discard 100 mL.

8) 13 fl oz Ensure + 13 fl oz water = 26 fl oz $\frac{1}{2}$ strength Ensure; one 12 fl oz can + one 4 fl oz can. Discard 3 fl oz (90 mL).

9) 1,000 mL needed for daily supply. 500 mL Sustacal + 500 mL water = 1,000 mL $\frac{1}{2}$ strength Sustacal; two 10 fl oz cans. Discard 100 mL.

10) 36 fl oz Isomil + 12 fl oz water = 48 fl oz $\frac{3}{4}$ strength Isomil; use three 12 fl oz cans. None discarded.

11) 4 fl oz Ensure + 2 fl oz water = 6 fl oz $\frac{2}{3}$ strength Ensure; use one 4 fl oz can. None discarded.

12) 4 fl oz Enusre + 12 fl oz water = 16 fl oz (1 pt) $\frac{1}{4}$ strength Ensure; use one 4 fl oz can. None discarded.

Solutions—Review Set 27

1) $D \times Q = \frac{1}{3} \times \overset{160}{\cancel{480}}$ mL = 160 mL (solute)

480 mL (quantity desired solution) − 160 mL (solute)

= 320 mL (solvent)

5) $D \times Q = \frac{1}{3} \times \overset{300}{\cancel{900}}$ mL = 300 mL (Ensure)

900 mL (total solution) − 300 mL (Ensure)

= 600 mL (water)

one 12 fl oz can = 30 mL/fl oz × 12 fl oz/can

= 360 mL/can

360 mL (full can) − 300 mL (Ensure needed)

= 60 mL (discarded)

6) 4 fl oz q.4h = 4 fl oz/feeding × 6 feedings

= 24 fl oz (total)

$D \times Q = \frac{1}{4} \times \overset{6}{\cancel{24}}$ fl oz = 6 fl oz (Isomil)

24 fl oz (solution) − 6 fl oz (Isomil) = 18 fl oz

(water); use one 6 fl oz can.

12) $D \times Q = \frac{1}{4} \times 16$ fl oz = $\frac{\overset{4}{\cancel{16}}}{\cancel{4}}$ = 4 fl oz (Ensure)

16 fl oz (solution) − 4 fl oz (Ensure) = 12 fl oz

(water); use one 4 fl oz can Ensure. No discard.

Practice Problems—Chapter 12 from pages 359–365

1) 3.375; 5; 3.7; 5 mL **2)** 2; 3 mL **3)** 1.5; 3 mL **4)** 9; 1; 10 mL **5)** 1.8; 3 mL; 2 (Dilute further for IV administration.)

> 2/6/xx, 0800, reconstituted as 280 mg/mL.
> Expires 2/13/xx, 0800. Keep refrigerated. G.D.P.

6) 3.8; 5 mL; 1 **7)** 2; 225; 1.3; 3 mL; 1; Yes **8)** 8; 500; 8; 62.5; 3.2; 5; 2; Yes **9)** 19.2; 100; 12.5; 20 mL; 1; Yes **10)** 3; 1,000,000; 0.5; 3 mL; 10; Yes **11)** 0.9; 250; 0.8; 3; 1; No, it would be too difficult to withdraw the small remainder for the next dose. **12)** 29; 20; 10; 5; Yes **13)** 2; 225; 1.8; 3 mL; 1; Yes **14)** 3.2; 1,000,000; 2; 3 mL; 2; Yes **15)** 1.8; 500,000; 2; 3 mL; 1; No

16) 2 fl oz hydrogen peroxide + 14 fl oz normal saline = 16 fl oz of the $\frac{1}{8}$ strength solution

17) 120 mL hydrogen peroxide + 200 mL normal saline = 320 mL of the $\frac{3}{8}$ strength solution

18) 50 mL hydrogen peroxide + 30 mL normal saline = 80 mL of the $\frac{5}{8}$ strength solution

19) 12 fl oz hydrogen peroxide + 6 fl oz normal saline = 18 fl oz of the $\frac{2}{3}$ strength solution

20) 14 fl oz hydrogen peroxide + 2 fl oz normal saline = 16 fl oz (1 pt) of the $\frac{7}{8}$ strength solution

21) 250 mL hydrogen peroxide + 750 mL normal saline = 1,000 mL (1 L) of the $\frac{1}{4}$ strength solution

22) 30 mL Enfamil + 90 mL water = 120 mL of the $\frac{1}{4}$ strength Enfamil; one 3 fl oz bottle. Discard 2 fl oz (60 mL).

23) 270 mL Sustacal + 90 mL water = 360 mL of the $\frac{3}{4}$ strength Sustacal; one 10 fl oz can. Discard 1 fl oz (30 mL).

24) 300 mL Ensure + 150 mL water = 450 mL of the $\frac{2}{3}$ strength Ensure; two 8 fl oz cans. Discard 6 fl oz (180 mL).

25) 36 fl oz Enfamil + 60 fl oz water = 96 fl oz of the $\frac{3}{8}$ strength Enfamil; six 6 fl oz bottles. None discarded.

26) 20 mL Ensure + 140 mL water = 160 mL of the $\frac{1}{8}$ strength Ensure; one 4 fl oz can. Discard 100 mL.

27) 275 mL Ensure + 275 mL water = 550 mL of the $\frac{1}{2}$ strength Ensure; one 12 fl oz can. Discard 85 mL.

28) 2 cans are needed; $1\frac{1}{2}$ cans are used (12 fl oz Enfamil)

29) 36

30) **Prevention:** This type of error could have been prevented had the nurse read the label carefully for the correct amount of diluent for the dosage of medication to be prepared. Had the nurse read the label carefully before the medication was prepared, medication charges, valuable time, and health care resources would have been saved. Additionally, if the nurse had used Step 2 (Think) of the Three-Step Approach, the nurse would have realized earlier (before preparing it) that 4 mL would be an unreasonable volume for an IM injection.

Solutions—Practice Problems—Chapter 12

1) Concentration is 3.375 g per 5 mL

Order: 2.5 g

Supply: 3.375 g per 5 mL

$\frac{D}{H} \times Q = \frac{2.5\ g}{3.375\ g} \times 5\ mL = \frac{12.5}{3.375}\ mL = 3.70\ mL$

$= 3.7\ mL$

4) Order: 900 mg

Supply: 100 mg/mL

$\frac{D}{H} \times Q = \frac{900\ mg}{100\ mg} \times 1\ mL = 9\ mL$

Vial has 1 g. Order is for 900 mg/dose.

1 g/vial = 1.000. = 1,000 mg/vial

1,000 mg/vial ÷ 900 mg/dose

$= 1,000\ mg/vial \times 1\ dose/900\ mg$

= 1.1 doses/vial = 1 full dose/vial

6) Order: 375 mg

Supply: 100 mg/mL

$\frac{D}{H} \times Q = \frac{375\ mg}{100\ mg} \times 1\ mL = 3.75\ mL = 3.8\ mL$

500 mg/vial ÷ 375 mg/dose

$= 500\ mg/vial \times 1\ dose/375\ mg = 1.3\ doses/vial$

= 1 full dose/vial

8) Order: 200 mg

Supply: 62.5 mg/mL

$\frac{D}{H} \times Q = \frac{200\ mg}{62.5\ mg} \times 1\ mL = 3.2\ mL$

500 mg/vial ÷ 200 mg/dose

$= 500\ mg/vial \times 1\ dose/200\ mg = 2.5\ doses/vial$

or 2 full doses/vial

9) Order: 1.25 g

Supply: 100 mg/mL

1 g = 1,000 mg (known equivalent)

1.25 g × 1,000 mg/g = 1.250. = 1,250 mg

$\frac{D}{H} \times Q = \frac{1,250\ mg}{100\ mg} \times 1\ mL = 12.5\ mL$

2,000 mg/vial ÷ 1,250 mg/dose

$= 2,000\ mg/vial \times 1\ dose/1,250\ mg$

= 1.6 doses/vial or 1 full dose/vial

11) Order: 200 mg

Supply: 250 mg/mL

$\frac{D}{H} \times Q = \frac{\overset{4}{200\ mg}}{\underset{5}{250\ mg}} \times 1\ mL = \frac{4}{5}\ mL = 0.8\ mL$

250 mg/vial ÷ 200 mg/dose

$= 250\ mg/vial \times 1\ dose/200\ mg = 1.25\ doses/vial$

or 1 full dose/vial

15) Order: 1,000,000 units

Supply: 50,000 units/mL

$\frac{D}{H} \times Q = \frac{\overset{20}{1,000,000\ units}}{\underset{1}{50,000\ units}} \times 1\ mL = 20\ mL$

(too much for IM dose)

Order: 1,000,000 units

Supply: 100,000 units/mL

$\frac{D}{H} \times Q = \frac{\overset{10}{1,000,000\ units}}{\underset{1}{100,000\ units}} \times 1\ mL = 10\ mL$

(too much for IM dose)

Order: 1,000,000 units

Supply: 250,000 units/mL

$\frac{D}{H} \times Q = \frac{\overset{4}{1,000,000\ units}}{\underset{1}{250,000\ units}} \times 1\ mL = 4\ mL$

(too much for IM dose—3 mL or less is preferable)

Order: 1,000,000 units

Supply: 500,000 units/mL

$\frac{D}{H} \times Q = \frac{\overset{2}{1,000,000\ units}}{\underset{1}{500,000\ units}} \times 1\ mL = 2\ mL$

(acceptable IM dose)

22) 12 mL every hour for

10 hours = 12 mL × 10 = 120 mL total

$D \times Q = \frac{1}{4} \times \overset{30}{120}\ mL = 30\ mL$ (Enfamil)

120 mL (solution) − 30 mL (Enfamil) = 90 mL

(water); one 3 fl oz bottle: 3 fl oz × 30 mL/fl oz

= 90 mL

90 mL (full bottle) − 30 mL (Enframil needed)

= 60 mL (2 fl oz discarded)

60 mL ÷ 30 mL/fl oz = 60 mL × 1 fl oz/30 mL

= 2 fl oz

28) $D \times Q = \frac{1}{\underset{1}{4}} \times \overset{12}{\cancel{48}}$ fl oz $= 12$ fl oz Enfamil;

$1\frac{1}{2}$ cans (8 fl oz each) of Enfamil is needed for each

infant.

29)   48 fl oz (solution) − 12 fl oz (Enfamil)

= 36 fl oz (water)

Review Set 28 from pages 379–385

1) 25; 312.5; 78.1; 625; 156.3; Yes **2)** 10 **3)** 2.2; 110; 55; Yes **4)** 0.55 **5)** 15; 120; Yes **6)** 6; 8 **7)** 320; 480; Yes **8)** 15

9) 20; 500; 125; 1,000; 250; Yes **10)** 5 **11)** 5; 7.5; 9.5; Yes

12) 0.8

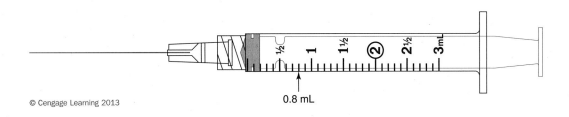

© Cengage Learning 2013

0.8 mL

13)   3.4; 51; 17; No

14)   The dosage of Kantrex 34 mg IV q.8h is higher than the recommended dosage. Therefore, the ordered dosage is not

safe. The prescribing practitioner should be called and the order questioned.

15)   120; 60; 7.5; Yes

16)   7.5; $1\frac{1}{2}$

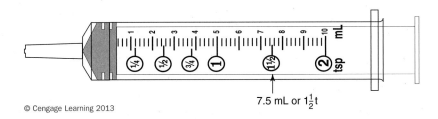

© Cengage Learning 2013

7.5 mL or $1\frac{1}{2}$ t

17)   1.8; 4.5; No

18)   The ordered dosage is too high and ordered to be given too frequently. The recommended dosage is 4.5 mg q.12h.

The ordered dosage is 40 mg q.8h. The prescribing practitioner should be notified and the order questioned.

19)   32.7; 818; 205; 1,635; 409; Yes

20)   1.6

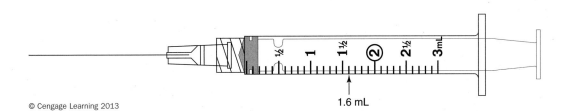

© Cengage Learning 2013

1.6 mL

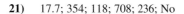

21) 17.7; 354; 118; 708; 236; No

22) The dosage ordered of 100 mg q.8h does not fall within the recommended dosage range of 118 to 236 mg/dose. It is an underdosage and would not produce a therapeutic effect. The physician should be called for clarification.

23) 25; 375; 125; 625; 208.3; No

24) The ordered dosage of 100 mg q.8h does not fall within the recommended dosage range of 125 to 208.3 mg q.8h. It is an underdosage, and the physician should be called for clarification.

25) No, the ordered dosage is not safe. The label states a maximum of 250 mg per single daily injection for children older than 8 years of age. This child is only 7 years old, so the order exceeds the maximum recommended dosage. The physician should be called to clarify the order.

26) 1 to 1.7 mg/kg IM/IV q.8h

27) 5 to 7 mg/kg IV q.24h

28) 59; 100

29) 296; 414

30) Yes

Solutions—Review Set 28

1) 1 kg = 2.2 lb; smaller $\uparrow$ larger $\rightarrow$ ($\div$)

55 lb $\div$ 2.2 lb/kg = 55 l̶b̶ $\times$ 1 kg/2.2 l̶b̶ = 25 kg

Minimum daily dosage:

12.5 mg/k̶g̶/day $\times$ 25 k̶g̶ = 312.5 mg/day

312.5 mg $\div$ 4 doses = 78.12 mg/dose = 78.1 mg/dose

Maximum daily dosage:

25 mg/k̶g̶/day $\times$ 25 k̶g̶ = 625 mg/day

625 mg $\div$ 4 doses = 156.25 mg/dose = 156.3 mg/dose

Yes, dosage is safe.

2) $\dfrac{D}{H} \times Q = \dfrac{\overset{2}{\cancel{125 \text{ mg}}}}{\underset{1}{\cancel{62.5 \text{ mg}}}} \times 5 \text{ mL} = 10 \text{ mL}$

3) Convert g to kg: 2,200 g = 2.200. = 2.2 kg

50 mg/k̶g̶/day $\times$ 2.2 k̶g̶ = 110 mg/day

110 mg $\div$ 2 doses = 55 mg/dose; yes dosage is safe

4) $\dfrac{D}{H} \times Q = \dfrac{55 \text{ m̶g̶}}{\underset{100}{\cancel{1,000 \text{ mg}}}} \times \overset{1}{\cancel{10}} \text{ mL} = \dfrac{55}{100} \text{ mL} = 0.55 \text{ mL}$

6) $\dfrac{D}{H} \times Q = \dfrac{\overset{6}{\cancel{120 \text{ mg}}}}{\underset{5}{\cancel{100 \text{ mg}}}} \times 5 \text{ mL} = \dfrac{\overset{6}{\cancel{30}}}{\underset{1}{\cancel{5}}} \text{ mL} = 6 \text{ mL}$

50 mL $\div$ 6 mL/dose = 50 m̶L̶ $\times$ 1 dose/6 m̶L̶

= 8.3 doses or 8 full doses

7) Minimum dosage: 10 mg/k̶g̶/dose $\times$ 32 kg = 320 mg/dose

Maximum dosage: 15 mg/k̶g̶/dose $\times$ 32 k̶g̶ = 480 mg/dose

Dosage is the *maximum* dosage (480 mg), and it is a safe dosage.

8) $\dfrac{D}{H} \times Q = \dfrac{\overset{3}{\cancel{480 \text{ mg}}}}{\underset{1}{\cancel{160 \text{ mg}}}} \times 5 \text{ mL} = 15 \text{ mL}$

13) 1 lb = 16 oz; 8 oz $\div$ 16 oz/lb = 8 o̶z̶ $\times$

1 lb/16 o̶z̶ = $\dfrac{1}{2}$ lb

7 lb 8 oz = $7\dfrac{1}{2}$ lb = 7.5 lb $\div$ 2.2 lb/kg

= 7.5 l̶b̶ $\times$ 1 kg/2.2 l̶b̶ = 3.40 kg = 3.4 kg

15 mg/k̶g̶/day $\times$ 3.4 k̶g̶ = 51 mg/day

51 mg $\div$ 3 doses = 17 mg/dose, if administered q.8h

Ordered dosage of 34 mg q.8h exceeds recommended dosage and is not safe.

19) 72 lb $\div$ 2.2 lb/kg = 72 l̶b̶ $\times$ 1 kg/2.2 l̶b̶ = 32.72 kg = 32.7 kg

Minimum daily dosage:

25 mg/k̶g̶/day $\times$ 32.7 k̶g̶ = 818 mg/day

Minimum single dosage:

818 mg $\div$ 4 doses = 204.5 mg/dose = 205 mg/dose

Maximum daily dosage:

50 mg/k̶g̶/day $\times$ 32.7 k̶g̶ = 1,635 mg/day

Maximum single dosage:

1,635 mg $\div$ 4 doses = 408.7 mg/dose = 409 mg/dose

Yes, dosage ordered is safe.

20) $\dfrac{D}{H} \times Q = \dfrac{400 \text{ m̶g̶}}{250 \text{ m̶g̶}} \times 1 \text{ mL} = 1.6 \text{ mL}$

21) 39 lb $\div$ 2.2 lb/kg = 39 l̶b̶ $\times$ 1 kg/2.2 l̶b̶ = 17.72 kg = 17.7 kg

Minimum daily dosage:

20 mg/k̶g̶/day $\times$ 17.7 k̶g̶ = 354 mg/day

Minimum single dosage:

354 mg $\div$ 3 doses = 118 mg/dose

Maximum daily dosage:

40 mg/k̶g̶/day $\times$ 17.7 k̶g̶ = 708 mg/day

Maximum single dosage:

708 mg $\div$ 3 doses = 236 mg/dose

The dosage of 100 mg q.8h is not safe. It is an underdosage and would not produce a therapeutic effect because the recommended dosage range is 118 to 236 mg/dose.

28) 130 lb ÷ 2.2 kg/lb = 130 l̶b̶ × 1 kg/2.2 l̶b̶

    = 59.09 kg = 59.1 kg

    1 mg/k̶g̶ × 59.1 k̶g̶ = 59.1 mg/dose = 59 mg/dose

    1.7 mg/k̶g̶ × 59.1 k̶g̶ = 100.4 mg/dose

    = 100 mg/dose

29) 5 mg/k̶g̶ × 59.1 k̶g̶ = 295.5 mg/dose = 296 mg/dose

    7 mg/k̶g̶ × 59.1 k̶g̶ = 413.7 mg/dose = 414 mg/dose

Practice Problems—Chapter 13 from pages 387–398

1) 5.5 **2)** 3.8 **3)** 1.6 **4)** 2.3 **5)** 15.5 **6)** 3 **7)** 23.6 **8)** 0.9 **9)** 240 **10)** 80 **11)** 19.5; 39; 48.8; Yes

12) 1

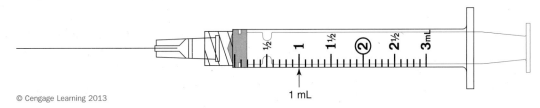

1 mL

© Cengage Learning 2013

13) 7.3; 3.7; 14.6; Yes

14) 1

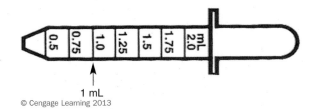

1 mL

© Cengage Learning 2013

15) 18.2; 182; 91; 364; 182; Yes

16) 7.5

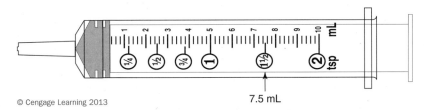

7.5 mL

© Cengage Learning 2013

17) 29.1; 291; 145.5; 1,746; 873; Yes

18) 3

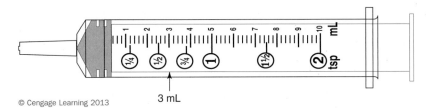

3 mL

© Cengage Learning 2013

19) 2.5; 125,000; 125,000; Yes

20) 18; 20; 250,000; 0.5

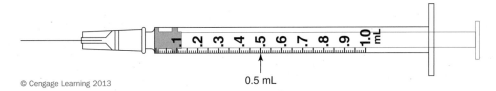

0.5 mL

© Cengage Learning 2013

21)   18.6; 372; 124; 744; 248; Yes

22)   6

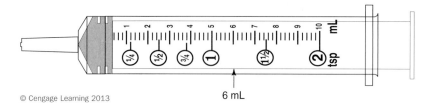

© Cengage Learning 2013

6 mL

23)   13.9; 556; 185.3; Yes, the ordered dosage is reasonably safe.

24)   5

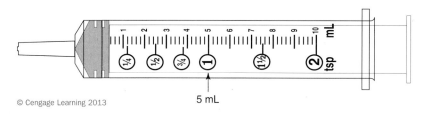

© Cengage Learning 2013

5 mL

25)   10; 0.1; Yes

26)   0.25

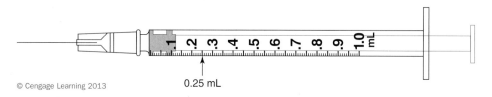

© Cengage Learning 2013

0.25 mL

27)   28; 35; Yes

28)   3.5

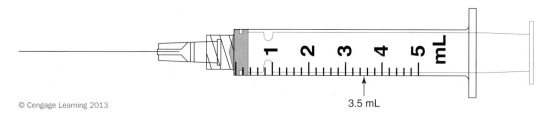

© Cengage Learning 2013

3.5 mL

29)   9.1; 455; 227.5; 682.5; 341.3; No

30)   The ordered dosage of 1 g is not safe. The recommended dosage range for a child of this weight is 227.5 to 341.3 mg/dose. Physician should be called for clarification.

31)   25.1; 0.05; Yes

32)   0.25

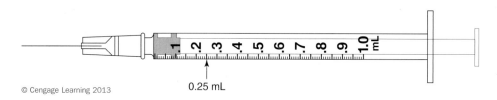

© Cengage Learning 2013

0.25 mL

Route is IM; may need to change needle to appropriate gauge and length.

33) 8.2; 1,200; 1.2; 410; 615; Yes

34) 9.6; 10; 100; 6

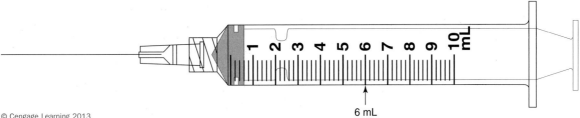

© Cengage Learning 2013

6 mL

35) 20.5; 512.5; 256.3; No

36) The dosage ordered is not safe. It is too low compared to the recommended dosage. Call the prescriber and clarify the order.

37) 8.2; 164; 54.7; No

38) Dosage ordered is not safe. Call prescriber for clarification, because ordered dosage is higher than the recommended dosage.

39) 20.5; 200; 400; No

40) Dosage ordered is not safe based on recommended maximum daily dosage and on the frequency of the order. Call prescriber for clarification.

41) 23.2; 348; 174; Yes, dosage is reasonably safe.

42) 3.5

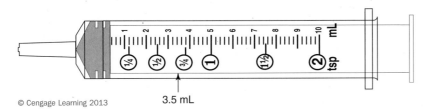

© Cengage Learning 2013

3.5 mL

43) 0.25

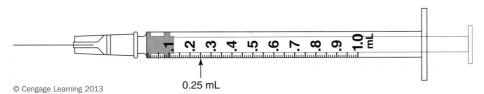

© Cengage Learning 2013

0.25 mL

44) 3.5

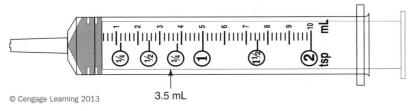

© Cengage Learning 2013

3.5 mL

45) 500,000; 0.9

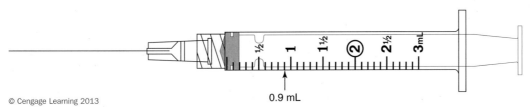

© Cengage Learning 2013

0.9 mL

46) Dosage is not safe; this child is ordered a total of 2 mg/day, which is too high. Prescriber should be called to clarify.

47) The ordered dosage of 1 mg IM stat is too high when compared to the recommended dosage range for a child of this weight. The order should be clarified with the prescriber.

48) 0.76; Route is IM; needle may need to be changed to appropriate gauge and length.

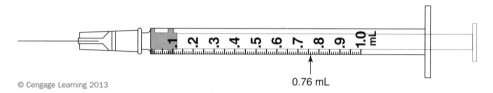

© Cengage Learning 2013   0.76 mL

49) #45 (penicillin G potassium) and #48 (cefazolin). (Note: #43 methylprednisolone is a single-dose vial. Check package insert to determine if storage after mixing is safe.)

50) **Prevention:** The child should have received 75 mg a day and no more than 25 mg per dose. The child received more than four times the safe dosage of tobramycin. Had the nurse calculated the safe dosage, the error would have been caught sooner, the resident would have been consulted, and the dosage could have been adjusted before the child ever received the first dose. The pharmacist also should have caught the error but did not. In this scenario, the resident, pharmacist, and nurse all committed medication errors. If the resident had not noticed the error, one can only wonder how many doses the child would have received. The nurse is the last safety net for the patient when it comes to a dosage error, because the nurse administers the drug.

In addition, the nurse has to reconcile the fact that she actually gave the overdose. The nurse is responsible for whatever dosage is administered and must verify the safety of the order and the patient's Six Rights. We are all accountable for our actions. Taking shortcuts in administering medications to children can be disastrous. The time the nurse saved by not calculating the safe dosage was more than lost in the extra monitoring, not to mention the cost of follow-up to the medication error and, *most importantly,* the risk to the child.

Solutions—Practice Problems—Chapter 13

1) 1 kg = 2.2 lb

12 lb ÷ 2.2 lb/kg = 12 l̶b̶ × 1 kg/2.2 l̶b̶

    = 5.45 kg = 5.5 kg

2) 8 lb 4 oz = $8\frac{4}{16}$ lb = $8\frac{1}{4}$ lb = 8.25 lb

8.25 lb ÷ 2.2 lb/kg = 8.25 l̶b̶ × 1 kg/2.2 l̶b̶

    = 3.75 kg = 3.8 kg

3) 1,570 g = 1.570. = 1.57 kg = 1.6 kg

6) 1 lb = 16 oz; 10 oz ÷ 16 oz/lb

= 10 o̶z̶ × 1 lb/16 o̶z̶ = $\frac{\overset{5}{\cancel{10}}}{\underset{8}{\cancel{16}}}$ lb = $\frac{5}{8}$ lb

6 lb 10 oz = $6\frac{5}{8}$ lb = 6.625 lb

6.625 lb ÷ 2.2 lb/kg = 6.625 l̶b̶ × 1 kg/2.2 l̶b̶

    = 3.01 kg = 3 kg

17) 64 lb ÷ 2.2 lb/kg = 64 l̶b̶ × 1 kg/2.2 l̶b̶

    = 29.09 kg = 29.1 kg

Minimum daily dosage:

10 mg/k̶g̶/day × 29.1 k̶g̶ = 291 mg/day

Minimum single dosage (based on b.i.d.):

291 mg/2 doses = 145.5 mg/dose

Maximum daily dosage (based on 60 mg/day):

60 mg/k̶g̶/day × 29.1 k̶g̶ = 1,746 mg/day

Maximum single dosage (based on b.i.d.):

1,746 mg ÷ 2 doses = 873 mg/dose

Dosage ordered is safe. Child will receive 300 mg in a 24-hour period in divided doses of 150 mg b.i.d. This falls within the allowable dosage range of 145.5 mg/dose to 873 mg/dose. Because the daily dosage exceeds 250 mg, the order is appropriately divided.

18) $\frac{D}{H} \times Q = \frac{\overset{3}{\cancel{150\ mg}}}{\underset{5}{\cancel{250\ mg}}} \times 5$ mL $= \frac{3}{5} \times \cancel{5}$ mL $= 3$ mL

19) 2,500 g = 2.500. = 2.5 kg

Recommended daily dosage:

50,000 units/k̶g̶/day × 2.5 k̶g̶ = 125,000 units/day

Recommended single dosage:

50,000 units/kg/dose × 2.5 kg = 125,000 units/dose

Ordered dosage is safe.

23) $30\frac{1}{2}$ lb = 30.5 lb ÷ 2.2 lb/kg = 30.5 lb × 1 kg/2.2 lb

= 13.86 kg = 13.9 kg

Recommended daily dosage:

40 mg/kg/day × 13.9 kg = 556 mg/day

Recommended single dosage:

556 mg ÷ 3 doses = 185.33 mg/dose = 185.3 mg/dose

The ordered dosage of 187 mg p.o. is reasonably safe for this child.

24) $\dfrac{D}{H} \times Q = \dfrac{\overset{1}{\cancel{187\ mg}}}{\underset{1}{\cancel{187\ mg}}} \times 5\ mL = 5\ mL$

If we used the recommended single dosage of 185 mg/dose, the calculation would be:

$\dfrac{D}{H} \times Q = \dfrac{185\ \cancel{mg}}{187\ \cancel{mg}} \times 5\ mL = \dfrac{925}{187}\ mL = 4.94\ mL = 4.9\ mL$

which we round to 5 mL to measure in the pediatric oral syringe; therefore, as stated earlier, the ordered dosage is reasonably safe.

25) 22 lb ÷ 2.2 lb/kg = 22 lb × 1 kg/2.2 lb = 10 kg

0.01 mg/kg/dose × 10 kg = 0.1 mg/dose

0.1 mg = 0.100. = 100 mcg

Ordered dosage is safe.

29) 20 lb ÷ 2.2 lb/kg = 20 lb × 1 kg/2.2 lb = 9.09 kg = 9.1 kg

Recommended minimum daily dosage:

50 mg/kg/day × 9.1 kg = 455 mg/day

Recommended minimum single dosage:

455 mg ÷ 2 doses = 227.5 mg/dose

Recommended maximum daily dosage:

75 mg/kg/day × 9.1 kg = 682.5 mg/day

Recommended maximum single dosage:

682.5 mg ÷ 2 doses = 341.25 mg/dose = 341.3 mg/dose

The dosage ordered (1 g q.12h) is not safe. The recommended dosage range for a child of this weight is 227.5 to 341.3 mg/dose. Physician should be called for clarification.

41) 51 lb ÷ 2.2 lb/kg = 51 lb × 1 kg/2.2 lb = 23.18 kg = 23.2 kg

Recommended daily dosage:

15 mg/kg/day × 23.2 kg = 348 mg/day

Recommended single dosage:

348 mg ÷ 2 doses = 174 mg/dose

Ordered dosage of 175 mg is reasonably safe as an oral medication and should be given.

43) 95 lb ÷ 2.2 lb/kg = 95 lb × 1 kg/2.2 lb = 43.18 kg = 43.2 kg

0.5 mg/kg/day × 43.2 kg = 21.6 mg/day

Because the recommended dosage is not less than 21.6 mg/day and the order is for 10 mg q.6h for a total of 40 mg/day, the order is safe.

$\dfrac{D}{H} \times Q = \dfrac{\overset{1}{\cancel{10\ mg}}}{\underset{4}{\cancel{40\ mg}}} \times 1\ mL = \dfrac{1}{4}\ mL = 0.25\ mL$

Review Set 29 from page 402

1) 0.05; 1 L = 1,000 mL **2)** 0.3; 1 kg = 1,000 g **3)** 38.18; 1 kg = 2.2 lb **4)** $2\frac{1}{2}$; 1 fl oz = 30 mL **5)** 0.75; 1 L = 1,000 mL

6) 45; 1 fl oz = 30 mL **7)** 0.625; 1 mg = 1,000 mcg **8)** $\frac{1}{2}$; 1 t = 5 mL **9)** 600; 1 kg = 1,000 g **10)** 3; 1 in = 2.5 cm

11) 16,000; 1 g = 1,000 mg **12)** $\frac{1}{2}$; 1 fl oz = 30 mL **13)** 0.2; 1 lb = 16 oz **14)** 2; 1 qt = 1 L **15)** 33; 1 kg = 2.2 lb

16) 5; 1 fl oz = 30 mL **17)** 1; 1 t = 5 mL **18)** 8; 1 L = 1,000 mL; 1 qt = 1 L; 1 qt = 32 fl oz **19)** 3; 1 t = 5 mL

20) 0.25; 1 mg = 1,000 mcg

Solutions—Review Set 29

3) $\dfrac{1\ kg}{2.2\ lb} \diagup\!\!\!\!\diagdown \dfrac{X\ kg}{84\ lb}$

2.2X = 84

$\dfrac{2.2X}{2.2} = \dfrac{84}{2.2}$

X = 38.18 kg

5) $\dfrac{1\ L}{1,000\ mL} \diagup\!\!\!\!\diagdown \dfrac{X\ L}{750\ mL}$

1,000X = 750

$\dfrac{1,000X}{1,000} = \dfrac{750}{1,000}$

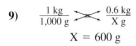

9) $\dfrac{1 \text{ kg}}{1{,}000 \text{ g}} \diagbox \dfrac{0.6 \text{ kg}}{\text{X g}}$

$\text{X} = 600 \text{ g}$

18) $1 \text{ L} = 1{,}000 \text{ mL}$

$\dfrac{1 \text{ L}}{1{,}000 \text{ mL}} \diagbox \dfrac{\text{X L}}{2{,}000 \text{ mL}}$

$1{,}000\text{X} = 2{,}000$

$\dfrac{1{,}000\text{X}}{1{,}000} = \dfrac{2{,}000}{1{,}000}$

$\text{X} = 2 \text{ L}$

$1 \text{ L} = 1 \text{ qt}; \ 2 \text{ L} = 2 \text{ qt}; \ 1 \text{ qt} = 32 \text{ fl oz}$

$\dfrac{1 \text{ qt}}{32 \text{ fl oz}} \diagbox \dfrac{2 \text{ qt}}{\text{X fl oz}}$

$\text{X} = 64 \text{ fl oz}$

$1 \text{ cup} = 8 \text{ oz}$

$\dfrac{1 \text{ cup}}{8 \text{ fl oz}} = \dfrac{\text{X cup}}{64 \text{ fl oz}}$

$8\text{X} = 64$

$\dfrac{8\text{X}}{8} = \dfrac{64}{8}$

$\text{X} = 8 \text{ cups or eight 8-fl oz-glasses}$

Review Set 30 from pages 405–406

1) 2 **2)** 2.5 **3)** 0.8 **4)** 1.3 **5)** 7.5 **6)** 0.6 **7)** $1\frac{1}{2}$ **8)** 3 **9)** 30 **10)** 1.6 **11)** 3 **12)** 0.5 **13)** $2\frac{1}{2}$ **14)** 250 mg; $\frac{1}{2}$ of 250 mg tab

15) 2.4 **16)** 2 **17)** 18 **18)** 1.3 **19)** 16 **20)** 7

Solutions—Review Set 30

2) $\dfrac{300 \text{ mg}}{5 \text{ mL}} \diagbox \dfrac{150 \text{ mg}}{\text{X mL}}$

$300\text{X} = 750$

$\dfrac{300\text{X}}{300} = \dfrac{750}{300}$

$\text{X} = 2.5 \text{ mL}$

5) $\dfrac{300 \text{ mg}}{5 \text{ mL}} \diagbox \dfrac{450 \text{ mg}}{\text{X mL}}$

$300\text{X} = 2.250$

$\dfrac{300\text{X}}{300} = \dfrac{2.250}{300}$

$\text{X} = 7.5 \text{ mL}$

6) $\dfrac{4 \text{ mg}}{1 \text{ mL}} \diagbox \dfrac{2.4 \text{ mg}}{\text{X mL}}$

$4\text{X} = 2.4$

$\dfrac{4\text{X}}{4} = \dfrac{2.4}{4}$

$\text{X} = 0.6 \text{ mL}$

9) $\dfrac{80 \text{ mg}}{15 \text{ mL}} \diagbox \dfrac{160 \text{ mg}}{\text{X mL}}$

$80\text{X} = 2{,}400$

$\dfrac{80\text{X}}{80} = \dfrac{2{,}400}{80}$

$\text{X} = 30 \text{ mL}$

13) $\dfrac{15 \text{ mg}}{1 \text{ tab}} \diagbox \dfrac{37.5 \text{ mg}}{\text{X tab}}$

$15\text{X} = 37.5$

$\dfrac{15\text{X}}{15} = \dfrac{37.5}{15}$

$\text{X} = 2.5 \text{ tab} = 2\frac{1}{2} \text{ tab}$

16) Convert mg to mcg:

$\dfrac{1 \text{ mg}}{1{,}000 \text{ mcg}} \diagbox \dfrac{0.15 \text{ mg}}{\text{X mcg}}$

$\text{X} = 150 \text{ mcg}$

$\dfrac{75 \text{ mcg}}{1 \text{ tab}} \diagbox \dfrac{150 \text{ mcg}}{\text{X}}$

$75\text{X} = 150$

$\dfrac{75\text{X}}{75} = \dfrac{150}{75}$

$\text{X} = 2 \text{ tab}$

18) $\dfrac{80 \text{ mg}}{1 \text{ mL}} \diagbox \dfrac{100 \text{ mg}}{\text{X mL}}$

$80\text{X} = 100$

$\dfrac{80\text{X}}{80} = \dfrac{100}{80}$

$\text{X} = 1.25 \text{ mL} = 1.3 \text{ mL (rounded to measure}$
$\text{in a 3 mL syringe)}$

19) $\dfrac{2.5 \text{ mg}}{5 \text{ mL}} \diagbox \dfrac{8 \text{ mg}}{\text{X mL}}$

$2.5\text{X} = 40$

$\dfrac{2.5 \text{ X}}{2.5} = \dfrac{40}{2.5}$

$\text{X} = 16 \text{ mL}$

Review Set 31 from pages 416–417

1) 0.5 **2)** 3 **3)** 34 **4)** 12 **5)** 10 **6)** 13 **7)** $1\frac{1}{2}$ **8)** 2 **9)** 2 **10)** 3 **11)** 1.7 **12)** 0.91 **13)** 0.3 **14)** 7.5 **15)** 0.75 **16)** 6 **17)** 3.2 **18)** 1.2 **19)** 4.4 **20)** 6.2

Solutions—Review Set 31

1) $X \text{ mL} = \dfrac{1 \text{ mL}}{10.000 \text{ units}} \times 5,000 \text{ units} = 0.5 \text{ mL}$

3) $X \text{ mL} = \dfrac{5 \text{ mL}}{250 \text{ mg}} \times \dfrac{15 \text{ mg}}{1 \text{ kg}} \times \dfrac{1 \text{ kg}}{2.2 \text{ lb}} \times 250 \text{ lb} = 34 \text{ mL}$

6) $X \text{ mL} = \dfrac{5 \text{ mL}}{250 \text{ mg}} \times \dfrac{1,000 \text{ mg}}{1 \text{ g}} \times \dfrac{0.01 \text{ g}}{1 \text{ kg}} \times \dfrac{1 \text{ kg}}{2.2 \text{ lb}} \times 143 \text{ lb} = 13 \text{ mL}$

11) $X \text{ mL} = \dfrac{1 \text{ mL}}{0.2 \text{ mg}} \times \dfrac{1 \text{ mg}}{1.000 \text{ mcg}} \times \dfrac{4 \text{ mcg}}{1 \text{ kg}} \times \dfrac{1 \text{ kg}}{2.2 \text{ lb}} \times 185 \text{ lb} = 1.68 \text{ mL} = 1.7 \text{ mL}$

12) $X \text{ mL} = \dfrac{1 \text{ mL}}{10.000 \text{ units}} \times \dfrac{150 \text{ units}}{1 \text{ kg}} \times \dfrac{1 \text{ kg}}{2.2 \text{ lb}} \times 133 \text{ lb} = 0.906 \text{ mL} = 0.91 \text{ mL}$

13) $X \text{ mL} = \dfrac{1 \text{ mL}}{2 \text{ mg}} \times \dfrac{1 \text{ mg}}{1.000 \text{ mcg}} \times \dfrac{50 \text{ mcg}}{1 \text{ kg}} \times \dfrac{1 \text{ kg}}{2.2 \text{ lb}} \times 27 \text{ lb} = 0.3 \text{ mL}$

15) $X \text{ mL} = \dfrac{1 \text{ mL}}{0.2 \text{ mg}} \times \dfrac{1 \text{ mg}}{1.000 \text{ mcg}} \times 150 \text{ mcg} = 0.75 \text{ mL}$

17) $X \text{ mL} = \dfrac{1 \text{ mL}}{2 \text{ mg}} \times \dfrac{1 \text{ mg}}{1.000 \text{ mcg}} \times \dfrac{80 \text{ mcg}}{1 \text{ kg}} \times 80 \text{ kg} = 3.2 \text{ mL}$

19) $X \text{ mL} = \dfrac{5 \text{ mL}}{375 \text{ mg}} \times \dfrac{990 \text{ mg}}{1 \text{ day}} \times \dfrac{1 \text{ day}}{24 \text{ h}} \times 8 \text{ h} = 4.4 \text{ mL (per dose)}$

Practice Problems—Chapter 14 from pages 419–422

1) 45 **2)** 2 **3)** 2 **4)** $\frac{1}{2}$ **5)** 2.5 **6)** 16 **7)** 1.4 **8)** 0.7 **9)** 2.3 **10)** 0.13 (measured in a 1 mL syringe) **11)** 1.6 **12)** 1.5 **13)** 1.3 **14)** 2.5 **15)** 1.6 **16)** 7.5 **17)** 1.6 **18)** 2 **19)** 8 **20)** 4.5 **21)** 30 **22)** 1.4 **23)** 0.4 **24)** 20 **25)** 12

26) Prevention: This type of calculation error occurred because the nurse set up the proportion incorrectly. In this instance, the nurse confused the **dosage supply** ratio with the **desired dosage** ratio. It is important to **think first** and then apply ratio-proportion to calculate the dosage. Remember: Ratio for the supply dosage you have on hand = ratio for the desired dosage. Thus, 125 mg per 5 mL is the correct supply dosage ratio.

$$\frac{125 \text{ mg}}{5 \text{ mL}} \diagdown\!\!\!\diagup \frac{50 \text{ mg}}{X \text{ mL}}$$

$$125X = 250$$

$$\frac{125X}{125} = \frac{250}{125}$$

$$X = 2 \text{ mL}$$

Solutions—Practice Problems—Chapter 14

1) ratio-proportion

$$\frac{3.33 \text{ g}}{5 \text{ mL}} \diagdown\!\!\!\diagup \frac{30 \text{ g}}{X \text{ mL}}$$

$$3.33X = 150$$

$$\frac{3.33X}{3.33} = \frac{150}{3.33}$$

$$X = 45 \text{ mL}$$

dimensional analysis

$$X \text{ mL} = \frac{5 \text{ mL}}{3.33 \text{ g}} \times 30 \text{ g} = 45 \text{ mL}$$

2) ratio-proportion

$$\frac{5,000,000 \text{ units}}{20 \text{ mL}} \diagdown\!\!\!\diagup \frac{500,000 \text{ units}}{X \text{ mL}}$$

$$5,000,000X = 10,000,000$$

$$\frac{5,000,000X}{5,000,000} = \frac{10,000,000}{5,000,000}$$

$$X = 2 \text{ mL}$$

dimensional analysis

$$X \text{ mL} = \frac{20 \text{ mL}}{5,000,000 \text{ units}} \times 500,000 \text{ units} = 2 \text{ mL}$$

6) ratio-proportion

$$\frac{12.5 \text{ mg}}{5 \text{ mL}} \diagdown\diagup \frac{40 \text{ mg}}{X \text{ mL}}$$

$$12.5X = 200$$

$$\frac{12.5X}{12.5} = \frac{200}{12.5}$$

$$X = 16 \text{ mL}$$

dimensional analysis

$$X \text{ mL} = \frac{5 \text{ mL}}{12.5 \text{ mg}} \times 40 \text{ mg} = 16 \text{ mL}$$

7) ratio-proportion

$$\frac{500,000 \text{ units}}{2 \text{ mL}} \diagdown\diagup \frac{350,000 \text{ units}}{X \text{ mL}}$$

$$500,000X = 700,000$$

$$\frac{500,000X}{500,000} = \frac{700,000}{500,000}$$

$$X = 1.4 \text{ mL}$$

dimensional analysis

$$X \text{ mL} = \frac{2 \text{ mL}}{500,000 \text{ units}} \times 350,000 \text{ units} = 1.4 \text{ mL}$$

8) ratio-proportion

$$\frac{10 \text{ mg}}{2 \text{ mL}} \diagdown\diagup \frac{3.5 \text{ mg}}{X \text{ mL}}$$

$$10X = 7$$

$$\frac{10X}{10} = \frac{7}{10}$$

$$X = 0.7 \text{ mL}$$

dimensional analysis

$$X \text{ mL} = \frac{2 \text{ mL}}{10 \text{ mg}} \times 3.5 \text{ mg} = 0.7 \text{ mL}$$

9) ratio-proportion

$$\frac{80 \text{ mg}}{2 \text{ mL}} \diagdown\diagup \frac{90 \text{ mg}}{X \text{ mL}}$$

$$80X = 180$$

$$\frac{80X}{80} = \frac{180}{80}$$

$$X = 2.25 \text{ mL} = 2.3 \text{ mL}$$

dimensional analysis

$$X \text{ mL} = \frac{2 \text{ mL}}{80 \text{ mg}} \times 90 \text{ mg} = 2.25 \text{ mL} = 2.3 \text{ mL}$$

13) ratio-proportion

Convert g to mg: 1 g = 1.000 mg

$$\frac{1,000 \text{ mg}}{2.5 \text{ mL}} \diagdown\diagup \frac{500 \text{ mg}}{X \text{ mL}}$$

$$1,000X = 1,250$$

$$\frac{1,000X}{1,000} = \frac{1,250}{1,000}$$

$$X = 1.25 \text{ mL} = 1.3 \text{ mL}$$

dimensional analysis

$$X \text{ mL} = \frac{2.5 \text{ mL}}{1 \text{ g}} \times \frac{1 \text{ g}}{1,000 \text{ mg}} \times 500 \text{ mg} = 1.25 \text{ mL} =$$

1.3 mL

16) ratio-proportion

$$\frac{20 \text{ mEq}}{15 \text{ mL}} \diagdown\diagup \frac{10 \text{ mEq}}{X \text{ mL}}$$

$$20X = 150$$

$$\frac{20X}{20} = \frac{150}{20}$$

$$X = 7.5 \text{ mL}$$

dimensional analysis

$$X \text{ mL} = \frac{15 \text{ mL}}{20 \text{ mEq}} \times 10 \text{ mEq} = 7.5 \text{ mL}$$

18) ratio-proportion

Convert mg to mcg:

$$\frac{1,000 \text{ mcg}}{1 \text{ mg}} \diagdown\diagup \frac{X \text{ mcg}}{0.075 \text{ mg}}$$

$$X = 75 \text{ mcg}$$

$$\frac{75 \text{ mcg}}{1 \text{ tab}} \diagdown\diagup \frac{150 \text{ mcg}}{X \text{ tab}}$$

$$75X = 150$$

$$\frac{75X}{75} = \frac{150}{75}$$

$$X = 2 \text{ tab}$$

dimensional analysis

$$X \text{ tab} = \frac{1 \text{ tab}}{0.075 \text{ mg}} \times \frac{1 \text{ mg}}{1.000 \text{ mcg}} \times 150 \text{ mcg} = \frac{150}{75} \text{ tab}$$

$$= 2 \text{ tab}$$

Section 3—Self-Evaluation from pages 423–436

1) C; 2 **2)** F; 1 **3)** G; 2 **4)** B; 2 **5)** H; 12 **6)** I; 2 **7)** E; 2 **8)** K; 1½ **9)** M; 1.25 **10)** L; 7.5 **11)** E; 4 **12)** C; 3.5 **13)** G; 0.2

14) A; 2 **15)** D; 1.5 **16)** F; 0.75 **17)** B; 0.75 **18)** H; 0.75

19)

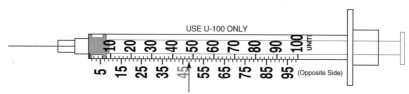

48 units

20)

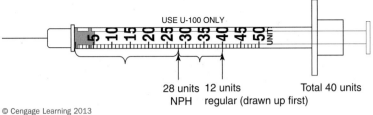

USE U-100 ONLY

28 units NPH   12 units regular (drawn up first)   Total 40 units

© Cengage Learning 2013

21) 4.8; 5; 100; 5

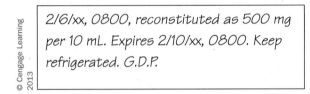

5 mL

© Cengage Learning 2013

22) 10; 10; 500; 10; 8; 1

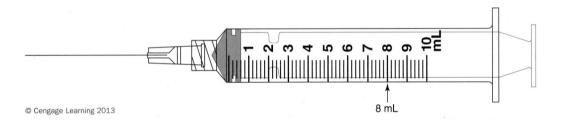

2/6/xx, 0800, reconstituted as 500 mg per 10 mL. Expires 2/10/xx, 0800. Keep refrigerated. G.D.P.

© Cengage Learning 2013

8 mL

© Cengage Learning 2013

23) 2.4; 2.5; 100; 1.5

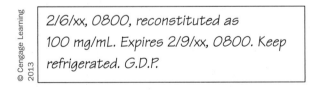

2/6/xx, 0800, reconstituted as 100 mg/mL. Expires 2/9/xx, 0800. Keep refrigerated. G.D.P.

© Cengage Learning 2013

1.5 mL

© Cengage Learning 2013

24) 2.5; 3; 330; 2.3

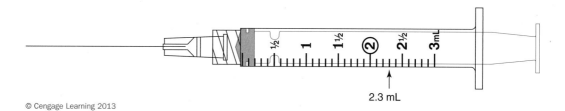

2/6/xx, 0800, reconstituted as 330 mg/mL. Expires 2/7/xx, 0800. Store at room temperature. G.D.P.

© Cengage Learning 2013

25) 8; 8; 62.5; 4; 2

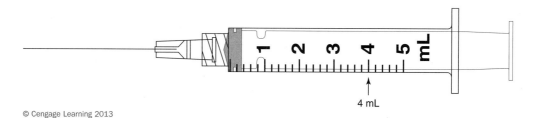

2/6/xx, 0800, reconstituted as 62.5 mg/mL. Expires 2/8/xx, 0800. Keep at controlled room temperature 20–25°C (66-77°F). G.D.P.

© Cengage Learning 2013

26) 29; 50; 100; 5; 20; 5

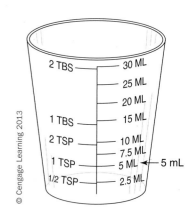

2/6/xx, 0800, reconstituted as 100 mg per 5 mL. Expires 2/20/xx, 0800. Keep refrigerated. G.D.P.

27) 10

28) No; the medication supplied will be used up before it expires. It is good for 14 days under refrigeration. The medication is to be given every 12 hours; therefore, 10 doses will be administered in 5 days.

29) 120; 240 **30)** 180; 60 **31)** 120 **32)** 1 **33)** 3 **34)** 540

35)   0.75

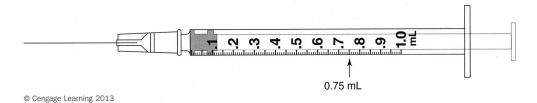

0.75 mL

© Cengage Learning 2013

36)   113; 150; 25; 3

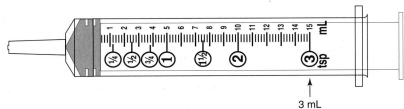

3 mL

© Cengage Learning 2013

37)   Order of 100 mg t.i.d. is too high, and the maximum recommended dosage is 100 mg/day for this child. The order is not safe. Physician should be called for clarification.

38)   Order is too high, and the maximum recommended dosage for this child is 292 mg/day. This order would deliver 748 mg/day. Recommended dosage is also 3 times daily, and this order is for 4 times/daily. This order is not safe. Physician should be called for clarification.

39)   a) Order is too high and is not safe. Recommended dosage is 109.5 mg/day or 36.5 mg/dose. Physician should be called for clarification.

   b) 500

40)   **Prevention:** This type of calculation error occurred because the nurse set up the $\frac{D}{H} \times Q$ formula method incorrectly.

   In this instance, the nurse mixed up the values for *desired* dosage and the dosage you *have* on hand.

   $$\frac{Desired}{Have} \times Quantity = X$$

   $$\frac{50 \text{ mg}}{\underset{25}{125 \text{ mg}}} \times \overset{1}{5} \text{ mL} = \frac{50}{25} \text{ mL} = 2 \text{ mL}$$

   In addition, **think first.** Then use the formula method to calculate the dosage.

41) 0.015; 1 g = 1,000 mg **42)** 52.3, 1 kg = 2.2 lb **43)** 0.625; 1 mg = 1,000 mcg **44)** 300; 1 g = 1,000 mg **45)** 7

46) 1.5 **47)** 10 **48)** 2 **49)** 3 **50)** 3.8 **51)** 1 mL **52)** a, b, c, d **53)** c

54)   Gather information about the drug.

   Inject 2 mL air into the vial of sterile water.

   Withdraw 2 mL sterile water.

   Add 2 mL sterile water to the antibiotic powder.

   Mix the powder and sterile water.

   Withdraw 1 mL antibiotic solution.

55)   B

Solutions—Section 3—Self-Evaluation

5) Order: 16 mEq

Supply: 20 mEq per 15 mL

$$\frac{D}{H} \times Q = \frac{\overset{4}{\cancel{16}\text{ mEq}}}{\underset{5}{\cancel{20}\text{ mEq}}} \times 15\text{ mL} = \frac{4}{\cancel{8}} \times \overset{3}{\cancel{15}}\text{ mL} = 12\text{ mL}$$

7) Order: 0.05 mg = 0.050. = 50 mcg

Supply: 25 mcg/tab

$$\frac{D}{H} \times Q = \frac{\overset{2}{\cancel{50}\text{ mcg}}}{\underset{1}{\cancel{25}\text{ mcg}}} \times 1\text{ tab} = 2\text{ tab}$$

Label N-Synthroid 100 mcg not selected because it is best to give whole tablets when possible rather than trying to split the tablet in half.

8) Order: 45 mg

Supply: 30 mg/tab

$$\frac{D}{H} \times Q = \frac{\overset{3}{\cancel{45}\text{ mg}}}{\underset{2}{\cancel{30}\text{ mg}}} \times 1\text{ tab} = \frac{3}{2}\text{ tab} = 1.5\text{ tab} = 1\tfrac{1}{2}\text{ tab}$$

9) Order: 12.5 mg

Supply: 10 mg/mL

$$\frac{D}{H} \times Q = \frac{12.5\text{ mg}}{10\text{ mg}} \times 1\text{ mL} = \frac{12.5}{10}\text{ mL} = 1.25\text{ mL}$$

Answer should be left at 1.25 mL because the dropper supplied with the medication will measure 1.25 mL. Notice the picture of the dropper on the label.

13) Order: 200 mcg

Supply: 1 mg/mL = 1,000 mcg/mL

$$\frac{D}{H} \times Q = \frac{\overset{2}{\cancel{200}\text{ mcg}}}{\underset{10}{\cancel{1,000}\text{ mcg}}} \times 1\text{ mL} = \frac{2}{10}\text{ mL} = 0.2\text{ mL}$$

17) Order: 7.5 mg

Supply: 10 mg/mL

$$\frac{D}{H} \times Q = \frac{7.5\text{ mg}}{10\text{ mg}} \times 1\text{ mL} = \frac{7.5}{10}\text{ mL} = 0.75\text{ mL}$$

22) Order: 400 mg

Supply: 500 mg per 10 mL

$$\frac{D}{H} \times Q = \frac{\overset{4}{\cancel{400}\text{ mg}}}{\underset{5}{\cancel{500}\text{ mg}}} \times 10\text{ mL} = \frac{40}{5}\text{ mL} = 8\text{ mL}$$

500 mg ÷ 400 mg/dose = 500 mg × 1 dose/400 mg

= 1.25 (doses, or 1 full dose)

25) Order: 250 mg

Supply: $\frac{500\text{ mg}}{8\text{ mL}}$ = 62.5 mg/mL

$$\frac{D}{H} \times Q = \frac{250\text{ mg}}{62.5\text{ mg}} \times 1\text{ mL} = \frac{250}{62.5}\text{ mL} = 4\text{ mL}$$

500 mg vial: 500 mg ÷ 250 mg/dose

= 500 mg × 1 dose/250 mg = 2 doses (full)

29) $D \times Q = \frac{1}{3} \times 360\text{ mL} = 120\text{ mL}$ (hydrogen peroxide); 360 mL (total) − 120 mL (solute) = 240 mL (solvent)

31) 8 fl oz × 30 mL/fl oz = 240 mL

$D \times Q = X$ (solve for Q)

$$\frac{2}{3} \times Q = 240$$

$$\frac{2}{3}Q = 240$$

$$\frac{\frac{2}{3}Q}{\frac{2}{3}} = \frac{240}{\frac{2}{3}}$$

$$Q = 240 \div \frac{2}{3} =$$

$$\frac{\overset{120}{\cancel{240}}}{1} \times \frac{3}{\underset{1}{\cancel{2}}} = 360\text{ mL (total quantity)}$$

360 mL (total) − 240 mL (Ensure) = 120 mL (water)

33) 9 infants require 4 fl oz each = 4 fl oz × 9

= 36 fl oz total

$D \times Q = X$

$\frac{1}{2} \times 36$ fl oz = 18 fl oz (Isomil)

18 fl oz ÷ 8 fl oz/can = 18 fl oz × 1 can/8 fl oz

= $2\tfrac{1}{4}$ cans (you would need to open 3 cans)

34) 36 fl oz total solution − 18 fl oz solute (Isomil) = 18 fl oz solvent (water)

18 fl oz × 30 mL/fl oz = 540 mL (water)

35) 67 lb ÷ 2.2 lb/kg = 67 lb × 1 kg/ 2.2 lb

= 30.45 = 30.5 kg

Recommended dosage:

100 mcg/kg/dose × 30.5 kg = 3.050 mcg (minimum)

200 mcg/kg/dose × 30.5 kg = 6,100 mcg (maximum)

Order: 6 mg; 6 mg = 6.000. = 6.000 mcg

This dosage is safe.

$$\frac{D}{H} \times Q = \frac{6\text{ mg}}{8\text{ mg}} \times 1\text{ mL} = \frac{6}{8}\text{ mL} = 0.75\text{ mL}$$

36) 15 lb ÷ 2.2 lb/kg = 15 lb × 1 kg/ 2.2 lb

= 6.81 kg = 6.8 kg

Minimum daily dosage:

20 mg/kg/day × 6.8 kg = 136 mg/day

Minimum single dosage:

136 mg ÷ 3 doses = 45.3 mg/dose

Maximum daily dosage:

40 mg/kg/day × 6.8 kg = 272 mg/day

Maximum single dosage:

272 mg ÷ 3 doses = 90.7 mg/dose

Dosage ordered is safe.

$$\frac{D}{H} \times Q = \frac{75 \text{ mg}}{125 \text{ mg}} \times 5 \text{ mL} = \frac{375}{125} \text{ mL} = 3 \text{ mL}$$

37) Recommended dosage:

5 mg/kg/day × 20 kg = 100 mg/day

100 mg ÷ 3 doses = 33.3 mg/dose

Order of 100 mg t.i.d. is not safe. It is higher than the recommended dosage of 33.3 mg/dose.

38) 16 lb ÷ 2.2 lb/kg = 16 lb × 1 kg/ 2.2 lb

= 7.27 kg = 7.3 kg

Recommended dosage:

40 mg/kg/day × 7.3 kg = 292 mg/day

Ordered dosage is not safe. The child would receive 187 mg × 4 doses, or a total of 748 mg/day, which is over the recommended dosage of 292 mg/day.

39 a) 16 lb ÷ 2.2 lb/kg = 16 lb × 1 kg/2.2 lb

= 7.27 kg = 7.3 kg

Recommended dosage:

15 mg/kg/day × 7.3 kg = 109.5 mg/day

109.5 mg ÷ 3 doses = 36.5 mg/dose

Dosage ordered is 60 mg q.8h, which is over the recommended dosage of 36.5 mg/dose. Although the total daily dosage is within limits, the q.8h dosage is too high and is not safe.

39 b) 275 lb ÷ 2.2 lb/kg = 275 lb × 1 kg/2.2 lb

= 125 kg

15 mg/kg/day × 125 kg = 1,875 mg/day

Because 1,875 mg/day or 1.9 g/day exceeds the recommended maximum dose of 1.5 g/day, you would expect the order for this adult to be the maximum recommended dosage of 1.5 g/day or 1,500 mg/day. That could be divided into 3 doses of 0.5 g q.8h or 500 mg q.8h.

41) Equivalent: 1 g = 1,000 mg

$$\frac{1 \text{ g}}{1,000 \text{ mg}} \diagdown\hspace{-1.6em}\diagup \frac{X \text{ g}}{15 \text{ mg}}$$

1,000X = 15

$$\frac{1,000X}{1,000} = \frac{15}{1,000}$$

X = 0.015 g

45) Order: 175 mg

Supply: 25 mg/mL

ratio-proportion

$$\frac{25 \text{ mg}}{1 \text{ mL}} \diagdown\hspace{-1.6em}\diagup \frac{175 \text{ mg}}{X \text{ mL}}$$

25X = 175

$$\frac{25X}{25} = \frac{175}{25}$$

X = 7 mL

dimensional analysis

$$X \text{ mL} = \frac{1 \text{ mL}}{25 \text{ mg}} \times 175 \text{ mg} = 7 \text{ mL}$$

48) Order: 600 mcg

Supply: 0.3 mg/tab

ratio-proportion

Convert: 1 mg = 1,000 mcg

$$\frac{1 \text{ mg}}{1,000 \text{ mcg}} \diagdown\hspace{-1.6em}\diagup \frac{0.3 \text{ mg}}{X \text{ mcg}}$$

X = 300 mcg

$$\frac{300 \text{ mcg}}{1 \text{ tab}} = \frac{600 \text{ mcg}}{X \text{ tab}}$$

300X = 600

$$\frac{300X}{300} = \frac{600}{300}$$

X = 2 tab

dimensional analysis

$$X \text{ tab} = \frac{1 \text{ tab}}{0.3 \text{ mg}} \times \frac{1 \text{ mg}}{1,000 \text{ mcg}} \times 600 \text{ mcg}$$

$$= \frac{600}{300} \text{ tab} = 2 \text{ tab}$$

Review Set 32 from pages 433–445

1) C; sodium chloride 0.9%, 0.9 g per 100 mL; 308 mOsm/L; isotonic

2) E; dextrose 5%, 5 g per 100 mL; 252 mOsm/L; isotonic

3) G; dextrose 5%, 5 g per 100 mL; sodium chloride 0.9%, 0.9 g per 100 mL; 560 mOsm/L; hypertonic

4) D; dextrose 5%, 5 g per 100 mL, sodium chloride 0.45%, 0.45 g per 100 mL; 406 mOsm/L; hypertonic

5) A; dextrose 5%, 5 g per 100 mL, sodium chloride 0.225%, 0.225 g per 100 mL; 329 mOsm/L; isotonic

6)   H; dextrose 5%, 5 g per 100 mL; sodium lactate 0.31 g per 100 mL, NaCl 0.6 g per 100 mL; KCl 0.03 g per 100 mL; CaCl 0.02 g per 100 mL; 525 mOsm/L; hypertonic

7)   B; dextrose 5%, 5 g per 100 mL; sodium chloride 0.45%; 0.45 g per 100 mL; potassium chloride 20 mEq per liter (0.149 g per 100 mL); 447 mOsm/L; hypertonic

8)   F; sodium chloride 0.45%, 0.45 g per 100 mL; 154 mOsm/L; hypotonic

Review Set 33 from page 447

1) 50; 9 **2)** 25; 2.25 **3)** 25 **4)** 6.75 **5)** 25; 1.125 **6)** 150; 27 **7)** 50; 1.125 **8)** 36; 2.7 **9)** 100; 4.5 **10)** 3.375

Solutions—Review Set 33

1) D_5NS = 5 g dextrose per 100 mL

and 0.9 g NaCl per 100 mL

Dextrose:

$$\frac{5\text{ g}}{100\text{ mL}} \diagdown\!\!\!\!\!\diagup \frac{X\text{ g}}{1,000\text{ mL}}$$

$$100X = 5,000$$

$$\frac{100X}{100} = \frac{5,000}{100}$$

$$X = 50\text{ g (dextrose)}$$

NaCl:

$$\frac{0.9\text{ g}}{100\text{ mL}} \diagdown\!\!\!\!\!\diagup \frac{X\text{ g}}{1,000\text{ mL}}$$

$$100X = 900$$

$$\frac{100X}{100} = \frac{900}{100}$$

$$X = 9\text{ g (NaCl)}$$

7) $D_{10}\frac{1}{4}NS$ = 10 g dextrose per 100 mL and 0.225 g NaCl per 100 mL

$$0.5\text{ L} = 0.5\text{ L} \times 1,000\text{ mL/L} = 500\text{ mL}$$

Dextrose:

$$\frac{10\text{ g}}{100\text{ mL}} \diagdown\!\!\!\!\!\diagup \frac{X\text{ g}}{500\text{ mL}}$$

$$100X = 5,000$$

$$\frac{100X}{100} = \frac{5,000}{100}$$

$$X = 50\text{ g (dextrose)}$$

NaCl:

$$\frac{0.225\text{ g}}{100\text{ mL}} \diagdown\!\!\!\!\!\diagup \frac{X\text{ g}}{500\text{ mL}}$$

$$100X = 112.5$$

$$\frac{100X}{100} = \frac{112.5}{100}$$

$$X = 1.125\text{ g (NaCl)}$$

Review Set 34 from pages 457–458

1) 100 **2)** 120 **3)** 83 **4)** 200 **5)** 120 **6)** 125 **7)** 125 **8)** 200 **9)** 75 **10)** 125 **11)** 63 **12)** 24 **13)** 150 **14)** 125 **15)** 42

Solutions—Review Set 34

1)   1 L = 1,000 mL

$$\frac{\text{Total mL}}{\text{Total h}} = \frac{1,000\text{ mL}}{10\text{ h}} = 100\text{ mL/h}$$

3) $\frac{\text{Total mL}}{\text{Total h}} = \frac{2,000\text{ mL}}{24\text{ h}} = 83.3\text{ mL/h} = 83\text{ mL/h}$

4) $\frac{100\text{ mL}}{\cancel{30\text{ min}}_{1}} \times \cancel{60\text{ min}}^{\,2}\text{/h} = 200\text{ mL/h}$

5) $\frac{30\text{ mL}}{\cancel{15\text{ min}}_{1}} \times \cancel{60\text{ min}}^{\,4}\text{/h} = 120\text{ mL/h}$

6)   2.5 L = 2.500 = 2,500 mL

$$\frac{\text{Total mL}}{\text{Total h}} = \frac{2,500\text{ mL}}{20\text{ h}} = 125\text{ mL/h}$$

Review Set 35 from pages 459–460

1) 15 **2)** 10 **3)** 60 **4)** 60 **5)** 10

Review Set 36 from pages 463–464

1) $\frac{V}{T} \times C = R$ **2)** 21 **3)** 50 **4)** 33 **5)** 25 **6)** 83 **7)** 42 **8)** 50 **9)** 50 **10)** 80 **11)** 20 **12)** 30 **13)** 17 **14)** 55 **15)** 40

Solutions—Review Set 36

1) $\frac{V}{T} \times C = R$ or $\frac{\text{Volume}}{\text{Time in min}} \times \text{Drop factor} = \text{Rate}$

Volume in mL divided by *time* in minutes, multiplied

by the *drop factor calibration* in drops per milliliter,

equals the flow *rate* in drops per minute.

2) $\frac{V}{T} \times C = \frac{125 \text{ mL}}{\overset{}{\underset{6}{60} \text{ min}}} \times \overset{1}{10} \text{ gtt/mL} = \frac{125 \text{ gtt}}{6 \text{ min}} = 20.8 \text{ gtt/min}$

$= 21 \text{ gtt/min}$

3) $\frac{V}{T} \times C = \frac{50 \text{ mL}}{\underset{1}{60} \text{ min}} \times \overset{1}{60} \text{ gtt/mL} = 50 \text{ gtt/min}$

Recall that when drop factor is 60 mL/h,

then number of mL/h = number of gtt/min.

4) $\frac{V}{T} \times C = \frac{100 \text{ mL}}{\underset{3}{60} \text{ min}} \times \overset{1}{20} \text{ gtt/mL} = \frac{100 \text{ gtt}}{3 \text{ min}} = 33.3 \text{ gtt/min}$

$= 33 \text{ gtt/min}$

6) Two 500 mL units of blood = 1,000 mL total

volume

$\text{mL/h} = \frac{1{,}000 \text{ mL}}{4 \text{ h}} = 250 \text{ mL/h}$

$\frac{V}{T} \times C = \frac{250 \text{ mL}}{\underset{3}{60} \text{ min}} \times \overset{1}{20} \text{ gtt/mL} = \frac{250 \text{ gtt}}{3 \text{ min}}$

$= 83.3 \text{ gtt/min} = 83 \text{ gtt/min}$

7) $\frac{\text{Total mL}}{\text{Total h}} = \frac{1{,}000 \text{ mL}}{6 \text{ h}} = 166.6 \text{ mL/h} = 167 \text{ mL/h}$

$\frac{V}{T} \times C = \frac{167 \text{ mL}}{\underset{4}{60} \text{ min}} \times \overset{1}{15} \text{ gtt/mL} = \frac{167 \text{ gtt}}{4 \text{ min}}$

$= 41.7 \text{ gtt/min} = 42 \text{ gtt/min}$

9) $\frac{150 \text{ mL}}{\underset{3}{45} \text{ min}} \times \overset{1}{15} \text{ gtt/mL} = \frac{\overset{50}{150} \text{ gtt}}{\underset{1}{3} \text{ min}} = 50 \text{ gtt/min}$

Review Set 37 from pages 466–467

1) 60 **2)** 1 **3)** 3 **4)** 4 **5)** 6 **6)** $\frac{\text{mL/h}}{\text{Drop factor constant}} = \text{gtt/min}$ **7)** 50 **8)** 42 **9)** 28 **10)** 60 **11)** 8 **12)** 31 **13)** 28
14) 25 **15)** 11

Solutions—Review Set 37

4) $\frac{60}{15} = 4$

7) $\frac{\text{mL/h}}{\text{Drop factor constant}} = \text{gtt/min};$ $\frac{200 \text{ mL/h}}{4} = 50 \text{ gtt/min}$

8) $\frac{\text{mL/h}}{\text{Drop factor constant}} = \text{gtt/min};$ $\frac{125 \text{ mL/h}}{3} = 41.6 \text{ gtt/min}$
$= 42 \text{ gtt/min}$

9) $\frac{\text{mL/h}}{\text{Drop factor constant}} = \text{gtt/min};$ $\frac{165 \text{ mL/h}}{6} = 27.5 \text{ gtt/min}$
$= 28 \text{ gtt/min}$

10) $\frac{\text{mL/h}}{\text{Drop factor constant}} = \text{gtt/min};$ $\frac{60 \text{ mL/h}}{1} = 60 \text{ gtt/min}$

(Set the flow rate at the same number of gtt/min as

the number of mL/h when the drop factor is 60 gtt/mL,

because the drop factor constant is 1.)

14) 0.5 L = 500 mL; $\frac{500 \text{ mL}}{20 \text{ h}} = 25 \text{ mL/h}$; because

when the drop factor is 60 gtt/mL, then number of

mL/h = number of gtt/min, so the rate is 25 gtt/min

15) $\frac{650 \text{ mL}}{10 \text{ h}} = 65 \text{ mL/h}$

$\frac{\text{mL/h}}{\text{Drop factor constant}} = \text{gtt/min};$ $\frac{65 \text{ mL/h}}{6} = 10.8 \text{ gtt/min}$
$= 11 \text{ gtt/min}$

Review Set 38 from pages 467–468

1) 125; 31 **2)** 100 **3)** 100; 33 **4)** 50 **5)** 125; 31 **6)** 125; 125 **7)** 35 **8)** 17 **9)** 25 **10)** 125 **11)** 83 **12)** 125 **13)** 200
14) 150 **15)** 200 **16)** 13.5 **17)** 20; 1.8 **18)** 22.5 **19)** 32.5; 2.925 **20)** 50; 2.25

Solutions—Review Set 38

1) $\dfrac{\text{Total mL}}{\text{Total h}} = \dfrac{3{,}000\text{ mL}}{24\text{ h}} = 125\text{ mL/h}$

$\dfrac{V}{T} \times C = \dfrac{125\ \cancel{\text{mL}}}{\cancelto{4}{60}\text{ min}} \times \cancelto{1}{15}\text{ gtt/}\cancel{\text{mL}} = \dfrac{125\text{ gtt}}{4\text{ min}} = 31.2\text{ gtt/min}$

$= 31\text{ gtt/min}$

7) $\dfrac{\text{mL/h}}{\text{Drop factor constant}} = \text{gtt/min};\ \dfrac{105\text{ mL/h}}{3} = 35\text{ gtt/min}$

8) $\dfrac{\text{mL/h}}{\text{Drop factor constant}} = \text{gtt/min};\ \dfrac{100\text{ mL/h}}{6} = 16.6\text{ gtt/min}$

$= 17\text{ gtt/min}$

10) $\dfrac{\text{Total mL}}{\text{Total h}} = \dfrac{1{,}000\text{ mL}}{8\text{ h}} = 125\text{ mL/h}$

13) $\dfrac{100\text{ mL}}{\cancelto{1}{30}\ \text{min}} \times \cancelto{2}{60}\ \text{min/h} = 200\text{ mL/h}$

15) $\dfrac{150\text{ mL}}{\cancelto{3}{45}\ \text{min}} \times \cancelto{4}{60}\ \text{min/h} = 200\text{ mL/h}$

16) $\frac{1}{2}\text{NS} = 0.45\% \text{ NaCl} = 0.45\text{ g NaCl per 100 mL}$

$\dfrac{0.45\text{ g}}{100\text{ mL}} \diagdown\!\!\!\!\diagup \dfrac{X\text{ g}}{3{,}000\text{ mL}}$

$100X = 1{,}350$

$\dfrac{100X}{100} = \dfrac{1{,}350}{100}$

$X = 13.5\text{ g (NaCl)}$

17) $D_{10} = 10\% \text{ dextrose} = 10\text{ g dextrose per 100 mL}$

Dextrose:

$\dfrac{10\text{ g}}{100\text{ mL}} \diagdown\!\!\!\!\diagup \dfrac{X\text{ g}}{200\text{ mL}}$

$100X = 2{,}000$

$\dfrac{100X}{100} = \dfrac{2{,}000}{100}$

$X = 20\text{ g (dextrose)}$

$NS = 0.9\% \text{ NaCl} = 0.9\text{ g NaCl per 100 mL}$

NaCl:

$\dfrac{0.9\text{ g}}{100\text{ mL}} \diagdown\!\!\!\!\diagup \dfrac{X\text{ g}}{200\text{ mL}}$

$100X = 180$

$\dfrac{100X}{100} = \dfrac{180}{100}$

$X = 1.8\text{ g (NaCl)}$

Review Set 39 from pages 471–474

1) 42; 6; 142; 47; 12%; reset to 47 gtt/min (12% increase is acceptable)

2) 42; 2; 180; 45; 7%; reset to 45 gtt/min (7% increase is acceptable)

3) 42; 4; 200; 67; 60%; recalculated rate is 67 gtt/min; 60% increase is unacceptable—consult physician

4) 28; 4; 188; 31; 11%; reset to 31 gtt/min (11% increase is acceptable)

5) 21; 4; 188; 31; 48%; 48% increase is unacceptable—consult physician

6) 31; 1,350; 10; 135; 34; 10%; reset to 34 gtt/min (10% increase is acceptable)

7) 50; 3; 233; 78; 56%; 56% increase is unacceptable—consult physician

8) 33; 3; 83; 28; −15%; −15% slower is acceptable, IV is ahead of schedule, slow rate to 28 gtt/min and observe patient's condition

9) 13; 10; 60; 15; 15%; reset to 15 gtt/min (15% increase is acceptable)

10) 100; 5; 100; 100; 0%; IV is on time, so no adjustment is needed

Solutions—Review Set 39

1) $\dfrac{V}{T} \times C = \dfrac{125\text{ mL}}{\underset{3}{\cancel{60}}\text{ min}} \times \overset{1}{\cancel{20}}\text{ gtt/mL} = \dfrac{125\text{ gtt}}{3\text{ min}} = 41.6\text{ gtt/min} = 42\text{ gtt/min (ordered rate)}$

$12\text{ h} - 6\text{ h} = 6\text{ h}$

$\dfrac{\text{Remaining volume}}{\text{Remaining hours}} = \text{Recalculated mL/h}; \ \dfrac{850\text{ mL}}{6\text{ h}} = 141.6\text{ mL/h} = 142\text{ mL/h}$

$\dfrac{V}{T} \times C = \dfrac{142\text{ mL}}{\underset{3}{\cancel{60}}\text{ min}} \times \overset{1}{\cancel{20}}\text{ gtt/mL} = \dfrac{142\text{ gtt}}{3\text{ min}} = 47.3\text{ gtt/min} = 47\text{ gtt/min (adjusted rate)}$

$\dfrac{\text{Adjusted gtt/min} - \text{Ordered gtt/min}}{\text{Ordered gtt/min}} = \%\text{ of variation}; \ \dfrac{47 - 42}{42} = \dfrac{5}{42} = 0.119 = 0.12 = 12\%$ (within the acceptable

% of variation); reset rate to 47 gtt/min

3) $\dfrac{V}{T} \times C = \dfrac{125\text{ mL}}{\underset{3}{\cancel{60}}\text{ min}} \times \overset{1}{\cancel{20}}\text{ gtt/mL} = \dfrac{125\text{ gtt}}{3\text{ min}} = 41.6\text{ gtt/min} = 42\text{ gtt/min (ordered rate)}$

$8\text{ h} - 4\text{ h} = 4\text{ h}$

$\dfrac{800\text{ mL}}{4\text{ h}} = 200\text{ mL/h}; \ \dfrac{V}{T} \times C = \dfrac{200\text{ mL}}{\underset{3}{\cancel{60}}\text{ min}} \times \overset{1}{\cancel{20}}\text{ gtt/mL} = \dfrac{200\text{ gtt}}{3\text{ min}} = 66.6\text{ gtt/min} = 67\text{ gtt/min (adjusted rate)}$

$\dfrac{\text{Adjusted gtt/min} - \text{Ordered gtt/min}}{\text{Ordered gtt/min}} = \%\text{ of variation}; \ \dfrac{67 - 42}{42} = \dfrac{25}{42} = 0.595 = 0.6 = 60\%$ faster;

unacceptable % of variation—call physician for a revised order

6) $\dfrac{V}{T} \times C = \dfrac{125\text{ mL}}{\underset{4}{\cancel{60}}\text{ min}} \times \overset{1}{\cancel{15}}\text{ gtt/mL} = \dfrac{125\text{ gtt}}{4\text{ min}} = 31.2\text{ gtt/min} = 31\text{ gtt/min (ordered rate)}$

$2{,}000\text{ mL} - 650\text{ mL} = 1{,}350\text{ mL remaining}; \ 16\text{ h} - 6\text{ h} = 10\text{ h}$

$\dfrac{1{,}350\text{ mL}}{10\text{ h}} = 135\text{ mL/h}; \ \dfrac{V}{T} \times C = \dfrac{135\text{ mL}}{\underset{4}{\cancel{60}}\text{ min}} \times \overset{1}{\cancel{15}}\text{ gtt/mL} = \dfrac{135\text{ gtt}}{4\text{ min}} = 33.7\text{ gtt/min} = 34\text{ gtt/min}$

$\dfrac{\text{Adjusted gtt/min} - \text{Ordered gtt/min}}{\text{Ordered gtt/min}} = \%\text{ of variation}; \ \dfrac{34 - 31}{31} = \dfrac{3}{31} = 0.096 = 0.10 = 10\%$

(within acceptable % of variation); reset rate to 34 gtt/min

8) $\dfrac{V}{T} \times C = \dfrac{100\text{ mL}}{\underset{3}{\cancel{60}}\text{ min}} \times \overset{1}{\cancel{20}}\text{ gtt/mL} = \dfrac{100\text{ gtt}}{3\text{ min}} = 33.3\text{ gtt/min} = 33\text{ gtt/min (ordered rate)}$

$5\text{ h} - 2\text{ h} = 3\text{ h}$

$\dfrac{250\text{ mL}}{3\text{ h}} = 83.3\text{ mL/h} = 83\text{ mL/h};$

$\dfrac{V}{T} \times C = \dfrac{83\text{ mL}}{\underset{3}{\cancel{60}}\text{ min}} \times \overset{1}{\cancel{20}}\text{ gtt/mL} = \dfrac{83\text{ gtt}}{3\text{ min}} = 27.6\text{ gtt/min} = 28\text{ gtt/min (adjusted rate)}$

$\dfrac{\text{Adjusted gtt/min} - \text{Ordered gtt/min}}{\text{Ordered gtt/min}} = \%\text{ of variation}; \ \dfrac{28 - 33}{33} = \dfrac{-5}{33} = -0.151 = -0.15 = -15\%$

(Remember that the minus sign indicates the IV is ahead of schedule and rate must be decreased.) Within the

acceptable % of variation. Slow IV to 28 gtt/min and closely monitor patient.

Review Set 40 from pages 479–480

1) 133 **2)** 133 **3)** 50 **4)** 200 **5)** 100 **6)** 25 **7)** 50 **8)** 200 **9)** 150 **10)** 167 **11)** 133 **12)** 25 **13)** 120 **14)** 56 **15)** 200
16) 12; 3; 1 **17)** 3; 3; 0.25 **18)** 0.6; 2.4; 0.06 **19)** 2; 18; 10; 2.5 **20)** 1.5; 0.75; 0.19

Solutions—Review Set 40

1) $\dfrac{V}{T} \times C = \dfrac{100 \text{ mL}}{\underset{3}{45} \text{ min}} \times \overset{4}{60} \text{ gtt/mL} = \dfrac{400 \text{ gtt}}{3 \text{ min}} = 133.3 \text{ gtt/min}$

   $= 133 \text{ gtt/min}$

2) $\dfrac{\text{Total mL ordered}}{\text{Total min ordered}} \times 60 \text{ min/h} = \text{mL/h}$

   $\dfrac{100 \text{ mL}}{\underset{3}{45} \text{ min}} \times \overset{4}{60} \text{ min/h} = \dfrac{400}{3} = 133.3 \text{ mL/h} = 133 \text{ mL/h}$

3) $\dfrac{V}{T} \times C = \dfrac{50 \text{ mL}}{\underset{1}{15} \text{ min}} \times \overset{1}{15} \text{ gtt/mL} = 50 \text{ gtt/min}$

4) $\dfrac{\text{Total mL ordered}}{\text{Total min ordered}} \times 60 \text{ min/h} = \text{mL/h}$

   $\dfrac{50 \text{ mL}}{\underset{1}{15} \text{ min}} \times \overset{4}{60} \text{ min/h} = 200 \text{ mL/h}$

11) $\dfrac{V}{T} \times C = \dfrac{100 \text{ mL}}{\underset{3}{15} \text{ min}} \times \overset{4}{20} \text{ gtt/mL} = \dfrac{400 \text{ gtt}}{3 \text{ min}} = 133.3 \text{ gtt/min}$

   $= 133 \text{ gtt/min}$

16) $\dfrac{D}{H} \times Q = \dfrac{120 \text{ mg}}{10 \text{ mg}} \times 1 \text{ mL} = 12 \text{ mL}$

   $\dfrac{D}{H} \times T = \dfrac{\overset{3}{120} \text{ mg}}{\underset{1}{40} \text{ mg}} \times 1 \text{ min} = 3 \text{ min}$

   Administer 12 mL over at least 3 min.

   1 min = 60 sec

   3 min × 60 sec/min = 180 sec

   $\dfrac{12 \text{ mL}}{180 \text{ sec}} \diagdown\!\!\!\!\!\diagup \dfrac{X \text{ mL}}{15 \text{ sec}}$

   $180X = 180$

   $\dfrac{180X}{180} = \dfrac{180}{180}$

   $X = 1 \text{ mL (per 15 sec)}$

17) $\dfrac{D}{H} \times Q = \dfrac{150 \text{ mg}}{\underset{50}{250} \text{ mg}} \times \overset{1}{5} \text{ mL} = \dfrac{\overset{3}{150}}{\underset{1}{50}} \text{ mL} = 3 \text{ mL}$

   $\dfrac{D}{H} \times T = \dfrac{\overset{3}{150} \text{ mg}}{\underset{1}{50} \text{ mg}} \times 1 \text{ min} = 3 \text{ min}$

   Administer 3 mL over 3 min.

   1 min = 60 sec

   3 min × 60 sec/min = 180 sec

   $\dfrac{3 \text{ mL}}{180 \text{ sec}} \diagdown\!\!\!\!\!\diagup \dfrac{X \text{ mL}}{15 \text{ sec}}$

   $180X = 45$

   $\dfrac{180X}{180} = \dfrac{45}{180}$

   $X = 0.25 \text{ mL (per 15 sec)}$

18) $\dfrac{D}{H} \times Q = \dfrac{6 \text{ mg}}{10 \text{ mg}} \times 1 \text{ mL} = \dfrac{6}{10} \text{ mL} = 0.6 \text{ mL}$

   $\dfrac{D}{H} \times T = \dfrac{6 \text{ mg}}{2.5 \text{ mg}} \times 1 \text{ min} = 2.4 \text{ min}$

   1 min = 60 sec

   2.4 min × 60 sec/min = 144 sec;

   $\dfrac{0.6 \text{ mL}}{144 \text{ sec}} \diagdown\!\!\!\!\!\diagup \dfrac{X \text{ mL}}{15 \text{ sec}}$

   $144X = 9$

   $\dfrac{144X}{144} = \dfrac{9}{144}$

   $X = 0.062 \text{ mL}$

   $X = 0.06 \text{ mL (per 15 sec)}$

Review Set 41 from pages 481–482

1) 5 h and 33 min **2)** 10 h **3)** 6 h and 24 min **4)** 12; 0400 the next morning **5)** 16; 0730 the next morning **6)** 3,000

7) 260 **8)** 300 **9)** 600 **10)** 360; 2400 (midnight)

Solutions—Review Set 41

1) Time $= \dfrac{\text{Total volume}}{\text{mL/h}} = \text{Total h}$

   $\dfrac{500 \text{ mL}}{90 \text{ mL/h}} = 5.55 \text{ h}$

   $0.55 \text{ h} \times 60 \text{ min/h} = 33 \text{ min}$

   $5.5 \text{ h} = 5 \text{ h and } 33 \text{ min}$

2) Time $= \dfrac{\text{Total volume}}{\text{mL/h}} = \text{Total h}$

   $\dfrac{\overset{10}{1,000} \text{ mL}}{\underset{1}{100} \text{ mL/h}} = 10 \text{ h}$

4) Time $= \dfrac{\text{Total volume}}{\text{mL/h}} = \text{Total h}$

   $\dfrac{1,200 \text{ mL}}{100 \text{ mL/h}} = 12 \text{ h}$

   2400 h − 1600 h = 8 h (until midnight)

   12 h − 8 h = 4 h (into next day)

   Completion time = 0400 (the next morning)

   Hint: Go back to Chapter 5, Figure 5-1, and look at the 24-hour clock.

5) $\text{Time} = \dfrac{\text{Total volume}}{\text{mL/h}} = \text{Total h}$

$\dfrac{2{,}000 \ \cancel{\text{mL}}}{125 \ \cancel{\text{mL}}/\text{h}} = 16 \text{ h}$

$$2400 \text{ h} = 23 \text{ h and } 60 \text{ min}$$

$$23 \text{ h } 60 \text{ min} - 15 \text{ h } 30 \text{ min} = 8 \text{ h } 30 \text{ min (until midnight)}$$

$$16 \text{ h} = 15 \text{ h and } 60 \text{ min}$$

$$15 \text{ h } 60 \text{ min} - 8 \text{ h } 30 \text{ min} = 7 \text{ h } 30 \text{ min (into the next day)}$$

$$\text{Completion time} = 0730 \text{ (the next morning)}$$

6)   Total hours $\times$ mL/h = Total volume

24 $\cancel{\text{h}}$ $\times$ 125 mL/$\cancel{\text{h}}$ = 3,000 mL

7)   Total hours $\times$ mL/h = Total volume

4 $\cancel{\text{h}}$ $\times$ 65 mL/$\cancel{\text{h}}$ = 260 mL

Practice Problems—Chapter 15 from pages 484–487

1) 17 **2)** 42 **3)** 42 **4)** 8 **5)** 125 **6)** Assess your patient and the pump. If the pump is programmed at 125 mL/h and is plugged in, discontinue the IV pump and confer with your supervisor to implement your backup plan. **7)** 31 **8)** 42
9) Assess patient. If stable, recalculate and reset to 50 gtt/min; observe patient closely. **10)** 3,000 **11)** Abbott Laboratories
12) 15 gtt/mL **13)** 4

14) $\text{mL/h} = \dfrac{500 \text{ mL}}{4 \text{ h}} = 125 \text{ mL/h}$

$\dfrac{\text{mL/h}}{\text{Drop factor constant}} = \text{gtt/min}: \ \dfrac{125 \text{ mL/h}}{4} = 31.2 \text{ gtt/min} = 31 \text{ gtt/min}$

15) $\dfrac{\text{V}}{\text{T}} \times \text{C} = \dfrac{125 \ \cancel{\text{mL}}}{\underset{4}{\cancel{60}} \text{ min}} \times \overset{1}{\cancel{15}} \text{ gtt/}\cancel{\text{mL}} = \dfrac{125 \text{ gtt}}{4 \text{ min}} = 31.2 \text{ gtt/min} = 31 \text{ gtt/min}$

16) 1930 (or 7:30 PM) **17)** 250 **18)** Recalculate 210 mL to infuse over remaining 2 hours. Reset IV to 26 gtt/min and observe patient closely. **19)** 125 **20)** 100 **21)** Dextrose 2.5% (2.5 g per 100 mL) and NaCl 0.45% (0.45 g per 100 mL)
22) 25; 4.5 **23)** A central line is a special catheter inserted to access a large vein in the chest. **24)** A primary line is the IV tubing used to set up a primary IV infusion. **25)** The purpose of a saline/heparin lock is to administer IV medications when the patient does not require continuous IV fluids. **26)** 10; 5; 0.5; 0.13 **27)** The purpose of the PCA pump is to allow the patient to safely self-administer IV pain medication without having to call the nurse for a p.r.n. medication.
28) Advantages of the syringe pump are that a small amount of medication can be delivered directly from the syringe and a specified time can be programmed in the pump. **29)** Phlebitis and infiltration **30)** every 30 min to 1 h, according to hospital policy **31)** This IV tubing has two spikes—one for blood, the other for saline—that join at a common drip chamber, or Y connection. **32)** 14 **33)** 21 **34)** 28 **35)** 83 **36)** 17 **37)** 25 **38)** 33 **39)** 100 **40)** 33 **41)** 50 **42)** 67 **43)** 200
44) 8 **45)** 11 **46)** 15 **47)** 45 **48)** 62.5 mL. The IV will finish in less than 30 minutes. IV will run out. Advise relief nurse to monitor IV, discontinue bag when complete, and plan to flush and cap the saline lock. **49)** 1250 (or 12:50 PM)
50) Prevention: This error could have been prevented had the nurse carefully inspected the IV tubing package to determine the drop factor. Every IV tubing set has the drop factor printed on the package, so it is not necessary to memorize or guess the drop factor. The IV calculation should have looked like this:

$\dfrac{\text{V}}{\text{T}} \times \text{C} = \dfrac{125 \ \cancel{\text{mL}}}{\underset{3}{\cancel{60}} \text{ min}} \times \overset{1}{\cancel{20}} \text{ gtt/}\cancel{\text{mL}} = \dfrac{125 \text{ gtt}}{3 \text{ min}} = 41.6 \text{ gtt/min} = 42 \text{ gtt/min}$

With the infusion set of 20 gtt/mL, a flow rate of 42 gtt/min would infuse 125 mL/h. At the 125 gtt/min rate the nurse calculated, the patient received three times the IV fluid ordered hourly. Thus, the patient actually received 375 mL/h of IV fluids.

Solutions—Practice Problems—Chapter 15

1) 100 mL/h = 100 mL per 60 min

$$\frac{V}{T} \times C = \frac{100 \ \cancel{mL}}{\underset{6}{\cancel{60}} \ min} \times \overset{1}{\cancel{10}} \ gtt/\cancel{mL} = \frac{100 \ gtt}{6 \ min} = 16.6 \ gtt/min$$

$$= 17 \ gtt/min$$

2) $\dfrac{Total \ mL}{Total \ h} = \dfrac{1{,}000 \ mL}{24 \ h} = 41.6 \ mL/h = 42 \ mL/h$

drop factor is 60 gtt/mL; 42 mL/h = 42 gtt/min

5) 1800 − 1000 = 800, or 8 h

$$\frac{Total \ mL}{Total \ h} = \frac{1{,}000 \ mL}{8 \ h} = 125 \ mL/h$$

6) After 1 h, there should be 875 mL remaining (1,000 mL − 125 mL = 875 mL). The IV is running too fast and is ahead of schedule. Assess your patient and the pump. Confirm that the IV pump is correctly programmed for 125 mL/h, and check to be sure that it is plugged in. If so, consider that it may need recalibration or that it has a mechanical or electrical failure. Discontinue the IV pump and confer with your supervisor to implement your backup plan: replace the IV pump with another one or with a straight gravity-flow IV system until another IV pump can be located.

7) 1,000 mL + 2,000 mL = 3,000 mL;

$$\frac{Total \ mL}{Total \ h} = \frac{3{,}000 \ mL}{24 \ h} = 125 \ mL/h$$

$$\frac{V}{T} \times C = \frac{125 \ \cancel{mL}}{\underset{4}{\cancel{60}} \ min} \times \overset{1}{\cancel{15}} \ gtt/\cancel{mL} = \frac{125 \ gtt}{4 \ min} = 31.2 \ gtt/min$$

$$= 31 \ gtt/min$$

8) $\dfrac{V}{T} \times C = \dfrac{125 \ \cancel{mL}}{\underset{3}{\cancel{60}} \ min} \times \overset{1}{\cancel{20}} \ gtt/\cancel{mL} = \dfrac{125 \ gtt}{3 \ min}$

$$= 41.6 \ gtt/min = 42 \ gtt/min$$

9) $\dfrac{Total \ mL}{Total \ h} = \dfrac{1{,}000 \ mL}{6 \ h} = 166.6 \ mL/h = 167 \ mL/h$

$$\frac{V}{T} \times C = \frac{167 \ \cancel{mL}}{\underset{4}{\cancel{60}} \ min} \times \overset{1}{\cancel{15}} \ gtt/\cancel{mL} = \frac{167 \ gtt}{4 \ min} = 41.7 \ gtt/min$$

$$= 42 \ gtt/min$$

6 h − 2 h = 4 h remaining; $\dfrac{Total \ mL}{Total \ h} = \dfrac{\overset{200}{\cancel{800}} \ mL}{\underset{1}{\cancel{4}} \ h}$

$$= 200 \ mL/h$$

$$\frac{V}{T} \times C = \frac{200 \ \cancel{mL}}{\underset{4}{\cancel{60}} \ min} \times \overset{1}{\cancel{15}} \ gtt/\cancel{mL} = \frac{\overset{50}{\cancel{200}} \ gtt}{\underset{1}{\cancel{4}} \ min}$$

$$= 50 \ gtt/min$$

$$\frac{Adjused \ gtt/min \ - \ Ordered \ gtt/min}{Ordered \ gtt/min} = \% \ variation:$$

$$\frac{50 - 42}{42} = \frac{8}{42} = 0.19 = 19\% \ increase;$$

within safe limits of 25% variance

Reset infusion rate to 50 gtt/min.

10) q.4h = 6 times per 24 h; 6 × 500 mL = 3,000 mL

13) $\dfrac{60}{15} = 4$

16) 1530 + 4 h = 1530 + 0400 = 1930; 1930 − 1200

$$= 7{:}30 \ \text{PM}$$

17) $\dfrac{Total \ mL}{Total \ h} = \dfrac{500 \ mL}{4 \ h} = 125 \ mL/h$

1730 − 1530 = 200, or 2 h

125 mL/$\cancel{h}$ × 2 $\cancel{h}$ = 250 mL

18) $\dfrac{Total \ mL}{Total \ h} = \dfrac{210 \ mL}{2 \ h} = 105 \ mL/h$

$$\frac{V}{T} \times C = \frac{105 \ \cancel{mL}}{\underset{4}{\cancel{60}} \ min} \times \overset{1}{\cancel{15}} \ gtt/\cancel{mL} = \frac{105 \ gtt}{4 \ min} = 26.2 \ gtt/min$$

$$= 26 \ gtt/min$$

$$\frac{Adjusted \ gtt/min \ - \ Ordered \ gtt/min}{Ordered \ gtt/min} = \% \ of \ variation:$$

$$\frac{26 - 31}{31} = \frac{-5}{31} = -0.161 = -0.16 = -16\% \ decrease;$$

within safe limits

Reset infusion rate to 26 gtt/min.

19) $\dfrac{Total \ mL}{Total \ h} = \dfrac{500 \ mL}{4 \ h} = 125 \ mL/h$

20) $\dfrac{Total \ mL \ ordered}{Total \ min \ ordered} \times 60 \ min/h = mL/h$

$$\frac{50 \ mL}{\underset{1}{\cancel{30}} \ \cancel{min}} \times \overset{2}{\cancel{60}} \ \cancel{min}/h = 100 \ mL/h$$

22) Dextrose 5% = 5 g per 100 mL; NaCl 0.9% = 0.9 g per 100 mL

Dextrose: NaCl:

$$\frac{5 \ g}{100 \ mL} \diagdown\!\!\!\!\diagup \frac{X \ g}{500 \ mL} \qquad \frac{0.9 \ g}{100 \ mL} \diagdown\!\!\!\!\diagup \frac{X \ g}{500 \ mL}$$

$$100X = 2{,}500 \qquad\qquad 100X = 450$$

$$\frac{100X}{100} = \frac{2{,}500}{100} \qquad\qquad \frac{100X}{100} = \frac{450}{100}$$

$$X = 25 \ g \ (dextrose) \qquad X = 4.5 \ g \ (NaCl)$$

26) $\dfrac{D}{H} \times T = \dfrac{\overset{10}{\cancel{50}} \ \cancel{mg}}{\underset{1}{\cancel{5}} \ \cancel{mg}} \times 1 \ min = \dfrac{10}{1} \ min = 10 \ min$

$$\frac{D}{H} \times Q = \frac{\overset{5}{\cancel{50}} \ \cancel{mg}}{\underset{1}{\cancel{10}} \ \cancel{mg}} \times 1 \ mL = \frac{5}{1} \ mL = 5 \ mL$$

$$\frac{5 \ mL}{10 \ min} \diagdown\!\!\!\!\diagup \frac{X \ mL}{1 \ min}$$

$$10X = 5$$

$$\frac{10X}{10} = \frac{5}{10}$$

$$X = 0.5 \ mL \ (per \ min)$$

Give 50 mg per 10 min, or 5 mL per 10 min;

0.5 mL/min

$$\frac{0.5 \ mL}{60 \ sec} \diagdown\!\!\!\!\diagup \frac{X \ mL}{15 \ sec}$$

$$60X = 7.5$$

$$\frac{60X}{60} = \frac{7.5}{60}$$

$$X = 0.125 \ mL = 0.13 \ mL \ (per \ 15 \ sec)$$

32) $\dfrac{\text{Total mL}}{\text{Total h}} = \dfrac{1{,}000 \text{ mL}}{12 \text{ h}} = 83.3 \text{ mL/h} = 83 \text{ mL/h};$

$\dfrac{V}{T} \times C = \dfrac{83 \cancel{\text{ mL}}}{\underset{6}{\cancel{60} \text{ min}}} \times \overset{1}{\cancel{10}} \text{ gtt/}\cancel{\text{mL}} = \dfrac{83 \text{ gtt}}{6 \text{ min}}$

$= 13.8 \text{ gtt/min} = 14 \text{ gtt/min}$

33) $\dfrac{V}{T} \times C = \dfrac{83 \cancel{\text{ mL}}}{\underset{4}{\cancel{60} \text{ min}}} \times \overset{1}{\cancel{15}} \text{ gtt/}\cancel{\text{mL}} = \dfrac{83 \text{ gtt}}{4 \text{ min}}$

$= 20.7 \text{ gtt/min} = 21 \text{ gtt/min}$

34) $\dfrac{V}{T} \times C = \dfrac{83 \cancel{\text{ mL}}}{\underset{3}{\cancel{60} \text{ min}}} \times \overset{1}{\cancel{20}} \text{ gtt/}\cancel{\text{mL}} = \dfrac{83 \text{ gtt}}{3 \text{ min}}$

$= 27.6 \text{ gtt/min} = 28 \text{ gtt/min}$

35) $\dfrac{V}{T} \times C = \dfrac{83 \cancel{\text{ mL}}}{\underset{1}{\cancel{60} \text{ min}}} \times \overset{1}{\cancel{60}} \text{ gtt/}\cancel{\text{mL}} = 83 \text{ gtt/min}$

Remember: If the drop factor is 60 gtt/mL,
then number of mL/h = number of gtt/min,
so 83 mL/h = 83 gtt/min.

48) Think: Flow rate is 125 mL/h. You will be gone 30 min, or $\frac{1}{2}$ hour.

$125 \text{ mL/}\cancel{\text{h}} \times 0.5 \cancel{\text{ h}} = 62.5 \text{ mL}$

Alert your relief nurse that the IV will likely run out before you return and to prepare to discontinue the bag and flush and cap the saline lock.

49) $\dfrac{400 \cancel{\text{ mL}}}{75 \cancel{\text{ mL}}\text{/h}} = 5\frac{1}{3}$ h or 5 h and 20 min

$0730 + 0520 = 1250$ (or 12:50 PM)

Review Set 42 from page 493

1) 0.68 **2)** 2.35 **3)** 0.69 **4)** 1.4 **5)** 2.03 **6)** 1 **7)** 1.67 **8)** 0.4 **9)** 1.69 **10)** 0.52 **11)** 1.11 **12)** 0.78 **13)** 0.15 **14)** 0.78 **15)** 0.39 **16)** 0.64 **17)** 0.25 **18)** 1.08 **19)** 0.5 **20)** 0.88

Solutions—Review Set 42

1) Household: BSA (m²) $= \sqrt{\dfrac{\text{ht (in)} \times \text{wt (lb)}}{3{,}131}} = \sqrt{\dfrac{36 \times 40}{3{,}131}} = \sqrt{\dfrac{1{,}440}{3{,}131}} = \sqrt{0.459\ldots} = 0.678 \text{ m}^2 = 0.68 \text{ m}^2$

2) Metric: BSA (m²) $= \sqrt{\dfrac{\text{ht (cm)} \times \text{wt (kg)}}{3{,}600}} = \sqrt{\dfrac{190 \times 105}{3{,}600}} = \sqrt{\dfrac{19{,}950}{3{,}600}} = \sqrt{5.541\ldots} = 2.354 \text{ m}^2 = 2.35 \text{ m}^2$

Review Set 43 from pages 495–497

1) 1,640,000 **2)** 5.9; 11.8 **3)** 735 **4)** 15.84; 63.36 **5)** 250 **6)** 0.49; 122.5; Yes; 2.5 **7)** 0.89; 2.9; Yes; 1.2 **8)** 66; 22; Yes **9)** 198; Yes; 990 **10)** 612; 612; 1,224; 2,448 **11)** 8.1; 24.7 **12)** 67–167.5; 33.5–83.8; Yes **13)** 8–14.4; Yes **14)** 0.82; 2,050; Yes; 2.7; 102.7; 51 **15)** 1.62; 4,050; Yes; 5.4; 105.4; 53

Solutions—Review Set 43

1) 2,000,000 units/$\cancel{\text{m}^2}$ × 0.82 $\cancel{\text{m}^2}$ = 1,640,000 units

2) 10 mg/$\cancel{\text{m}^2}$/day × 0.59 $\cancel{\text{m}^2}$ = 5.9 mg/day
(minimum safe dosage)
20 mg/$\cancel{\text{m}^2}$/day × 0.59 $\cancel{\text{m}^2}$ = 11.8 mg/day
(maximum safe dosage)

3) 500 mg/$\cancel{\text{m}^2}$ × 1.47 $\cancel{\text{m}^2}$ = 735 mg

4) 6 mg/$\cancel{\text{m}^2}$/day × 2.64 $\cancel{\text{m}^2}$ = 15.84 mg/day
15.84 mg/$\cancel{\text{day}}$ × 4 $\cancel{\text{days}}$ = 63.36 mg

6) Household: BSA (m²) $= \sqrt{\dfrac{\text{ht (in)} \times \text{wt (lb)}}{3{,}131}} =$

$\sqrt{\dfrac{30 \times 25}{3{,}131}} = \sqrt{\dfrac{750}{3{,}131}} = \sqrt{0.239\ldots} =$

0.489 m² = 0.49 m²

250 mg/$\cancel{\text{m}^2}$ × 0.49 $\cancel{\text{m}^2}$ = 122.5 mg; dosage is safe

$\dfrac{D}{H} \times Q = \dfrac{122.5 \cancel{\text{ mg}}}{50 \cancel{\text{ mg}}} \times 1 \text{ mL} = 2.45 \text{ mL} = 2.5 \text{ mL}$

8) 150 mg/$\cancel{\text{m}^2}$/day × 0.44 $\cancel{\text{m}^2}$ = 66 mg/day

$\dfrac{66 \text{ mg}}{3 \text{ doses}} = 22 \text{ mg/dose}$; dosage is safe

9) $900 \text{ mg/m}^2\text{/day} \times 0.22 \text{ m}^2 = 198 \text{ mg/day}$;

dosage is safe

$198 \text{ mg/day} \times 5 \text{ days} = 990 \text{ mg}$

10) $600 \text{ mg/m}^2 \times 1.02 \text{ m}^2 = 612 \text{ mg}$, initially

$300 \text{ mg/m}^2 \times 1.02 \text{ m}^2 = 306 \text{ mg}$ (per q.4h dose):

$306 \text{ mg} \times 2 \text{ doses} = 612 \text{ mg}$ (for 2 q.4h doses)

q.12 h is 2 doses/day and

2 doses/day $\times$ 2 days = 4 doses

$306 \text{ mg} \times 4 \text{ doses} = 1{,}224 \text{ mg}$ (for 4 q.12h doses)

$612 \text{ mg} + 612 \text{ mg} + 1{,}224 \text{ mg} = 2{,}448 \text{ mg}$ (total)

11) $10 \text{ mg/m}^2 \times 0.81 \text{ m}^2 = 8.1 \text{ mg}$ (bolus)

$30.5 \text{ mg/m}^2\text{/day} \times 0.81 \text{ m}^2 = 24.7 \text{ mg/day}$

14) Metric: BSA $(\text{m}^2) = \sqrt{\dfrac{\text{ht (cm)} \times \text{wt (kg)}}{3{,}600}} =$

$\sqrt{\dfrac{100 \times 24}{3{,}600}} = \sqrt{\dfrac{2{,}400}{3{,}600}} = \sqrt{0.666\ldots} =$

$0.816 \text{ m}^2 = 0.82 \text{ m}^2$

$2{,}500 \text{ units/m}^2 \times 0.82 \text{ m}^2 = 2{,}050 \text{ units}$;
dosage is safe

$\dfrac{\text{D}}{\text{H}} \times \text{Q} = \dfrac{2{,}050 \text{ units}}{750 \text{ units}} \times 1 \text{ mL} = \dfrac{2{,}050}{750} \text{ mL} = 2.73 \text{ mL}$

$= 2.7 \text{ mL}$

2.7 mL (Oncaspar) + 100 mL $(D_5W) =$

102.7 mL (total volume)

$\dfrac{102.7 \text{ mL}}{2 \text{ h}} = 51.3 \text{ mL/h} = 51 \text{ mL/h}$

15) Metric: BSA $(\text{m}^2) = \sqrt{\dfrac{\text{ht (cm)} \times \text{wt (kg)}}{3{,}600}} =$

$\sqrt{\dfrac{162 \times 58.2}{3{,}600}} = \sqrt{\dfrac{9{,}428.4}{3{,}600}} = \sqrt{2.619} =$

$1.618 \text{ m}^2 = 1.62 \text{ m}^2$

$2{,}500 \text{ units/m}^2 \times 1.62 \text{ m}^2 = 4{,}050 \text{ units}$;

dosage is safe

$\dfrac{\text{D}}{\text{H}} \times \text{Q} = \dfrac{4{,}050 \text{ units}}{750 \text{ units}} \times 1 \text{ mL} = \dfrac{4{,}050}{750} \text{ mL} = 5.4 \text{ mL}$

5.4 mL (Oncaspar) + 100 mL $(D_5W) =$

105.4 mL (total volume)

$\dfrac{105.4 \text{ mL}}{2 \text{ h}} = 52.7 \text{ mL/h} = 53 \text{ mL/h}$

Review Set 44 from pages 500–501

1) 87; 2; 48 **2)** 75; 3; 57 **3)** 120; 3; 22 **4)** 80; 6; 44 **5)** 60; 1; 31; 180 **6)** 2; 23 **7)** 2; 8 **8)** 12; 45 **9)** 7.2; 36.8
10) 7.5; 88.5

Solutions—Review Set 44

1) Total volume: 50 mL + 15 mL = 65 mL

$\dfrac{\text{V}}{\text{T}} \times \text{C} = \dfrac{65 \text{ mL}}{45 \text{ min}} \times \overset{4}{\cancel{60}} \text{ gtt/mL} =$

$\dfrac{260 \text{ gtt}}{3 \text{ min}} = 86.6 \text{ gtt/min} = 87 \text{ gtt/min}$

$\dfrac{\text{D}}{\text{H}} \times \text{Q} = \dfrac{60 \text{ mg}}{60 \text{ mg}} \times 2 \text{ mL} = 2 \text{ mL}$ (medication)

Volume IV fluid to add to chamber:

50 mL − 2 mL = 48 mL

4) Total volume: 50 mL + 30 mL = 80 mL

80 mL per 60 min = 80 mL/h

$\dfrac{\text{D}}{\text{H}} \times \text{Q} = \dfrac{0.6 \text{ g}}{1 \text{ g}} \times 10 \text{ mL} =$

6 mL (medication)

Volume IV fluid to add to chamber:

50 mL − 6 mL = 44 mL

6) $\dfrac{50 \text{ mL}}{60 \text{ min}} \diagdown \dfrac{\text{X mL}}{30 \text{ min}}$

$60\text{X} = 1{,}500$

$\dfrac{60\text{X}}{60} = \dfrac{1{,}500}{60}$

$\text{X} = 25 \text{ mL}$ (total volume)

$\dfrac{\text{D}}{\text{H}} \times \text{Q} = \dfrac{250 \text{ mg}}{125 \text{ mg}} \times 1 \text{ mL} = 2 \text{ mL}$ (medication)

Volume IV fluid to add to chamber:

25 mL − 2 mL = 23 mL

8) $\dfrac{85 \text{ mL}}{60 \text{ min}} \diagdown \dfrac{\text{X mL}}{40 \text{ min}}$

$60\text{X} = 3{,}400$

$\dfrac{60\text{X}}{60} = \dfrac{3{,}400}{60}$

$\text{X} = 56.6 \text{ mL} = 57 \text{ mL}$ (total volume)

$\dfrac{\text{D}}{\text{H}} \times \text{Q} = \dfrac{600 \text{ mg}}{50 \text{ mg}} \times 1 \text{ mL} = 12 \text{ mL}$ (medication)

Volume IV fluid to add to chamber:

57 mL − 12 mL = 45 mL

9)

$$\frac{66 \text{ mL}}{60 \text{ min}} \diagdown \frac{X \text{ mL}}{40 \text{ min}}$$

$$60X = 2,640$$

$$\frac{60X}{60} = \frac{2,640}{60}$$

$$X = 44 \text{ mL (total volume)}$$

$$\frac{D}{H} \times Q = \frac{720 \text{ mg}}{\underset{100}{1,000 \text{ mg}}} \times \overset{1}{10} \text{ mL} = \frac{720}{100} \text{ mL}$$

$$= 7.2 \text{ mL (medication)}$$

Volume IV fluid to add to chamber:

$$44 \text{ mL} - 7.2 \text{ mL} = 36.8 \text{ mL}$$

Hint: Add the medication to the volume control chamber, and fill with IV fluid to the 44 mL mark. The chamber measures whole (not fractional) mL.

10) $48 \text{ mL/h} \times 2 \text{ h} = 96 \text{ mL (total volume)}$

$$\frac{D}{H} \times Q = \frac{75 \text{ mg}}{\underset{10}{100 \text{ mg}}} \times \overset{1}{10} \text{ mL} = \frac{75}{10} \text{ mL} = 7.5 \text{ mL}$$

Volume IV fluid to add to chamber:

$$96 \text{ mL} - 7.5 \text{ mL} = 88.5 \text{ mL}$$

Review Set 45 from page 505

1) 4 **2)** 25 **3)** 1,600; 67 **4)** 1,150; 48 **5)** 1,800; 75 **6)** 350; 15 **7)** 3.5 or 4; 11.6 or 12 **8)** 2.6 or 3; 65 **9)** 2.3 or 2; 35

10) This order should be questioned, because normal saline is an isotonic solution and appears to be a continuous infusion for this child. This solution does not contribute enough electrolytes for the child, and water intoxication may result.

Solutions—Review Set 45

1)

$$\frac{100 \text{ mg}}{1 \text{ mL}} \diagdown \frac{400 \text{ mg}}{X \text{ mL}}$$

$$100X = 400$$

$$\frac{100X}{100} = \frac{400}{100}$$

$$X = 4 \text{ mL}$$

3)

$$100 \text{ mL/kg/day} \times 10 \text{ kg} = 1,000 \text{ mL/day for first 10 kg}$$

$$50 \text{ mL/kg/day} \times 10 \text{ kg} = 500 \text{ mL/day for next 10 kg}$$

$$20 \text{ mL/kg/day} \times 5 \text{ kg} = \underline{100 \text{ mL/day for remaining 5 kg}}$$

$$\text{Total} = 1,600 \text{ mL/day or per 24 h}$$

$$\frac{1,600 \text{ mL}}{24 \text{ h}} = 66.6 \text{ mL/h} = 67 \text{ mL/h}$$

4)

$$100 \text{ mL/kg/day} \times 10 \text{ kg} = 1,000 \text{ mL/day for first 10 kg}$$

$$50 \text{ mL/kg/day} \times 3 \text{ kg} = \underline{150 \text{ mL/day for next 10 kg}}$$

$$\text{Total} = 1,150 \text{ mL/day or per 24 h}$$

$$\frac{1,150 \text{ mL}}{24 \text{ h}} = 47.9 \text{ mL/h} = 48 \text{ mL/h}$$

5)

$$77 \text{ lb} \div 2.2 \text{ lb/kg} = 77 \text{ lb} \times 1 \text{ kg}/2.2 \text{ lb} = 35 \text{ kg}$$

$$100 \text{ mL/kg/day} \times 10 \text{ kg} = 1,000 \text{ mL/day for first 10 kg}$$

$$50 \text{ mL/kg/day} \times 10 \text{ kg} = 500 \text{ mL/day for next 10 kg}$$

$$20 \text{ mL/kg/day} \times 15 \text{ kg} = \underline{300 \text{ mL/day for remaining 15 kg}}$$

$$\text{Total} = 1,800 \text{ mL/day or per 24 h}$$

$$\frac{1,800 \text{ mL}}{24 \text{ h}} = 75 \text{ mL/h}$$

7)

$$\frac{100 \text{ mg}}{1 \text{ mL}} \diagdown \frac{350 \text{ mg}}{X \text{ mL}}$$

$$100X = 350$$

$$\frac{100X}{100} = \frac{350}{100}$$

$$X = 3.5 \text{ or } 4 \text{ mL (min. dilution volume)}$$

$$\frac{30 \text{ mg}}{1 \text{ mL}} \diagdown \frac{350 \text{ mg}}{X \text{ mL}}$$

$$30X = 350$$

$$\frac{30X}{30} = \frac{350}{30}$$

$$X = 11.6 \text{ or } 12 \text{ mL (max. dilution volume)}$$

Practice Problems—Chapter 16 from pages 507–512

1) 1.17; 1.8–2.3; Yes; 2; 0.5 **2)** 0.51; 41; 0.82 **3)** 0.43; 108 **4)** 2.2 **5)** 0.7 **6)** 350 **7)** one of each (one 100 mg capsule and one 250 mg capsule) **8)** 0.8; 2,000 **9)** 2.7 **10)** No **11)** 1.3; 26 **12)** 13 **13)** 1.69 **14)** 1.11 **15)** 0.32 **16)** 1.92 **17)** 1.63 **18)** 0.69 **19)** 1.67 **20)** 0.52 **21)** 560,000 **22)** 1,085; 1.09 **23)** 1.9–3.8 **24)** 8 **25)** 40 **26)** 45; 90; 4.2; 25.8 **27)** 58.8 **28)** 60; 60; 1.9; 43.1 **29)** 22.8 **30)** 10; 33 **31)** 200 **32)** 6.2; 37.8 **33)** 130.2 **34)** 1,000; 42 **35)** 1,520; 63 **36)** 1,810; 75 **37)** 1,250; 52 **38)** 240; 10 **39)** 1,500–1,875; 250–312.5; Yes; 2.8 **40)** 35; 2.8; 32.2 **41)** 12.3; 1,230; 308; Yes; 6.2 **42)** 23; 6.2; 16.8 **43)** 330–495; 110–165; Yes; 3.3 **44)** 25; 3.3; 21.7 **45)** 1,800–2,700; 300–450; No; exceeds maximum dose; do not give dosage ordered. **46)** Consult physician before further action. **47)** 25; 2,500,000–6,250,000; 416,667–1,041,667 **48)** Yes; 2.6 **49)** 20; 2.6; 17.4

50) Prevention: The nurse made several assumptions in trying to calculate and prepare this chemotherapy quickly. The recording of the weights as 20/.45 was confusing. The nurse interpreted the 20/.45 notation to indicate the patient's weight in pounds or kilograms, as was done in the adult unit. Notice the period before the 45, which later the physician stated was the calculated BSA, 0.45 m². Because no unit of measure was identified, it was unclear what those numbers really meant. Never assume; always ask for clarification when notation is unclear. Additionally, the actual volume drawn up was probably small in comparison to most adult dose volumes that this nurse prepares. The amount of 1.6 mL likely seemed reasonable to the nurse. Finally, this is an instance in which the person giving the medication, the physician, prevented a medication error by stopping and thinking what was a reasonable amount for this child and questioning the actual calculation of the dose. Remember: The person who administers the medication is the last point at which a potential error can be avoided.

Solutions—Practice Problems—Chapter 16

1) Household: $BSA\ (m^2) = \sqrt{\dfrac{ht\ (in) \times wt\ (lb)}{3,131}} = \sqrt{\dfrac{50 \times 85}{3,131}}$

$$= \sqrt{\dfrac{4,250}{3,131}} = \sqrt{1.357\ldots} = 1.165\ m^2 = 1.17\ m^2$$

Recommended dosage range:

$1.5\ mg/m^2 \times 1.17\ m^2 = 1.8\ mg$

$2\ mg/m^2 \times 1.17\ m^2 = 2.3\ mg$

Ordered dosage is safe.

$\dfrac{1\ mg}{1\ mL} \diagdown\!\!\!\!\diagup \dfrac{2\ mg}{X\ mL}$

$X = 2\ mL$

Give 2 mL/min

$\dfrac{2\ mL}{60\ sec} \diagdown\!\!\!\!\diagup \dfrac{X\ mL}{15\ sec}$

$60X = 30$

$\dfrac{60X}{60} = \dfrac{30}{60}$

$X = 0.5\ mL$ (per 15 sec)

2) $BSA = 0.51\ m^2$

$80\ mg/m^2/day \times 0.51\ m^2 = 40.8\ mg/day$

$= 41\ mg/day$

$\dfrac{D}{H} \times Q = \dfrac{41\ mg}{50\ mg} \times 1\ mL = \dfrac{41}{50}\ mL = 0.82\ mL$

3) $BSA = 0.43\ m^2$

$250\ mcg/m^2/day \times 0.43\ m^2 = 107.5\ mcg/day$

$= 108\ mcg/day$

4) $\dfrac{D}{H} \times Q = \dfrac{108\ mcg}{500\ mcg} \times 10\ mL = \dfrac{1,080}{500}\ mL$

$= 2.16\ mL = 2.2\ mL$

6) $0.5\ g/m^2 \times 0.7\ m^2 = 0.35\ g$

$0.35\ g = 0.350. = 350\ mg$

8) $BSA = 0.8\ m^2$

$2,500\ units/m^2 \times 0.8\ m^2 = 2,000\ units$

9) $\dfrac{D}{H} \times Q = \dfrac{2,000\ units}{750\ units} \times 1\ mL = \dfrac{2,000}{750}\ mL$

$= 2.66\ mL = 2.7\ mL$

10) Dose amount exceeds child maximum IM volume per injection site; give in 2 injections.

11) Metric: $BSA\ (m^2) = \sqrt{\dfrac{ht\ (cm) \times wt\ (kg)}{3,600}} =$

$\sqrt{\dfrac{140 \times 43.5}{3,600}} = \sqrt{\dfrac{6.090}{3,600}} = \sqrt{1.691\ldots} =$

$1.30\ m^2 = 1.3\ m^2$

$20\ mg/m^2 \times 1.3\ m^2 = 26\ mg$

12) $\dfrac{D}{H} \times Q = \dfrac{\overset{13}{\cancel{26}\text{ mg}}}{\underset{1}{\cancel{2}\text{ mg}}} \times 1 \text{ mL} = 13 \text{ mL}$

13) 1 ft = 12 in

$\dfrac{1 \text{ ft}}{12 \text{ in}} \diagdown\!\!\!\!\diagup \dfrac{5 \text{ ft}}{X \text{ in}}$

$X = 60 \text{ in}$

Convert 5 ft 6 in to total in: 60 in + 6 in = 66 in

Household: BSA (m²) $= \sqrt{\dfrac{\text{ht (in)} \times \text{wt (lb)}}{3.131}} =$

$\sqrt{\dfrac{66 \times 136}{3,131}} = \sqrt{\dfrac{8.976}{3,131}} = \sqrt{2.866\ldots} =$

1.693 m² = 1.69 m²

15) Metric: BSA (m²) $= \sqrt{\dfrac{\text{ht (cm)} \times \text{wt (kg)}}{3,600}} =$

$\sqrt{\dfrac{60 \times 6}{3,600}} = \sqrt{\dfrac{360}{3,600}} = \sqrt{0.1} =$

0.316 m² = 0.32 m²

19) 1 in = 2.5 cm

$\dfrac{1 \text{ in}}{2.5 \text{ cm}} = \dfrac{64 \text{ in}}{X \text{ cm}}$

$X = 160 \text{ cm}$

Metric: BSA (m²) $= \sqrt{\dfrac{\text{ht (cm)} \times \text{wt (kg)}}{3,600}} =$

$\sqrt{\dfrac{160 \times 63}{3,600}} = \sqrt{\dfrac{10,080}{3,600}} = \sqrt{2.8} =$

1.673 m² = 1.67 m²

22) 500 mg/m² × 2.17 m² = 1,085 mg

1,085 mg = 1.085. = 1.085 g = 1.09 g

24) 6 mg/m² × 1.34 m² = 8.04 mg = 8 mg

25) 8 mg/day × 5 days = 40 mg

26) Total volume = 30 mL + 15 mL = 45 mL

IV pump flow rate if time is less than 1 h:

$\dfrac{\text{Total mL ordered}}{\text{Total min ordered}} \times 60 \text{ min/h} = \text{mL/h}$

Flow rate: $\dfrac{45 \text{ mL}}{\underset{1}{\cancel{30}\text{ min}}} \times \overset{2}{\cancel{60}} \text{ min/h} = 90 \text{ mL/h}$

$\dfrac{D}{H} \times Q = \dfrac{420 \text{ mg}}{\underset{100}{\cancel{500}\text{ mg}}} \times \overset{1}{\cancel{5}} \text{ mL} = \dfrac{420}{100} \text{ mL}$

$= 4.2 \text{ mL (medication)}$

30 mL (total solution) − 4.2 mL (med)

$= 25.8 \text{ mL (D}_5\text{NS)}$

Note: Add 4.2 mL med. to chamber and fill with D₅NS to 30 mL.

27) 4.2 mL/dose × 2 doses/day = 8.4 mL/day

8.4 mL/day × 7 days = 58.8 mL (total)

28) Total volume: 45 mL + 15 mL = 60 mL

Flow rate: $\dfrac{60 \text{ mL}}{60 \text{ min}} \times 60 \text{ min/h} = 60 \text{ mL/h}$; or more

simply, 60 mL/60 min = 60 mL/h

$\dfrac{D}{H} \times Q = \dfrac{285 \text{ mg}}{75 \text{ mg}} \times 0.5 \text{ mL} = \dfrac{142.5}{75} \text{ mL}$

$= 1.9 \text{ mL (med)}$

Volume of IV fluid: 45 mL − 1.9 mL = 43.1 mL

29) 1.9 mL/dose × 3 doses/day = 5.7 mL/day

5.7 mL/day × 4 days = 22.8 mL (total)

30) $\dfrac{D}{H} \times Q = \dfrac{\overset{10}{\cancel{500}\text{ mg}}}{\underset{1}{\cancel{50}\text{ mg}}} \times 1 \text{ mL} = 10 \text{ mL (med)}$

$\dfrac{65 \text{ mL}}{60 \text{ min}} \diagdown\!\!\!\!\diagup \dfrac{X \text{ mL}}{40 \text{ min}}$

$60X = 2,600$

$\dfrac{60X}{60} = \dfrac{2,600}{60}$

$X = 43.3 \text{ mL} = 43 \text{ mL}$

43 mL (total solution) − 10 mL (med) =

33 mL (D₅ 0.33% NaCl)

31) 10 mL/dose × 4 doses/day = 40 mL/day

40 mL/day × 5 days = 200 mL

35) 100 mL/kg/day × 10 kg = 1,000 mL/day for first 10 kg

50 mL/kg/day × 10 kg = 500 mL/day for next 10 kg

20 mL/kg/day × 1 kg = 20 mL/day for remaining 1 kg

Total = 1,520 mL/day or per 24 h

$\dfrac{1,520 \text{ mL}}{24 \text{ h}} = 63.3 \text{ mL/h} = 63 \text{ mL/h}$

36) 78 lb ÷ 2.2 lb/kg = 78 lb × 1 kg/2.2 lb = 35.45 kg = 35.5 kg

100 mL/kg/day × 10 kg = 1,000 mL/day for first 10 kg

50 mL/kg/day × 10 kg = 500 mL/day for next 10 kg

20 mL/kg/day × 15.5 kg = 310 mL/day for remaining 15.5 kg

Total = 1,810 mL/day or per 24 h

$\dfrac{1,810 \text{ mL}}{24 \text{ h}} = 75.4 \text{ mL/h} = 75 \text{ mL/h}$

38) 2,400 g = 2.400. = 2.4 kg

100 mL/kg/day × 2.4 kg = 240 mL/day

$\dfrac{240 \text{ mL}}{24 \text{ h}} = 10 \text{ mL/h}$

39) Safe daily dosage range:

100 mg/kg × 15 kg = 1,500 mg

125 mg/kg × 15 kg = 1,875 mg

Safe single dosage range:

$\dfrac{1,500}{6 \text{ doses}} = 250 \text{ mg/dose}$

$\dfrac{1,875}{6 \text{ doses}} = 312.5 \text{ mg/dose}$

Yes, the dosage is safe.

1 g = 1,000 mg

$\dfrac{D}{H} \times Q = \dfrac{275 \text{ mg}}{1,000 \text{ mg}} \times 10 \text{ mL} = \dfrac{2,750}{1,000} \text{ mL} = 2.75 \text{ mL} = 2.8 \text{ mL}$

40) IV fluid volume:

$\dfrac{53 \text{ mL}}{60 \text{ min}} \diagdown\!\!\!\!\diagup \dfrac{X \text{ mL}}{40 \text{ min}}$

$60X = 2,120$

$\dfrac{60X}{60} = \dfrac{2,120}{60}$

$X = 35.3 \text{ mL} = 35 \text{ mL}$

35 mL (total) − 2.8 mL (med) = 32.2 mL (D₅ 0.45% NaCl)

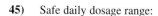

45) Safe daily dosage range:

200 mg/kg × 9 kg = 1,800 mg

300 mg/kg × 9 kg = 2,700 mg

Safe single dosage range:

$\frac{1,800 \text{ mg}}{6 \text{ doses}} = 300$ mg/dose

$\frac{2,700 \text{ mg}}{6 \text{ doses}} = 450$ mg/dose

Dosage is *not* safe; exceeds maximum safe dosage.

Do not give dosage ordered; consult with

physician.

47) 55 lb ÷ 2.2 lb/kg = 55 lb × 1 kg/2.2 lb = 25 kg

Safe daily dosage:

100,000 units/kg × 25 kg = 2,500,000 units

250,000 units/kg × 25 kg = 6,250,000 units

Safe single dosage:

$\frac{2,500,000 \text{ units}}{6 \text{ doses}} = 416,666.6$ units/dose

= 416,667 units/dose

$\frac{6,250,000 \text{ units}}{6 \text{ doses}} = 1,041,666.6$ units/dose

= 1,041,667 units/dose

48) Yes, dosage is safe.

$\frac{D}{H} \times Q = \frac{525,000 \text{ units}}{200,000 \text{ units}} \times 1 \text{ mL} = 2.62 \text{ mL} = 2.6 \text{ mL}$

49) $\frac{60 \text{ mL}}{60 \text{ min}} \diagdown \frac{X \text{ mL}}{20 \text{ min}}$

60X = 1,200

$\frac{60X}{60} = \frac{1,200}{60}$

X = 20 mL

20 mL (total) − 2.6 mL (med) = 17.4 mL (D₅NS)

Review Set 46 from pages 528–529

1) 40 **2)** 14 **3)** 10 **4)** 19 **5)** 48; Consult physician; per policy, you may be directed to stop this infusion if physician does not respond immediately. **6)** 16 **7)** 75; 6,000; 6; 1,350; 14 **8)** 6,000; 6; 300; 3; 17 **9)** 3,000; 3; 150; 1.5; 19 **10)** Continue the rate at 19 mL/h. **11)** Yes; 10 **12)** 25 **13)** no bolus required **14)** 8 **15)** Hold insulin infusion × 60 min and check blood glucose every 15 min until greater than or equal to 80 mg/dL.

Solutions—Review Set 46

1) $\frac{D}{H} \times Q = \frac{1,000 \text{ units/h}}{25,000 \text{ units}} \times 1,000 \text{ mL} = \frac{1,000}{25} \text{ mL/h}$

= 40 mL/h

4) $\frac{D}{H} \times Q = \frac{1,500 \text{ units/h}}{40,000 \text{ units}} \times 500 \text{ mL} = \frac{1,500}{80} \text{ mL/h}$

= 18.7 mL/h = 19 mL/h

5) $\frac{D}{H} \times Q = \frac{1,200 \text{ units/h}}{25,000 \text{ units}} \times 1,000 \text{ mL} = \frac{1,200}{25} \text{ mL/h} = 48 \text{ mL/h}$

The IV is infusing too rapidly. The physician should be called immediately for further action.

6) $\frac{D}{H} \times Q = \frac{800 \text{ units/h}}{25,000 \text{ units}} \times 500 \text{ mL} = \frac{800}{50} \text{ mL/h} = 16 \text{ mL/h}$

7) 165 lb ÷ 2.2 lb/kg = 165 lb × 1 kg/2.2 lb = 75 kg

Initial heparin bolus: 80 units/kg × 75 kg = 6,000 units

$\frac{D}{H} \times Q = \frac{6,000 \text{ units}}{1,000 \text{ units}} \times 1 \text{ mL} = 6 \text{ mL}$

Initial heparin infusion rate: 18 units/kg/h × 75 kg
= 1,350 units/h

$\frac{D}{H} \times Q = \frac{1,350 \text{ units/h}}{25,000 \text{ units}} \times 250 \text{ mL} = \frac{1,350}{100} \text{ mL/h}$

= 13.5 mL/h = 14 mL/h

8) Rebolus: 80 units/kg × 75 kg = 6,000 units

$\frac{D}{H} \times Q = \frac{6,000 \text{ units}}{1,000 \text{ units}} \times 1 \text{ mL} = 6 \text{ mL}$

Reset infusion rate: 4 units/kg/h × 75 kg
= 300 units/h (increase)

$\frac{D}{H} \times Q = \frac{300 \text{ units/h}}{25,000 \text{ units}} \times 250 \text{ mL} = \frac{300}{100} \text{ mL/h}$

= 3 mL/h

14 mL/h + 3 mL/h = 17 mL/h

Reset infusion rate to 17 mL/h

9) Rebolus: 40 units/kg × 75 kg = 3,000 units

$\frac{D}{H} \times Q = \frac{3,000 \text{ units}}{1,000 \text{ units}} \times 1 \text{ mL} = 3 \text{ mL}$

Reset infusion rate: 2 units/kg/h × 75 kg
= 150 units/h (increase)

$\frac{D}{H} \times Q = \frac{150 \text{ units/h}}{25,000 \text{ units}} \times 250 \text{ mL} = \frac{150}{100} \text{ mL/h}$

= 1.5 mL/h

17 mL/h + 1.5 mL/h = 18.5 mL/h = 19 mL/h

Reset infusion rate to 19 mL/h

12) $\frac{D \text{ (units/h)}}{H \text{ (units)}} \times Q \text{ (mL)} = R \text{ (mL/h)}$

$\frac{25 \text{ units/h}}{100 \text{ units}} \times 100 \text{ mL} = 25 \text{ mL/h}$

14) $\frac{D \text{ (units/h)}}{H \text{ (units)}} \times Q \text{ (mL)} = R \text{ (mL/h)}$

$\frac{8 \text{ units/h}}{100 \text{ units}} \times 100 \text{ mL} = 8 \text{ mL/h}$

Review Set 47 from pages 536–537

1) 2; 120 **2)** 1; 60 **3)** 1.5; 90 **4)** 90; 360; 0.4; 24 **5)** 1,050; 0.66; 39.6 **6)** 142–568 **7)** 0.14–0.57 **8)** Yes **9)** 4

10) Yes **11)** 100; 25 **12)** 1 **13)** 0.025 **14)** 25 **15)** Yes

Solutions—Review Set 47

1) $\dfrac{D}{H} \times Q = \dfrac{4 \text{ mg/min}}{2,000 \text{ mg}} \times 1,000 \text{ mL} = \dfrac{2}{1} \text{ mL/min} = 2 \text{ mL/min}$

$2 \text{ mL/min} \times 60 \text{ min/h} = 120 \text{ mL/h}$

2) $\dfrac{D}{H} \times Q = \dfrac{2 \text{ mg/min}}{500 \text{ mg}} \times 250 \text{ mL} = \dfrac{2}{1} \text{ mL/min} = 1 \text{ mL/min}$

$1 \text{ mL/min} \times 60 \text{ min/h} = 60 \text{ mL/h}$

3) $\dfrac{D}{H} \times Q = \dfrac{6 \text{ mcg/min}}{2,000 \text{ mcg}} \times 500 \text{ mL} = \dfrac{6}{4} \text{ mL/min}$

$= 1.5 \text{ mL/min}$

$1.5 \text{ mL/min} \times 60 \text{ min/h} = 90 \text{ mL/h}$

4) $198 \text{ lb} \div 2.2 \text{ lb/kg} = 198 \text{ lb} \times 1 \text{ kg}/2.2 \text{ lb} = 90 \text{ kg};$

$4 \text{ mcg/kg/min} \times 90 \text{ kg} = 360 \text{ mcg/min}$

$360 \text{ mcg/min} = .360. = 0.36 \text{ mg/min}$

$\dfrac{D}{H} \times Q = \dfrac{0.36 \text{ mg/min}}{450 \text{ mg}} \times 500 \text{ mL} = \dfrac{3.6}{9} \text{ mL/min}$

$= 0.4 \text{ mL/min}$

$0.4 \text{ mL/min} \times 60 \text{ min/h} = 24 \text{ mL/h}$

5) $15 \text{ mcg/kg/min} \times 70 \text{ kg} = 1,050 \text{ mcg/min}$

$1,050 \text{ mcg/min} = 1.050. = 1.05 \text{ mg/min}$

$\dfrac{D}{H} \times Q = \dfrac{1.05 \text{ mg/min}}{800 \text{ mg}} \times 500 \text{ mL} = \dfrac{5.25}{8} \text{ mL/min}$

$= 0.656 \text{ mL/min} = 0.66 \text{ mL/min}$

$0.66 \text{ mL/min} \times 60 \text{ min/h} = 39.6 \text{ mL/h}$

6) $125 \text{ lb} \div 2.2 \text{ lb/kg} = 125 \text{ lb} \times 1 \text{ kg}/2.2 \text{ lb} = 56.81 \text{ kg}$

$= 56.8 \text{ kg}$

Minimum: $2.5 \text{ mcg/kg/min} \times 56.8 \text{ kg} = 142 \text{ mcg/min}$

Maximum: $10 \text{ mcg/kg/min} \times 56.8 \text{ kg} = 568 \text{ mcg/min}$

7) Minimum: $142 \text{ mcg/min} = .142. = 0.142 \text{ mg/min}$

$= 0.14 \text{ mg/min}$

Maximum: $568 \text{ mcg/min} = .568. = 0.568 \text{ mg/min}$

$= 0.57 \text{ mg/min}$

8) $\dfrac{D}{H} \times Q = R$

$\dfrac{D \text{ mg/h}}{500 \text{ mg}} \times 500 \text{ mL} = 15 \text{ mL/h}$

$\dfrac{D}{500} \times 500 = \dfrac{15}{1}$

$\dfrac{500D}{500} \times\!\!\!\!\diagup\!\!\!\!\times \dfrac{15}{1}$

$500D = 7,500$

$\dfrac{500D}{500} = \dfrac{7,500}{500}$

$D = 15 \text{ mg/h}$

$\dfrac{15 \text{ mg/h}}{60 \text{ min/h}} = 0.25 \text{ mg/min}$

Yes, the order is within the safe range of 0.14 to 0.57 mg/min.

9) $\dfrac{D}{H} \times Q = R$

$\dfrac{D \text{ mg/h}}{2,000 \text{ mg}} \times 500 \text{ mL} = 60 \text{ mL/h}$

$\dfrac{D}{2,000} \times 500 = 60$

$\dfrac{500D}{2,000} \times\!\!\!\!\diagup\!\!\!\!\times \dfrac{60}{1}$

$500D = 120,000$

$\dfrac{500D}{500} = \dfrac{120,000}{500}$

$D = 240 \text{ mg/h}$

$\dfrac{240 \text{ mg/h}}{60 \text{ min/h}} = 4 \text{ mg/min}$

10) Yes, 4 mg/min is within the normal range of 2 to 6 mg/min.

11) Bolus:

$\dfrac{D}{H} \times Q = \dfrac{2 \text{ g}}{20 \text{ g}} \times 500 \text{ mL} = \dfrac{1000}{20} \text{ mL} = 50 \text{ mL}$

$\dfrac{\text{Total mL}}{\text{Total min}} \times 60 \text{ min/h} = \dfrac{50 \text{ mL}}{30 \text{ min}} \times 60 \text{ min/h}$

$= 100 \text{ mL/h}$

Continuous: You know that 50 mL contains 2 g; therefore,

$\dfrac{D}{H} \times Q = R$

$\dfrac{1 \text{ g/h}}{2 \text{ g}} \times 50 \text{ mL} = \dfrac{50}{2} \text{ mL/h} = 25 \text{ mL/h}$

12) 1 milliunit = 0.001. = 0.001 units

$$\frac{D}{H} \times Q = \frac{0.001 \text{ units/min}}{15 \text{ units}} \times 250 \text{ mL} = \frac{0.25}{15} \text{ mL/min}$$

$$= 0.0166 \text{ mL/min} = 0.017 \text{ mL/min}$$

$$0.017 \text{ mL/min} \times 60 \text{ min/h} = 1.02 \text{ mL/h} = 1 \text{ mL/h}$$

$$\frac{1{,}000D}{10} = \frac{150}{1}$$

$$1{,}000D = 1{,}500$$

$$\frac{1{,}000D}{1{,}000} = \frac{1{,}500}{1{,}000}$$

$$D = 1.5 \text{ mg/h}$$

13) $\frac{D}{H} \times Q = R$

$$\frac{D \text{ mg/h}}{10 \text{ mg}} \times 1{,}000 \text{ mL} = 150 \text{ mL/h}$$

$$\frac{1.5 \text{ mg/h}}{60 \text{ min/h}} = 0.025 \text{ mg/min}$$

14) 0.025 mg/min = 0.025. = 25 mcg/min

Review Set 48 from pages 540–541

1) 33; 19 **2)** 40; 42 **3)** 25; 32 **4)** 50; 90 **5)** 50; 40 **6)** 100; 100 **7)** 200; 76 **8)** 200; 122 **9)** 17; 21 **10)** 120; 112

Solutions—Review Set 48

1) **Step 1** IV PB rate: $\frac{V}{T} \times C = \frac{100 \text{ mL}}{\overset{}{\underset{3}{30 \text{ min}}}} \times \overset{1}{10} \text{ gtt/mL} =$

$$\frac{100}{3} \text{ gtt/min} = 33.3 \text{ gtt/min} = 33 \text{ gtt/min}$$

Step 2 Total IV PB time: q.4h = 6 times per 24h; 6 × 30 min = 180 min;

180 min ÷ 60 min/h = 180 min × 1 h/60 min = 3 h

Step 3 Total IV PB volume: 6 × 100 mL = 600 mL

Step 4 Total regular IV volume: 3,000 mL − 600 mL = 2,400 mL

Step 5 Total regular IV time: 24 h − 3 h = 21 h

Step 6 Regular IV rate:

$$\frac{2{,}400 \text{ mL}}{21 \text{ h}} = 114.2 \text{ mL/h} = 114 \text{ mL/h}$$

$$\frac{\text{mL/h}}{\text{Drop factor constant}} = \text{gtt/min}; \ \frac{114 \text{ mL/h}}{6} = 19 \text{ gtt/min}$$

2) **Step 1** IV PB rate: When drop factor is 60 gtt/mL, then mL/h = gtt/min. Rate is 40 gtt/min.

Step 2 Total IV PB time: q.i.d = 4 times per 24h; 4 × 1 h = 4 h

Step 3 Total IV PB volume: 4 × 40 mL = 160 mL

Step 4 Total regular IV volume: 1,000 mL − 160 mL = 840 mL

Step 5 Total regular IV time: 24 h − 4 h = 20 h

Step 6 Total regular IV rate: mL/h = $\frac{840 \text{ mL}}{20 \text{ h}}$ = 42 mL/h. When drop factor is 60 gtt/mL, then

mL/h = gtt/min. Rate is 42 gtt/min.

3) **Step 1** IV PB rate: $\frac{V}{T} \times C = \frac{50 \text{ mL}}{\overset{}{\underset{2}{30 \text{ min}}}} \times \overset{1}{15} \text{ gtt/mL} = \frac{\overset{25}{50}}{\overset{}{\underset{1}{2}}} \text{ gtt/min} = 25 \text{ gtt/min}$

Step 2 Total IV PB time: q.6h = 4 times per 24h; 4 × 30 min = 120 min;

120 min ÷ 60 min/h = 120 min × 1 h/60 min = 2 h

Step 3 Total IV PB volume: 4 × 50 mL = 200 mL

Step 4 Total regular IV volume: 3,000 mL − 200 mL = 2,800 mL

Step 5 Total regular IV time: 24 h − 2 h = 22 h

Step 6 Total regular IV rate:

$$\frac{2{,}800 \text{ mL}}{22 \text{ h}} = 127.2 \text{ mL/h} = 127 \text{ mL/h}$$

$$\frac{\text{mL/h}}{\text{Drop factor constant}} = \text{gtt/min}; \ \frac{127 \text{ mL/h}}{4} = 31.7 \text{ gtt/min} = 32 \text{ gtt/min}$$

4) **Step 1**   IV PB rate: 50 mL/h or 50 gtt/min (because drop factor is 60 gtt/mL)

   Step 2   Total IV PB time: q.6h = 4 times per 24 h; 4×1 h = 4 h

   Step 3   Total IV PB volume: 4×50 mL = 200 mL

   Step 4   Total regular IV volume: 2,000 mL − 200 mL = 1,800 mL

   Step 5   Total regular IV time: 24 h − 4 h = 20 h

   Step 6   Regular IV rate: $\frac{1,800 \text{ mL}}{20 \text{ h}}$ = 90 mL/h or 90 gtt/min (because drop factor is 60 gtt/mL)

5) **Step 1**   IV PB rate: 50 mL/h or 50 gtt/min (because drop factor is 60 gtt/mL)

   Step 2   IV PB time: q.8h = 3 times per 24h; 3×1 h = 3 h

   Step 3   IV PB volume: 3×50 mL = 150 mL

   Step 4   Total regular IV volume: 1,000 mL − 150 mL = 850 mL

   Step 5   Total regular IV time: 24 h − 3 h = 21 h

   Step 6   Regular IV rate: $\frac{850 \text{ mL}}{21 \text{ h}}$ = 40.4 mL/h = 40 mL/h or 40 gtt/min (because drop factor is 60 gtt/mL)

6) **Step 1**   IV PB rate

   $\frac{50 \text{ mL}}{30 \text{ min}} \underset{\nearrow}{\searrow} \frac{X \text{ mL}}{60 \text{ min}}$

   $30X = 3,000$

   $\frac{30X}{30} = \frac{3,000}{30}$

   $X = 100$ mL; 100 mL per 60 min = 100 mL/h

   Step 2   IV PB time: q.6h = 4 times per 24h; 4×30 min = 120 min;

   120 min ÷ 60 min/h = 120 m̶i̶n̶ × 1 h/60 m̶i̶n̶ = 2 h

   Step 3   IV PB volume: 4×50 mL = 200 mL

   Step 4   Total regular IV volume: 2,400 mL − 200 mL = 2,200 mL

   Step 5   Total regular IV time: 24 h − 2 h = 22 h

   Step 6   Regular IV rate: $\frac{2,200 \text{ mL}}{22 \text{ h}}$ = 100 mL/h

7) **Step 1**   IV PB rate:

   $\frac{100 \text{ mL}}{30 \text{ min}} \underset{\nearrow}{\searrow} \frac{X \text{ mL}}{60 \text{ min}}$

   $30X = 6,000$

   $\frac{30X}{30} = \frac{6,000}{30}$

   $X = 200$ mL; 200 mL per 60 min = 200 mL/h

   Step 2   IV PB time: q.8h = 3 times per 24h; 3×30 min = 90 min;

   90 min ÷ 60 min/h = 90 m̶i̶n̶ × 1 h/60 m̶i̶n̶ = $1\frac{1}{2}$ h

   Step 3   IV PB volume: 3×100 mL = 300 mL

   Step 4   Total regular IV volume: 2,000 mL − 300 mL = 1,700 mL

   Step 5   Total regular IV time: 24 h − $1\frac{1}{2}$ h = $22\frac{1}{2}$ h

   Step 6   Regular IV rate: $\frac{1,700 \text{ mL}}{22.5 \text{ h}}$ = 75.5 mL/h = 76 mL/h

8) **Step 1**   IV PB rate

   $\frac{50 \text{ mL}}{15 \text{ min}} \underset{\nearrow}{\searrow} \frac{X \text{ mL}}{60 \text{ min}}$

   $15X = 3,000$

   $\frac{15X}{15} = \frac{3,000}{15}$

   $X = 200$ mL; 200 mL per 60 min = 200 mL/h

Step 2	IV PB time: q.6h = 4 times per 24h; 4 × 15 min = 60 min = 1 h
Step 3	IV PB volume: 4 × 50 mL = 200 mL
Step 4	Total regular IV volume: 3,000 mL − 200 mL = 2,800 mL
Step 5	Total regular IV time: 24 h − 1 h = 23 h
Step 6	Regular IV rate: $\frac{2,800\ mL}{23\ h}$ = 121.7 mL/h = 122 mL/h

Practice Problems—Chapter 17 from pages 543–548

1) 60 2) 5 3) 20 4) 50 5) 1 6) 12 7) 50 8) 63 9) 35 10) 6; 15 11) 60 12) 45 13) 60 14) 24 15) Yes 16) 17; 22
17) 100; 127 18) 102 19) 8 mEq 20) 2 21) 15 22) 50 23) 25 24) 7.4 25) 12; 18 26) 150; 50 27) 2 28) 35 29) 8
30) 63 31) 80 32) 0.4 33) 4 34) 4 35) 100 36) 0.2; 200 37) 30 38) 200; 50 39) 5 40) 550 41) 2,450 42) 19 43) 129
44) 13; 39 45) 100; 80 46) 8,000; 1,000; 8 47) 18; 1,800; 100; 18 48) 6; 40; 4,000; 4; increase; 2; 200; 2; 20
49) Decrease rate by 2 units/kg/h; 18

STANDARD WEIGHT-BASED HEPARIN PROTOCOL WORKSHEET

Round patient's total body weight to nearest 10 kg: _100_ kg.
DO NOT change the weight based on daily measurements.

FOUND ON THE ORDER FORM
Initial Bolus (80 units/kg): _8,000_ units _8_ mL
Initial Infusion Rate (18 units/kg/h): _1,800_ units/h _18_ mL/h

Make adjustments to the heparin drip rate as directed by the order form.
ALL DOSES ARE ROUNDED TO THE NEAREST 100 UNITS.

Date	Time	aPTT	Bolus	Rate Change Units/h	mL/h	New Rate	RN 1	RN 2
5/10/xx	1730	37 sec	4,000 units (4 mL)	+200 units/h	+2 mL/h	20 mL/h	G.P.	M.S.
5/10/xx	2330	77 sec		−200 units/h	−2 mL/h	18 mL/h	G.P.	M.S.

Signatures	Initials
G. Pickar, R.N.	G.P.
M. Smith, R.N.	M.S.

---

50) **Prevention:** The nurse who prepares any IV solution with an additive should *carefully* compare the order and medication three times: before beginning to prepare the dose, after the dosage is prepared, and just before it is administered to the patient. Further, the nurse should verify the safety of the dosage using the Three-Step Approach (convert, think, and calculate). It was clear that the nurse realized the error when a colleague questioned what was being prepared and the nurse verified the actual order. Also, taking the time to do the calculation on paper helps the nurse to "see" the answer and avoid a potentially life-threatening error. The precriber should also write out units and milliunits (U and mU are not permitted abbreviations). The nurse should contact the prescriber to clarify an order when unacceptable notation is used.

Solutions—Practice Problems—Chapter 17

1) Volume control sets are microdrop infusion sets calibrated for 60 gtt/mL.

2) 1 g is ordered and it is prepared as a supply dosage of 1 g per 5 mL. Add 5 mL.

3) $\dfrac{50 \text{ mL}}{60 \text{ min}} \underset{\times}{\times} \dfrac{X \text{ mL}}{30 \text{ min}}$

$\qquad 60X = 1{,}500$

$\qquad \dfrac{60X}{60} = \dfrac{1{,}500}{60}$

$\qquad X = 25 \text{ mL}$ (total volume)

$\qquad 25 \text{ mL (total)} - 5 \text{ mL (med)} = 20 \text{ mL (D}_5\text{W)}$

4) $\dfrac{\text{mL/h}}{\text{Drop factor constant}} = \dfrac{50 \text{ mL/h}}{1} = 50 \text{ gtt/min};$

when drop factor is 60 gtt/mL, then mL/h = gtt/min

5) once (at 1200 hours)

6) $\dfrac{D}{H} \times Q = \dfrac{1{,}200 \text{ units/h}}{25{,}000 \text{ units}} \times \overset{1}{250} \text{ mL} = \dfrac{\overset{12}{1{,}200}}{\underset{1}{100}} \text{ mL/h}$

$\qquad = 12 \text{ mL/h}$

7) $\dfrac{D}{H} \times Q = \dfrac{5 \text{ mg/h}}{100 \text{ mg}} \times \overset{10}{1{,}000} \text{ mL} = 50 \text{ mL/h}$

8) $\dfrac{D}{H} \times Q = \dfrac{500 \text{ mg/h}}{4{,}000 \text{ mg}} \times \overset{1}{500} \text{ mL} = \dfrac{500}{8} \text{ mL/h} = 62.5 \text{ mL/h}$

$\qquad = 63 \text{ mL/h}$

9) $\dfrac{D}{H} \times Q = \dfrac{1{,}400 \text{ units/h}}{20{,}000 \text{ units}} \times \overset{1}{500} \text{ mL} = \dfrac{1{,}400}{40} \text{ mL/h} = 35 \text{ mL/h}$

10) $1.5 \text{ L} = 1.500. = 1{,}500 \text{ mL}$

$\qquad \dfrac{4 \text{ mL}}{1 \text{ min}} \underset{\times}{\times} \dfrac{1{,}500 \text{ mL}}{X \text{ min}}$

$\qquad\quad 4X = 1{,}500$

$\qquad\quad \dfrac{4X}{4} = \dfrac{1{,}500}{4}$

$\qquad\quad\ X = 375 \text{ min}$

$\qquad \dfrac{60 \text{ min}}{1 \text{ h}} \underset{\times}{\times} \dfrac{375 \text{ min}}{X \text{ h}}$

$\qquad\quad 60X = 375$

$\qquad\quad \dfrac{60X}{60} = \dfrac{375}{60}$

$\qquad\qquad X = 6.25 = 6\tfrac{1}{4} \text{ h} = 6 \text{ h } 15 \text{ min}$

11) $\dfrac{D}{H} \times Q = \dfrac{4 \text{ mg/min}}{2{,}000 \text{ mg}} \times \overset{1}{500} \text{ mL} = \dfrac{\overset{4}{4}}{\underset{1}{4}} \text{ mL/min} = 1 \text{ mL/min},$

which is the same as 60 mL per 60 min or 60 mL/h

12) $\dfrac{D}{H} \times Q = \dfrac{3 \text{ mg/min}}{1{,}000 \text{ mg}} \times \overset{1}{250} \text{ mL} = \dfrac{3}{4} \text{ mL/min} = 0.75 \text{ mL/min}$

$\qquad 0.75 \text{ mL/min} \times 60 \text{ min/h} = 45 \text{ mL/h}$

13) $\dfrac{D}{H} \times Q = \dfrac{2 \text{ mg/min}}{1{,}000 \text{ mg}} \times \overset{1}{500} \text{ mL} = \dfrac{\overset{2}{2}}{\underset{1}{2}} \text{ mL/min} = 1 \text{ mL/min},$

which is the same as 60 mL per 60 min or 60 mL/h

14) $5 \text{ mcg/kg/min} \times 80 \text{ kg} = 400 \text{ mcg/min}$

$\qquad 400 \text{ mcg/min} = .400. = 0.4 \text{ mg/min}$

$\qquad \dfrac{D}{H} \times Q = \dfrac{0.4 \text{ mg/min}}{250 \text{ mg}} \times \overset{1}{250} \text{ mL} = 0.4 \text{ mL/min}$

$\qquad 0.4 \text{ mL/min} \times 60 \text{ min/h} = 24 \text{ mL/h}$

15) $\dfrac{D}{H} \times Q = R$

$\qquad \dfrac{D \text{ mg/h}}{2{,}000 \text{ mg}} \times 1{,}000 \text{ mL} = 75 \text{ mL/h}$

$\qquad \dfrac{D}{2{,}000} \times 1{,}000 = 75$

$\qquad \dfrac{1{,}000D}{2{,}000} = \dfrac{75}{1}$

$\qquad 1{,}000D = 150{,}000$

$\qquad \dfrac{1{,}000D}{1{,}000} = \dfrac{150{,}000}{1{,}000}$

$\qquad D = 150 \text{ mg/h}$

$\qquad 150 \text{ mg/h} \div 60 \text{ min/h} = 150 \text{ mg/h} \times 1 \text{ h}/60 \text{ min}$

$\qquad = 2.5 \text{ mg/min};$ within normal range of 1 to 4 mg/min

16) IV PB flow rate: $\dfrac{\text{mL/h}}{\text{Drop factor constant}} = \dfrac{100 \text{ mL/h}}{6} =$

16.6 gtt/min = 17 gtt/min

Total IV PB time: q.6h = 4 times per 24h;

$4 \times 1 \text{ h} = 4 \text{ h}$

Total IV PB volume: $4 \times 100 \text{ mL} = 400 \text{ mL}$

Total regular IV volume: $3{,}000 \text{ mL} - 400 \text{ mL} =$

2,600 mL

Total regular IV time: 24 h − 4 h = 20 h

Regular IV rate: mL/h $= \dfrac{2{,}600 \text{ mL}}{20 \text{ h}} = 130 \text{ mL/h};$

$\dfrac{\text{mL/h}}{\text{Drop factor constant}} = \dfrac{130 \text{ mL/h}}{6} = 21.6 \text{ gtt/min}$

= 22 gtt/min

17) IV PB rate

$\qquad \dfrac{50 \text{ mL}}{30 \text{ min}} \underset{\times}{\times} \dfrac{X \text{ mL}}{60 \text{ min}}$

$\qquad\quad 30X = 3{,}000$

$\qquad\quad \dfrac{30X}{30} = \dfrac{3{,}000}{30}$

$\qquad\qquad X = 100 \text{ mL}; 100 \text{ mL per } 60 \text{ min} = 100 \text{ mL/h}$

Total IV PB time: q.i.d = 4 times per 24h; ordered for

30 min per administration; $4 \times 30 \text{ min} = 120 \text{ min};$

$120 \text{ min} \div 60 \text{ min/h} = 120 \text{ min} \times 1 \text{ h}/60 \text{ min} = 2 \text{ h}$

Total IV PB volume: $4 \times 50 \text{ mL} = 200 \text{ mL}$

Total regular IV volume:

3,000 mL − 200 mL = 2,800 mL

Total regular IV time: 24 h − 2 h = 22 h

Regular IV rate: $\frac{2,800 \text{ mL}}{22 \text{ h}}$ = 127.2 mL/h = 127 mL/h

18) 125 lb ÷ 2.2 lb/kg = 125 l̶b̶ × 1 kg/2.2 l̶b̶

  = 56.81 kg = 56.8 kg

  3 mcg/k̶g̶/min × 56.8 k̶g̶ = 170.4 mcg/min

  170.4 mcg/min = .170.4 = 0.1704 = 0.17 mg/min

  $\frac{D}{H} \times Q = \frac{0.17 \text{ m̶g̶/min}}{50 \text{ m̶g̶}} \times 500 \text{ mL}$ = 1.7 mL/min

  1.7 mL/min × 60 m̶i̶n̶/h = 102 mL/h

19) 1,000 mL − 800 mL = 200 mL infused

  $\frac{40 \text{ mEq}}{1,000 \text{ mL}} \diagdown\diagup \frac{X \text{ mEq}}{200 \text{ mL}}$

  1,000X = 8,000

  $\frac{1,000X}{1,000} = \frac{8,000}{1,000}$

  X = 8 mEq

20) $\frac{125 \text{ mL}}{60 \text{ min}}$ = 2.08 mL/min = 2 mL/min

21) 1,500 mL ÷ 100 mL/h = 1,500 m̶L̶ × 1 h/100 m̶L̶

  = 15 h

22) $\frac{D}{H} \times Q = \frac{2 \text{ m̶E̶q̶/h/}}{40 \text{ m̶E̶q̶}} \times 1,000 \text{ mL}$ = 50 mL/h

23) $\frac{D}{H} \times Q = \frac{1,250 \text{ u̶n̶i̶t̶s̶/h}}{50,000 \text{ u̶n̶i̶t̶s̶}} \times 1,000 \text{ mL} = \frac{1,250}{50}$ mL/h

  = 25 mL/h

24) $\frac{5 \text{ mg}}{1 \text{ mL}} \diagdown\diagup \frac{37 \text{ mg}}{X \text{ mL}}$

  5X = 37

  $\frac{5X}{5} = \frac{37}{5}$

  X = 7.4 mL

25) 10 units = 10.000. = 10,000 milliunits

  $\frac{D}{H} \times Q = \frac{4 \text{ m̶i̶l̶l̶i̶u̶n̶i̶t̶s̶/min}}{10,000 \text{ m̶i̶l̶l̶i̶u̶n̶i̶t̶s̶}} \times 500 \text{ mL} =$

  $\frac{4}{20}$ mL/min = $\frac{1}{5}$ mL/min =

  0.2 mL/min (for first 20 min)

  0.2 mL/m̶i̶n̶ × 60 m̶i̶n̶/h = 12 mL/h

  $\frac{D}{H} \times Q = \frac{6 \text{ m̶i̶l̶l̶i̶u̶n̶i̶t̶s̶/min}}{10,000 \text{ m̶i̶l̶l̶i̶u̶n̶i̶t̶s̶}} \times 500 \text{ mL}$

  $= \frac{6}{20}$ mL/min = $\frac{3}{10}$ mL/min =

  0.3 mL/min (for next 20 min)

  0.3 mL/m̶i̶n̶ × 60 m̶i̶n̶/h = 18 mL/h

26) Bolus:

  $\frac{D}{H} \times Q = \frac{3 \text{ g̶}}{20 \text{ g̶}} \times 500 \text{ mL} = \frac{1,500}{20}$ mL =

  75 mL (per 30 min)

  $\frac{75 \text{ mL}}{30 \text{ m̶i̶n̶}} \times 60 \text{ m̶i̶n̶/h}$ = 150 mL/h

  Continuous:

  $\frac{D}{H} \times Q = \frac{2 \text{ g̶/h}}{20 \text{ g̶}} \times 500 \text{ mL} = \frac{500}{10}$ mL/h = 50 mL/h

29) $\frac{4,000 \text{ mg}}{500 \text{ mL}}$ = 8 mg/mL

30) $\frac{D}{H} \times Q = \frac{500 \text{ m̶g̶/h}}{4,000 \text{ m̶g̶}} \times 500 \text{ mL} = \frac{500}{8}$ mL/h = 62.5 mL/h

  = 63 mL/h

31) 80 units = 80.000. = 80,000 milliunits

  $\frac{80,000 \text{ milliunits}}{1,000 \text{ mL}}$ = 80 milliunits/mL

33) 4 mg = 4.000. = 4,000 mcg

  $\frac{4,000 \text{ mcg}}{1,000 \text{ mL}}$ = 4 mcg/mL

36) $\frac{20 \text{ mg}}{100 \text{ mL}} = \frac{2}{10}$ mg/mL = 0.2 mg/mL

  0.2 mg/mL = 0.200. = 200 mcg/mL

37) 1 mcg/kg/min × 100 k̶g̶ = 100 mcg/min

  $\frac{D}{H} \times Q = \frac{100 \text{ m̶c̶g̶/min}}{20,000 \text{ m̶c̶g̶}} \times 100 \text{ mL} = \frac{100}{200}$ mL/min

  = 0.5 mL/min

  0.5 mL/m̶i̶n̶ × 60 m̶i̶n̶/h = 30 mL/h

38) IV PB rates:

  $\frac{100 \text{ mL}}{30 \text{ min}} \diagdown\diagup \frac{X \text{ mL}}{60 \text{ min}}$

  30X = 6,000

  $\frac{30X}{30} = \frac{6,000}{30}$

  X = 200 mL (per 60 min)

  or 200 mL/h (ampicillin) gentamicin: 50 mL/h

39) ampicillin: q.6h = 4 times per day; ordered 30 min per administration; 4 × 30 min = 120 min;

  120 min ÷ 60 min/h = 120 m̶i̶n̶ × 1 h/60 m̶i̶n̶ = 2 h

  gentamicin: q.8h = 3 times per day; ordered 1 h per administration; 3 × 1 h = 3 h

  Total IV PB time: 2 h + 3 h = 5 h

40) ampicillin: 4 d̶o̶s̶e̶s̶ × 100 mL/d̶o̶s̶e̶ = 400 mL

  gentamicin: 3 d̶o̶s̶e̶s̶ × 50 mL/d̶o̶s̶e̶ = 150 mL

  Total IV PB volume: 400 mL + 150 mL = 550 mL

41) 3,000 mL − 550 mL = 2,450 mL

42) $24\,h - 5\,h = 19\,h$

43) $\dfrac{2{,}450\,\text{mL}}{19\,h} = 129\,\text{mL/h}$

44) $190\,\text{lb} \div 2.2\,\text{lb/kg} = 190\,\cancel{\text{lb}} \times 1\,\text{kg}/2.2\,\cancel{\text{lb}}$

$= 86.36\,\text{kg} = 86.4\,\text{kg}$

$4\,\text{mcg/}\cancel{\text{kg}}\text{/min} \times 86.4\,\cancel{\text{kg}} = 345.6\,\text{mcg/min}$

$345.6\,\text{mcg/}\cancel{\text{min}} \times 60\,\cancel{\text{min}}\text{/h} = 20{,}736\,\text{mcg/h} =$

$20{,}736\,\text{mcg/h} = 20.736. = 20.736\,\text{mg/h} = 21\,\text{mg/h}$

$\dfrac{D}{H} \times Q = \dfrac{21\,\cancel{\text{mg/h}}}{\underset{8}{800}\,\cancel{\text{mg}}} \times \overset{5}{\cancel{500}}\,\text{mL} = \dfrac{105}{8}\,\text{mL/h} =$

$13.1\,\text{mL/h} = 13\,\text{mL/h}$ (initial rate)

$12\,\text{mcg/}\cancel{\text{kg}}\text{/min} \times 86.4\,\cancel{\text{kg}} = 1{,}036.8\,\text{mcg/min}$

$1{,}036.8\,\text{mcg/}\cancel{\text{min}} \times 60\,\cancel{\text{min}}\text{/h} = 62{,}208\,\text{mcg/h}$

$62{,}208\,\text{mcg/h} = 62.208. = 62.208\,\text{mcg/h} = 62\,\text{mg/h}$

$\dfrac{D}{H} \times Q = \dfrac{62\,\cancel{\text{mg/h}}}{\underset{8}{800}\,\cancel{\text{mg}}} \times \overset{5}{\cancel{500}}\,\text{mL} = \dfrac{310}{8}\,\text{mL/h} =$

$38.7\,\text{mL/h} = 39\,\text{mL/h}$ (after titration)

45) $225\,\text{lb} \div 2.2\,\text{lb/kg} = 225\,\cancel{\text{lb}} \times 1\,\text{kg}/2.2\,\cancel{\text{lb}} = 102.2\,\text{kg}$

$= 100\,\text{kg}$ (rounded to the nearest 10 kg)

80 units/kg bolus dosage

46) $80\,\text{units/}\cancel{\text{kg}} \times 100\,\cancel{\text{kg}} = 8{,}000\,\text{units}$

1,000 units/mL

$\dfrac{D}{H} \times Q = \dfrac{\overset{8}{\cancel{8{,}000}}\,\cancel{\text{units}}}{\underset{1}{\cancel{1{,}000}}\,\cancel{\text{units}}} \times 1\,\text{mL} = 8\,\text{mL}$

47) 18 units/kg/h

$18\,\text{units/}\cancel{\text{kg}}\text{/h} \times 100\,\cancel{\text{kg}} = 1{,}800\,\text{units/h}$

25,000 units per 250 mL, or 100 units/mL

$\dfrac{D}{H} \times Q = \dfrac{\overset{18}{\cancel{1{,}800}}\,\cancel{\text{units/h}}}{\underset{1}{\cancel{100}}\,\cancel{\text{units}}} \times 1\,\text{mL} = 18\,\text{mL/h}$

48) q.6h

$40\,\text{units/}\cancel{\text{kg}} \times 100\,\cancel{\text{kg}} = 4{,}000\,\text{units}$

$\dfrac{D}{H} \times Q = \dfrac{4{,}000\,\cancel{\text{units}}}{1{,}000\,\cancel{\text{units}}} \times 1\,\text{mL} = 4\,\text{mL}$

Increase rate: $2\,\text{units/}\cancel{\text{kg}}\text{/h} \times 100\,\cancel{\text{kg}} = 200\,\text{units/h}$

Increase rate: $\dfrac{\overset{2}{\cancel{200}}\,\cancel{\text{units/h}}}{\underset{1}{\cancel{100}}\,\cancel{\text{units}}} \times 1\,\text{mL} = 2\,\text{mL/h}$

$18\,\text{mL/h} + 2\,\text{mL/h} = 20\,\text{mL/h}$ (new infusion rate)

49) Decrease rate by 2 units/kg/h.

$2\,\text{units/}\cancel{\text{kg}}\text{/h} \times 100\,\cancel{\text{kg}} = 200\,\text{units/h}$

$\dfrac{D}{H} \times Q = \dfrac{200\,\cancel{\text{units/h}}}{100\,\cancel{\text{units}}} \times 1\,\text{mL} = 2\,\text{mL/h}$

$20\,\text{mL/h} - 2\,\text{mL/h} = 18\,\text{mL/h}$ (new infusion rate)

Section 4—Self-Evaluation from pages 549–555

1) 0.9% NaCl **2)** 0.9 g NaCl per 100 mL **3)** 0.45 g NaCl per 100 mL **4)** 50 **5)** 4.5 **6)** 2.25 **7)** 75 **8)** 6.75 **9)** mL/h **10)** 21 **11)** 83 **12)** 1940 **13)** 1,536 **14)** Give a total of 3,000 mL IV solution per day, to include normal saline (0.9% NaCl) with 20 milliequivalents of potassium chloride added per liter (1,000 mL) *and* an IV piggyback solution of 250 mg cefazolin added to 100 mL of normal saline (0.9% NaCl) over 30 min administered every 8 hours. To administer the order each day, give 900 mL NS with KCl over $7\frac{1}{2}$ hours × 3 administrations and 100 mL NS with cefazolin over $\frac{1}{2}$ hour × 3 administrations **15)** 120 **16)** 200 **17)** Reset rate to 118 gtt/min, if policy and patient's condition permit. **18)** 1,410 **19)** 59 **20)** 120 **21)** 5 **22)** 0.48 **23)** 1.3 **24)** 1.04 **25)** 0.5 **26)** 18.5–37.5 **27)** Yes **28)** 18.5 **29)** 37 mL **30)** 120 **31)** 18.5 **32)** 0.8 **33)** 1.6 **34)** Yes **35)** 1.6 **36)** 18; 2 **37)** 7.5 **38)** 43 **39)** 200 **40)** 43 **41)** 200 **42)** 50 **43)** 12 **44)** 15 **45)** 0.13 **46)** 8 **47)** 80 **48)** 20.5 **49)** 61.4 **50)** 37.5 **51)** protamine sulfate **52)** a, c, and d **53)** b

54)   1—Record weight in kilograms.

   2—Check aPTT test results.

   3—Administer bolus, if required.

   4—Start continuous infusion, if required.

   5—Check aPTT test results.

   6—Administer rebolus, if required.

   7—Adjust infusion rate, if required.

55)   10,000 units/mL best choice. 5,000 units/mL would work but would need multiple vials.

Solutions—Section 4—Self-Evaluation

4) D_5 0.45% NaCl = 5% dextrose =

5 g dextrose per 100 mL

$$\frac{5\ g}{100\ mL} \diagdown\!\!\!\!\diagup \frac{X\ g}{1{,}000\ mL}$$

$$100X = 5{,}000$$

$$\frac{100X}{100} = \frac{5{,}000}{100}$$

$$X = 50\ g$$

5) D_5 0.45% NaCl = 0.45% NaCl =

0.45 g NaCl per 100 mL

$$\frac{0.45\ g}{100\ mL} \diagdown\!\!\!\!\diagup \frac{X\ g}{1{,}000\ mL}$$

$$100X = 450$$

$$\frac{100X}{100} = \frac{450}{100}$$

$$X = 4.5\ g$$

10) $\dfrac{2{,}000\ mL}{24\ h} = 83.3\ mL/h = 83\ mL/h$

$$\frac{mL/h}{Drop\ factor\ constant} = gtt/min$$

$$\frac{83\ mL/h}{4} = 20.7 = 21\ gtt/min$$

12) $\dfrac{V}{T} \times C = R:\ \dfrac{400\ mL}{T\ min} \times 15\ gtt/mL = 24\ gtt/min$

$$\frac{400}{T} \times 15 = 24$$

$$\frac{6{,}000}{T} \diagdown\!\!\!\!\diagup \frac{24}{1}$$

$$24T = 6{,}000$$

$$\frac{24T}{24} = \frac{6{,}000}{24}$$

$$T = 250\ min$$

$$250\ min \div 60\ min/h = 250\ min \times 1\ h/60\ min$$

$$= 4.16\ h = 4\tfrac{1}{6}\ h = 4\ h\ 10\ min$$

$$\begin{array}{r} 1530\ hours \\ +\ \ 410\ hours \\ \hline 1940\ hours \end{array}$$

13) $\dfrac{V}{T} \times C = R$

$$\frac{V\ mL}{60\ min} \times 10\ gtt/mL = 32\ gtt/min$$

$$\frac{10V}{60} \diagdown\!\!\!\!\diagup \frac{32}{1}$$

$$10V = 1{,}920$$

$$\frac{10V}{10} = \frac{1{,}920}{10}$$

V = 192 mL per 60 min, or

V = 192 mL/h; 192 mL/h × 8 h = 1,536 mL
(administered during your 8 h shift)

15) On fluid restriction of 3,000 mL/day

IV PB total volume: 100 mL × 3 = 300 mL

IV PB total time: 30 min × 3 = 90 min = $1\tfrac{1}{2}$ h

Regular IV total volume: 3,000 mL − 300 mL = 2,700 mL

Regular IV total time: 24h − $1\tfrac{1}{2}$ h = $22\tfrac{1}{2}$ h (22.5 h)

$$\frac{2{,}700\ mL}{22.5\ h} = 120\ mL/h$$

16) $\dfrac{100\ mL}{\overset{}{\underset{1}{30\ min}}} \times \overset{2}{60}\ min/h = 200\ mL/h$

17) $1{,}200\ mL \div 100\ mL/h = 1{,}200\ mL \times 1\ h/100\ mL = 12\ h$

$$\tfrac{1}{6}\ h \times 60\ min/h = 10\ min$$

$4\tfrac{1}{6}$ h = 4 h 10 min (total time ordered to infuse 1,200 mL)

$$\begin{array}{r} 2200\ hours\ (current\ time) \\ -1530\ hours\ (start\ time) \\ \hline 0630 = 6\ h\ 30\ min\ (elapsed\ time) \end{array}$$

6 h 30 min = $6\tfrac{1}{2}$ h = 6.5 h;

6.5 h × 100 mL/h = 650 mL (expected to be infused)

1,200 mL − 650 mL = 550 mL (should be remaining)

After $6\tfrac{1}{2}$ h, 650 mL should have been infused, with 550 mL remaining. IV is behind schedule.

$$\frac{Remaining\ volume}{Remaining\ time} = \frac{650\ mL}{5.5\ h} = 118\ mL/h\ (adjusted\ rate)$$

$$\frac{Adjusted\ gtt/min - Ordered\ gtt/min}{Ordered\ gtt/min} = \%\ of\ variation;$$

$$\frac{118 - 100}{100} = \frac{18}{100} = 0.18 = 18\%\ (variance\ is\ safe)$$

If policy and patient's condition permit, reset rate to 118 mL/h.

18) $40\ lb \div 2.2\ lb/kg = 40\ lb \times 1\ kg/2.2\ lb$

$$= 18.18\ kg = 18.2\ kg$$

First 10 kg: 100 mL/kg/day × 10 kg = 1,000 mL/day

Remaining 8.2 kg: 50 mL/kg/day × 8.2 kg = $\underline{410\ mL/day}$

1,410 mL/day

19) $\dfrac{1{,}410\ mL}{24\ h} = 58.7\ mL/h = 59\ mL/h$

20) 1,185 g = 1.185. = 1.185 kg = 1.2 kg

First 10 kg: 100 mL/kg/day × 1.2 kg = 120 mL/day

21) $\dfrac{120\ mL}{24\ h} = 5\ mL/h$

22) Household:

$$BSA\ (m^2) = \sqrt{\frac{ht\ (in)\ \times\ wt\ (lb)}{3{,}131}} = \sqrt{\frac{30 \times 24}{3{,}131}} = \sqrt{\frac{720}{3{,}131}}$$

$$= \sqrt{0.229\ldots} = 0.479\ m^2 = 0.48\ m^2$$

23) Metric:

$$BSA\ (m^2) = \sqrt{\frac{ht\ (cm)\ \times\ wt\ (kg)}{3{,}600}} = \sqrt{\frac{155 \times 39}{3{,}600}} =$$

$$\sqrt{\frac{6{,}045}{3{,}600}} = \sqrt{1.679\ldots} = 1.295\ m^2 = 1.3\ m^2$$

26) Minimum safe dosage: 37 mg/m² × 0.5 m² = 18.5 mg

Maximum safe dosage: 75 mg/m² × 0.5 m² = 37.5 mg

28) $\dfrac{D}{H} \times Q = \dfrac{18.5 \text{ m\cancel{g}}}{1 \text{ m\cancel{g}}} \times 1 \text{ mL} = 18.5 \text{ mL}$

29) $\dfrac{1 \text{ mg}}{2 \text{ mL}} \diagdown\diagup \dfrac{18.5 \text{ mg}}{X \text{ mL}}$

$X = 37 \text{ mL}$

30) $\dfrac{D}{H} \times Q = \dfrac{1 \text{ m\cancel{g}/min}}{18.5 \text{ m\cancel{g}}} \times 37 \text{ mL} = \dfrac{37}{18.5} \text{ mL/min} =$

2 mL/min

$2 \text{ mL/\cancel{min}} \times 60 \text{ \cancel{min}/h} = 120 \text{ mL/h}$

31) Think: At 1 mg/min, 18.5 mg will infuse in 18.5 min.

$\dfrac{1 \text{ mg}}{1 \text{ min}} \diagdown\diagup \dfrac{18.5 \text{ mg}}{X \text{ min}}$

$X = 18.5 \text{ min}$

33) $2 \text{ mg/\cancel{m}}^2 \times 0.8 \text{ \cancel{m}}^2 = 1.6 \text{ mg}$

36) $\dfrac{D}{H} \times Q = \dfrac{\overset{2}{\cancel{250}} \text{ mg}}{\underset{1}{\cancel{125}} \text{ mg}} \times 1 \text{ mL} = 2 \text{ mL (Ancef)}$

$\dfrac{40 \text{ mL}}{60 \text{ min}} \diagdown\diagup \dfrac{X \text{ mL}}{30 \text{ min}}$

$60X = 1{,}200$

$\dfrac{60X}{60} = \dfrac{1{,}200}{60}$

$X = 20 \text{ mL}$

$20 \text{ mL (total IV solution)} - 2 \text{ mL(Ancef)} =$

18 mL (NS)

37) $\dfrac{100 \text{ mg}}{1 \text{ mL}} \diagdown\diagup \dfrac{750 \text{ mg}}{X \text{ mL}}$

$100X = 750$

$\dfrac{100X}{100} = \dfrac{750}{100}$

$X = 7.5 \text{ mL}$

7.5 mL IV solution is to be used with the 750 mg of

Timentin for minimal dilution.

38) Total IV PB volume: $100 \text{ mL} \times 6 = 600 \text{ mL}$

Regular IV volume: $1{,}500 \text{ mL} - 600 \text{ mL} = 900 \text{ mL}$

Total IV PB time of q.4h = 6 times per 24h;

$6 \times 30 \text{ min} = 180 \text{ min}$;

$180 \text{ min} \div 60 \text{ min/h} = 180 \text{ \cancel{min}} \times 1 \text{ h/60 \cancel{min}} = 3 \text{ h}$

Total regular IV time: $24 \text{ h} - 3 \text{ h} = 21 \text{ h}$

Regular IV rate: $\text{mL/h} = \dfrac{900 \text{ mL}}{21 \text{ h}} = 42.8 \text{ mL/h}$

$= 43 \text{ mL/h or } 43 \text{ gtt/min (because drop factor is}$

60 gtt/mL)

$\dfrac{\text{mL/h}}{\text{Drop factor constant}} = \text{gtt/min};$

$\dfrac{42.8 \text{ mL/h}}{1} = 42.8 \text{ gtt/min} = 43 \text{ gtt/min}$

39) $\dfrac{V}{T} \times C = \dfrac{100 \text{ m\cancel{L}}}{\underset{1}{\cancel{30}} \text{ min}} \times \overset{2}{\cancel{60}} \text{ gtt/m\cancel{L}} = 200 \text{ gtt/min}$

40) See #38. Regular IV rate calculated at 43 mL/h.

41) See #39. Because the flow rate is 200 gtt/min with a drop

factor of 60 gtt/mL, the infusion pump flow rate

would be set at 200 mL/h.

42) $\dfrac{D}{H} \times Q = \dfrac{\overset{1}{\cancel{2}} \text{ m\cancel{Eq}/h}}{\underset{20}{\cancel{40}} \text{ m\cancel{Eq}}} \times 1{,}000 \text{ mL} = \dfrac{\overset{50}{\cancel{1{,}000}}}{\underset{1}{\cancel{20}}} \text{ mL/h} = 50 \text{ mL/h}$

43) $\dfrac{25 \text{ mg}}{1 \text{ L}} = \dfrac{25.000.}{1.000.} = \dfrac{25{,}000 \text{ mcg}}{1{,}000 \text{ mL}} = \dfrac{25{,}000 \text{ mcg}}{1{,}000 \text{ mL}} = 25 \text{ mcg/mL}$

$\dfrac{D}{H} \times Q = \dfrac{\overset{1}{\cancel{5}} \text{ m\cancel{cg}/min}}{\underset{5}{\cancel{25}} \text{ m\cancel{cg}}} \times 1 \text{ mL} = \dfrac{1}{5} \text{ mL/min} =$

0.2 mL/min

$0.2 \text{ mL/\cancel{min}} \times 60 \text{ \cancel{min}/h} = 12 \text{ mL/h}$

44) $\dfrac{15 \text{ units}}{1 \text{ L}} = \dfrac{15.000.}{1.000.} = \dfrac{15{,}000 \text{ milliunits}}{1{,}000 \text{ mL}} = 15 \text{ milliunits/mL}$

45) $\dfrac{D}{H} \times Q = \dfrac{2 \text{ milliun\cancel{its}/min}}{15 \text{ milliun\cancel{its}}} \times 1 \text{ mL} = \dfrac{2}{15} \text{ mL/min}$

$= 0.133 \text{ mL/min} = 0.13 \text{ mL/min}$

46) $0.13 \text{ mL/\cancel{min}} \times 60 \text{ \cancel{min}/h} = 7.8 = 8 \text{ mL/h}$

47) $\dfrac{D}{H} \times Q = \dfrac{\overset{4}{\cancel{20}} \text{ milliun\cancel{its}/min}}{\underset{3}{\cancel{15}} \text{ milliun\cancel{its}}} \times 1 \text{ mL} = \dfrac{4}{3} \text{ mL/min}$

$= 1.33 \text{ mL/min}$

$1.33 \text{ mL/\cancel{min}} \times 60 \text{ \cancel{min}/h} = 79.8 \text{ mL/h} = 80 \text{ mL/h}$

48) $150 \text{ lb} \div 2.2 \text{ lb/kg} = 150 \text{ \cancel{lb}} \times 1 \text{ kg/2.2 \cancel{lb}}$

$= 68.18 \text{ kg} = 68.2 \text{ kg};$

$4 \text{ mcg/kg/min} \times 68.2 \text{ \cancel{kg}} = 272.8 = 273 \text{ mcg/min}$

$273 \text{ mcg/\cancel{min}} \times 60 \text{ \cancel{min}/h} = 16{,}380 \text{ mcg/h}$

$0.5 \text{ L} = 0.500. = 500 \text{ mL}$

$\dfrac{400 \text{ mg}}{0.5 \text{ L}} = \dfrac{400 \text{ mg}}{500 \text{ mL}}$

$= 0.8 \text{ mg/mL}$

$0.8 \text{ mg/mL} = 0.800. = 800 \text{ mcg/mL}$

$\dfrac{D}{H} \times Q = \dfrac{16{,}380 \text{ m\cancel{cg}/h}}{800 \text{ m\cancel{cg}}} \times 1 \text{ mL} =$

$\dfrac{16{,}380}{800} \text{ mL/h} = 20.47 \text{ mL/h} = 20.5 \text{ mL/h}$

49) $12 \text{ mcg/kg/min} \times 68.2 \text{ \cancel{kg}} = 818.4 \text{ mcg/min} =$

818 mcg/min

$818 \text{ mcg/\cancel{min}} \times 60 \text{ \cancel{min}/h} = 49{,}080 \text{ mcg/h}$

$\dfrac{D}{H} \times Q = \dfrac{49{,}080 \text{ m\cancel{cg}/h}}{800 \text{ m\cancel{cg}}} \times 1 \text{ mL} = \dfrac{49{,}080}{800} \text{ mL/h} =$

$61.35 \text{ mL/h} = 61.4 \text{ mL/h}$

50) $\dfrac{D}{H} \times Q = \dfrac{750 \text{ un\cancel{its}/h}}{\underset{20}{\cancel{10{,}000}} \text{ un\cancel{its}}} \times \overset{1}{\cancel{500}} \text{ mL} = \dfrac{750}{20} \text{ mL/h} =$

37.5 mL/h

Comprehensive Skills Evaluation from pages 565–580

1) 80 **2)** 0500; 09/04/xx **3)** 1,920 **4)** 0.8; 19.2 **5)** a) immediately b) one time only

6) a) 1; 4; 5; 1; 0.25

b) Fill syringe with 1 mL of digoxin and 4 mL of normal saline.

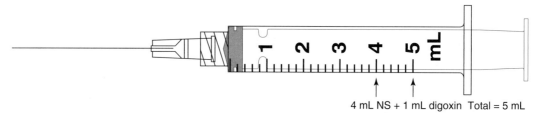

4 mL NS + 1 mL digoxin Total = 5 mL

© Cengage Learning 2013

7) e

8) a) 2; 2; 0.5

b)

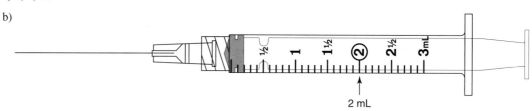

2 mL

© Cengage Learning 2013

9) $\frac{1}{2}$ **10)** 1 **11)** 2 **12)** a) 2 b) 4 hours later, if she complains again of a headache **13)** digoxin for injection and tablets, furosemide for injection, nitroglycerin **14)** 80

15) a) 5

b)

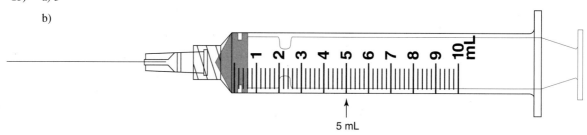

5 mL

© Cengage Learning 2013

16) 30

17) a) Yes; dosage ordered is at the maximum of the recommended range of 250 mcg/min to 500 mcg/min for Mrs. Smith, who weighs 110 lb, or 50 kg.

b) 5

c)

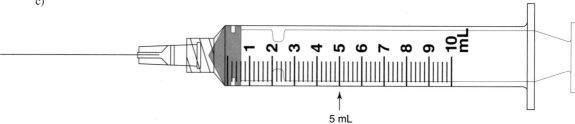

5 mL

© Cengage Learning 2013

18) 18.6 **19)** 30,000; 30 **20)** 60 **21)** a) Yes, the recommended dosage for this child is 225 mg/day in 3 divided doses, or 75 mg/dose. This is the same as the order. b) 2; 23; 40 **22)** Yes, safe dosage for this child is 300 mg/dose, which is the same as the order. **23)** a) 6 b) 44 c) 1,200 **24)** a) 1,700 b) 70.8 c) No. The ordered rate of 50 mL per hour is less than the recommended hourly maintenance IV rate. **25)** 3.2

26)

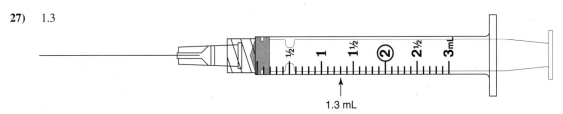

2/6/xx, 0800, reconstituted as 1.5 g in 4 mL. Expires 2/9/xx, 0800, keep refrigerated. G.D.P.

© Cengage Learning 2013

27)   1.3

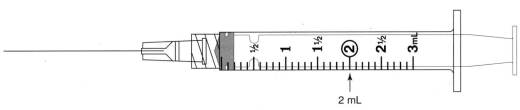

1.3 mL

© Cengage Learning 2013

28)   102

29)   a) 2

        b) 60

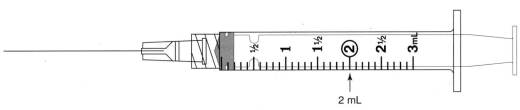

2 mL

© Cengage Learning 2013

30) a) 56.8 b) 4,544 c) 4.5 d) 1,022; 10.2 **31)** a) Decrease rate by 2 units/kg/h. b) 114; 1 c) 9.1

32) 8; 0.08; Insulin should be administered with an insulin syringe. This question and answer are provided to evaluate your understanding of the insulin syringe and insulin concentration. 8 units of U-100 insulin equals a volume of 0.08 mL.

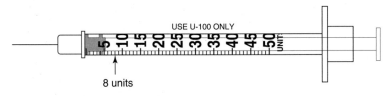

8 units

© Cengage Learning 2013

33) a) 60

b)

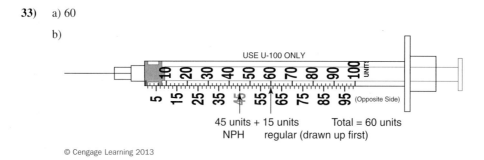

USE U-100 ONLY

(Opposite Side)

45 units + 15 units   Total = 60 units
NPH   regular (drawn up first)

© Cengage Learning 2013

34) 20 **35)** 720; 960 **36)** 730; 30 **37)** 1.43 **38)** a) 14.3–28.6 b) Yes; the dosage ordered is within the allowable range.
39) a) 0.5 b) 56; 5.6; 1.4 **40)** 50; 4.5 **41)** 6; 44 **42)** Yes; the recommended amount of IV fluid to safely dilute this med is
15–60 mL. The order calls for 50 mL total, or 44 mL of IV fluid. **43)** a) 1,600,000 b) Yes, the minimum daily dosage is
1,500,000 units/day, and the maximum is 2,500,000 units/day. The ordered dosage falls within this range. c) 1.8; 500,000
d) 0.8 e) Contact the prescriber.

> 1/14/xx; 0800, reconstituted as
> 500,000 units/mL. Expires 1/21/xx; 0800.
> Keep refrigerated. G.D.P.

© Cengage Learning 2013

44) 101 **45)** 2145 **46)** 0.5; 0.13 **47)** 15 **48)** 230

49) Prevention: The frequency of this order is missing and the route is unclear. If the student actually gave this
medication in the eye, it would cause a severe reaction. The medication particles could scratch the eyes or cause a worse
reaction, such as blindness.

To prevent this from occurring, the student nurse should always ensure that each medication order is complete.
Every order should include the name of the drug, the dose, the route, and the time (with the patient, prescriber, and
licensure identified). When any of these are missing, the order should be clarified. Further, the "O.D." abbreviation is
obsolete and discouraged by The Joint Commission. The student nurse should also look up medications and know the safe
use for each medication ordered. Had this student looked up Lanoxin in a drug guide, the student would have discovered
that the medication is never given in the eye.

50) Prevention: The student nurse took the correct action with this order. The nurses who had given the medication
previously should have looked up the medication if they were unfamiliar with it, to safely identify whether it was ordered
with an appropriate route, correct dosage, and correct frequency. There was also an error made by the pharmacist who
supplied the medication to the nursing unit. It is extremely important to be familiar with the medications being given. If
there's a question or any doubt, the medication should be looked up in a drug guide and/or the prescriber should be
questioned. Also, close reading of the label and matching it to the order is extremely important. Remember the Six Rights
of medication administration. Ideally, packaging by the pharmacy using "Tall Man" lettering would further enhance
patient safety and alert the nurse to select the correct drug.

Solutions—Comprehensive Skills Evaluation

1) $\dfrac{mL/h}{\text{Drop factor constant}} = gtt/min$

$\dfrac{80\ mL/h}{1} = 80\ gtt/min$ or

$80\ mL/h = 80\ gtt/min$ (because drop factor is

$60\ gtt/mL$)

2) $\dfrac{1,000\ \cancel{mL}}{80\ \cancel{mL}/h} = 12.5\ h = 12\ h\ 30\ min$

$1630\ hours + 12\ h\ 30\ min\ later = 0500\ hours$

the next day (09/04/xx)

3) $80\ mL/\cancel{h} \times 24\ \cancel{h} = 1,920\ mL$

4) The total fluid volume is:

$1,000\ mL\ (D_5\tfrac{1}{2}NS) + 5\ mL\ (KCl) = 1,005\ mL$

$\dfrac{D}{H} \times Q = X$

$\dfrac{D\ mEq/h}{10\ mEq} \times 1,005\ mL = 80\ mL/h$

$\dfrac{D}{10} \times 1,005 = 80$

$\dfrac{1,005D}{10} = \dfrac{80}{1}$

$1,005D = 800$

$\dfrac{1,005D}{1005} = \dfrac{800}{1,005}$

$D = 0.79\ mEq/h = 0.8\ mEq/h$

$0.8\ mEq/\cancel{h} \times 24\ \cancel{h} = 19.2\ mEq$ (per day)

6) $0.25\ mg$ is ordered and the supply dosage is

$0.25\ mg/mL$. It is obvious that the nurse should give 1

mL. 1 mL added to 4 mL NS = 5 mL total solution.

$\dfrac{\overset{1}{\cancel{5}}\ mL}{\underset{1}{\cancel{5}}\ min} = 1\ mL/min$

$\dfrac{1\ mL}{60\ sec} \diagdown\!\!\!\diagup \dfrac{X\ mL}{15\ sec}$

$60X = 15$

$\dfrac{60X}{60} = \dfrac{15}{60}$

$X = 0.25\ mL$ (per 15 sec)

7) The total amount of fluid is too small for an IV PB.

8) $\dfrac{D}{H} \times Q = \dfrac{\overset{2}{\cancel{20}}\ mg}{\underset{1}{\cancel{10}}\ mg} \times 1\ mL = 2\ mL$

$\dfrac{\overset{20}{\cancel{40}}\ mg}{\underset{1}{\cancel{2}}\ min} = 20\ mg/min$

Give 2 mL over 1 min.

$\dfrac{2\ mL}{60\ sec} \diagdown\!\!\!\diagup \dfrac{X\ mL}{15\ sec}$

$60X = 30$

$\dfrac{60X}{60} = \dfrac{30}{60}$

$X = 0.5\ mL$ (per 15 sec)

9) $0.125\ mg = 0.125. = 125\ mcg$

$\dfrac{D}{H} \times Q = \dfrac{\overset{1}{\cancel{125}\ mcg}}{\underset{2}{\cancel{250}\ mcg}} \times 1\ tab = \dfrac{1}{2}\ tab$

$0.125\ mg$ ordered daily means you will need $\dfrac{1}{2}$ tab

per 24 h.

10) $\dfrac{D}{H} \times Q = \dfrac{\overset{1}{\cancel{20}\ mg}}{\underset{1}{\cancel{20}\ mg}} \times 1\ tab = 1\ tab$

11) $\dfrac{D}{H} \times Q = \dfrac{\overset{2}{\cancel{13}\ mg}}{\underset{1}{\cancel{6.5}\ mg}} \times 1\ cap = 2\ cap$

12) $1\ g = 1,000\ mg$

$\dfrac{D}{H} \times Q = \dfrac{\overset{2}{\cancel{1,000}\ mg}}{\underset{1}{\cancel{500}\ mg}} \times 1\ tab = 2\ tab$

14) Order is for 80 mL/h—this is the setting for the

controller.

15) $\dfrac{D}{H} \times Q = \dfrac{\overset{5}{\cancel{50}\ mg}}{\underset{1}{\cancel{10}\ mg}} \times 1\ mL = 5\ mL$

16) $\dfrac{D}{H} \times Q = \dfrac{2\ mg/min}{\underset{4}{\cancel{2,000}\ mg}} \times \overset{1}{\cancel{500}}\ mL = \dfrac{\overset{1}{\cancel{2}}}{\underset{2}{\cancel{4}}} = 0.5\ mL/min$

$0.5\ mL/\cancel{min} \times 60\ \cancel{min}/h = 30\ mL/h$

17) $110\ lb \div 2.2\ lb/kg = 110\ \cancel{lb} \times 1\ kg/2.2\ \cancel{lb} = 50\ kg$

Minimum: $5\ mcg/\cancel{kg}/min \times 50\ \cancel{kg} = 250\ mcg/min$

Maximum: $10\ mcg/\cancel{kg}/min \times 50\ \cancel{kg} = 500\ mcg/min$

Ordered dosage is safe.

$\dfrac{D}{H} \times Q = \dfrac{\overset{5}{\cancel{400}\ mg}}{\underset{1}{\cancel{80}\ mg}} \times 1\ mL = 5\ mL$

18) $500\ mcg/min = .500. = 0.5\ mg/min$

$\dfrac{D}{H} \times Q = \dfrac{0.5\ mg/min}{\underset{8}{\cancel{400}\ mg}} \times \overset{5}{\cancel{250}}\ mL = \dfrac{2.5\ mL}{8\ min}$

$= 0.312\ mL/min = 0.31\ mL/min$

$0.31\ mL/\cancel{min} \times 60\ \cancel{min}/h = 18.6\ mL/h$

(program in tenths of mL)

19) $500\ mcg/\cancel{min} \times 60\ \cancel{min}/h = 30,000\ mcg/h$

$30,000\ mcg/h = 30.000. = 30\ mg/h$

20) $\dfrac{D}{H} \times Q = \dfrac{4\ mg/min}{\underset{4}{\cancel{2,000}\ mg}} \times \overset{1}{\cancel{500}}\ mL = \dfrac{\overset{1}{\cancel{4}}}{\underset{1}{\cancel{4}}} = 1\ mL/min$

$1\ mL/\cancel{min} \times 60\ \cancel{min}/h = 60\ mL/h$

21) $33\ lb \div 2.2\ lb/kg = 33\ \cancel{lb} \times 1\ kg/2.2\ \cancel{lb} = 15\ kg$

$15\ mg/\cancel{kg}/day \times 15\ \cancel{kg} = 225\ mg/day$

Maximum: $\dfrac{\overset{75}{\cancel{225}}\ mg}{\underset{1}{\cancel{3}}\ doses} = 75\ mg/dose$

The order is safe. It is obvious that 2 mL should be given.

$25\ mL$ (total IV solution) $- 2\ mL$ (Kantrex) $= 23\ mL$

$(D_5\tfrac{1}{2}NS)$

25 mL (total solution) + 15 mL (flush) = 40 mL
(total in 1 h)

40 mL over 1 h is 40 mL/h.

22) 66 lb ÷ 2.2 lb/kg = 66 l̶b̶ × 1kg/2.2 l̶b̶ = 30 kg

40 mg/kg/day × 30 k̶g̶ = 1,200 mg/day

$$\dfrac{\overset{300}{\cancel{1200}}\ \text{mg}}{\underset{1}{\cancel{4}}\ \text{doses}} = 300\ \text{mg/dose}$$

23) $\dfrac{\text{D}}{\text{H}} \times \text{Q} = \dfrac{300\ \cancel{\text{mg}}}{\underset{50}{\cancel{500}}\ \cancel{\text{mg}}} \times \overset{1}{\cancel{10}}\ \text{mL} = \dfrac{\overset{6}{\cancel{300}}}{\underset{1}{\cancel{50}}}\ \text{mL} = 6\ \text{mL}$

50 mL (total IV volume) − 6 mL (vancomycin) =

44 mL (D$_5\frac{1}{2}$NS); 50 mL/h̶ × 24 h̶ = 1,200 mL

24) Child weighs 30 kg.

100 mL/kg/day × 10 k̶g̶ = 1,000 mL/day
(for first 10 kg)

50 mL/kg/day × 10 k̶g̶ = 500 mL/day
(for next 10 kg)

20 mL/kg/day × 10 k̶g̶ = 200 mL/day
(for remaining 10 kg)

Total: 1,000 mL/day + 500 mL/day + 200 mL/day
= 1,700 mL/day or per 24 h

1,700 mL/day ÷ 24 h/day

= 1,700 mL/d̶a̶y̶ × 1 d̶a̶y̶/24 h = 70.8 mL/h

The ordered rate is less than the recommended daily rate of maintenance fluids. The nurse should consider possible clinical reasons for the difference and consult the physician as needed for clarification.

25) The vial size is 1.5 g. Choose the diluent that corresponds to the vial chosen. Adding 3.2 mL will yield a total of 4.0 mL containing 1.5 g.

27) $\dfrac{\text{D}}{\text{H}} \times \text{Q} = \dfrac{\overset{1}{\cancel{500}}\ \cancel{\text{mg}}}{\underset{3}{\cancel{1,500}}\ \cancel{\text{mg}}} \times 4\ \text{mL} = \dfrac{4}{3}\ \text{mL}$
= 1.33 mL = 1.3 mL

28) 50 mL (IV PB fluid) + 1.3 mL (med) = 51.3 mL (total fluid to infuse in 30 min) Round 51.3 to 51 for the purpose of calculating the infusion rate.

$\dfrac{51\ \text{mL}}{\underset{1}{\cancel{30}}\ \cancel{\text{min}}} \times \overset{2}{\cancel{60}}\ \cancel{\text{min}}/\text{h} = 102\ \text{mL/h}$

29) $\dfrac{\text{D}}{\text{H}} \times \text{Q} = \dfrac{\overset{2}{\cancel{10,000}}\ \cancel{\text{units}}}{\underset{1}{\cancel{5,000}}\ \cancel{\text{units}}} \times 1\ \text{mL} = 2\ \text{mL}$

$\dfrac{\text{D}}{\text{H}} \times \text{Q} = \dfrac{1,200\ \cancel{\text{units}}/\text{h}}{\underset{20}{\cancel{10,000}}\ \cancel{\text{units}}} \times \overset{1}{\cancel{500}}\ \text{mL} = \dfrac{\overset{60}{\cancel{1,200}}}{\underset{1}{\cancel{20}}}\ \text{mL/h}$
= 60 mL/h

30) 125 lb ÷ 2.2 lb/kg = 125 l̶b̶ × 1 kg/2.2 l̶b̶
= 56.81 kg = 56.8 kg

80 units/k̶g̶ × 56.8 k̶g̶ = 4,544 units

$\dfrac{\text{D}}{\text{H}} \times \text{Q} = \dfrac{4,544\ \cancel{\text{units}}}{1,000\ \cancel{\text{units}}} \times 1\ \text{mL} = \dfrac{4,544}{1,000}\ \text{mL}$
= 4.54 mL = 4.5 mL

18 units/kg/h × 56.8 k̶g̶ = 1,022.4 units/h
= 1,022 units/h

$\dfrac{\text{D}}{\text{H}} \times \text{Q} = \dfrac{1,022\ \cancel{\text{units}}/\text{h}}{\underset{100}{\cancel{25,000}}\ \cancel{\text{units}}} \times \overset{1}{\cancel{250}}\ \text{mL} = \dfrac{1,022}{100}\ \text{mL/h}$
= 10.22 mL/h = 10.2 mL/h

31) Decrease rate by 2 units/kg/h.

2 units/kg/h × 56.8 k̶g̶ = 113.6 units/h = 114 units/h

1,022 units/h − 114 units/h = 908 units/h

$\dfrac{\text{D}}{\text{H}} \times \text{Q} = \dfrac{908\ \cancel{\text{units}}/\text{h}}{\underset{100}{\cancel{25,000}}\ \cancel{\text{units}}} \times \overset{1}{\cancel{250}}\ \text{mL} = \dfrac{908}{100}\ \text{mL/h}$
= 9.08 mL/h = 9.1 mL/h

32) $\dfrac{\text{D}}{\text{H}} \times \text{Q} = \dfrac{8\ \cancel{\text{units}}}{100\ \cancel{\text{units}}} \times 1\ \text{mL} = \dfrac{8}{100}\ \text{mL} = 0.08\ \text{mL}$

U-100 insulin should only be administered with a U-100 insulin syringe. This question and solution are provided to evaluate your understanding of the insulin syringe and insulin concentration. 8 units of U-100 insulin equals a dose volume of 0.08 mL.

33) 15 units + 45 units = 60 units

34) $\dfrac{\text{D}}{\text{H}} \times \text{Q} = \dfrac{\overset{3}{\cancel{300}}\ \cancel{\text{units}}}{\underset{1}{\cancel{100}}\ \cancel{\text{units}}} \times 1\ \text{mL} = 3\ \text{mL}$

Total IV volume: 150 mL (NS) + 3 mL (insulin)
= 153 mL

$\dfrac{\text{D}}{\text{H}} \times \text{Q} = \text{R}$

$\dfrac{\text{D}\ \cancel{\text{units}}/\text{h}}{300\ \cancel{\text{units}}} \times 153\ \text{mL} = 10\ \text{mL/h}$

$\dfrac{\text{D}}{300} \times 153 = 10$

$\dfrac{153\text{D}}{300} = \dfrac{10}{1}$

$153\text{D} = 3,000$

$\dfrac{153\text{D}}{153} = \dfrac{3,000}{153}$

D = 19.6 units/h = 20 units/h

35) 8 f̶l̶ ̶o̶z̶ × 30 mL/f̶l̶ ̶o̶z̶ = 240 mL

D × Q = X

$\dfrac{1}{4} \times \text{Q} = 240\ \text{mL}$

$\dfrac{1}{4}\text{Q} = 240\ \text{mL}$

$\dfrac{\frac{1}{4}\text{Q}}{\frac{1}{4}} = \dfrac{240}{\frac{1}{4}}$

$\text{Q} = 240 \times \dfrac{4}{1}$

Q = 960 mL (total volume of reconstituted $\frac{1}{4}$ strength Isomil)

960 mL (total solution) − 240 mL (solution or Isomil)
= 720 mL solvent or water

36) $16 \text{ lb} \div 2.2 \text{ lb/kg} = 16 \text{ lb} \times 1 \text{ kg}/2.2 \text{ lb}$

$= 7.27 \text{ kg} = 7.3 \text{ kg}$

$100 \text{ mL/kg/day} \times 7.3 \text{ kg} = 730 \text{ mL/day}$

$730 \text{ mL/day} \div 24 \text{ h/day} = 30.4 = 30 \text{ mL/h}$

37) $5 \text{ ft} \times 12 \text{ in/ft} = 60 \text{ in}; 60 \text{ in} + 2 \text{ in} = 62 \text{ in}$

Household:

$$\text{BSA (m}^2) = \sqrt{\frac{\text{ht (in)} \times \text{wt (lb)}}{3{,}131}} = \sqrt{\frac{62 \times 103}{3{,}131}} = \sqrt{\frac{6{,}386}{3{,}131}}$$

$$= \sqrt{2.039 \ldots} = 1.428 \text{ m}^2 = 1.43 \text{ m}^2$$

38) $10 \text{ mg/m}^2 \times 1.43 \text{ m}^2 = 14.3 \text{ mg}$

$20 \text{ mg/m}^2 \times 1.43 \text{ m}^2 = 28.6 \text{ mg}$

Yes, the order is safe.

39) Concentration: $40 \text{ mg}/80 \text{ mL} = 0.5 \text{ mg/mL}$

$$\frac{D}{H} \times Q = \frac{28 \text{ mg}}{0.5 \text{ mg}} \times 1 \text{ mL} = \frac{28}{0.5} \text{ mL} = 56 \text{ mL}$$

$$\frac{56 \text{ mL}}{10 \text{ min}} = 5.6 \text{ mL/min (or 5.6 mL per 60 sec)}$$

$$\frac{5.6 \text{ mL}}{60 \text{ sec}} \diagdown\!\!\!\!\diagup \frac{\text{X mL}}{15 \text{ sec}}$$

$60X = 84$

$\dfrac{60X}{60} = \dfrac{84}{60}$

$X = 1.4 \text{ mL (per 15 sec)}$

40) Dextrose:

$$\frac{5 \text{ g}}{100 \text{ mL}} \diagdown\!\!\!\!\diagup \frac{\text{X g}}{1{,}000 \text{ mL}}$$

$100X = 5{,}000$

$\dfrac{100X}{100} = \dfrac{5{,}000}{100}$

$X = 50 \text{ g}$

NaCl:

$$\frac{0.45 \text{ g}}{100 \text{ mL}} \diagdown\!\!\!\!\diagup \frac{\text{X g}}{1{,}000 \text{ mL}}$$

$100X = 450$

$\dfrac{100X}{100} = \dfrac{450}{100}$

$X = 4.5 \text{ g}$

41) $\dfrac{D}{H} \times Q = \dfrac{600 \text{ mg}}{100 \text{ mg}} \times 1 \text{ mL} = \dfrac{\overset{6}{600}}{\underset{1}{100}} \text{ mL} = 6 \text{ mL}$

$50 \text{ mL (total fluid)} - 6 \text{ mL (med)} = 44 \text{ mL (IV}$

fluid). Note: Add the medicine to the chamber and

then add IV fluid up to 50 mL.

42) $\dfrac{10 \text{ mg}}{1 \text{ mL}} \diagdown\!\!\!\!\diagup \dfrac{600 \text{ mg}}{\text{X mL}}$

$10X = 600$

$\dfrac{10X}{10} = \dfrac{600}{10}$

$X = 60 \text{ mL (per 600 mg) minimum dilution}$

$\dfrac{40 \text{ mg}}{1 \text{ mL}} \diagdown\!\!\!\!\diagup \dfrac{600 \text{ mg}}{\text{X mL}}$

$40X = 600$

$\dfrac{40}{40} = \dfrac{600}{40}$

$X = 15 \text{ mL (per 600 mg) maximum dilution}$

43) $400{,}000 \text{ units/dose} \times 4 \text{ doses/day} =$

$1{,}600{,}000 \text{ units/day}$

Minimum: $150{,}000 \text{ units/kg/day} \times 10 \text{ kg} =$

$1{,}500{,}000 \text{ units/day}$

Maximum: $250{,}000 \text{ units/kg/day} \times 10 \text{ kg} =$

$2{,}500{,}000 \text{ units/day}$

Reconstitute with 1.8 mL for a concentration of

500,000 units/mL. This concentration is selected

because it will be further diluted.

$$\frac{D}{H} \times Q = \frac{\overset{4}{400{,}000 \text{ units}}}{\underset{5}{500{,}000 \text{ units}}} \times 1 \text{ mL} = \frac{4}{5} \text{ mL}$$

$= 0.8 \text{ mL penicillin G potassium}$

44) $100 \text{ mL (NS)} + 0.8 \text{ mL (penicillin G potassium)} =$

$100.8 \text{ or } 101 \text{ mL (to be infused in 60 min, or 1 h)}.$

Set IV pump at 101 mL/h.

45) $1{,}000 \text{ mL} \div 125 \text{ mL/h} =$

$1{,}000 \text{ mL} \times 1 \text{ h}/125 \text{ mL} = 8 \text{ h}$

The primary IV will infuse for 8 hours. The IV PB

will infuse for 30 minutes. Therefore, the primary IV

will be interrupted by the IV PB and then will resume.

The IV will be completely infused in 8 hours and

30 min.

$(1315 + 8 \text{ h } 30 \text{ min} = 1315 + 0830 = 2145)$

46) $\dfrac{D}{H} \times Q = \dfrac{12.5 \text{ mg}}{25 \text{ mg}} \times 1 \text{ mL} = \dfrac{12.5}{25} \text{ mL} = 0.5 \text{ mL}$

Think: Although the recommendation is "not to exceed

25 mg/min," which is 1 mL of the dosage you have on

hand, you don't have to give it that rapidly. The order

requires 12.5 mg or half the maximum allowable

amount to give in 1 min. Use the dose amount

(0.5 mL) and administer that over 1 min (60 sec).

Give 0.5 mL/min or

$\dfrac{0.5 \text{ mL}}{60 \text{ sec}} \diagdown\!\!\!\!\diagup \dfrac{\text{X mL}}{15 \text{ sec}}$

$60X = 7.5$

$\dfrac{60X}{60} = \dfrac{7.5}{60}$

$X = 0.125 \text{ mL} = 0.13 \text{ mL (per 15 sec)}$

47) $\dfrac{D}{H} \times Q = \dfrac{\overset{15}{1{,}500 \text{ mg}}}{\underset{1}{100 \text{ mg}}} \times 1 \text{ mL} = \dfrac{15}{1} \text{ mL} = 15 \text{ mL}$

48) $100 \text{ mL (IV PB)} + 15 \text{ mL (med)} = 115 \text{ mL}$

(total to infuse in 30 min)

$\dfrac{115 \text{ mL}}{\underset{1}{30 \text{ min}}} \times \overset{2}{60 \text{ min}}/\text{h} = 230 \text{ mL/h}$

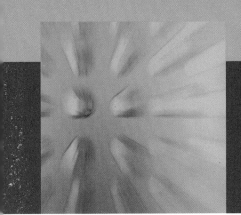

Appendix A: Study Guide

Base Units in the Metric System

Weight: gram (g)
Volume: liter (L)
Length: meter (m)

Metric Prefixes

micro-   one millionth *or* 0.000001 *or* $\frac{1}{1,000,000}$ of the base unit

milli-   one thousandth *or* 0.001 *or* $\frac{1}{1,000}$ of the base unit

centi-   one hundredth *or* 0.01 *or* $\frac{1}{100}$ of the base unit

deci-   one tenth *or* 0.1 *or* $\frac{1}{10}$ of the base unit

kilo-   one thousand *or* 1,000 times the base unit

SI Metric System

	Unit	Abbreviation	Equivalent
Weight	**gram** (base unit)	g	**1 g** = 1,000 mg = 1,000,000 mcg
	milligram	mg	0.001 g = **1 mg** = 1,000 mcg
	microgram	mcg	0.000001 g = 0.001 mg = **1 mcg**
	kilogram	kg	**1 kg** = 1,000 g
Volume	**liter** (base unit)	L	**1 L** = 1,000 mL
	deciliter	dL	0.1 L = **1 dL**
	milliliter	mL	0.001 L = **1 mL**
Length	**meter** (base unit)	m	**1 m** = 100 cm = 1,000 mm
	centimeter	cm	0.01 m = **1 cm** = 10 mm
	millimeter	mm	0.001 m = 0.1 cm = **1 mm**

Frequently Used Household Units

gtt	drop
t (or tsp)	teaspoon
T (or tbs)	tablespoon
fl oz	fluid ounce
cup	cup
pt	pint
qt	quart
oz	ounce (weight)
lb	pound
in	inch

CHAPTER 4—CONVERSIONS

Approximate Equivalents: Metric and Household

1 t = 5 mL

$1 \text{ T} = 3t = 15 \text{ mL} = \frac{1}{2} \text{ fl oz}$

1 fl oz = 30 mL = 6 t

1 L = 1 qt = 32 fl oz = 2 pt = 4 cups

1 pt = 16 fl oz = 2 cups

1 cup = 8 fl oz = 240 mL

1 kg = 2.2 lb

1 in = 2.5 cm

Conversion Factor Method

To convert from a larger to a smaller unit, multiply by the conversion factor:

Larger ↓ Smaller → Multiply (×)   2 mg × 1,000 mcg/mg = 2.000. = 2,000 mcg

To convert from a smaller to a larger unit, divide by the conversion factor:

Smaller ↑ Larger → Divide (÷)   450 g ÷ 1,000 g/kg = 450 g × 1 kg/1,000 g = .450. = 0.45 kg

CHAPTER 5—CONVERSIONS FOR TIME AND TEMPERATURE

Converting Between Traditional and International Time

- International time is designated by 001 through 1259 for 12:01 AM through 12:59 PM and 1300 through 2400 for 1:00 PM through 12:00 midnight.

- Between the hours of 1:00 PM (1300) and 12:00 AM (2400), **add 1200** to traditional time to find the equivalent international time; **subtract 1200** from international time to convert to equivalent traditional time.

Comparison of Traditional and International Time

AM	Int'l. Time	PM	Int'l. Time
12:00 midnight	2400	12:00 noon	1200
1:00	0100	1:00	1300
2:00	0200	2:00	1400
3:00	0300	3:00	1500
4:00	0400	4:00	1600
5:00	0500	5:00	1700
6:00	0600	6:00	1800
7:00	0700	7:00	1900
8:00	0800	8:00	2000
9:00	0900	9:00	2100
10:00	1000	10:00	2200
11:00	1100	11:00	2300

Converting Between Celsius and Fahrenheit Temperature Scales

$$°C = \frac{°F - 32}{1.8}$$

$$°F = 1.8°C + 32$$

CHAPTER 7—INTERPRETING DRUG ORDERS

Seven Parts of a Drug Order:

1. Name of **patient**
2. Name of **drug**
3. **Dosage** of drug
4. **Route** by which the drug is to be administered
5. **Frequency, time, and special instructions** related to administration of drug
6. **Date and time** the order was written
7. **Signature and licensure** of the person writing the order

Medical Abbreviations

Route

IM	intramuscular
IV	intravenous
IV PB	intravenous piggyback
subcut	subcutaneous
SL	sublingual, under the tongue
ID	intradermal
GT	gastrostomy tube
NG	nasogastric tube
NJ	nasojejunal tube
p.o.	by mouth, orally
p.r.	per rectum, rectally

Frequency

a.c.	before meals
p.c.	after meals
ad. lib.	as desired, freely
p.r.n.	when necessary
stat	immediately
b.i.d.	twice a day
t.i.d.	three times a day
q.i.d.	four times a day
min	minute
h	hour
q.h	every hour
q.2h	every 2 hours
q.4h	every 4 hours
q.6h	every 6 hours
q.8h	every 8 hours
q.12h	every 12 hours

General

$\bar{a}$	before
$\bar{p}$	after
$\bar{c}$	with
$\bar{s}$	without
q	every
qs	quantity sufficient
aq	water
NPO	nothing by mouth
gtt	drop
tab	tablet
cap	capsule
et	and
noct	night

CHAPTER 9—PREVENTING MEDICATION ERRORS

"Do Not Use" List of Medical Abbreviations

U, u
IU
Q.D., QD, q.d., qd
Q.O.D., QOD, q.o.d., qod
Trailing zero (X.0 mg)
Lack of leading zero (.X mg)
MS
MSO_4 and $MgSO_4$

Six Rights of Safe and Accurate Medication Administration

The *right patient* must receive the *right drug* in the *right amount* by the *right route* at the *right time* followed by the *right documentation.*

CHAPTERS 10 & 11—ORAL AND PARENTERAL DOSAGE OF DRUGS

Three-Step Approach to Dosage Calculations

Step 1: **Convert**—Ensure that all measurements are in the same system of measurement.
Step 2: **Think**—Estimate what is a *reasonable amount* of the drug to administer.
Step 3: **Calculate**—Apply the formula method to find the amount to give.

Dosage Calculations: Formula Method

$$\frac{D}{H} \times Q = X \qquad \frac{D \text{ (desired)}}{H \text{ (have)}} \times Q \text{ (quantity)} = X \text{ (amount)}$$

CHAPTER 12—RECONSTITUTION OF SOLUTIONS

Important Definitions

- **Reconstitution:** the process of mixing and diluting solutions
- **Solute:** a substance to be dissolved or diluted
- **Solvent:** a substance (liquid) that dissolves another substance to prepare a solution; diluent
- **Solution:** the resulting mixture of a solute plus a solvent

Fractions That Express the Strength of a Solution

- The numerator of the fraction expresses the number of parts of the solute.
- The denominator of the fraction is the total number of parts of the solution.
- The difference between the denominator (total solution) and the numerator (parts of the solute) is the number of parts of the solvent.

Formulas for Preparing Solutions

1. **D × Q = X**
   D (Desired solution strength) × **Q** (Quantity of desired solution) = **X** (Amount of solute)
2. Quantity of desired solution − Amount of solute = Amount of solvent

CHAPTER 13—PEDIATRIC AND ADULT DOSAGES BASED ON BODY WEIGHT

Body Weight Method for Calculating Safe Dosages

1. Convert the patient's weight from pounds to kilograms (rounded to nearest tenths): 1 kg = 2.2 lb
2. Calculate the safe dosage in mg/kg for a patient of this weight:
   Multiply mg/kg by patient's weight in kg: **mg/kg × kg = X mg**

3. Compare the ordered dosage to the recommended dosage, and decide if dosage is safe.

4. If safe, calculate the amount to give and administer the dose; if the dosage seems unsafe, consult with the prescribing practitioner before administering the drug.

Note: The dosage per kg may be **mg/kg, mcg/kg, g/kg, mEq/kg, units/kg, milliunits/kg.**

CHAPTER 14—ALTERNATIVE DOSAGE CALCULATION METHODS: RATIO-PROPORTION AND DIMENSIONAL ANALYSIS

Converting with Ratio-Proportion

In a proportion, the ratio for a known equivalent equals the ratio for an unknown equivalent. To use ratio-proportion to convert from one unit to another:

1. Recall the equivalents.

2. Set up a proportion of two equivalent ratios.

3. Cross-multiply to solve for an unknown quantity, X. Label the units to match the unknown X.

Dosage Calculations: Ratio-Proportion Method

$$\frac{\text{Dosage on hand}}{\text{Amount on hand}} = \frac{\text{Dosage desired}}{\text{X Amount desired}}$$

Dosage Calculations: Dimensional Analysis Method

Amount to give ratio = Supply dosage ratio × Conversion factor ratio × Ordered dosage ratio

1. Write the unknown X and the unit of measure for *amount to give ratio* on the left side of the equation, followed by equal sign (=).

2. Units in the numerator on the left side of the equal sign are the same units that are placed in the numerator of the first ratio on the right side of the equation.

3. When the units in the numerator and the units in the denominator are the same, they cancel each other out.

4. Set up the rest of the ratios so that the units cancel out, leaving only the *amount to give* unit.

CHAPTER 15—INTRAVENOUS SOLUTIONS, EQUIPMENT, AND CALCULATIONS

Common IV Component Abbreviations

D = Dextrose
W = Water
S = Saline
NaCl = Sodium Chloride
NS = Normal Saline (0.9% NaCl)
RL = Ringer's Lactate
LR = Lactated Ringer's

Solution strength expressed as a percent (%) indicates the number of g per 100 mL:

$$\frac{\text{\# of g solute}}{\text{100 mL solution}}$$

Osmolarity of Solutions

Hypotonic: <250 mOsm/L
Isotonic: 250–375 mOsm/L
Hypertonic: >375 mOsm/L

IV Rate by Electronic Infusion Pump (mL/h)

$$\frac{\text{Total mL ordered}}{\text{Total h ordered}} = \textbf{mL/h (rounded to a whole number or tenths depending on equipment)}$$

If infusion time is less than 1 hour: $\frac{\text{Total mL ordered}}{\text{Total min ordered}} \times \textbf{60 min/h} = \textbf{mL/h}$

Flow Rate for Manually-Regulated IV (gtt/min)

Drop factor = gtt/mL
Macrodrop factors: 10, 15, or 20 gtt/mL
Microdrop factor: 60 gtt/mL

Calculating IV Flow Rate for Manually-Regulated IV in gtt/min: Formula Method

$$\frac{\text{V}}{\text{T}} \times \textbf{C} = \textbf{R} \qquad \frac{\text{Volume (mL)}}{\text{Time (min)}} \times \text{Calibration or drop factor (\textbf{gtt/mL})} = \text{Rate (\textbf{gtt/min})}$$

Shortcut Method to Calculate IV Flow Rate in gtt/min

To use shortcut method, remember drop factor constants: $10 \text{ gtt/mL} = \frac{60}{10} = \textbf{6}$

$$15 \text{ gtt/mL} = \frac{60}{15} = \textbf{4}$$

$$20 \text{ gtt/mL} = \frac{60}{20} = \textbf{3}$$

$$60 \text{ gtt/mL} = \frac{60}{60} = \textbf{1}$$

$$\frac{\text{mL/h}}{\text{Drop factor constant}} = \textbf{gtt/min} \qquad \textit{(Do not use shortcut method if time is less than 1 hour.)}$$

Adjusting IV Flow Rates (as allowed by agency policy)

Step 1: $\frac{\textbf{Remaining volume}}{\textbf{Remaining hours}} = \textbf{Recalculated mL/h}$

Step 2: $\frac{\text{V}}{\text{T}} \times \textbf{C} = \textbf{R (gtt/min)}$

Step 3: $\frac{\textbf{Adjusted rate} - \textbf{Ordered rate}}{\textbf{Ordered rate}} = \textbf{\%Variation (maximum 25\%variation)}$

Calculating IV Infusion Time

$$\frac{\text{Total mL}}{\text{mL/h}} = \text{Total hours}$$

Calculating IV Infusion Volume

Total hours × mL/h = Total mL

CHAPTER 16—BODY SURFACE AREA AND ADVANCED PEDIATRIC CALCULATIONS

Calculating Body Surface Area (BSA): Formula Method

Using **metric** measurement of height and weight: $\text{BSA (m}^2) = \sqrt{\dfrac{\text{ht (cm)} \times \text{wt (kg)}}{3{,}600}}$

Using **household** measurement of height and weight: $\text{BSA (m}^2) = \sqrt{\dfrac{\text{ht (in)} \times \text{wt (lb)}}{3{,}131}}$

Dosage Calculations Using BSA

1. Determine BSA in m²

2. Calculate safe dosage based on BSA: **mg/m² × m² = X mg**

3. Compare the ordered dosage to the recommended dosage, and decide if dosage is safe

4. If the dosage is safe, calculate the amount to give and administer dose. If dosage seems unsafe, consult with the ordering practitioner before administering the drug.

Note: The dosage per m² may be **mg/m², mcg/m², g/m², mEq/m², units/m², milliunits/m².**

Calculation of Daily Volume for Pediatric Maintenance Fluids

- 100 mL/kg/day for first 10 kg of body weight

- 50 mL/kg/day for next 10 kg of body weight

- 20 mL/kg/day for each kg above 20 kg of body weight

CHAPTER 17—ADVANCED ADULT INTRAVENOUS CALCULATIONS

Actions for the Administration of Critical Intravenous Medications (e.g., Heparin and Insulin)

Action 1: Calculate bolus
Action 2: Calculate initial continuous infusion flow rate
Action 3: Calculate re-bolus and/or adjust continuous infusion flow rate

Action 1: Calculation of the Heparin Bolus

1. Calculate the dosage (units) of the heparin bolus based on patient's weight (kg):

   units/kg × kg = units

2. Calculate the volume (mL) of the bolus to prepare using the dosage calculation formula:

   $$\frac{D}{H} \times Q = X$$

Action 2: Calculation of Initial Continuous Flow Rate of the IV Heparin Solution (mL/h)

1. Calculate the dosage (units/h) of the initial continuous infusion based on patient's weight (kg):

   units/kg/h × kg = units/h

2. Calculate the continuous infusion rate (mL/h) using a version of the dosage calculation formula:

   $$\frac{D \text{ (units/h desired)}}{H \text{ (units you have available)}} \times Q \text{ (mL you have available)} = R \text{ (mL/h rate)}$$

Action 3: Calculation of the Heparin Re-bolus and Adjustment of Continuous Infusion Rate

1. Calculate the dose (units) of the heparin bolus based on aPTT results and patient's weight (kg):
   units/kg × kg = units

2. Calculate the volume (mL) of the bolus to prepare using the dosage calculation formula:

   $$\frac{D}{H} \times Q = X$$

3. Calculate the dosage (units/h) of the continuous infusion adjustment based on aPTT results and patient's weight (kg): **units/kg/h × kg = units/h**

4. Calculate the adjustment to the hourly infusion rate (mL/h) using a version of the dosage calculation formula:

   $$\frac{D \text{ (units/h desired)}}{H \text{ (units you have available)}} \times Q \text{ (mL you have available)} = R \text{ (mL/h rate)}$$

5. Calculate the new hourly infusion rate (mL/h):

   Current rate (mL/h) ± adjustment (mL/h) = new rate (mL/h)

Calculation of the Insulin Bolus and Continuous Flow Rate

The insulin bolus is based on blood glucose level.

$$\frac{D \text{ (units/h desired)}}{H \text{ (units you have available)}} \times Q \text{ (mL you have available)} = R \text{ (mL/h rate)}: \frac{D}{H} \times Q = R$$

Note: This rule applies to other drugs ordered in **units/h, milliunits/h, mg/h, mcg/h, g/h, or mEq/h.**

Calculation of the Flow Rate for IV Medications Ordered in mg/min

Step 1:   Calculate the dosage in mL/min: $\frac{D \text{ (mg/min)}}{H \text{ (mg)}} \times Q \text{ (mL)} = R \text{ (mL/min)}$

Step 2:   Calculate the flow rate in mL/h of the volume to administer per minute:

   mL/min × 60 min/h = mL/h

Calculation of the Flow Rate for IV Medications Ordered in mg/kg/min

Step 1:   Convert to like units (mg to mcg, lb to kg)

Step 2:   Calculate desired dosage per minute: **mg/kg/min × kg = mg/min**

Step 3:   Calculate the dosage flow rate in mL/min: $\dfrac{\textbf{D (mg/min)}}{\textbf{H (mg)}} \times \textbf{Q (mL)} = \textbf{R (mL/min)}$

Step 4:   Calculate the flow rate in mL/h of the volume to administer per minute:
mL/min × 60 min/h = mL/h

Calculation of Flow Rate for IV Medications Ordered Over a Specific Time Period (mg/min)

Step 1:   Calculate mg/mL

Step 2:   Calculate mL/h

Steps to Verify Safe Dosage of IV Medications Recommended in mg/min and Ordered in mL/h

Step 1:   Calculate mg/h

Step 2:   Calculate mg/min

Step 3:   Compare recommended dosage and ordered dosage to decide if the dosage is safe.

Steps to Verify Safe Dosage of IV Medications Recommended in mg/kg/min and Ordered in mL/h

Step 1:   Convert to like units

Step 2:   Calculate recommended mg/min

Step 3:   Calculate ordered mg/h

Step 4:   Calculate ordered mg/min

Step 5:   Compare ordered and recommended dosages to decide if the dosage is safe.

Calculation of Flow Rate for IV Medications That Include IV Piggyback

Step 1:	IV PB flow rate	$\dfrac{V}{T} \times C = R$
Step 2:	Total IV PB time	Time for 1 dose × # of doses in 24 h
Step 3:	Total IV PB volume	Volume of 1 dose × # of doses in 24 h
Step 4:	Total regular IV volume	Total volume − IV PB volume = Regular IV volume
Step 5:	Total regular IV time	Total time − IV PB time = Regular IV time
Step 6:	Regular IV flow rate	$\dfrac{V}{T} \times C = R$

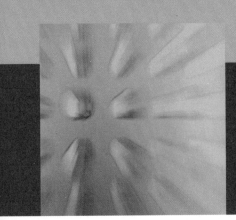

Appendix B: Apothecary System

The apothecary system was introduced in Chapter 3. The following units, abbreviations, symbols, and equivalents describe the remnants of this ancient method of measuring medication dosages. Because it is less accurate than the metric system, it is no longer recommended for safe practice. The basic units are the weight measure *grain (15 grains is approximately equivalent to 1 gram)* and the liquid volume measures of *dram* (similar to a teaspoon and still found on some medicine cups), *ounce* (same as household *fluid ounce*), and *minim* (like a drop). You can compare apothecary and metric measures with the following tables and figure.

Apothecary Units

Measure	Apothecary Unit	Abbreviation	Symbol
Weight	grain	gr	N/A
Volume	ounce	oz	℥
Volume	dram	dr	ʒ
Volume	minim	min	♏

Apothecary-Metric Approximate Equivalents

Volume				Weight			
oz	**mL**	**min**	**mL**	**gr**	**mg**	**gr**	**mg**
1	= 30	45 = 3		15 = 1,000		$\frac{1}{4}$ = 15	
$\frac{1}{2}$	= 15	30 = 2		10 = 600		$\frac{1}{6}$ = 10	
		15 = 1		$7\frac{1}{2}$ = 500		$\frac{1}{8}$ = 7.5	
dr	**mL**	12 = 0.75		5 = 300		$\frac{1}{10}$ = 6	
$2\frac{1}{2}$	= 10	10 = 0.6		4 = 250		$\frac{1}{15}$ = 4	
2	= 8	8 = 0.5		3 = 200		$\frac{1}{20}$ = 3	
$1\frac{1}{4}$	= 5	5 = 0.3		$2\frac{1}{2}$ = 150		$\frac{1}{30}$ = 2	
1	= 4	4 = 0.25		2 = 120		$\frac{1}{40}$ = 1.5	
		3 = 0.2		$1\frac{1}{2}$ = 100		$\frac{1}{60}$ = 1	
1 minim	= 1 gtt	$1\frac{1}{2}$ = 0.1		1 = 60		$\frac{1}{100}$ = 0.6	
		1 = 0.06		$\frac{3}{4}$ = 45		$\frac{1}{120}$ = 0.5	
		$\frac{3}{4}$ = 0.05		$\frac{1}{2}$ = 30		$\frac{1}{150}$ = 0.4	
		$\frac{1}{2}$ = 0.03		$\frac{1}{3}$ = 20		$\frac{1}{200}$ = 0.3	
						$\frac{1}{250}$ = 0.25	

Apothecary-Metric Approximate Equivalent "Conversion Clock"

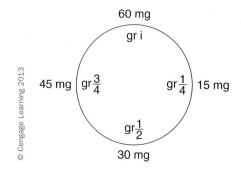

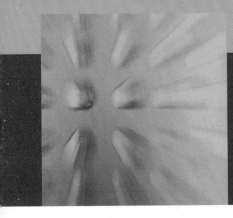

Index

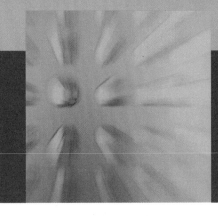

Drug Label Index

Boldface indicates generic drug name

A

Acetaminophen, 240–241
Acyclovir, 339
Albuterol sulfate, 235, 396
Aldactone (**spironolactone**), 98, 164, 251
Aluminum magnesium and **simethicone oral suspension** (Antacid Plus), 99
Amiodarone HCl injection, 273
Amoxicillin and **clavulanate potassium**, 5, 17, 394
Amoxicillin oral suspension, 16, 235, 373, 383, 390
Amphotericin B, 337
Ampicillin, 340, 383
Ampicillin sodium/sulbactam sodium (Unasyn), 346
Antacid Plus (**aluminum magnesium** and **simethicone oral suspension**), 99
Apidra (**insulin glulisine**), 282
Ativan (**lorazepam**), 204, 266, 269
Atomoxetine HCl (Strattera), 4
Azithromycin (Zithromax), 9, 161, 322, 326, 341
Azulfidine (**sulfasalazine**), 223

B

Biaxin (**clarithromycin**), 167, 211, 395
Bumetanide, 173, 273
Butorphanol tartrate injection, 6

C

Calan SR (**verapamil hydrochloride**), 4, 223
Carafate (**sucralfate**), 14, 158, 210, 250
Carbamazepine (Tegretol), 163, 167, 223, 250, 388
Cefaclor, 228–229, 235, 372, 391, 394
Cefadroxil monohydrate (Duricef), 225
Cefazolin, 324, 350, 363, 398
Cefepime injection, 349
Cefotaxime (Claforan), 168, 499
Cefpodoxime proxetil (Vantin), 161, 168, 171, 363, 395
Ceftriaxone, 392
Ceftriaxone injection, 18, 334, 348, 359, 362, 393
Cephradine (Velosef), 350
Ciprofloxacin injection, 162
Claforan (**cefotaxime**), 168, 499

Clarithromycin (Biaxin), 167, 211, 395
Clindamycin, 209, 271, 404
Clonazepam, 163, 167, 209, 212, 215, 251, 397
Clonazepam (Klonopin), 4
Clonidine HCl, 209, 212, 215
Continu-Flo solution set, 460
Continu-Flo solution set with duo-vent spike, 448, 460
Co-Trimoxazole (**trimethoprim** and **sulfamethoxazole**), 382
Cytarabine, 345

D

DCL (**ceftriaxone**), 392
Depakene (**valproic acid**), 235, 389
Depo-Provera (**medroxyprogesterone acetate**), 126, 172, 269
Dexamethasone sodium phosphate, 261, 413
Dextromethorphan hydrobromide (Robitussin), 376
Dextrose 5% injection, 441, 445
Dextrose 5% injection and **0.9% sodium chloride**, 442, 445
Dextrose 5% injection and **0.45% sodium chloride**, 444
Dextrose 5% injection and **0.225% sodium chloride**, 444
Digoxin, 319, 407
Digoxin injection, 8, 240, 251, 261, 268
Digoxin tablets, 223
Dilantin (**phenytoin sodium**), 10
Diltiazem HCl injection, 263, 273, 319
Diphenhydramine HCl injection, 263, 268
Doxycycline injection, 9, 341, 342
Droperidol (Inapsine), 160, 318
Duricef (**cefadroxil monohydrate**), 225

E

Enfamil formulas, 354
Epinephrine injection, 166

F

Famotidine, 158, 173, 260, 318
Feldene (**piroxicam**), 250
Flagyl (**metronidazole**), 250
Fluoxetine (Prozac), 219
Folic acid injection, 269

Fosphenytoin sodium injection, 264, 273
Furosemide, 161, 239
Furosemide (Lasix), 219, 251
Furosemide oral solution, 124, 388

G

Gabapentin (Neurontin), 222
Gemfibrozil (Lopid), 159, 223, 251, 404
Gentamicin, 7, 209, 271, 318, 379, 382, 385, 387, 403, 499
Glycopyrrolate (Robinul), 8, 165, 262, 268, 392

H

Halcion (**triazolam**), 98
Haloperidol decanoate, 318, 413
HEMA II Y-Type Blood Set, 460
Heparin Lock Flush, 170, 277–278, 303, 305
Heparin sodium injection, 92, 160, 170, 201, 278, 303, 305–308, 516, 555
Humalog (**insulin lispro injection**), 282, 289, 299, 304
Humalog Mix 75/25 (**insulin lispro protamine suspension/insulin lispro injection**), 284
Human insulin injection/rDNA (Novolin 70/30), 284, 318
Human insulin injection/rDNA (Novolin R), 11, 14, 161, 283, 294, 319
Human insulin isophane suspension (Humulin 70/30 Pen), 295
Human insulin isophane suspension/rDNA (Novolin N), 11, 163, 283, 290, 304, 319
Human insulin rDNA origin (Humulin N), 283
Humulin 70/30 Pen (**human insulin isophane suspension**), 295
Humulin N (**human insulin rDNA origin**), 283
Humulin R (**insulin human injection**), 277, 282–283, 289, 299, 304, 306, 318, 525
Hydrochloride (Promethazine), 6, 240, 318
Hydrochlorothiazide, 224
Hydrocodone bitartrate and **acetaminophen** (Lortab), 5, 165, 173, 226

Claire 25